The AIDS Pandemic

Michael Merson • Stephen Inrig

The AIDS Pandemic

Searching for a Global Response

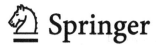 Springer

Michael Merson
Wolfgang Joklik Professor of Global Health
Duke Global Health Institute
Duke University
Durham, NC, USA

Stephen Inrig
Director, Health Policy and Management
  Program
Mount Saint Mary's University
Los Angeles, CA, USA

ISBN 978-3-319-47132-7 (hardcover)   ISBN 978-3-319-47133-4 (eBook)
ISBN 978-3-319-48431-0 (softcover)
DOI 10.1007/978-3-319-47133-4

Library of Congress Control Number: 2017938580

Cover picture: Woman laborers carry water to sprinkle on a sand sculpture, created by sand artist Sudarshan Pattnaik, on the eve of World AIDS Day on a beach in Konark, about 60 kilometers (38 miles) from Bhubaneswar, India, Friday, Nov. 30, 2012. (AP Photo/Biswaranjan Rout).

Printed on acid-free paper

This Springer imprint is published by Springer Nature
The registered company is Springer International Publishing AG
The registered company address is: Gewerbestrasse 11, 6330 Cham, Switzerland

Acknowledgments

Mike: To my wife, Kathy Sikkema, and son, Jonathan, who encouraged me to tell this story and patiently supported my writing and completion of this book. Also, to my grandchildren, Patrick and Elaine, with the hope that their generation can learn from our response to AIDS how best to confront global pandemics in the future.

Stephen: To my wife, Jula, who is to me a Knight of Faith and who has, more than anyone else, modeled for me and my children what unconditional love looks like; to my immediate family—Gary, Elizabeth, Heather, Evan, McKenna, and Lawson—for their limitless love; and to Craig Shearer, Brad McDermott, Mark Maines, John Van Dyck, Nat Stine, Chris Lillis, and Kevin Markle, who have embodied for me the depths of true friendship.

Introduction

Jose Esparza was despondent. The program in which he was working at the World Health Organization (WHO) was closing; worse yet, for Esparza personally at least, his job was going away, too. A physician, virologist, and cell biologist, the Venezuelan had worked since 1986 in WHO and since 1988 in WHO's Global Programme on AIDS (GPA), rising to become Chief of the Vaccine Development Unit. And now, in the waning months of 1995, this was all coming to an end.

Esparza's job had not been abolished because acquired immune deficiency syndrome (AIDS)[1] had ceased to be a threat or because the disease no longer demanded a vaccine. Quite the opposite: in many ways the AIDS pandemic was at its worst. Indeed, as he placed his desk mementos into a box, Esparza reflected on the numbers his colleagues had projected for global AIDS just months earlier: they estimated that as many as 4.5 million people had already developed AIDS across the globe, and that an additional 15 million were HIV-infected, even though they weren't showing symptoms.[2] Worse still, Esparza thought as he put on his jacket, 30–40 million people would go on to acquire the virus by the end of the decade.[3] Those fighting AIDS needed a vaccine immediately … AIDS was anything but over.

Esparza checked his ticket again. He was on his way to Canada to explore a job opportunity. He wished he could stay where he was, in Geneva, and continue battling the pandemic, but that seemed unlikely now. As he walked to the elevator, he knew several things: that clinicians caring for people with AIDS still lacked a drug regimen to reduce AIDS-related mortality; that people were still not using the effective prevention tools that existed—like condoms and clean needles—and that a

---

Within this chapter the singular pronouns *I* and *my* refer to Michael Merson alone, whereas the plural pronouns *we* and *us* generally refer to Michael Merson and Stephen Inrig jointly. Where *we* or *us* refers to Michael Merson and his colleagues at WHO, the object of the pronoun is clarified by context.

[1] AIDS is often referred to as HIV/AIDS; for the purposes of this text, we use the general term AIDS unless otherwise specified.

[2] "United Nations Forms Program to Combat AIDS," *Vaccine Weekly*, June 12, 1995, 12–13.

[3] Ibid.

vaccine … well, that was his area of expertise and he knew better than most just how far researchers were from finding an effective candidate. With the situation the way it was, the fight against AIDS needed people like him. But along with about half of his colleagues at GPA, Esparza had been encouraged to find employment elsewhere, maybe even outside the field of AIDS.

Riding down on the elevator, Esparza reflected on the team of people who were all in the same position as him, all looking for work. WHO, from the mid-1980s to the mid-1990s, had been the most prominent international agency fighting AIDS across the globe, and what a difficult fight it had been.

AIDS, perhaps more than any other disease since the influenza pandemic of 1918, speaks to the challenges the global health community faces in responding to pandemics in our modern era. AIDS emerged at a time when many global health experts considered global health to be transitioning from infectious to chronic diseases. First discovered in 1981 as an atypical set of cases of *Pneumocystis Carinii* pneumonia among homosexual men living in Los Angeles, this unusual syndrome quickly expanded to include other immune deficiency diseases in different populations in many countries. The United States Centers for Disease Control and Prevention (CDC), working with other agencies, developed a case definition for this disease and researchers began investigating its cause. In May 1983, French scientists isolated a retrovirus (later to be termed Human Immunodeficiency Virus or HIV) from a patient with the early symptoms of AIDS. Twenty-two months later, the United States Food and Drug Administration (FDA) approved a commercial test to detect the virus. By that time, HIV had infected more than 2 million people in sub-Saharan Africa alone.

As the world is now well aware, the AIDS pandemic has had, and continues to have, an enormous impact locally and globally, far beyond that of a mere "illness." Fear, stigma, cruelty, and death have spread along with the disease. Much has been written elsewhere about the horrific magnitude of the human toll of AIDS. The discrimination, extreme suffering, and human rights violations that occurred and continue to occur have reached far beyond the disease itself. AIDS has inflicted tragedy throughout the world: families torn apart; women stoned to death; people driven into poverty; health care and housing denied to the sick; orphans left to fend for themselves after their communities shunned them; people denied entry into other countries and rejected by their own. AIDS has torn at the very fabric of our societies, our economies, our ethics, and our values as a global community.

It is under these difficult and challenging circumstances that the world has attempted to stem the tide of both the disease and the stigma and denial it caused. Just as the AIDS pandemic has been unique, so too has been the global response, a response that in the early years was led by GPA. In 1984, WHO, under the direction of Fakhry Assaad and (soon thereafter) Jonathan Mann, assumed leadership of the global response by establishing its Control Programme on AIDS (CPA), later to be called GPA. During its meteoric expansion under Mann's leadership, GPA raised awareness of the pandemic's potential spread, mobilized substantial resources, provided much-needed strategic and technical direction under its Global AIDS Strategy, and supported development of national control efforts in more than 120 countries.

By 1995, GPA led the global fight against AIDS on several fronts: it had crafted global guidelines for issues ranging from securing national blood supplies to combating AIDS-related discrimination; it had supported AIDS control programs in essentially all low-and middle-income countries; it had provided millions of condoms and promoted harm reduction programs; it had established HIV vaccine testing sites; it had supported research on the interruption of perinatal transmission with antiretroviral drugs and on the development of microbicides and female condoms; it had deployed hundreds of AIDS professionals and indirectly supported several thousand more across the globe; and it had distributed almost $750 million towards the global fight against AIDS. In the process, GPA had become the largest and most prominent program in WHO's history. And yet, come December 1995, WHO was closing down the program—Esparza and dozens of others were on their own.

Why, then, did WHO close one of its most prominent and imperative programs at the height of the pandemic? Why were Jose Esparza and so many others who had dedicated years of their lives to fighting AIDS losing their jobs? Put simply, WHO closed GPA because the larger global health community—donor governments, Member States, intergovernmental agencies, and non-governmental organizations (NGOs)—concluded that the program was insufficient to the task of leading the global response to a complex pandemic like AIDS. They had a number of concerns: the continued expansion of the pandemic; WHO's performance at country level, competition among United Nations (UN) agencies; discontent with the WHO Director-General Hiroshi Nakajima; and the declining availability of donor resources in the post-Cold War years. Moreover, AIDS encompassed so many factors beyond health, issues for which observers felt other UN agencies had greater expertise and more appropriate organizational mandates. This led the global health community to call, in 1993, for a more multidisciplinary and coordinated global response. In GPA's place, these global health stakeholders created a new intergovernmental agency: the Joint United Nations Programme on HIV/AIDS (more popularly known as UNAIDS). This program became operational on January 1, 1996, the day after GPA closed its doors.

UNAIDS, many donors believed, would stand as an independent UN entity that could function as a consultative mechanism that included all the relevant UN agencies, along with bilateral donors, low- and middle-income countries, and international NGO networks.[4] It would be leaner and more efficient than GPA. It would leave much of the biomedical research—the work scientists like Esparza lead—to other entities and focus on what it could do best: coordinate the UN agencies in their efforts to support national AIDS programs, raise funds, and address a broad array of social, behavioral, and demographic factors that drive the spread this complex disease. These developments—the formation, evolution, and dissolution of GPA, the launch and subsequent course of UNAIDS, and the subsequent global response to the pandemic since the turn of the last century—are the topic of this book.

---

[4] Health and Population Directorate, "AIDS Program Coordination, or: Should we be here if we want to get there?" Internal Memorandum from Josef Decosas to Cathy Mains, *Health and Population Directorate*, 13 January 1993, 2.

This story of GPA serves as a case study on the way the global health community responds to pandemics of global magnitude. The AIDS pandemic is admittedly a unique pandemic, and yet there are several experiences—strategies adopted, roads taken and not taken, lessons learned—that can inform the global health community's response to other global health challenges. As we follow the course of these developments, we will explore a series of questions: How and why did WHO assume leadership of the global response? How did GPA develop? What were its strategies for raising awareness, mobilizing resources, providing direction, and supporting the formation of national AIDS programs? What drove the pandemic's expansion? What hindered WHO performance at country level? What led to the competition between WHO and other UN agencies and bilateral programs for the diminishing pot of donor resources in the 1990s? What were the factors leading to the multidisciplinary and coordinated global response known as UNAIDS? What impact did the closure of GPA have on the global response? What impact did it have on WHO? What have been some of the challenges that UNAIDS has faced since its inception? What have these changes meant for non-governmental, bilateral, and global health efforts? How much more coordinated is the global response to AIDS today? Is it still fragmented? We hope that in answering these and other related questions, we will offer a "useful history" of the global response to the AIDS pandemic and, in doing so, provide experience and guidance that will be helpful to the global health community as it continues to tackle AIDS and other present and potential pandemics in the future.

[Authors' note: In order to better understand GPA's response to the pandemic, we have provided background on the formation of WHO and its structure in Appendix 1.]

A Note About Authorship

The reader will likely have recognized that we have used the pronoun "we" or "us" in the text above. That is because this book is the product of two authors: Michael Merson and Stephen Inrig. Michael Merson (Mike) is the founding Director of the Duke University Global Health Institute and the Wolfgang Joklik Professor of Global Health and Professor of Medicine, Community and Family Medicine, and Public Policy at Duke University. As we relate later in the book, Mike worked at WHO between 1978 and 1995. He knows this story well because he was part of it. He did not start WHO's AIDS program, but in 1990, after 10 years serving as Director of WHO's Diarrheal Diseases Control Programme (CDD) and 3 years serving concurrently as the Director of WHO's Acute Respiratory Infections Control (ARI) Programme, he accepted the appointment from WHO Director-General Hiroshi Nakajima to serve as Director of GPA. In this capacity, for 5 years, he led the effort to mobilize and coordinate the global response to the AIDS pandemic. He was also intimately involved in the transition from GPA to UNAIDS. After leaving

WHO, between 1995 and 2004, he served as the first Dean of Public Health at Yale University and also as Director of the Center for Interdisciplinary Research on AIDS. Mike has been at Duke since 2006.

Stephen Inrig, a trained medical historian and health policy researcher, is Associate Professor of Health Policy and Management and Director of the Graduate Program in Health Policy and Management at Mount Saint Mary's University in Los Angeles. Stephen trained in retrospective policy analysis and qualitative research at Duke University and University of North Carolina—Chapel Hill, and then served as a health policy and health outcomes professor and researcher at University of Texas Southwestern Medical School from 2008 to 2014. He has been at Mount Saint Mary's University since 2014. Stephen has written on the history of AIDS in North Carolina, the American South, the greater United States, and Africa, and he has served as a co-investigator on research related to social health determinants and health systems interventions in Texas, California, North Carolina, and across the United States.

Mike and Stephen initially met not long after Mike arrived at Duke, while Stephen was finishing up his doctorate there in the history of medicine. Mike had been planning to write a book about his time at GPA soon after he moved from WHO to Yale in the mid-1990s. Beginning in 2000, he pulled together his documents and interviewed key informants to fill the gaps about his time in WHO. However, the demands of Mike's position at Yale and then at Duke kept him from progressing further on this task, and he realized he needed a skilled historian to complete the project. In 2008, Mike began discussing collaboration with Stephen, who by then had moved to the University of Texas Southwestern Medical School working on the history of HIV/AIDS. Stephen agreed to join the project with the understanding that the work involve original research and mutual collaboration, and serve not merely as a memoir, which aligned with Mike's goals and to which he readily concurred. The result is this work, which goes beyond Mike's time at GPA and covers the first three decades of the global response to the AIDS pandemic in great detail and with (we hope) substantive fairness. Our goal has been to blend memoir and historical analysis in a way that students of history will find rigorous and engaging and students of global health will find interesting, informative, and sufficiently motivating to pursue a career in global health.

This has been a highly collaborative project in research and writing. While Stephen has been the primary writer, each chapter has generated numerous discussions and multiple drafts, with both of us making numerous edits, corrections, and amendments along the way. While it has been a mutual process, much of this story covers periods of time where Mike was a participant, and not just an observer. Consequently, throughout this book, the singular pronouns *I* and *my* refer to Mike alone, whereas plural pronouns *we* and *us* generally refer to Mike and Stephen jointly. Where *we* or *us* refers to Mike and his colleagues at WHO, the object of the pronoun is clarified by context. Throughout the whole book, however, the writing is ours (Stephen and Mike).

A Note About Sources

As we explained above, our aim has been to present a book that is an amalgam of historical monograph and personal memoir. To the extent that it is a memoir, it is a limited memoir at best, as we devote very little attention to Mike's years in WHO prior to directing the AIDS program or to his career since leaving the Organization. Mike began collecting much of the records undergirding this book in 2000. Shortly thereafter Mike was awarded a grant by the Kaiser Family Foundation to work on the project while on sabbatical during the 2001–2002 academic year. During that time Mike gathered four types of data: his own recollections (including his calendar, diary, and written documents); official documents stored in WHO's archives; interviews with major AIDS-related stakeholders active during his tenure; and related secondary literature on HIV/AIDS and global health governance. Mike spent a month working in the WHO archives, where with the tireless assistance of Gillian Mignon, he copied much of the documentation that served as background to this study.[5] After gathering this information, Mike then spent a month at the Rockefeller Foundation Center in Bellagio, Italy, where he prepared a synopsis of the book he thought he was going to write. Mike then spent the rest of his sabbatical conducting approximately 100 interviews in person and by phone, which were transcribed by Mignon (we have listed these in Appendix 3), and working on the book's initial structure, which focused mainly on his tenure. During the subsequent years, he continued to conduct additional interviews as presented in the appendix.

After Mike had gathered much of the original source material, Stephen joined him with the objective of providing an even more academically rigorous account and leading the analytical and writing process of the project. Stephen revisited the interviews Mike had conducted, creating an inductive coding schema, and coding the transcripts using NVivo software. Stephen then conducted his own interviews, approved by the UT Southwestern IRB, between 2009 and 2015 (see Appendix 3). These interviews provided additional information on key figures and events to the story, including criticisms of decisions made by Mike while he was Director of GPA. Along with these interviews, Stephen organized over 60,000 pages of primary source material, used Adobe software to organize these data chronologically, and used NVivo qualitative software to analyze the data. By the late 2000s, WHO had put a substantial number of additional documents in its online archive, and Stephen drew on these resources to add a significant amount of additional primary and secondary source material to the documents and interviews Mike had already

---

[5] Obtaining access to these documents proved more difficult than Michael originally had expected, because WHO initially declined him access to the relevant WHO registry files so he could obtain memoranda, correspondence, and other pertinent documents and information. It reversed this policy after Michael appealed to the US State Department for assistance. Several of the important notes included in this book came from the data gleaned from the registry.

collected.[6] As Stephen researched and wrote the first draft, we engaged in numerous hours of conversation and discussion, much of which Stephen recorded and included in this monograph.

This work has taken a substantial amount of time and effort, and it would not have been possible without a tremendous team of research assistants and administrators. Jennifer Simmen Lewin at Yale and Caroline Hope Griffiths, Erin Escobar, and Lizzy Do Lee at Duke provided important background information at the beginning and towards the end of the project. Michelle Pender at Duke worked tirelessly in the last year of the project, editing and fact-checking drafts of the manuscript. Mary Catherine Crowley from Southern Methodist University and Heather Isfan from CIRE Research Services helped Stephen organize the thousands of pages of archival material and transcripts, while Simon Craddock Lee, Jasmin Tiro, and the UT Southwestern staff gave him the room and resources to succeed. Finally, we have been aided by reviewers who provided insightful corrections and comments during the writing process.

---

[6] This amounted to a collection of over 3500 cubic feet of space and an in-depth analysis of about 20,000 pages of primary source documents.

Endorsements

Tom Quinn, Director of Johns Hopkins Center for Global Health

"Merson and Inrig provide us with a rare and unique insider's view of the politics and science behind WHO's initial response to the massive and deadly rise of HIV/ AIDS across the globe. During the early years of this epidemic, HIV spread relentlessly from country to country and person to person. Confronted with overwhelming stigma, governmental denial, personal shame, millions of deaths, and no effective treatment in sight, WHO formed the Global Programme on AIDS (GPA) and tried to mount an effective response to counter the forces that propelled the epidemic forward. Following in the footsteps of Jonathan Mann, the first Director of GPA, Mike Merson became the second Director, and his story in this book reveals the difficulties, successes, and failures of the WHO-led response. The story provides us with enumerable lessons that the world needs to heed in mounting global responses to the current and future pandemics."

Stef Bertozzi, Dean of the University of California, Berkeley, School of Public Health

"Mike Merson had a front-row seat on the global response to AIDS during most of its crucial early years, from the day the charismatic Jonathan Mann was fired by World Health Organization Director-General Hiroshi Nakajima to the folding of WHO's Global Programme on AIDS and the birth of UNAIDS under Peter Piot's leadership. Merson and Inrig's unique perspective and insights not only bring to life a fascinating period in our history, they also offer many lessons for current and future international efforts to combat global pandemics and health inequity."

Kathleen Cravero, President of Oak Foundation (Formerly Deputy Executive Director UNAIDS)

"To someone who lived through the transition from GPA to UNAIDS, this is a fascinating account of who did what, when, and how. The complex web of personalities, politics, and events - set against a raging epidemic - makes for a fascinating read. For anyone interested in the UN, global health, or human rights, this book is a must.

On the one hand, this book is about how the World Health Organization tried - and ultimately failed - to take on one of the greatest public health threats of our time. On the other, it is a fascinating tale of the people, the politics, and events that shaped the global response to AIDS and the factors that will continue to hinder how the world approaches epidemics. For anyone interested in understanding the complexities of responding to global public health threats, this book is a must. Merson and Inrig provide a fascinating account of what WHO did or didn't do, how the rest of the UN got involved, the role of civil society and human rights activists, and the impact it all had on the people and communities being ravaged by AIDS. The highs and lows of the global response to HIV/AIDS are described with remarkable honesty and insight from one of its main protagonists."

Contents

Part I
Global Mobilization in a Pandemic

Chapter 1
The Response Before the Global Response

On November 20, 1986, in a press conference at the United Nations (UN) in New York, Halfdan Mahler announced to the world that the AIDS[1] pandemic was worse than he had thought. As many as 100,000 people were already living with AIDS, Mahler explained, while another 100 million people could become infected with the HIV virus over the next 5 years. Mahler, the third Director-General of the World Health Organization (WHO), acknowledged to the reporters present that he had ignored earlier warning signs: "I thought 'wait and see—maybe it is not as hot as some are making it appear.'" But by then, at the end of 1986, the evidence clearly showed how quickly AIDS was spreading, and Mahler admitted he had grossly underestimated the disease. "We stand nakedly in front of a very serious pandemic as mortal as any pandemic there ever has been," he forewarned the press. "I don't know of any greater killer than AIDS ... Everything is getting worse and worse in AIDS and all of us have been underestimating it." And so Mahler declared that WHO would prioritize AIDS, treating it with the same vigor it had devoted to small-pox eradication. This commitment would require $1.5 billion a year by the early 1990s, Mahler confessed, but the world had little choice. "[I] cannot imagine a worse health problem in this century," he concluded.[2]

Mahler's frank admission represents an important turning point in the history of AIDS: his announcement propelled WHO to the forefront of the global fight against

---

Within this chapter the singular pronouns *I* and *my* refer to Michael Merson alone, whereas the plural pronouns *we* and *us* generally refer to Michael Merson and Stephen Inrig jointly. Where *we* or *us* refers to Michael Merson and his colleagues at WHO, the object of the pronoun is clarified by context.

[1] For the purposes of this text, we will use the term AIDS to encompass both AIDS and HIV unless otherwise specified.

[2] Halfdan Mahler, "20 November 1986—Press Briefing on AIDS," World Health Organization, 1877F/MED/CPA, p. 1 and Lawrence K. Altman, "Global Program Aims To Combat AIDS 'Disaster'" *The New York Times,* November 21, 1986, A1. Mann and Mahler calculated this budget on the back of an envelope on the flight they took together to NYC.

© Springer International Publishing AG 2018
M. Merson, S. Inrig, *The AIDS Pandemic,* DOI 10.1007/978-3-319-47133-4_1

AIDS for the next decade. Yet his statement also raises some important questions. It was 1986, after all, over 5 years since the first reports of AIDS and at least 2 years since the world was stunned by news of widespread infection in sub-Saharan Africa. Why had it taken so long for Mahler and WHO to act on AIDS? What threshold of urgency needs to be breached before the world's primary health entity recognizes and responds to a global health emergency? In the next three chapters, we will explore the story of WHO's response to AIDS during the first years of the pandemic. We will chronicle the ways that WHO staff and others came to perceive the severity of AIDS, and follow the path taken by organization leaders from the first reports of the disease through Mahler's frank admission to those reporters in 1986 and the launch of WHO's high-priority AIDS program. The key question we will try to address is why WHO did not launch its global program on AIDS sooner.

Historians and journalists have, by now, comprehensively documented the discovery of HIV and AIDS.[3] On June 5, 1981, the United States Centers for Disease Control and Prevention (CDC) in Atlanta, Georgia, reported five cases of *Pneumocystis carinii* pneumonia (a kind of pneumonia that occurs in persons with compromised immune systems) in five homosexual men living in Los Angeles.[4] Shortly thereafter, more cases were reported in homosexual men living in New York and California, and among Haitians living in the United States, hemophiliacs, women, and newborns.[5] In these early years, the extent of AIDS's reach outside of developed nations was not immediately apparent.

We now know that doctors in Africa and Haiti had been observing cases of AIDS for some time, however. Beginning in 1975, for example, physicians in Kinshasa, Zaire (now the Democratic Republic of Congo) began seeing persistent diarrhea and dramatic weight loss among their patients; these symptoms were joined, after 1981, by cases of severe cryptococcal meningitis. During this same period, doctors in Zambia and Uganda began tracking dramatic cases of enteropathy, while physicians in Rwanda recorded spikes in oral and esophageal thrush.[6] At about the same time, across the globe in Haiti, dermatologists began recording unusual cases of Kaposi's

---

[3] Randy Shilts, *And the Band Played On: Politics, People, and the AIDS Epidemic*. New York: Penguin Books, 1988; Mirko Grmek, *History of AIDS: Emergence and Origin of a Modern Pandemic*, Princeton, NJ: Princeton University Press, 1990.

[4] "*Pneumocystis* pneumonia—Los Angeles," *MMWR*, 30, 250–2, 1981.

[5] "Kaposi's sarcoma and *Pneumocystis pneumonia* among homosexual men—New York City and California," *MMWR Morb Mortal Wkly Rep*, 30, 305–8, 1981; "Opportunistic infections and Kaposi's sarcoma among Haitians in the United States," *MMWR Morb Mortal Wkly Rep*, 31, 353–4, 360–1, 1982; "*Pneumocystis carinii* pneumonia among persons with hemophilia A," *MMWR Morb Mortal Wkly Rep*, 31, 365–7, 1982; H. Masur, M.A. Michelis, G.P. Wormser,, et al., "Opportunistic infection in previously healthy women: initial manifestations of a community-acquired cellular immunodeficiency," *Ann Intern Med*, 97, 533–9, 1982; "Unexplained immuno-deficiency and opportunistic infections in infants—New York, New Jersey, California," *MMWR Morb Mortal Wkly Rep*, 31, 665–7, 1982.

[6] Mirko Grmek, *History of AIDS: Emergence and Origin of a Modern Pandemic*, Princeton, NJ: Princeton University Press, 1990, pp. 21–30, 172–173.

sarcoma.[7] After similar cases began emerging in the North American medical literature, Haitian doctors recognized their experience might have larger salience and launched, in May 1982, the Haitian Study Group on Kaposi's Sarcoma and Opportunistic Infections (GHESKIO).[8] As examples like these proliferated, researchers scrambled to grasp how these regional instances connected to a larger global pattern.

With so many unusual disease clusters occurring in various countries across the globe, by mid-1982, researchers began taking note of the global extent of the pandemic and started piecing together the patterns of its spread. Many in Europe were the first to make these connections. In France, clinical immunologist Jacques Leibowitch and other members of the *Group de Travail Français sur le SIDA* (French AIDS Task Force) recalled several earlier cases whose symptoms resembled the American cases. Since some of those patients were from Africa, Leibowitch hypothesized that the disease originated there, and he spent the remainder of 1982 searching for corroborating evidence.[9] As reports about the Haitian cases became known, Leibowitch and his team began hypothesizing that AIDS was in fact a "French-speaking African phenomenon."[10] Throughout the spring of 1983, in academic symposia and medical journals, Leibowitch and his colleagues began promoting this perspective.[11]

In Belgium, around the same time, researchers were making similar connections. In Antwerp, the strange American cases brought to mind several patients Peter Piot and his colleagues had seen in the late 1970s. Piot was a Belgian infectious disease doctor who had made an early name for himself by co-discovering the Ebola virus in 1976 and, with supplemental training at the CDC and the University of Washington in Seattle, had launched a career in sexually transmitted diseases (STDs)[12] that, while based in Antwerp, had several ongoing African connections.[13] As the United

---

[7] Ibid, pp. 34–36; Paul Farmer, *Infections and Inequalities: The Modern Plagues.* Berkeley: University of California Press, 1999, pp. 101–102; Laurie Garrett, *The Coming Plague: Newly Emerging Diseases in a World Out of Balance.* New York: Farrar, Strauss and Giroux: 1994, pp. 307–308.

[8] Paul Farmer, *Infections and Inequalities: The Modern Plagues.* Berkeley: University of California Press, 1999.

[9] Laurie Garrett, *The Coming Plague: Newly Emerging Diseases in a World Out of Balance.* New York: Farrar, Strauss and Giroux: 1994, pp. 319–320.

[10] Mirko Grmek, *History of AIDS: Emergence and Origin of a Modern Pandemic*, Princeton, NJ: Princeton University Press, 1990, pp. 21–30. See also Laurie Garrett, *The Coming Plague: Newly Emerging Diseases in a World Out of Balance.* New York: Farrar, Strauss and Giroux: 1994, pp. 319–320.

[11] Mirko Grmek, *History of AIDS: Emergence and Origin of a Modern Pandemic*, Princeton, NJ: Princeton University Press, 1990, pp. 21–30; J. B. Brunet, E. Bouvet, J. Chaperon, J. C. Gluckman, S. Kernbaum, D. Klatzmann, D. Lachiver, J. Leibowitch, C. Mayaud, O. Picard, J. Revuz, W. Rozenbaum, J. Villalonga, C. Wesselberg, "Acquired Immunodeficiency Syndrome In France," *The Lancet,* 26 March 1983, 321(8326):700–701; Cristine Russell, "Body's Immune System Disease Seen Occurring Also in Equatorial Africa," *The Washington Post*, April 2, 1983, A7.

[12] For the purposes of this text we use the term sexually transmitted disease(s) and the abbreviation STD rather than the other term sexually transmitted infection(s) or STIs.

[13] Peter Piot, *No Time to Lose: A Life in Pursuit of Deadly Viruses.* New York: Norton, 2012,. 17.

States cases became public, Piot found his interest piqued and, by early 1983, he had identified at least four local cases with similar symptoms, all of which had connections to Zaire.[14] At the same time, 30 miles to the south in Brussels, infectious disease specialist Nathan Clumeck and his colleagues began treating five African patients also stricken with the disease. In the spring of 1983, Clumeck published a letter in the journal *The Lancet* suggesting "black Africans" might be at risk for AIDS.[15] Similarly in Denmark, I.C. Bygbjerg recalled "an AIDS-like disease of probably African origin" from 1976 and published his findings in *The Lancet*.[16] Over the next few weeks, other European researchers published similar findings in a Belgian medical journal and the *New England Journal of Medicine*.[17]

For their part, American researchers had also picked up on the international patterns of AIDS in their hemisphere. Specifically, after clinicians in Miami and Brooklyn reported several cases of AIDS among recent Haitian immigrants, the CDC dispatched Alain Roisin—a Belgian physician who spoke Creole—to link up with GHESKIO in Port-au-Prince to explore their cases.[18]

All this attention on the international scope of AIDS meant that, by 1983, a consensus began emerging among researchers that AIDS had probably originated in Africa. Leibowitch and other members of the *Group de Travail Français sur le SIDA* (including Jean Baptiste Brunet and Odile Picard) elucidated their hypothesis at a Boston seminar in February 1983 that AIDS was a "French-speaking African phenomenon," repeating it again at a New York symposium in March 1983. [19] That same month, the Belgians published their "African Origin" theory in European,

---

[14]Laurie Garrett, *The Coming Plague: Newly Emerging Diseases in a World Out of Balance*. New York: Farrar, Strauss and Giroux: 1994, pp. 290–291.

[15]N. Clumeck, F. Mascart-Lemone, J. De Maubeuge, D. Brenez, L. Marcelis, "Acquired Immune Deficiency Syndrome In Black Africans," *The Lancet,* 19 March 1983, 321(8325):642; Laurie Garrett, *The Coming Plague: Newly Emerging Diseases in a World Out of Balance*. New York: Farrar, Strauss and Giroux: 1994, pp. 319–320; Laurie Garrett, "Deadly Virus Spread Quietly Across Nations," *Newsday*, December 26, 1988.

[16]I.C. Bygbjerg, "AIDS in a Danish surgeon (Zaire, 1976)." *Lancet. 1983* Apr 23;1(8330):925; I.C. Bygbjerg and J.O. Nielsen, "AIDS from Central Africa in a Heterosexual Danish Male," *NIAID: AIDS Memorandum*, October 1983, 1(2):9–10.

[17]H Taelman, J Dasnoy, E Van Marck, L Eyckmans. "Acquired immune deficiency syndrome in 3 patients from Zaire," *Annales De La Societe Belgue De Medecine Tropicale*. 1983 Mar; 63(1):73–4; G. Offenstadt, et al., "Multiple opportunistic infection due to AIDS in a previously healthy black woman from Zaire," *New England Journal of Medicine,* March 31, 1983, 308(13): 775.

[18]Laurie Garrett, *The Coming Plague: Newly Emerging Diseases in a World Out of Balance*. New York: Farrar, Strauss and Giroux: 1994, pp. 307–308; Mirko Grmek, *History of AIDS: Emergence and Origin of a Modern Pandemic*, Princeton, NJ: Princeton University Press, 1990, pp. 34–36.

[19]Mirko Grmek, *History of AIDS: Emergence and Origin of a Modern Pandemic*, Princeton, NJ: Princeton University Press, 1990, pp. 21–30. See also Laurie Garrett, *The Coming Plague: Newly Emerging Diseases in a World Out of Balance*. New York: Farrar, Strauss and Giroux: 1994, pp. 319–320.

British, and American medical journals.[20] Then, in the summer of 1983, American researcher Robert Gallo proposed in the *Journal of the American Medical Association* that AIDS cases in the United States had causal links with Haiti and Africa, while an internal National Institute of Allergy and Infectious Diseases (NIAID) newsletter suggested "that 'Africans' be included in the list of risk groups" for AIDS.[21]

This growing consensus about the African origin of AIDS had yet to translate into concern about the problem AIDS might pose to the nations on that continent, however. Indeed, few staff members at WHO were paying it much attention. I was directing the WHO Diarrheal Diseases Control Programme (CDD) at the time, which was organizationally located within the Division of Communicable Diseases. We had weekly divisional staff meetings, for example, but AIDS was almost never discussed. At times, some of us in the meetings would ask about AIDS, but the Division leadership felt it fell outside of WHO's main concerns. In fact, the WHO staffers closest to the burgeoning pandemic largely considered AIDS a disease confined to the United States and other industrialized nations, and that it belonged in the capable hands of domestic agencies like the CDC. As Fakhry Assaad, head of WHO's Communicable Diseases Division explained to Mahler in July 1983, "[AIDS] is being very well taken care of by some of the richest countries in the world where there is the manpower and know-how and where most of the patients are to be found.'"[22] However, WHO staff did give the disease some attention in WHO's *Weekly Epidemiological Record* (WER) and the Pan American Health Organization (PAHO) *Epidemiological Bulletin* (EB) which, throughout 1983, published a total of eight articles on the problem (WER-6, EB-2).[23] The initial response seemed somewhat perfunctory to individuals like CDC's Walt Dowdle, who later told us.

> I was often the person who delivered the presentations on HIV that nobody believed at the time. It was the usual story: WHO was not interested in this—this was a gay problem, a US problem, and all these stories were not interesting—they had bigger fish to fry, this was another legionnaire's disease that nobody believed. Another cock and bull story that these US people dreamed up. …I happened to be … making a presentation about the blood borne HIV—at the time AIDS was associated with blood—of course you know that the blood community just fought us tooth and nail. Unbelievable. Disbelief. They just didn't

---

[20] N. Clumeck, F. Mascart-Lemone, J. De Maubeuge, D. Brenez, L. Marcelis, "Acquired Immune Deficiency Syndrome In Black Africans," *The Lancet,* 19 March 1983, 321(8325):642; G. Offenstadt et al., "Multiple opportunistic infection due to AIDS in a previously healthy black woman from Zaire," *New England Journal of Medicine,* March 31, 1983, 308(13): 775; H Taelman, J Dasnoy, E Van Marck, L Eyckmans. "Acquired immune deficiency syndrome in 3 patients from Zaire," *Annales De La Societe Belgue De Medecine Tropicale.* 1983 Mar; 63(1):73–4.

[21] On the Gallo comment, see Laurie Garrett, *The Coming Plague: Newly Emerging Diseases in a World Out of Balance.* New York: Farrar, Strauss and Giroux: 1994, pp. 321; on the internal NIAIDS newsletter, see I.C. Bygbjerg and J.O. Nielsen, "AIDS from Central Africa in a Heterosexual Danish Male," *NIAID: AIDS Memorandum,* October 1983, 1(2):9–10.

[22] Memorandum of Fakhry Assaad, Director of WHO Communicable Diseases Division to Halfdan Mahler, Director-General of the WHO, July 1983. cited in Katarina Tomasevski, Sofia Gruskin, Zita Lazzarini, and Aart Hendriks, "AIDS and Human Rights," in Jonathan Mann, Daniel J. M. Tarantola, and Thomas W. Netter, eds., *AIDS in the World: A Global Report,* Cambridge, MA: Harvard University Press, 1992, p. 567.

[23] See *Weekly Epidemiological Report* 1983, 58(14):101–108; 58(21):157–164; 58(40):305–312; 58(42):321–328; 58(45):345–352; 58(48):369–376.

accept it. So here's [a] Brit who gets up and really just tears into me—'it's another swine flu, legionnaires disease; these crazy Americans!' That was the type of thing you were putting up with at the time—in WHO. ... Nobody believed it.[24]

However, as data on the reality of AIDS mounted, a few staff in the WHO regional offices and headquarters in Geneva did begin taking greater responsibility for the regional and global response to AIDS.

As early as April 1983, for example, WHO's regional office for Europe, in Copenhagen, launched a voluntary AIDS-surveillance program for Western European Member States and requested each country to send them information on AIDS cases being "recorded by health administrators and/or institutions" in the region.[25] In August 1983, as cases in the Western Hemisphere climbed, PAHO invited researchers and health officials to "discuss the spread of AIDS in the Americas."[26] Of particular interest and contention was the incidence of AIDS in Haiti and the island nation's alleged role in the spread of AIDS into North America.[27] Finally, in November 1983, WHO headquarters convened a meeting of 38 experts in Geneva to "review the world occurrence of AIDS ... and identify risk factors for the disease and data about its cause."[28] Not only did this meeting prove to be the first WHO conference exploring the global impact of AIDS, but it was at this meeting that the earliest data coming from Central African countries suggested AIDS might pose a bigger threat to "less developed areas of the world" than researchers had previously thought.[29] Coming out of the meeting, participants recommended that WHO "coordinate [the] exchange of information between regions of the world" through the Collaborating Center on AIDS that WHO had recently established at the *Institut de Medicine et d'epidemiologie Tropicales* at the Hospital Claude Bernard in Paris.[30]

Despite these promising actions at the end of 1983, WHO's leadership still largely considered AIDS an inconsequential threat to developing nations (that is low- and middle-income countries) as compared to other diseases. As Mahler would later admit (in 1986), "most of us have somehow been satisfied that for once this was a rich man's disease and look[ed] at the very affluent societies, saying, 'well, they can afford it, they asked for it, and they can cope with it.'"[31]

---

[24] Walt Dowdle, Interview by Michael Merson, New Haven, CT, August, 2002.

[25] WHO, "Acquired Immune Deficiency Syndrome (AIDS)," *WER*, April 8, 1983, 58(14):101–102.

[26] Lawrence K. Altman, "The Confusing Haitian Connection To AIDS," *The New York Times*, August 16, 1983, C2.

[27] John Wilke, "Haitian Says Economy Hurt by AIDS Fear," *The Washington Post*, August 10, 1983, A9.

[28] Lawrence K. Altman, "Concern Over AIDS Grows Internationally," *The New York Times*, May 24,1983, C1; Margot Slade and Wayne Biddle, "Immune Disease Given Priority," *The New York Times*, May 29, 1983, 4:8.

[29] Lawrence K. Altman, "AIDS Now Seen As A Worldwide Health Problem," *The New York Times*, November 29, 1983, C1.

[30] "Acquired immunodeficiency syndrome – an assessment of the present situation in the world: Memorandum from a WHO Meeting," *Bulletin of the WHO*, 62 no. 3, 419–432, 1984.

[31] Transcript of Halfdan Mahler Press conference, New York, November 20, 1986.

With WHO leaders slow to grasp the potential enormity of the problem, it fell to researchers in France, Belgium, and the United States to begin exploring the implications of the African AIDS cases. Piot was one of the first to take up the African AIDS connection. Having now uncovered even more Belgian AIDS cases linked to Zaire, in early 1983 he began seeking financial support to conduct a research study on AIDS in Central Africa. According to Piot, neither the Belgian government nor CDC seemed interested, however.[32] Fortuitously for Piot, Richard Krause, Director of NIAID, delivered a lecture on AIDS at an international conference on infectious diseases in Vienna in the summer of 1983. Through a colleague, infectious disease expert Tom Quinn, Piot was able to secure a small grant from Krause for a collaborative research project in Zaire between Belgium's Institute of Tropical Medicine (ITM) and NIAID.[33]

That same summer, at an infectious diseases conference in Virginia, CDC's Joseph McCormick learned from a Belgian colleague, Jan Desmyter, about numerous Zairian AIDS patients he had been treating in Belgium. McCormick was an American pediatrician and epidemiologist who had spent time teaching math and science in Kinshasa before becoming a physician. Trained in CDC's Epidemic Intelligence Service and the National Institutes for Health (NIH) Preventive Medicine program, McCormick had gained renown for his work in the mid-1970s on meningococcal meningitis in Brazil, Lassa fever in Sierra Leone, and Ebola in Zaire and Sudan. In 1979 he had become Chief of CDC's Special Pathogens Branch.[34] In light of his broad experience with African infectious diseases, McCormick immediately understood the implications of the cases mentioned by Desmyter: "All kinds of lightbulbs began flashing above my head," McCormick later recalled, "AIDS was global."[35] McCormick returned to Atlanta and made the

[32] Peter Piot *No Time to Lose: A Life in Pursuit of Deadly Viruses*. New York: Norton, 2012, 127–128; Laurie Garrett, *The Coming Plague: Newly Emerging Diseases in a World Out of Balance*. New York: Farrar, Strauss and Giroux: 1994, pp. 345–347. For his part, James Curran did not "recall Peter ever requesting money from CDC (we didn't have any for international work)." Curran personal communication, April 11, 2016.

[33] Peter Piot *No Time to Lose: A Life in Pursuit of Deadly Viruses*. New York: Norton, 2012,128.; Laurie Garrett, *The Coming Plague: Newly Emerging Diseases in a World Out of Balance*. New York: Farrar, Strauss and Giroux: 1994, pp. 345–347; Jon Cohen, "The rise and fall of Projet SIDA," *Science*; 11/28/97, 278 (5343): 1565–1569; Richard Krause, Interview by Victoria A. Harden, Bethesda, MD: National Institutes of Health, November 17, 1988; Thomas Quinn, Interview with Michael Merson, 2002; Thomas Quinn, Interview with Victoria Harden and Caroline Hannaway, Baltimore, MD: Johns Hopkins University, December 5, 1996.

[34] Joseph B. McCormick and Susan Fisher-Hoch, *Level 4: Virus Hunters of the CDC*. New York: Barnes & Noble Books, 1999; Frontline, "Interview: Joseph McCormick, January 18, 2005," Boston: WGBH Educational Foundation, 2006, http://www.pbs.org/wgbh/pages/frontline/aids/interviews/mccormick.html, accessed December 6, 2012; "Instructor Profile: Joseph McCormick, MD," Ann Arbor, MI: University Of Michigan School of Public Health, 2011, https://practice.sph.umich.edu/practice/dynamic/site.php?module=courses_one_instructor&id=140.   Accessed December 6, 2012.

[35] Greg Behrman, *The Invisible People: How the U.S. Has Slept Through the Global AIDS Pandemic, the Greatest Humanitarian Catastrophe of Our Time*. New York: Free Press, 2004. pp. 3–5.

case to the CDC AIDS Task Force head, Jim Curran, that it needed to probe the extent of the disease in Africa. His research team had proven unable to determine the "disease's origins, its incubation period, and … mode(s) of transmissibility," and the European "African hypothesis" had grown increasingly convincing in the ensuing months.[36] Curran pledged his full support and McCormick set about securing permission from the Zairian Health Ministry for his project.[37]

Weeks before either team left for Zaire, the United States Health and Human Services Secretary realized there were two foreign travel notifications for AIDS research in Zaire—one from NIH and the other from CDC—and demanded that the two teams collaborate.[38] In mid-October 1983, the joint NIH/CDC/ITM project team arrived in Kinshasa, Zaire.[39] The team, led by Piot, worked with Bela Kapita at the Mama Yemo and University Hospitals in Kinshasa.[40] For 3 weeks the group collected specimens and determined that, although the disease was "predominately heterosexually transmitted, [it] had the same clinical features as those described in the United States and … Haiti."[41] In mid-November 1983, while Piot and McCormick continued their research in Zaire, Quinn (who was also part of the team) traveled to Aarhus, Denmark, where he delivered the preliminary results of the team's work at an AIDS conference. Quinn then traveled to the United States, where he again shared the preliminary data.[42] At the end of November, the Zaire team's preliminary

---

[36] On the emerging evidence for the "African Hypothesis," see Mirko Grmek, *History of AIDS: Emergence and Origin of a Modern Pandemic*, Princeton, NJ: Princeton University Press, 1990, pp. 21–30; N. Clumeck, F. Mascart-Lemone, J. De Maubeuge, D. Brenez, L. Marcelis, "Acquired Immune Deficiency Syndrome In Black Africans," *The Lancet*, 19 March 1983, 321(8325):642; G. Offenstadt et al., "Multiple opportunistic infection due to AIDS in a previously healthy black woman from Zaire," *New England Journal of Medicine*, March 31, 1983, 308(13): 775; H Taelman, J Dasnoy, E Van Marck, L Eyckmans. "Acquired immune deficiency syndrome in 3 patients from Zaire," *Annales De La Societe Belgue De Medecine Tropicale*. 1983 Mar; 63(1):73–4; Laurie Garrett, "Deadly Virus Spread Quietly Across Nations," *Newsday*, December 26, 1988; J. B. Brunet, E. Bouvet, J. Chaperon, J. C. Gluckman, S. Kernbaum, D. Klatzmann, D. Lachiver, J. Leibowitch, C. Mayaud, O. Picard, J. Revuz, W. Rozenbaum, J. Villalonga, C. Wesselberg, "Acquired Immunodeficiency Syndrome In France," *The Lancet*, 26 March 1983, 321(8326):700–701. On Curran's decision, see Greg Behrman, *The Invisible People: How the U.S. Has Slept Through the Global AIDS Pandemic, the Greatest Humanitarian Catastrophe of Our Time*. New York: Free Press, 2004. pp. 7–8.

[37] Joseph B. McCormick and Susan Fisher-Hoch, *Level 4: Virus Hunters of the CDC*. New York: Barnes & Noble Books, 1999, p. 162.

[38] Peter Piot *No Time to Lose: A Life in Pursuit of Deadly Viruses*. New York: Norton, 2012, 128–129.

[39] Thomas Quinn, Interview with Victoria Harden and Caroline Hannaway, Baltimore, MD: Johns Hopkins University, December 5, 1996; Greg Behrman, *The Invisible People: How the U.S. Has Slept Through the Global AIDS Pandemic, the Greatest Humanitarian Catastrophe of Our Time*. New York: Free Press, 2004. pp. 7–8; Jon Cohen, "The rise and fall of Projet SIDA," *Science*; 11/28/97, 278 (5343): 1565–1569; Richard Krause, Interview by Victoria A. Harden, Bethesda, MD: National Institutes of Health, November 17, 1988.

[40] Jon Cohen, "The rise and fall of Projet SIDA," *Science*; 11/28/97, 278 (5343): 1565–1569.

[41] Thomas Quinn, Interview by Michael Merson, New Haven, CT, August, 2002.

[42] Thomas Quinn, Interview with Victoria Harden and Caroline Hannaway, Baltimore, MD: Johns Hopkins University, December 5, 1996, p. 24.

data was shared with 38 researchers meeting at WHO's headquarters to discuss the global impact of AIDS.[43] Both in Europe and the United States, Quinn found little resistance to the notion that HIV might be transmitted heterosexually: "Everyone got all excited," Quinn recalled. "There was no credibility problem that we were seeing what we thought was a heterosexually transmitted disease or a disease that affected both men and women. ... None of it was published, so it was not in any literature yet. But I did not have any negative feedback."[44] Still, as we have noted, WHO staff did not find this preliminary data sufficient enough to respond more aggressively to AIDS.

Soon, however, the findings of Quinn, Piot, and McCormick were joined by similarly alarming evidence from other researchers. Clumeck, the Brussels-based physician who had treated several Zairois with AIDS in 1982 and 1983, mailed a questionnaire to physicians in Kigali, Rwanda, to determine if they were seeing AIDS patients. When dozens of affirmative responses came back, Clumeck and his colleagues traveled to Kigali in January 1984 to carry out more definitive tests. One month later, in February, they returned to Belgium convinced "AIDS could be endemic in urban areas of Central Africa."[45] At the same time, the French Pasteur Group also began exploring AIDS in Rwanda and the Central African Republic in 1983 and early 1984 and obtained blood samples from patients in those countries. The analyses they ran showed that many samples carried cell count patterns very similar to blood taken from people with AIDS, suggesting "alarming rates of ... infection in the general population."[46]

With evidence mounting about the threat of AIDS in developing countries, but with no further move by WHO leadership to take up the problem, other groups clamored to lead the response. In November 1983, soon after Quinn, Piot, and McCormick returned from Zaire, they held a conference call to revisit their findings and chart their next steps. "We said, 'we have got to do something,'" recalled Quinn, "... we have got to set up a prospective program." The three agreed to return to their respective institutions and scrounge together financial support for the project. Each institution would assign one person to the jointly sponsored program.[47]

McCormick's report convinced Curran that CDC needed to involve itself more thoroughly in the global aspects of the epidemic. "[Curran] actually took over Joe McCormick's aspects of it," Quinn recalled. "He said, 'this is AIDS, it fits under my task force.'"[48] Part of this switch came from McCormick himself: "I had established

---

[43] Lawrence K. Altman, "AIDS Now Seen As A Worldwide Health Problem," *The New York Times*, November 29, 1983, C1.

[44] Thomas Quinn, Interview with Victoria Harden and Caroline Hannaway, Baltimore, MD: Johns Hopkins University, December 5, 1996, p. 24.

[45] Laurie Garrett, *The Coming Plague: Newly Emerging Diseases in a World Out of Balance*. New York: Farrar, Strauss and Giroux: 1994, pp. 319–320, 344–345.

[46] Ibid, pp. 349–350.

[47] Thomas Quinn, Interview with Victoria Harden and Caroline Hannaway, Baltimore, MD: Johns Hopkins University, December 5, 1996, p. 24–27.

[48] Thomas Quinn, Interview by Michael Merson, New Haven, CT, August, 2002.

myself in viral hemorrhagic fevers; I was developing a program I loved and was excited by the research I was doing," McCormick would later explain, "I wasn't interested in abandoning my field of interest to work on AIDS." Still, McCormick had been the one to recommend that CDC support a long-term AIDS study in Zaire. Curran and CDC's Walt Dowdle gave him the task of setting up the program and finding a project director.[49] In the meantime, Piot and Quinn set about securing funds and support from NIAID and ITM.[50]

Tasked with setting up CDC's long-term research project in Zaire, McCormick set about recruiting the project's director. His leading candidate was the French-speaking, State Epidemiologist and Assistant Director of the Health Department in New Mexico, Jonathan Mann. Mann—who had earned his medical degree from Washington University at St. Louis in 1974 and his Master of Public Health from Harvard University in 1980, and who had served in various public health roles in New Mexico for a decade—had been looking for a new challenge.[51] "After almost 10 years," Mann would later recall, "… I felt that I had really pretty much done everything I could [in New Mexico] … I decided it was really time to move on … I felt that professionally there was a risk of stagnation if I stayed."[52] Towards the end of January 1984, McCormick called Mann and pitched the Zairian research job to him.[53] Mann, who had a young family and two other job offers on the table—one in Washington, DC, the other in Massachusetts—took some time to weigh his options. Despite the change it might mean for his family and potential loss of other career opportunities, Mann accepted the position in Zaire.[54]

While McCormick considered Mann an excellent fit for the job, others needed to be certain. Curran had first considered Mann after Lyle Conrad at CDC approached him about the idea, and—having McCormick's support and after meeting and interviewing Mann himself—Curran became convinced of his scientific and leadership potential. Since Mann had never been to Africa, and Kapita and staff in the United States embassy had never met him, Curran was reluctant to assign him there until after Mann spent some time in Zaire: "[Mann] had actually never been to Africa, so I insisted, before we hired him, that he take a trip to Kinshasa to see what it was like."[55] Dutifully, McCormick took Mann to Zaire to provide him with an on-site

[49] Joseph B. McCormick and Susan Fisher-Hoch, *Level 4: Virus Hunters of the CDC*. New York: Barnes & Noble Books, 1999, pp. 178–179.

[50] Jon Cohen, "The rise and fall of Projet SIDA," *Science*; 11/28/97, 278 (5343): 1565–1569.

[51] Ofelia T. Monzon, "Profiles of Famous Educators: Jonathan Mann, 1947–98," UNESCO International Bureau of Education, 2001. http://www.ibe.unesco.org/fileadmin/user_upload/ archive/publications/ThinkersPdf/manne.pdf Accessed on July 29, 2009.

[52] Jonathan M. Mann Oral History, Interviewed by Jake Spidle, New Mexico Health Historical Collection, UNM Health Sciences Library and Informatics Center, 1996.

[53] Joseph B. McCormick and Susan Fisher-Hoch, *Level 4: Virus Hunters of the CDC*. New York: Barnes & Noble Books, 1999, pp. 178–179.

[54] Ibid; Jonathan M. Mann Oral History, Interviewed by Jake Spidle, New Mexico Health Historical Collection, UNM Health Sciences Library and Informatics Center, 1996.

[55] James Curran, Interview by Michael Merson, 2002; James Curran, Interview by Victoria A. Harden, Bethesda, MD: National Institutes of Health,

overview of the situation and lay the groundwork for the long-term project.[56] Curran then contacted Quinn and Piot and informed them that he had identified Mann to lead CDC's part of the project. Quinn had already identified an American who had been working in the NIAID Laboratory of Parasitic Diseases, Henry "Skip" Francis, to establish the immunology aspect of the project. Piot identified Robert Colebunders to run the clinical component, and sent him to train with Francis and Quinn so they could design consistent clinical research protocols. Both Piot and Quinn initially expressed concern about Mann's lack of experience with AIDS, but Curran reassured them. "Jim said, 'He is great.'" Quinn recalled. "'He's a very good epidemiologist. He'll do a good job.' So I said, 'Fine. He's your selection. Here's my selection. Here's Peter's selection.' And off it went."[57]

Mann and McCormick traveled through Europe on their way back and forth to Zaire.[58] In the process, Mann visited Piot in Belgium and indicated that CDC planned to launch its own project. "Being a pragmatic guy," Piot later recalled, "I said let's work together and see how we can collaborate."[59] CDC "wanted to do their own thing [in Zaire]," remembered Krause. "[They] did not see why NIAID had to get involved. As far as I was concerned, we had to be involved because, by congressional mandate, CDC can only take research a certain distance."[60] Curran consequently contacted Quinn, who was establishing the NIH laboratory investigations in Zaire and suggested that CDC and NIH work together.[61] "So we ended up with a compromise," explained Krause, "… the CDC representative was the director of the project and the NIH person was the director of the laboratory."[62] Belgium's ITM would direct the clinical core of the project. Thereafter, CDC became the project's major funder: of its final $4 million budget, roughly $2.5 million came from CDC, $1 million from NIAID, and $0.5 million from ITM.[63]

Having resolved the initial coordination issues, the project began in the summer of 1984. Mann arrived first and, along with two Zairian physicians—Bosenga Ngali and Nzilambi Nzila—established the program, known as *Projet SIDA* (French for Project AIDS). Francis soon joined them, followed by Colebunders.[64] As journalist

---

[56] Joseph B. McCormick and Susan Fisher-Hoch, *Level 4: Virus Hunters of the CDC*. New York: Barnes & Noble Books, 1999, pp. 178–179.

[57] Thomas Quinn, Interview with Victoria Harden and Caroline Hannaway, Baltimore, MD: Johns Hopkins University, December 5, 1996, p. 24–27.

[58] Richard Krause, Interview by Victoria A. Harden, Bethesda, MD: National Institutes of Health, November 17, 1988; Jonathan M. Mann Oral History, Interviewed by Jake Spidle, New Mexico Health Historical Collection, UNM Health Sciences Library and Informatics Center, 1996; Jon Cohen, "The rise and fall of Projet SIDA," *Science*; 11/28/97, 278 (5343): 1565–1569.

[59] Jon Cohen, "The rise and fall of Projet SIDA," *Science*; 11/28/97, 278 (5343): 1565–1569.

[60] Richard Krause, Interview by Victoria A. Harden, Bethesda, MD: National Institutes of Health, November 17, 1988.

[61] Thomas Quinn, Interview by Michael Merson, New Haven, CT, August, 2002.

[62] Richard Krause, Interview by Victoria A. Harden, Bethesda, MD: National Institutes of Health, November 17, 1988.

[63] Jon Cohen, "The rise and fall of Projet SIDA," *Science*; 11/28/97, 278 (5343): 1565–1569.

[64] Ibid.; Thomas Quinn, Interview with Victoria Harden and Caroline Hannaway, Baltimore, MD:

Jon Cohen notes, *Projet SIDA* quickly "began addressing the most fundamental of epidemiological questions: How many people were infected? Who got the disease? Was AIDS the same in Zaire as seen elsewhere?"[65] Indeed, *Projet SIDA* would become an early and important contributor in the global response to AIDS.

The story of *Projet SIDA* throws into sharp relief the fact that WHO had yet to accept responsibility for global leadership on the AIDS pandemic. In these early years, the Americans vied with the French and the Belgians to assume primacy in understanding the spread of AIDS and sculpting a response. Moreover, American agencies frequently sparred with each other to see who would become the lead agency to craft that response. WHO leaders, however, had yet to consider AIDS of significant global import, and consequently they continued to opt not to leverage their resources against AIDS. "[N]obody was paying any attention to AIDS or HIV," Dowdle later told us. "I was doing a lot of reporting [on AIDS to the WHO Division of Communicable Diseases] at the time because of my connection with the communicable disease group, and …WHO was not interested in this."[66] Curran met with a similar response.[67] It is impossible to know, of course, what impact early and aggressive efforts might have had on the spread of AIDS, particularly in Africa. What is clear, however, is that it would be at least 3 more years before some countries even acknowledged they had an AIDS problem, much less began taking steps to contain the pandemic. Three years is a lot of time when it comes to the global spread of a disease.

Johns Hopkins University, December 5, 1996, p. 24–27.

[65] Jon Cohen, "The rise and fall of Projet SIDA," *Science*; 11/28/97, 278 (5343): 1565–1569.

[66] Walt Dowdle, Interview by Michael Merson, New Haven, CT, August, 2002.

[67] James Curran, personal communication, April 11, 2016.

Chapter 2
The Launch of the Control Programme on AIDS

Fakhry Assaad was taken aback: he had not put AIDS[1] on the agenda for this meeting, but here they were, talking about AIDS. Arguing about AIDS was more like it. It was the end of 1984, and Fakhry Assaad (Picture 2.1)—then Director of the World Health Organization's (WHO) Division of Communicable Diseases—had gathered with a small group of WHO staff and advisors to discuss immunization and communicable diseases in Karlsbad, Czechoslovakia.[2] The morning session had centered on pertussis and the afternoon was spent on WHO's China program. And now, it was evening, and the discussion had somehow turned to AIDS.

Since Assaad had omitted AIDS from the agenda, he found himself on the defensive and felt he needed to explain his position. He did not plan on engaging all of the Communicable Diseases Division on the problem, he explained; it was something for high-income countries to handle. At this point in the meeting, one of the attendees challenged Assaad's stance: "You think you are WHO, you are talking as if you were WHO, but you *have* to take into consideration AIDS!" A heated discussion then broke out between the various participants over whether WHO should engage more fully in AIDS, and Assaad found himself on the losing end of the argument.

Perhaps Assaad should not have been surprised. By the end of 1984, a growing body of evidence indicated that AIDS would be a much greater problem than originally imagined. Consequently, key leaders both inside and outside WHO had finally awakened to the fact that the agency needed to address AIDS more aggressively. But the main catalyst for substantive change would have to be Assaad.

Within this chapter the singular pronouns *I* and *my* refer to Michael Merson alone, whereas the plural pronouns *we* and *us* generally refer to Michael Merson and Stephen Inrig jointly. Where *we* or *us* refers to Michael Merson and his colleagues at WHO, the object of the pronoun is clarified by context.

[1] For the purposes of this text, we will use the term AIDS to encompass both AIDS and HIV unless otherwise specified.

[2] Meeting attendees included Vilimirovic, Dittman, Aswall, Ralph Henderson, and Assaad, among others. Fawsia Assaad, Interview by Michael Merson, New Haven, CT, July, 2002.

© Springer International Publishing AG 2018

M. Merson, S. Inrig, *The AIDS Pandemic*, DOI 10.1007/978-3-319-47133-4_2

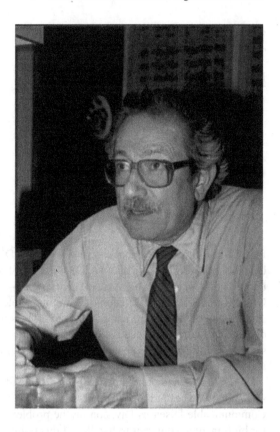

An Egyptian primary care physician who had worked with WHO as an Egyptian government counterpart, Assaad formally joined the organization in late 1959. First stationed in Taiwan, conducting epidemiological research on trachoma, Assaad moved to WHO headquarters in Geneva in the summer of 1964 as a medical officer in the communicable diseases area. In 1981, just as AIDS emerged, Assaad became Chief of Virus Diseases; less than a year later, following the retirement of his predecessor, Albert Zahra, Assaad became Director of WHO's Division of Communicable Diseases.[3]

While Assaad would eventually play an important role crafting WHO's first response to AIDS, initially (as we have suggested) he paid AIDS only scant attention. His division and the WHO regional offices did begin tracking and reporting on AIDS in late 1982 and early 1983,[4] but at this early date, Assaad committed little engagement from his division. He believed that WHO's mandate was to address the diseases of poorer nations and AIDS, he felt, was a Western disease that the affected

---

[3] Ibid.

[4] "Acquired Immune Deficiency Syndrome (AIDS)," *Weekly Epidemiological Record*, April 8, 1983, 58(14):1–2.

"rich" nations could handle adequately on their own.[5] Even after *Projet SIDA* and other observers began reporting the pandemic's spread in Africa in 1984, Assaad felt AIDS did not merit the attention of other global health concerns: "Fakhry, for some reason, after this group had done the studies in Africa, didn't want to deal with this. He said he had enough on his plate" recalled Joshua "Joe" Cohen, who had joined WHO in the early 1970s and who in the mid-1980s was serving as Senior Health Policy Advisor to Director-General Halfdan Mahler.[6]

Admittedly, some of Assaad's reluctance sprang in part from his ambivalence about the morality associated with AIDS: "[Assaad] was a deep puritan," his wife, Fawsia (a long time human rights advocate), explained, "and he had the feeling that [AIDS] was a first world disease for very dissolute people."[7] More importantly, Assaad and many of his WHO colleagues did not think that WHO could do much to address AIDS. In 1984, renowned University of Washington epidemiologist and sexually transmitted disease (STD)[8] specialist, King Holmes, approached Assaad "to motivate him to create an AIDS program" at WHO. According to Holmes, Assaad explained WHO's inaction with an analogy to a tuberculosis screening program that Assaad had launched in Egypt: "[Assaad] had identified a large number of people who had tuberculosis and [his boss asked] 'Now that you are finding all these people with tuberculosis, what are you going to do with them?'"[9] Assaad appeared to be saying that WHO's initial decision not to start an AIDS program was based on the belief that, even if AIDS was a growing problem, it would be unhelpful to identify all those infected since WHO had little to offer them.

Assaad seems not to have been comfortable with that position for very long, however. Sometime in 1984, Assaad changed his mind about WHO's approach to AIDS. We suspect there were a number of reasons for this. Assaad had a keen interest in virology, so perhaps the change started in May of that year, when Robert Gallo and his team at the National Institutes for Health (NIH) clearly showed a virus to be the causative agent for AIDS. Assaad had a deep commitment to fighting diseases in low- and middle-income countries, so maybe a more definitive shift came that summer when he met Jonathan Mann for the first time in Geneva while Mann was engaged in the early stages of *Projet SIDA* in Zaire.[10] Additionally, Assaad during this time was very much in touch with the staff at the Centers for Disease Control

---

[5] Memorandum of Fakhry Assaad, Director of WHO Communicable Diseases Division to Halfdan Mahler, Director-General of the WHO, July 1983, cited in Katarina Tomasevski, Sofia Gruskin, Zita Lazzarini, and Aart Hendriks, "AIDS and Human Rights," in Jonathan Mann, Daniel J. M. Tarantola, and Thomas W. Netter, eds., *AIDS in the World: A Global Report*, Cambridge, MA: Harvard University Press, 1992, p. 567.

[6] Joshua Cohen, Interviewed by Michael Merson, New Haven, CT, August, 2002.

[7] Fawsia Assaad, Interview by Michael Merson, New Haven, CT, July, 2002.

[8] For the purposes of this text we use the term sexually transmitted disease(s) and the abbreviation STD rather than the other term sexually transmitted infection(s) or STIs.

[9] King Holmes, Interview by Michael Merson, New Haven, CT, September, 2002.

[10] Jonathan M. Mann Oral History, Interviewed by Jake Spidle, New Mexico Health Historical Collection, UNM Health Sciences Library and Informatics Center, 1996.

and Prevention (CDC), so perhaps his concern emerged gradually throughout the year as Walt Dowdle kept him abreast of the latest information on the pandemic.[11]

Whatever the reason, the tipping point appears to have occurred at that meeting in Karlsbad towards the end of 1984. Jo Asvall, a Norwegian and the Regional Director for the European Office of WHO from 1985 to 2000, remembers being struck that Assaad had not put AIDS on the agenda; that Assaad and WHO had essentially ignored it or avoided it.[12] It was Professor S. Dittman, the famous virologist from the Institute of Hygiene, Microbiology and Epidemiology in Berlin, who had first broached the subject of AIDS that evening, highlighting the tremendous concern health care providers in his country and elsewhere had about AIDS. As we have explained, Assaad at this stage seems to have grown concerned about AIDS, though he still largely considered it a problem for high-income countries. He had not wanted to involve his Communicable Diseases Division in Geneva in a problem he considered to be of such limited scope, but he had been willing for "EURO [WHO's Regional Office for Europe] to take over AIDS."[13]

As we noted above, at some point in the meeting Assaad found his position assailed by the other infectious disease specialists. They argued vociferously over the relative merits of WHO's modest approach on AIDS; none considered Assaad's decision to limit WHO involvement satisfactory. Coming out of the meeting (according to Assaad's wife), the argument about AIDS had a transformative effect on him: "then he got involved himself. It was sudden: after this big fight, the following day he took over AIDS. After this fight at the end of 1984 ... in Karlsbad, he did not wait, he just ground himself into AIDS."[14] Assaad had made a decision; thereafter he would become a key champion, dragging WHO into the global fight against AIDS.[15]

The largest problem for Assaad was WHO's ongoing inertia regarding AIDS. "Fakhry was the only one interested in anything—he was a dynamo," Dowdle explained, "... he was very keen on what was happening and was following through on everything but couldn't get anyone else in WHO interested." Assaad put himself on a steep learning curve, staying in constant touch with CDC as the pandemic expanded.[16] In particular, he began relying heavily on CDC's McCormick and Dowdle for advice about how WHO should respond. Dowdle became a standing participant in Assaad's Collaborative Center meetings, and McCormick became one of Assaad's regular correspondents on global AIDS policy.[17] By mid-1985, Assaad had become such an expert on global AIDS that some in the media took to labeling him "Mr. AIDS" or "*Monsieur SIDA.*"[18] Media briefings on AIDS now became

---

[11] Walt Dowdle, Interview by Michael Merson, New Haven, CT, August, 2002.

[12] Joe Asvall, Interview by Michael Merson, January, 2002.

[13] Fawsia Assaad, Interview by Michael Merson, New Haven, CT, July, 2002.

[14] Ibid.

[15] Ibid.

[16] Walt Dowdle, Interview by Michael Merson, New Haven, CT, August, 2002.

[17] Ibid; Joseph B. McCormick and Susan Fisher-Hoch, *Level 4: Virus Hunters of the CDC.* New York: Barnes & Noble Books, 1999, p. 187.

[18] Fawsia Assaad, Interview by Michael Merson, New Haven, CT, July, 2002.

marathons, with Assaad sometimes answering questions for up to 2 h as reporters from various countries sought answers about the expanding pandemic.[19]

Despite Assaad's increased attention to AIDS, he had yet to convince WHO leadership that the organization needed to make AIDS a greater priority. "[Assaad] had already become convinced that he needed to get a program started under the auspices of WHO," McCormick later explained, "but his chief, Dr. Halfdan Mahler, was more difficult to persuade and was slower to grasp the significance of what was happening."[20] "Between 1984 and 1985 ..." recalled then Director-General of the Swedish National Institute for Infectious Disease Control, Lars Kallings, "Fakhry Assaad called on me to convince Mahler that AIDS was indeed a problem."[21] According to Dowdle, Mahler largely ignored Assaad's concerns about AIDS, to Assaad's tremendous aggravation: "He didn't listen—neither did anyone else ... [Assaad's] frustration was profound."[22] Indeed, in September 1985, Mahler told reporters in Zambia that "if African countries continued to make AIDS a 'front-page' issue, the objectives of Health for All by the Year 2000 would be lost." Mahler agreed that WHO should help others strategize and mobilize against the pandemic, but he did not think it should make the disease a high priority: "AIDS is not spreading like a bush fire in Africa," Mahler concluded. "It is malaria and other tropical diseases that are killing millions of children every day."[23]

Mahler's reluctance to prioritize AIDS stemmed both from his professional commitments and organizational prejudices. Born in 1923, raised by his father (a Danish Baptist preacher) and mother (a German woman from a family of physicians), and educated as a physician in Denmark, Mahler led an antituberculosis campaign for the Red Cross in Ecuador immediately before joining WHO as a tuberculosis officer in the early 1950s. He was initially attached to the tuberculosis control program in India and in 1962 became Chief of the Tuberculosis Unit in WHO in Geneva. In 1969 he headed up WHO's Project Systems Analysis before being elected for the first of his three terms as Director-General in 1973. A visionary and charismatic man with passionate views and a minister's oratory, Mahler believed fervently in his 'primary health care' model—the Global Strategy for Health for All by the Year 2000—and the decentralized, local-level responsibility structure that went with it.

Launched at the International Conference on Primary Health Care in Alma-Ata, USSR in 1978, the Global Strategy proposed by Mahler and his Senior Health Policy Advisor, Joe Cohen, called for a peripheral, nonphysician-based, health infrastructure that would provide basic prevention and care services for the world's poor using appropriate technologies, in contrast to one focusing on vertical, disease-control approaches that produced in their eyes only short-term gains. In Mahler's mind, another global, "vertical" program like the one that had recently eradicated

---

[19] Ibid.

[20] Joseph B. McCormick and Susan Fisher-Hoch, *Level 4: Virus Hunters of the CDC*. New York: Barnes & Noble Books, 1999, p. 187.

[21] Lars Kallings, Interview by Michael Merson, New Haven, CT, September, 2002.

[22] Walt Dowdle, Interview by Michael Merson, New Haven, CT, August, 2002.

[23] *Times of Zambia*, 11 September 1985, cited in John Iliffe, *The AIDS Epidemic: A History* p. 68.

smallpox—particularly for a disease that seemed disproportionately to affect high-income nations like AIDS—would distract from the importance of primary health care as a global health priority. Cohen himself was not convinced that AIDS deserved attention, telling Suzanne Cherney, editor at the time of the WHO *Chronicle*, "not to make too much of the epidemic as it stigmatized Africans and any way 'it's not going to spread like wildfire through Africa.'"[24]

Also, Mahler had hoped WHO could avoid taking on the global responsibilities for a socially complex disease like AIDS. Mahler felt that WHO had a dismal record when it came to helping countries establish STD prevention programs, and he doubted it would do any better with AIDS. Mahler believed that such diseases were primarily "social problems," and therefore were not WHO's forte. WHO should focus on what it did well, he concluded. Despite Assaad's petitions for an aggressive AIDS program at WHO, Mahler remained unconvinced.[25]

Mahler's disengagement and reluctance notwithstanding, Assaad recognized he needed to move forward and establish an AIDS program within WHO. His first major step was to partner with the United States' CDC to host the first major International Conference on Acquired Immunodeficiency Syndrome (AIDS) on April 15–17, 1985 in Atlanta. The conference drew more than 3000 participants from 50 countries and included 392 presentations on aspects of this new disease.[26] For 3 days in Atlanta, participants tried to wrap their minds around this emerging problem that was simultaneously scientifically exciting, therapeutically discouraging, and politically controversial. Perhaps most disturbing for conference participants was the revelation that the virus causing AIDS had a longer incubation period than previously thought, sparking the growing realization that "many of those dying [from AIDS] in 1985 had been infected before 1981."[27] As the unique and interesting epidemiological data emerged from across the globe, the conference left the clear impression that AIDS was not just a real and potentially devastating problem, but that it was a worldwide problem.[28]

Immediately following the conference, Assaad convened a WHO consultation group to assess and make recommendations emanating from the conference findings. Led by Assaad and Dowdle, 38 participants from 21 countries recommended WHO establish an AIDS Collaborating Centers network; generate a common reporting format and case definition for AIDS; coordinate global AIDS surveillance; facil-

[24] Suzanne Cherney, Interview (email) by Michael Merson, August 13, 2013.

[25] Halfdan Mahler, Interview by Michael Merson, Geneva, October, 2001.

[26] "The Acquired immunodeficiency syndrome (AIDS): Memorandum from a WHO Meeting," *Bulletin of the WHO*, 63 no. 4, 667–672, 1985; Boris Bytchenko. "Travel Report Summary on World Health Organization European Consultation on AIDS," Atlanta Georgia, 18–19 April 1985; WHO Division of Communicable Diseases, "WHO Consultation on AIDS, 18–19 April 1985, Atlanta, Georgia, USA," WHO Unpublished document, p. 1.

[27] Katherine E. Bliss. *The International AIDS Conference Returns to the United States: Lessons from the past and opportunities for July 2012*. Washington, DC: Center for Strategic and International Studies, 2012, 5.

[28] Boris Bytchenko. "Travel Report Summary on World Health Organization European Consultation on AIDS," Atlanta Georgia, 18–19 April 1985.

itate the development of an effective vaccine, and assist in the development of effective control strategies.[29] The group also called on countries to inform their citizens on how AIDS was spread, establish surveillance systems, set up blood screening programs, develop guidelines for counseling and care of infected patients, and maintain the confidentiality of positive results of serological testing and the identity of AIDS patients.[30] Over the next several months, Assaad designated five institutes as WHO Collaborating Centers on AIDS: the Division of Viral Diseases, CDC, Atlanta; *Institut de Medicine et d'Epidemiologie Tropicales*, Hospital Clande Bernard, Paris; Department of Hygiene and Medical Microbiology, Max von Pettenkofer Institute, Munich; Virus Laboratory, Fairfield Hospital, Fairfield, Victoria; and the *Unité d'Oncologie Virale, Institut Pasteur*, Paris. Each of these centers had extensive experience in laboratory diagnosis of viral infections, and each was to provide advice in its areas of expertise to assist WHO in formulating AIDS policies.

The conference only heightened the demand for more information about AIDS, and WHO Member States began calling on Assaad and his WHO colleagues to coordinate regional and global AIDS control activities more aggressively.[31] Each of WHO's six Regional Committees traditionally met annually in the months just after the conference had ended, so Assaad found himself peppered with questions at each of these meetings for information and assistance on AIDS.[32] Addressing these requests put a tremendous administrative burden on Assaad and his staff.[33] "At this point the Member States [began] to pose questions," Assaad's senior operations officer at the time, Bill Parra remembered.

And these cables are beginning to come in because we didn't have... any internet. There was no way of communicating except through cables.... So we would come in everyday and we had these long tables in the workroom, we would lay out these cables and we would try to figure out what we were able to respond to quickly. There were just more questions than we could answer... My job to help Fakhry was to say, 'ok what can we do, how can we lay out this process? How can we get this answer? What does WHO require, what can I do to help you?' So we would sit down and chart them.[34]

Consequently, Assaad became even more determined that WHO needed to have "a major AIDS program" run from its headquarters in Geneva that "would concentrate its efforts on the developing world," and over the summer and early fall of 1985

---

[29] "The Acquired immunodeficiency syndrome (AIDS): Memorandum from a WHO Meeting," *Bulletin of the WHO*, 63 no. 4, 667–672, 1985; Control Programme on AIDS, "Global WHO Strategy For the Prevention And Control of Acquired Immunodeficiency Syndrome: Projected Needs For 1986–1987," World Health Organization AIDS/CPA/86.2, June 1986, p. 5.

[30] "The Acquired immunodeficiency syndrome (AIDS): Memorandum from a WHO Meeting," *Bulletin of the WHO*, 63 no. 4, 667–672, 1985.

[31] Control Programme on AIDS, "Global WHO Strategy For the Prevention And Control of Acquired Immunodeficiency Syndrome: Projected Needs For 1986–1987," World Health Organization AIDS/CPA/86.2, June 1986, p. 6.

[32] Ibid.

[33] William Parra, Interview with Stephen Inrig, October 14, 2010.

[34] Ibid.

he began calling "several people to solicit ideas about who might set [it] up."[35] "We are concerned about a disease which is still spreading," Assaad told reporters in mid-September, explaining his evolving plans. "We don't have any treatment that we can validate, and we don't have a vaccine. And one of the things that can be done to prevent AIDS is to spread information as widely as possible. We cannot just wait until it spreads throughout the entire world. ... When we began to realize that it was spreading in other countries, we decided we must make sure we have the means available, all the tools for handling it." Assaad also laid out what he considered to be the foundational components of a larger WHO plan: "We foresee using WHO as the organization that would be a coordinator for the exchange of information. ... the organization would probably also coordinate research and provide support to countries in the developing world.'"[36]

In lieu of such a global program, Assaad began relying heavily on the directors of the AIDS Collaborating Centers for advice and guidance. By this time, Assaad had expanded the list of Centers to 12 (five in the United States, two in Britain, two in France, and one each in West Germany, Australia, and the Central African Republic).[37] In late September, 1985, Assaad convened a meeting in Geneva of the center directors to review the status of the pandemic, define their responsibilities, and recommend priority actions WHO should take. On the technical front, the directors called for the development of an international panel of anti-LAV/HTLV-III (the former name for HIV)[38] reference sera and distribution of standard preparations of the LAV/HTLV-III virus; collection and characterization of viral isolates; and provision of epidemiological data on LAV/HTLV-III infection. They also recommended 12 priority actions for WHO that focused on laboratory diagnosis, epidemiological surveillance, and blood safety. Finally, at the end of the meeting, the group affirmed the important role WHO could play in the prevention and control of AIDS, particularly in developing countries, and backed Assaad's idea that WHO should develop a global AIDS program.[39] This latter point was prescient, because by the time of this

---

[35] Joseph B. McCormick and Susan Fisher-Hoch, *Level 4: Virus Hunters of the CDC*. New York: Barnes & Noble Books, 1999, p. 189–190.

[36] Thomas W. Netter, "U.N. Agency Announces Steps To Coordinate Fight Against AIDS," *The New York Times*, September 23, 1985, A14.

[37] Ibid.; Alan McGregor, "World experts meet to reassess Aids data The Times of London, September 25 1985. The new centers included the National Institute for Biological Standards and Control, London; Faculty of Medicine, University of Singapore, Singapore; Laboratory Centre for Disease Control, Ottawa; Institut Pasteur, Bangui; Central Public Health Laboratory, London's Institute for Viral Research, Kyoto University, Kyoto; National Bacteriological Laboratory, Stockholm; and the Center for Drugs and Biologics, Food and Drug Administration (FDA) in Bethesda.

[38] Before being assigned the universally agreed upon designation of HIV, the virus that causes AIDS had at least two designations, depending on who the designee considered the discoverer of the virus to be. Those supporting the French called the virus. *Lymphadenopathy Associated Virus* (LAV), while those supporting the Americans called it the *human T-lymphotropic virus* (HTLV)-III.

[39] Control Programme on AIDS, "Global WHO Strategy For the Prevention And Control of Acquired Immunodeficiency Syndrome: Projected Needs For 1986–1987," World Health

meeting, WHO had received over 15,000 reports of AIDS cases; more than 2000 of which had come from 40 countries outside the United States.[40] We should note, at this point, that the shape of WHO's early AIDS program was largely focused on the technical aspects of AIDS control: securing the blood supply, establishing diagnostic criteria, and setting up viral collection and repository standards. Activities related to the prevention of sexual transmission—behavior change, educational programs, and the like—and the formation of national action plans or concerns about the human rights of people with AIDS were not yet in play or even under consideration.

Assaad began working with CDC's McCormick to develop a clinical case definition of AIDS that low- and middle-income countries could utilize, as participants at April's post International AIDS Conference consultation meeting had recommended. McCormick had continued to press the concern in the ensuing months and consequently, in late October, 1985, Assaad organized a workshop in Bangui, Central African Republic to develop a clinical case definition for AIDS in adolescents and adults for clinicians to use for surveillance when a laboratory diagnosis was impossible.[41] Clinicians from nine African countries who had treated AIDS patients joined WHO representatives to draft the provisional clinical definition and to elucidate ways that WHO could further collaborate with Member States in its use, particularly those countries struggling with AIDS.[42] With a case definition in place and the Coordinating Centers providing advice and support, Assaad felt he could begin taking the next steps towards developing a full-fledged WHO program.

Launching such a program was no simple task, however, and by the closing months of 1985 the demands for AIDS programs were becoming unwieldy for Assaad and his team. First, there were new diplomatic sensitivities associated with the pandemic, most prominently in Africa. As researchers traced the origins of AIDS back to different countries in Africa, epidemiological data mixed with anthropological conjecture fostered several unwarranted speculations that allegedly unique aspects of "African culture" played a role in the spread of the disease. The conjectures that made it into the academic and popular press often seemed to blame Africans for AIDS, or assigned the origins of AIDS to allegedly taboo sexual prac-

Organization AIDS/CPA/86.2, April 1986, p. 5. Alan McGregor, "World experts meet to reassess AIDS data." *The Times*, September 25 1985; Ibid, "Health experts attempt to lessen fear of Aids," *The Times*, September 27 1985.

[40]Thomas W. Netter, "U.N. Agency Announces Steps To Coordinate Fight Against AIDS," *The New York Times*, September 23, 1985, A14.

[41]DCS Control Programme on AIDS, "Global WHO Strategy For the Prevention And Control of Acquired Immunodeficiency Syndrome: Projected Needs For 1986–1987," World Health Organization AIDS/CPA/86.2, April 1986, p. 6; Joseph B. McCormick and Susan Fisher-Hoch, *Level 4: Virus Hunters of the CDC*, New York: Barnes & Noble Books, 1996, 1999, p. 188.

[42]WHO, "Workshop on AIDS in Central Africa: Bangui, Central African Republic," WHO/CDS/ AIDS/85.1, 22–25 October 1985; "Revision of the case definition of AIDS for national reporting— United States," *MMWR*, 1985, 34(25):373–375; DCS Control Programme on AIDS, "Global WHO Strategy For the Prevention And Control of Acquired Immunodeficiency Syndrome: Projected Needs For 1986–1987," World Health Organization AIDS/CPA/86.2, April 1986, p. 6; "WHO/CDC Case definition for AIDS," *WER*, 1986, 61:69–76.

tices in African countries. Assaad found himself in a precarious position. On the one hand, he wanted to silence speculations that drew on negative or colonial-era stereotypes of Africans. On the other hand, he wanted to safeguard against African leaders becoming so sensitive to these unfounded theories that they ignored the very real epidemiology of the pandemic. Kenya and South Africa were the only African countries reporting AIDS cases to WHO by year's end, so Assaad realized he needed to approach this conundrum very carefully if he wanted to ensure maximum buy-in from other affected countries.[43]

Second, Assaad faced several logistical issues. He had to begin planning in the fall of 1985 to place the topic of AIDS on the agenda of the next WHO Executive Board meeting in January, 1986. That meant he needed to convince the Executive Board's Program Committee in October of the importance of the full Board making recommendations on the needed response to the pandemic at its January meeting.[44] WHO's Executive Board is composed of members (31 at the time) technically qualified in the field of health who are elected for 3-year terms (see Appendix 1 for more on WHO structure). The Executive Board meets twice a year. It holds its main meeting, at which resolutions are adopted to be forwarded to the World Health Assembly (WHA) every January, while it convenes its second (and much shorter) meeting in May, immediately after the WHA (where it considers mainly administrative matters). With AIDS numbers climbing across the globe, getting AIDS as an item on the January meeting agenda was imperative.

Assuming he succeeded in placing AIDS onto the agenda, Assaad then had to prepare relevant documentation for the members of the Board—this would be the first official discussion of AIDS held by WHO's Executive Board. So, in the fall of 1985, Assaad drafted a background paper for a proposed WHO AIDS program that would be distributed to Executive Board members in November 1985. Assaad based the document on recommendations made during the AIDS consultations and meetings in which he had participated during the previous year.[45] He called for a six-point WHO AIDS program that included: preparing and distributing technical guidelines; coordinating the exchange of AIDS information; providing direct technical support to developing countries; advising governments on safeguarding their blood supplies; guiding the deployment of commercially available antibody test kits; and coordination of research on development of therapeutic agents and vaccines. After formulating his proposal, Assaad continued fleshing out the details in mid-December when he met again with the heads of his Collaborating Centers to

---

[43] "Rwanda: In Brief: AIDS not yet a public health problem," *BBC Summary of World Broadcasts*, January 24, 1986; "African AIDS Conference Ends," *The Associated Press*, January 24, 1986; "Is nobody safe from AIDS?" *The Economist*, February 1, 1986, p. 91; Lawrence K. Altman, "New Fear On Drug Use And AIDS," *The New York Times*, April 6, 1986, 1:1.

[44] DCS Control Programme on AIDS, "Global WHO Strategy For the Prevention And Control of Acquired Immunodeficiency Syndrome: Projected Needs For 1986–1987," World Health Organization AIDS/CPA/86.2, April 1986, p. 6.

[45] WHO Executive Board, "WHO activities for the prevention and control of AIDS: Report by the Director-General," EB77/42, 25 November 1985.

discuss further the ways that WHO could meet the needs of Member States.[46] Among other things, the group agreed on coordinating their antibody testing and epidemiological assessment efforts and antiviral/vaccine research. They also committed to developing diagnostic kits that low- and middle-income countries could employ.[47]

Finally, Assaad began helping Member States establish national AIDS programs. In late December 1985, for example, Assaad flew to India to help the government establish its AIDS program. By this time, several cases of AIDS had already surfaced in the country. Assaad met with India's Health Ministry officials and helped them open seven HIV testing facilities. In conjunction with his Collaborating Center directors, he also helped India establish 25 technical teams and distribute AIDS alerts in all 106 of the nation's medical schools.[48]

The India trip proved successful, but it exhausted Assaad. India was but one example of the demands AIDS was now making on his calendar in the last half of 1985. During those last months, his schedule had erupted with AIDS-related travel, planning, diplomacy, and technical advising. These new demands began crowding out the time Assaad had previously spent running his division effectively. Assaad did not want any part of his divisional program to suffer from his absence, so as his schedule began ramping up around AIDS in the summer and fall of 1985, he began searching for someone to lead the AIDS program.[49]

In his preliminary search for a potential program leader, Assaad again sought the opinion of McCormick. McCormick recommended Jonathan Mann. As we noted earlier, Assaad had initially met Mann in 1984, as Mann passed through Geneva on his way to *Projet SIDA* in Zaire.[50] That meeting was premature, of course, as Assaad had only started thinking about WHO's role in AIDS and the prospect of a global AIDS program remained months away. But McCormick extolled Mann to Assaad: "I couldn't imagine a better candidate for the position," McCormick recalled.[51] As it turned out, Assaad "would have a chance … [to] sound him out" with relative ease when the two would meet in Bangui in late October at the meeting to develop the clinical case definition for AIDS.[52] "[Assaad] and [Mann] hit it off well," McCormick recalled, "But

[46] Control Programme on AIDS, "Global WHO Strategy For the Prevention And Control of Acquired Immunodeficiency Syndrome: Projected Needs For 1986–1987," World Health Organization AIDS/CPA/86.2, April 1986, p. 5.

[47] "Second Meeting of the WHO Collaborating Centres on AIDS," 2nd draft, December 16–18, 1985, Geneva.

[48] Fawsia Assaad, Interview by Michael Merson, New Haven, CT, July, 2002; "India launches AIDS education campaign," *United Press International*, May 9, 1986.

[49] Joseph B. McCormick and Susan Fisher-Hoch, *Level 4: Virus Hunters of the CDC*. New York: Barnes & Noble Books, 1999, p. 189.

[50] Jonathan M. Mann Oral History, Interviewed by Jake Spidle, New Mexico Health Historical Collection, UNM Health Sciences Library and Informatics Center, 1996. p. 3.

[51] Joseph B. McCormick and Susan Fisher-Hoch, *Level 4: Virus Hunters of the CDC*, New York: Barnes & Noble Books, 1996, 1999, pp. 189–190.

[52] CDS Control Programme on AIDS, "Global WHO Strategy For the Prevention And Control of Acquired Immunodeficiency Syndrome: Projected Needs For 1986–1987," World Health Organization AIDS/CPA/86.2, April 1986, p. 6; Joseph B. McCormick and Susan Fisher-Hoch, *Level 4: Virus Hunters of the CDC*, New York: Barnes & Noble Books, 1996, 1999, p. 188.

when [Assaad] asked him whether he'd have any interest in setting up a WHO program on AIDS, [Mann] didn't immediately agree, although he did tell [Assaad] that he would help him put together some ideas for the new organization."[53]

While Mann initially seemed ambivalent about the venture, Assaad returned from the Bangui meeting largely convinced Mann was his candidate. "He came back saying that he wanted to get Jonathan," Assaad's wife later remembered.[54] Consequently, Assaad called Dowdle at CDC to discuss his hopes for a new AIDS program and Mann as the potential program leader. Was Mann available? Assaad asked Dowdle.[55] It turned out, Mann was available and, more importantly, interested. Despite his initial ambivalence during his meeting with Assaad in October, Mann had quickly come around to the idea of heading WHO's AIDS program. "I noticed ... that his fervor increased," recalled Tom Quinn, Mann's partner at *Projet SIDA*.

> He became more passionate, much more. ... I noticed that 3 months before he announced he was leaving. ... I do think that [Mann], having lived [in Zaire] for 2 years, saw that this was a disaster in the making and no one was doing anything. So he became more impassioned – something had to be done, a leader had to go out there and make the predictions and the acknowledgement that this was a tremendous epidemic with global proportions. That's what he wanted to do. ... [Mann] was saying this is going to be the worst epidemic of all times, of our times ... about a month later, he called me and said, I'm going to be leaving *Projet SIDA*, the WHO wants to form a global program—just a unit maybe—and I need to take this on. I think ... he had to take this to a different level. I think he thought WHO was the place to go ... he was religious in his fervor on this topic.[56]

In January, 1986, Assaad and Mahler formally offered Mann the job. Mann agreed and joined WHO on a secondment from CDC assigned out of the office of Jim Curran, who was directing CDC's AIDS efforts.[57] WHO announced Mann's new position on January 16, 1986, though he would not begin his official duties until later in the year.[58] For his part, Mann was not unmindful of the fact this opportunity had arisen through strategic contacts and some serendipitous encounters along the way, particularly his initial meeting with Assaad in Geneva in 1984. "I know perfectly well," Mann told an interviewer in 1996, reflecting on that initial encounter with Assaad in Geneva, "that if, in 1986, there'd been an open application for a job as a head of that AIDS program at WHO, I really doubt I would have been chosen, because there would have been people who are older, who had more of this

[53] Joseph B. McCormick and Susan Fisher-Hoch, *Level 4: Virus Hunters of the CDC*, New York: Barnes & Noble Books, 1996, 1999, pp. 189–190.

[54] Fawsia Assaad, Interview by Michael Merson, New Haven, CT, July, 2002.

[55] Walt Dowdle, Interview by Michael Merson, New Haven, CT, August, 2002.

[56] Thomas Quinn, Interview by Michael Merson, New Haven, CT, August, 2002.

[57] James Curran, Interviewed by Michael Merson, September 3, 2002; Walt Dowdle, Interview by Michael Merson, New Haven, CT, August, 2002.

[58] "More than 20,000 Cases Worldwide, U.N. Agency Reports," *The Associated Press*, January 16, 1986.

experience or that experience."[59] Mann would bring more to the task than Assaad could ever have imagined.

Mann's recruitment was just part of Assaad's greater effort to launch a large, global AIDS program at WHO. Even as Assaad and Mahler were wooing Mann to join the new venture, the two of them were placing Assaad's AIDS program proposal before WHO's Executive Board. On January 17, 1986, Mahler walked the Board through the six-point AIDS program plan that Assaad had provided the Program Committee in written form the previous November.[60] It had taken four and a half years from the initial discovery for AIDS to make it onto the agenda of WHO's Executive Board.

In response to Assaad's proposed plan, the Board passed its first resolution on AIDS.[61] In Resolution EB 77.R12, the Board acknowledged that AIDS and other manifestations of HIV infection were becoming a major public health concern in many areas of the world and urgently required global alertness and preparedness from the global health community.[62] Since public information, education, and a safe blood supply were, at that stage, the only measures available to limit the spread of AIDS, the resolution urged countries to share information on AIDS incidence and called on WHO to expand its information exchange on the disease, to develop a simple and inexpensive test for the virus, and to advise countries on the provision of a safe blood supply.[63] The Board called on governments "to maintain vigilance and carry out as necessary public health strategies for the prevention and control of AIDS," and requested the Director-General to seek additional funds (of an unspecified amount) to support "national and collective programs of surveillance and epidemiology, laboratory service, clinical support, and prevention and control."[64]

Following this call from WHO's Executive Board, Assaad continued convening various WHO constituencies to move the AIDS program forward. Working with the assistance of Karen Esteves, a technical officer from Sweden, Assaad organized a meeting of AIDS test-kit manufacturers soon after the Board meeting to encourage a new generation of screening tests, ones that would make HIV testing accessible to low-and middle-income countries. The participants agreed to fast-track kits that were "simple, inexpensive, and capable of being performed and read with minimal laboratory equipment ... under a wide range of conditions in the field."[65] Then, 2 months

[59] Jonathan M. Mann Oral History, Interviewed by Jake Spidle, New Mexico Health Historical Collection, UNM Health Sciences Library and Informatics Center, 1996. pp. 3–4.

[60] World Health Organization, "Executive Board, Seventy-Seventh Session Agenda, Geneva, 8 January 1986." EB 77/1.

[61] WHO Executive Board, "WHO activities for the prevention and control of AIDS," EB77/12, Geneva, 8–17 January 1986.

[62] John Iliffe, *The African AIDS Epidemic: A History*. Ohio University Press, 2006, p. 68.

[63] "Acquired Immunodeficiency Syndrome (AIDS): WHO Programme on AIDS," *Weekly Epidemiology Record,* January 31, 1986, 5:35; See also "WHO board reviews 'health for all by year 2000' strategy," *UN Chronicle*, April 1, 1986, 23:88–90.

[64] WHO Executive Board, "WHO activities for the prevention and control of AIDS," EB77/12, Geneva, 8–17 January 1986.

[65] WHO, "Summary of financial requirements for the WHO strategy for the prevention and control

later, in early March, Assaad participated in a WHO meeting of 41 African governments in Brazzaville, the location of the WHO regional office for Africa.[66] Following extensive debates, the group unanimously approved "Recommendations for a Plan of Action for AIDS Control in the African Region of WHO," which proposed that every government commence public education, institute a surveillance system, develop its laboratory facilities, form a national AIDS committee, and perform an epidemiological assessment.[67]

By April 1986, Assaad had his WHO AIDS program—dubbed the Control Programme on AIDS (CPA)—on its way. He had a small budget: WHO's Executive Board had allocated $1.15 million from its 1986–1987 regular budget for AIDS activities.[68] He had put together a small team: two permanent staff (Hiko Tamashiro, a Japanese epidemiologist, and Edith Bernard, an experienced WHO administrative assistant), a patch-work of part-time support from other WHO programs (about six full time employee equivalents), and Jonathan Mann, seconded from CDC to serve as the responsible officer.[69] He also had Coordinating Centers throughout the world providing improved and economical antibody kits and updated blood safety guidelines for low- and middle-income countries to protect their blood supply and conduct surveillance.[70] The WHO program was small, but it was a very real and important start.

of AIDS," AIDS/CPA/86.2, June 1986.

[66] John Iliffe, *The African AIDS Epidemic: A History*. Ohio University Press, 2006, p. 68. WHO, "Summary of financial requirements for the WHO strategy for the prevention and control of AIDS," AIDS/CPA/86.2, June 1986; "AIDS: Plan of action for control in the African region," *WER*, 61, 93, 1986.

[67] John Iliffe, *The African AIDS Epidemic: A History*. Ohio University Press, 2006, p. 68; DCS Control Programme on AIDS, "Global WHO Strategy For the Prevention And Control of Acquired Immunodeficiency Syndrome: Projected Needs For 1986–1987," World Health Organization AIDS/CPA/86.2, April 1986, p. 6; WHO, "Summary of financial requirements for the WHO strategy for the prevention and control of AIDS," AIDS/CPA/86.2, June 1986; "AIDS: Plan of action for control in the African region," *WER*, 61, 93, 1986.

[68] CDS Control Program on AIDS, "Meeting of Donors For the Prevention and Control of Acquired Immunodeficiency Syndrome, Geneva, 21–22 April 1986." World Health Organization, AIDS/CPA/86.1, 5.

[69] Ibid.; Ofelia T. Monzon, "Profiles of Famous Educators: Jonathan Mann, 1947–98," UNESCO International Bureau of Education, 2001. http://www.ibe.unesco.org/fileadmin/user_upload/archive/publications/ThinkersPdf/manne.pdf Accessed on July 29, 2009; DCD Control Programme on AIDS, "Meeting on Educational Strategies for the Prevention and Control of AIDS, Geneva, 17–19 June 1986," World Health Organization, AIDS/CPA/86.4, Annex 1, p. 12.

[70] WHO Executive Board, "WHO Activities for the Prevention and Control of Acquired Immunodeficiency Syndrome, Seventy-ninth Session, Provisional agenda item 7.2," World Health Organization, November 25, 1986, EB79/12, p. 7; "New Test Developed for AIDS Detection," *Japan Economic Newswire*, April 16, 1986.

Chapter 3
Creating a Global Response

In early 1986 the World Health Organization (WHO) launched its Control Programme on AIDS (CPA), but this event was clearly overshadowed by the growing AIDS[1] pandemic. By early April, 83 countries had reported between 22,000 and 25,000 cases of AIDS to WHO, and WHO epidemiologists were estimating that between 2 million and 3 million people had already acquired the infection.[2] Research at the time was showing that HIV had a much longer latency period than originally thought—upwards of 5 years at that stage—and suggested—ominously—that HIV was much more lethal than originally suspected. At least 40% of people with the virus could expect to develop AIDS and, barring some new intervention, would die from their illness.[3] Better comprehension, both of risk groups and risk behaviors, indicated that the task of prevention and control would be a long and difficult process. Many observers were publicly fretting over the all-but-inevitable and explosive spread of the pandemic into Asia, the Caribbean, and Latin America. "The disease has also started to reach epidemic proportions in parts of Latin America and Africa," noted one reporter.[4] "AIDS in the industrialized world is spreading with 'controlled acceleration,'" noted Diagnostics Pasteur Chairman, Christian Policard, "but in countries like Brazil it is 'catastrophic.'"[5] What made this prospect all the

---

Within this chapter the singular pronouns *I* and *my* refer to Michael Merson alone, whereas the plural pronouns *we* and *us* generally refer to Michael Merson and Stephen Inrig jointly. Where *we* or *us* refers to Michael Merson and his colleagues at WHO, the object of the pronoun is clarified by context.

[1] For the purposes of this text, we will use the term AIDS to encompass both AIDS and HIV unless otherwise specified.

[2] David Marsh, "The Billion Dollar Squabble," *Financial Times* (London), June 23, 1986, Monday, 13.

[3] Philip M. Boffey, "AIDS in the Future: Experts Say Deaths Will Climb Sharply," *New York Times*, January 14, 1986.

[4] David Marsh, "The Billion Dollar Squabble," *Financial Times* (London), June 23, 1986, Monday, 13.

[5] Ibid.

© Springer International Publishing AG 2018

M. Merson, S. Inrig, *The AIDS Pandemic*, DOI 10.1007/978-3-319-47133-4_3

more bleak was the fact that AIDS's complexity appeared to be putting to rest any premature promises of a quick vaccine and even threatened the prospect of a treatment or cure. At that point in time, no credible drug existed to ward off the relentless progression of the virus. Moreover, although at least one company had made significant advances on at least one promising drug—the reverse transcriptase inhibitor known as azidothymidine (AZT)—clinical trials would not show its efficacy for several months. Thus, even as many hailed the launch of WHO's $1.15 million AIDS program, with its small but motivated staff, many observers were keenly aware that the devastating potential of the global pandemic made these efforts appear far from sufficient to the task. A truly global response would demand substantial donor funding; it would require visionary leadership; and it would depend on strong institutional backing.

For WHO's Fakhry Assaad and Jonathan Mann, obtaining government and donor support required them to convince governments of the severity of the problem, persuade donors they had a material interest in AIDS prevention and that CPA had a credible plan for stopping or even controlling the pandemic. Assaad and Mann hoped to use the May 1986 World Health Assembly (WHA) as their first major platform from which to raise global AIDS awareness and announce the formation of CPA.[6] Assaad and Mann (who the Centers for Disease Control and Prevention [CDC] did not formally second to WHO until June 1986) spent time before the Assembly securing support for CPA from various governments, and drafted a summary report of the new program that Director-General Halfdan Mahler distributed to WHA Member States prior to the event.[7] Nine high-income countries offered strong support of WHO's efforts, and Sweden and the United States specifically called on WHO to establish an "action program" in Geneva.[8] The United States announced it would commit $2.5 million towards the program's establishment.[9]

Other countries were more ambivalent, however, when they took the floor of the Assembly to discuss both the AIDS situation and the formation of CPA. Some Southeast Asian countries, for example, considered AIDS only a threat from outside their borders: Thailand assured others that "there had been only six cases of AIDS in the country and "all had been imported from abroad"; China announced it had taken steps to prevent the disease, including reinforcing "monitoring and screening points" in "provinces which were open to foreigners"; and North Korea asked WHO to encourage "international and national organizations responsible for international tourism and sports travel" not to "organize their work in areas where AIDS had occurred and spread."[10] Other countries displayed similar hesitancy, downplaying

[6] John Iliffe, *The African AIDS Epidemic: A History*. Ohio University Press, 2006, p. 68.

[7] World Health Assembly, "WHO activities for the prevention and control of AIDS: Report by the Director-General," A39/16, 4 April 1986.

[8] Committee A. "WHO Activities for the Prevention and Control of Acquired Immunodeficiency Syndrome (Report by the Director-General: Item 28 of the Agenda (Resolution EB77.R12; Document A39/16)." Thirty-Ninth World Health Assembly, Final Summary Records of Committee A, May 1986, pp. 215–216.

[9] Ibid, pp. 216.

[10] Ibid.

the extent or severity of their epidemics: India claimed they had identified only six women with the disease; Cameroon's Minister of Health suggested "the situation in Cameroon was not alarming"; and Ghana's Minister concluded "the disease did not really merit all the clamor and notoriety it had attracted in such a short time."[11] Many African countries took umbrage at suggestions that AIDS had originated in their continent, or to the idea of sending HIV-infected African expats back to their country of origin: Cameroon's Minister asked WHO to "take action to repair the moral prejudice done to black Africa" because of "allegations from Western countries that AIDS had originated in Central Africa"; Ghana's delegate found it "unacceptable that persons infected with AIDS be expelled and returned to countries which were less capable of handling the situation"; while Zaire's representative maintained that the "dispute about the origins of diseases such as AIDS...only distracted attention from the main priority—the fight against the disease."[12]

It was in this context of denial and ambivalence that the representative from Uganda, Samuel Okware, surprised the WHA audience by admitting AIDS was a problem in his country and by offering Uganda's support to CPA. Okware acknowledged that, in recent years, the country had observed cases very similar to AIDS.[13] I was attending the Assembly during this discussion and remember this moment vividly. The room filled with an eerie silence as Okware related the spread of AIDS in his country. The first cases had appeared among "peasants and rural inhabitants ... between 1982 and 1985, and since then the number of new cases had steadily increased—as had the overall mortality rate." While the "disease appeared to have started in two border districts in 1982," Okware explained, it "had now spread to four adjacent districts." Okware called on WHO to "develop more reliable and specific serological tests which would take into account the ecological and environmental background of the population concerned ... [and also] to conduct applied research in less developed countries." Okware maintained that "his country preferred to concentrate its limited resources on more widespread diseases, such as measles, malaria, gastroenteritis, and respiratory diseases ... [but it] had to acknowledge that AIDS was not confined to affluent Western countries."[14] As he sat down, I remember being struck by how quiet the room had become.

Why did Okware's speech hush the Assembly so definitively? Because in that one speech, Okware had finally broken the silence around AIDS in Africa and, we believe, this proved to be one of the key turning points in the early global response to the pandemic. In the ensuing years, Uganda would go on to develop a very

---

[11] Ibid, pp. 218, 221.

[12] Ibid., pp. 218–221.

[13] John Iliffe, *The African AIDS Epidemic: A History*. Ohio University Press, 2006, p. 68, 71. Indeed, not only was this speech surprising, in many ways it was also historical. It was the first time a country frankly admitted to having many AIDS cases. I (Michael Merson) attended this session at the Assembly....and one could have heard a pin drop when he spoke...it broke the silence by Africans about AIDS in Africa.

[14] Committee A. "WHO Activities for the Prevention and Control of Acquired Immunodeficiency Syndrome (Report by the Director-General: Item 28 of the Agenda (Resolution EB77.R12; Document A39/16)." Thirty-Ninth World Health Assembly, Final Summary Records of Committee A, May 1986, pp. 215.

forthright and aggressive national AIDS program (see Chapter 10).[15] At the end of
the debate that day, Uganda joined the other delegations in unanimously passing
Resolution WHA 39.29. It was the first resolution addressing what was now a
5-year-old pandemic of a fatal disease; over 2 million adults in over half the countries in the world were already affected.

Bolstered by this strong showing of support, Assaad and Mann took their message of global pandemic awareness to the 2nd International Conference on AIDS in
June 1986. More than 2000 participants journeyed to Paris for the meeting, which
WHO, the French Ministry of Health, the Pasteur Institute, and France's National
Institute for Health and Medical Research (INSERM) sponsored jointly.[16] The
importance of the conference for CPA was that it helped shape the discourse around
the global pandemic. Drawing on Assaad and Mann's AIDS strategy, Mahler opened
the conference by highlighting the severity of the pandemic. After listing the multiple diseases by which millions of people across the globe were afflicted, Mahler
concluded:

> Now AIDS comes along, and risks overshadowing all the other communicable diseases.
> AIDS, the syndrome, is only the tip of the iceberg; for every AIDS case there are three to
> five cases of the less severe AIDS-related complex and anything between 50 to 100 silent
> carriers. Giving a cumulative total of five to ten million infected persons, capable of trans-
> mitting the virus. … AIDS is a universal problem. …In recent history, there is hardly any
> disease that has taken humanity in its grip as AIDS has.[17]

Adding to Mahler's point, Mann expressed concerns over the emerging threat
AIDS posed and the futile efforts the global community had exerted against the
pandemic thus far: "We're still foundering," he explained in his report to the conference. "The disease is showing clear signs of spreading in areas where it never
existed before and growing in areas where it already existed."[18] Since researchers
were only in the early stages of comprehending the full impact of its transmission
and infection, "the evidence suggest[ed] that the risk appears relatively stable and
[did not] appear to be declining."[19] While Mann and Assaad sought to ameliorate
concerns about blood safety, particularly in high-income countries, WHO staff

---

[15] "Uganda admits widespread AIDS outbreak," *United Press International*, May 28, 1986; Blaine
Harden "Uganda Battles AIDS Epidemic; Disease Reported Rampant Among Promiscuous
Heterosexuals," *The Washington Post*, June 2, 1986, A1.

[16] Paul Treuthardt, "World Conference To Highlight Vaccine, Africa, Children," *The Associated
Press*, June 22, 1986.

[17] Halfdan Mahler, "International Conference on AIDS, Paris, 23–25 June 1986: Opening Speech."
World Health Organization, 9992F/o399H/29.5.86, p. 2, 4–5. See also Matt Clark, Ann McDaniel,
Michael Reese, Ruth Marshall, and Mark Starr, "AIDS in the Workplace," *Newsweek,* July 7, 1986,
p. 62; Andrew Veitch, "'Up to 10 million' have AIDS virus: Comment by World Health Organisation
head Mahler," *The Guardian*, June 24, 1986; Richard A. Knox, "Scourge of AIDS Spreads
Worldwide," *Boston Globe*, June 22, 1986, 1.

[18] Richard Z. Chesnoff with Sophie Roquelle, "6 Percent of Africans Estimated to Have AIDS
Virus; Fighting a world epidemic," *U.S. News & World Report,* July 7, 1986, 72; Steve Holland,
"Doctors say up to 100,000 suffering from AIDS," *United Press International,* June 23, 1986.

[19] Richard A. Knox, "Scourge of AIDS Spreads Worldwide," *Boston Globe*, June 22, 1986, 1.

wanted to stress the vulnerability of resource-poor nations.[20] "AIDS is a universal problem," Mahler explained in his speech,

> However, the world can be divided into three areas. ... The first group includes the developed countries ... The second group of countries includes those that are apparently free, or nearly free, of LAV/HTLV-III infection. ... Finally, in the third group are the many countries in the developing world which currently face an AIDS crisis. ... These countries must confront a complex LAV/HTLV-III problem superimposed upon the already severe public health problems of the developing world ...[21]

Given the complexity of the pandemic in these vulnerable nations, WHO's strategy aimed to tackle the long-term reality before them: "We can't just pour in money and equipment," Assaad told reporters in a telephone interview, "We have to start training and build up the whole health infrastructure in these developing nations. But in the long run for a country to maintain this will not be an easy thing."[22]

Assaad's emphasis on infrastructure highlights the second task he and Mann had before them: providing a coherent strategy to address the mounting crisis. Assaad had already drafted WHO's preliminary AIDS control strategy in the fall of 1985 to gain WHO approval for CPA. Now, he and Mann had to fill out the program in greater detail. In mid-June, 1986, the two hosted a meeting with science and public health experts in Geneva to explore the most effective educational strategies available for the prevention and control of AIDS. The group pushed for WHO's program to base its AIDS educational strategy on the chronic-disease response model, one that combined "rapid diffusion of information with well-designed programs to achieve life-style changes," and particularly to identify the most effective ways "to use modern communications to address [AIDS] at national and local levels."[23] Policy-makers, the WHO advisors suggested, needed to understand their national epidemic within a global perspective. WHO therefore should take the lead in this endeavor, Assaad's advisors recommended "standardizing the core concepts of AIDS, and coordinat[ing global] AIDS prevention research and implementation strategies."[24]

In response to these requests, Assaad and Mann began funding small pilot studies on behavioral change. "The nature of AIDS" Assaad explained to reporters, "... is uniformly fatal among those who get the full-blown form of the disease, mak[ing] it different from any other sexually transmitted illness." The virus's long incubation period meant people could easily miss the cause and effect relationship between

[20] Steve Holland, "Doctors report on experimental AIDS treatment," *United Press International*, June 24, 1986.

[21] Halfdan Mahler, "International Conference on AIDS, Paris, 23–25 June 1986: Opening Speech." World Health Organization, 9992F/o399H/29.5.86, p. 2, 4–5.

[22] Richard A. Knox, "Scourge of AIDS Spreads Worldwide," *Boston Globe*, June 22, 1986, 1.

[23] CDS Control Programme on AIDS, "Meeting on Educational Strategies for the Prevention and Control of AIDS, Geneva, 17–19 June 1986," World Health Organization, AIDS/CPA/86.4, pp. 3–5.

[24] Ibid.

high risk behavior and infection. Nations had to start stressing behavior change, and the pilot projects—one in Africa and one "elsewhere"—were meant to demonstrate "what might be done." "We have to start small and learn as we go," Assaad told reporters. "If we have to change behavior, we will do it. If this is the only thing to do, we will do it. That's my attitude."[25]

Unrolling such a complex health intervention on such a broad scale raised a host of logistical questions. How would CPA support national AIDS control programs? How would it relate to other parts of WHO and other United Nations (UN) agencies? What would be the criteria by which CPA would select countries receiving assistance? To what extent would CPA "fund non-governmental AIDS organizations?"[26]Assaad and Mann were scrambling to develop answers to these questions, since WHO had never so quickly had to design and implement a program of the magnitude required to confront the AIDS pandemic. Rather than addressing the particular ways WHO would coordinate with countries and with other UN agencies, Assaad and Mann concentrated on securing WHO's central role of coordinating the global response to the disease and providing support to Member States. This, they believed, would reduce competition with other agencies and help secure donor dollars to support national efforts. To meet the burgeoning Member States' demand for information on AIDS, Assaad and Mann produced and broadly distributed AIDS information to countries (and other health organizations) through the WHO regional offices.[27] This included a weekly update of reported AIDS cases, a monthly update of the most recent AIDS information, and biweekly AIDS articles (written by Mann) in WHO's *Weekly Epidemiological Record*. CPA staff also compiled information on AIDS legislation and policies that Assaad and Mann disseminated for governments to use. They also leveraged the media—Mann particularly excelled at this—to promote their message through press briefings and interviews.

Raising awareness and designing a strategy were almost meaningless without appropriate financial support, so Assaad and Mann spent a considerable amount of time that year raising funds for CPA. To begin with, on April 21–22, 1986, Assaad spearheaded WHO's first Meeting of Donor Agency Representatives (later to be called Interested Parties) on the Prevention and Control of Acquired Immunodeficiency Syndrome (AIDS) in Geneva to present its financial needs.[28] Mahler and Assaad had agreed to launch CPA as an "extrabudgetary" program

[25] Richard A. Knox, "Worldwide Campaign Launched Against AIDS; UN Unit Presses For Funds," *Boston Globe*, June 29, 1986, p.15.

[26] WHO, "Report of meeting of participating parties for the prevention and control of AIDS," AIDS/CPA/86.3, Geneva, 28 June 1986. WHO, "WHO Programme on AIDS: Projected Plans and Needs 1986-1987," April 1986; CDS Control Programme on AIDS, "Report of [the] Meeting of Participating Parties for the Prevention and Control of Acquired Immunodeficiency Syndrome, Geneva, 28 June 1986." World Health Organization, AIDS/CPA/86.3, p. 2.

[27] WHO Executive Board, "WHO activities for the prevention and control of AIDS," EB79/12, 25 November 1986.

[28] CDS Control Programme on AIDS, "Meeting of Donors For the Prevention and Control of Acquired Immunodeficiency Syndrome, Geneva, 21–22 April 1986." World Health Organization, AIDS/CPA/86.1, pp. 2, 8–9; CDS Control Programme on AIDS, "WHO Programme on AIDS: Projected Plans and Needs 1986–1987," World Health Organization, April 1986.

under the auspices of Assaad's Division of Communicable Diseases, so such a fundraising effort was imperative.

What is an "extrabudgetary program"? In WHO parlance, it is a program supported through resources outside WHO's regular budget (which consisted of assessed contributions from Member States). Since the mid-1970s, WHO had successfully launched a number of such programs. These extrabudgetary programs included The Special Programme of Research, Development and Research Training in Human Reproduction (HRP) (it used to be known as the Special Programme of Research in Human Reproduction), the Special Programme for Research and Training in Tropical Diseases, the Expanded Programme on Immunization, and the Diarrheal Diseases Control Programme (which I directed from 1980 to 1990). In the 1986–1987 biennium, HRP alone received $37 million in extrabudgetary support (WHO's total Regular Budget in 1986–1987 was $300 million).[29] These programs had their own management oversight committees, allowing them to operate with less political constraints than programs that were supported mainly through WHO's Regular Budget. Assaad and Mahler felt confident that CPA needed the independence and flexibility inherent in an extrabudgetary program. What they were unclear about, at this stage, was whether CPA would exist as a free-standing program or remain under the Division of Communicable Diseases.[30]

Assaad, along with Ingar Brueggemann, led the first meeting of Interested Parties (Mann had not yet been formally seconded to WHO). Brueggemann, a highly respected German woman who had worked at WHO for many years, was the Organization's Director of External Coordination for Health and Social Development. The meeting, which included scientists and donor representatives from 15 countries and two international agencies, discussed Assaad and Mann's "Global WHO Strategy for the Prevention and Control of AIDS: Projected Needs for 1986–1987." This Strategy summarized the worldwide epidemiological situation of HIV infections, spelled out WHO's planned activities for the 1986–1987 biennium, and identified areas towards which the extrabudgetary funds would be directed.[31] Assaad asked for $13.8 million in donor support over the 2 years, 80% of which would be provided to 25 high-incidence, low-resource countries to help them establish an AIDS surveillance, prevention, and control program. The remaining 20% were to be used for WHO staff, technical meetings, and support to WHO's Collaborating

[29] Fiona Godlee, "The World Health Organisation: WHO's special programmes: undermining from above," *BMJ* 1995;310:178–182 (21 January).

[30] On whether the AIDS program should have been "in communicable diseases or … be a separate thing," see Walt Dowdle, Interview by Michael Merson, New Haven, CT, August, 2002.

[31] The countries and agencies involved included Australia, Austria, Belgium, Canada, Denmark, Finland, France, the Federal Republic of Germany, Japan, the Netherlands, Norway, Sweden, Switzerland, the United Kingdom, and the United States as well as from the Commission of European Communities (CEC) and the World Bank attended the meeting. See CDS Control Programme on AIDS, "Meeting of Donors For the Prevention and Control of Acquired Immunodeficiency Syndrome, Geneva, 21–22 April 1986." World Health Organization, AIDS/CPA/86.1, p. 2; WHO, "WHO Programme on AIDS: Projected Plans and Needs 1986-1987," April 1986; CDS Control Programme on AIDS, "Meeting of Donors For the Prevention and Control of Acquired Immunodeficiency Syndrome, Geneva, 21–22 April 1986." World Health Organization, AIDS/CPA/86.1, pp. 8–9.

Centers. The participants concluded that all Member States should work together to control the pandemic with WHO coordinating both multilateral and bilateral assistance. They also agreed that the initial financial outlays would help WHO mobilize personnel and resources, but that CPA would need additional resources beyond 1987. In light of the longer term commitments expected, the donors requested that WHO develop mechanisms to verify program implementation, monitor program elements, and ensure fiscal accountability.[32]

As 1986 unfolded and the scope of the pandemic increased, Assaad and Mann were forced to revise their cost estimates upwards. They had already secured about $2.6 million in pledged extrabudgetary support (mostly from the United States), which they had on top of the regular budget resources WHO's Executive Board had already approved, as well as Mann's salary (from the United States government) and the part-time effort of WHO staff donated from five WHO programs to CPA.[33] Looking at the needs of the various countries requesting help, Assaad and Mann estimated that each country would "require between US$ 320,000 and US$ 700,000" to start up and implement the first year of a program.[34] While not every country would need that level of support (the average would be about $400,000), the two expected that at least 20 resource-poor countries would require full assistance establishing their AIDS programs. This pushed their projected costs for CPA in the first year to almost $10 million, with $17 million required over the first 2 years.[35]

The early donor response somewhat disappointed Assaad and Mann. By the end of June, 1986, only the United States and Sweden had pledged support to the program. Assaad later admitted that he and Mann had hoped to secure all the financial support at the donor agencies meeting. Having fallen far short of that, they urged the other nations to return home and secure funds "to combat the burgeoning problem

---

[32] CDS Control Programme on AIDS, "Meeting of Donors For the Prevention and Control of Acquired Immunodeficiency Syndrome, Geneva, 21–22 April 1986." World Health Organization, AIDS/CPA/86.1, pp. 8–9.

[33] Assaad and Mann budgeted the first $1.15 million accordingly: $238,000 for two CPA posts, $212,000 for support for exchange of Information, $650,000 for Regional program support, $35,000 for Research, and $15,000 for Data Processing Equipment. They also expected $2.6 million in extrabudgetary support from the United States and other sources, which they budgeted accordingly: $112,500 for exchange of information, $160,000 for preparation and distribution of guidelines, $415,000 for assessment of diagnostic methodology, $1,811,000 for cooperation with Member States, $20,000 for coordination of research, and $78,000 for administrative support for the CPA. See CDS Control Programme on AIDS, "Summary of Financial Requirements For the WHO Strategy for the Prevention and Control of AIDS," World Health Organization, AIDS/CPA/86.2 Add.1, June 1986, pp. 1–4.

[34] CDS Control Programme on AIDS, "Summary of Financial Requirements For the WHO Strategy for the Prevention and Control of AIDS," World Health Organization, AIDS/CPA/86.2 Add.1, June 1986, pp. 1–4.

[35] The initial budgetary and extrabudgetary costs were for the 1986–1987 biennium, while the $8 million start-up funds were for the "initial implementation and first year operation" costs. See CDS Control Programme on AIDS, "Summary of Financial Requirements For the WHO Strategy for the Prevention and Control of AIDS," World Health Organization, AIDS/CPA/86.2 Add.1, June 1986, pp. 1–4. Richard A. Knox, "Scourge of AIDS Spreads Worldwide," *Boston Globe*, June 22, 1986, 1.

of AIDS."[36] In the meantime, they tried to frame the situation optimistically: The lack of immediate commitment from other nations "may be very encouraging," Assaad told a reporter, "because it may mean they will go back and negotiate harder with their government."[37] Indeed, by the end of October, the United Kingdom and Norway joined the United States and Sweden in giving to the program, bringing the total from those four countries to $4.5 million. Only six African nations had attended the donors' meeting, although at least ten were facing an imminent threat from the pandemic. Each of those six had little money to pledge, and "every (donor) country is waiting for the other to start," Assaad explained.[38]

Fundraising for CPA proved initially challenging, in part, because the new program had entered into the funding stream at precisely the time when donors, the United States in particular, were reducing their contributions to WHO. In July 1986 for example, the United States government had stripped $35 million from its expected commitment to the UN and its affiliated agencies because of overall displeasure with the direction of the UN. According to the United States Government Accounting Office (GAO), the Reagan Administration only planned to give 60–70% of the requested $426 million for the 1986–1987 biennium.[39] WHO bore much of the brunt of the United States cuts, and the reductions meant WHO would need to cut its own $544 million dollar regular budget by 6% over the next 2 years, with programs in Africa, Southeast Asia, the Eastern Mediterranean, as well as administrative services, taking the largest hits. Most of the budget cuts came after Senator Nancy Kassebaum, a Republican from Kansas, sponsored an amendment that mandated a 20% reduction in American contributions to any UN organization that made decisions on a "one-country, one-vote" basis. According to the GAO study, Congress adopted the amendment "after years of congressional complaints that international organizations routinely make anti-American decisions and then implement them with money supplied by the United States."[40] The cutbacks "appeared to single out WHO as less responsive to United States interests than other specialized agencies," concluded Mahler, and he felt they would "be particularly damaging to WHO's reputation and its ability to maintain expected funding levels from other key contributors."[41] For CPA to thrive in this environment, Assaad and Mann knew they could not rely only on support from WHO's regular budget to fund the fight against AIDS.

Increasingly, the burden and responsibility of directing CPA fell to Mann. By the late spring of 1986, Mann had transitioned from being a special consultant on loan to CPA to the Responsible Officer for the Program. His fledgling CPA budget afforded him a two-module office on the sixth floor of the main WHO building

---

[36] Richard A. Knox, "Worldwide Campaign Launched Against AIDS; UN Unit Presses For Funds," *Boston Globe*, June 29, 1986, p.15.

[37] Ibid.

[38] Ibid.

[39] Ibid.

[40] "U.N. Agency for Health Facing Cuts," *The Dallas Morning News*, July 27, 1986, 31A.

[41] Ibid.

across from Assaad's office. There, he and his two staff set to work distributing, for example, WHO's new guidelines on AIDS prevention in health care settings and organizing an expert consultation on educational strategies for preventing sexually transmitted HIV.[42] Having addressed these and other tasks, Mann turned to his most pressing one: organizing the Second Meeting of Interested Parties (Assaad and Brueggemann having led the first meeting), scheduled for June. In May, Mann drafted and distributed a background document for that meeting, which he titled "Global WHO Strategy for the Prevention and Control of Acquired Immunodeficiency Syndrome."[43] In the document, Mann spelled out, for the first time, his own initial vision of a Global AIDS Strategy.

Mann's strategy revolved around two main components: national AIDS control programs and WHO's coordinating role. Mann's national AIDS control program strategy largely mirrored the one Assaad had earlier articulated: surveillance; blood safety; laboratory support; epidemiological assessment; and education of the general public, high-risk groups, and health care workers. In later years, when Mann reflected on this stage of development, he would describe this part of the strategy as the "individual risk reduction" model, one mainly gauged to alert individuals about AIDS.[44] In the strategy document, Mann articulated ways that CPA could promote "the more complex tasks of informing, educating, and providing specific health and social services to help stimulate, support, and sustain individual behavioral change."[45] This included social marketing strategies to promote sexual behavior change. As for CPA's role in the global fight against AIDS, Mann reiterated Mahler and Assaad's stance: WHO would provide "global coordination as well as assistance to the national (operational) level."[46]

Mann added two more components to the strategy beyond the ones that he and Assaad had already developed: he encouraged the formation of national AIDS committees in each country, and he called for the inclusion of "ethical dimensions of LAV/HTLV-III infection." In the appeal for national AIDS committees, Mann was following the traditional WHO approach of organizing these groups under each nation's Ministry of Health, though he also called for structuring them to obtain input from "representatives from health, social services, education and other relevant sectors" in each nation.[47] Thus, from the outset, Mann's approach anticipated what observers would later call the "multisectoral response" to AIDS.

---

[42] See CDS, "Guidelines for the Prevention and Control of Infection with LAV/HTLV III," World Health Organization, May 1986, WHO/CDS/AIDS/86.1.

[43] Control Programme on AIDS, "Global WHO Strategy for the Prevention and Control of AIDS: Projected Needs for 1986–1987," AIDS/CPA/86.2, June 1986.

[44] Jonathan Mann, "Human Rights and AIDS: The Future of the Pandemic," in Jonathan Mann, Sofia Gruskin, Michael Grodin, and George Annas, eds., *Health and Human Rights: A Reader*. New York: Routledge, 1999, p. 217.

[45] Ibid.

[46] Control Programme on AIDS, "Global WHO Strategy for the Prevention and Control of AIDS: Projected Needs for 1986–1987," AIDS/CPA/86.2, June 1986.

[47] Ibid.

As to his concern for ethics, Mann stressed in the strategy document that ethics was "vitally important" to achieve effective "public health action," focusing mainly on the prevention of "discrimination toward those infected with HIV."[48] Mann's emphasis on ethics was relatively nascent at this point, but it was an approach he would later champion and for which he would become famous: the health and human rights framework. Mann's "public health ethics rationale" was pragmatic at this stage; it did not "reflect any ideological or philosophical commitment to human rights per se," Mann would later write, "but rather [it] arose from an appreciation for the instrumental value of respecting the rights and dignity of HIV-infected and ill people."[49] Mann's more robust emphasis on human rights still lay in the future.

At the June 1986 Meeting of Interested Parties, Member States and agencies endorsed the WHO's Global AIDS Strategy. Mann's new role at WHO in the summer of 1986 now positioned him as an increasingly prominent advocate in the global fight against AIDS.[50] He brought considerable assets to the program: keen intelligence, great energy, deep knowledge about the pandemic, and firsthand experience working with the disease in Kinshasa. His previous experience in public health gave him great facility working with government officials, public health professionals, and researchers. His fluency in French allowed him to converse easily with policy-makers and scientists from francophone countries. As an American paid by the CDC, Mann was well positioned to attract extrabudgetary resources from the United States and other high-income countries to WHO. Most importantly, as someone given to ethical reflection on matters of policy, Mann quickly bonded with the WHO Director-General Mahler, who shared Mann's humanistic concerns and perspectives.[51]

Mann's deftness with the media accelerated his emergence as WHO's spokesperson on global AIDS. Mann was adept, for example, at helping the media put the promise of new therapies in global perspective. A case in point came in September 1986, when news that clinical trials showing azidothymidine (AZT) to be a potentially promising AIDS therapy set the medical world and AIDS community abuzz.[52] To donor nations, Mann tried to remain circumspect about the drug's effects: "[it] did not directly attack the virus already present nor eliminate it from the body." To reporters he proved equally cautious: "[the new therapy was] no breakthrough of the kind that lets us say 'we have now seen the light at the end of the tunnel.'"[53]

---

[48] Ibid.

[49] Ibid.

[50] CDS Control Programme on AIDS, "Meeting on Educational Strategies for the Prevention and Control of AIDS, Geneva, 17–19 June 1986," World Health Organization, AIDS/CPA/86.4, Annex 1, p. 12.

[51] Importantly, Mann also developed a very close relationship with Joe Cohen, an Israeli who served as Mahler's chief administrator. Like Jon, Cohen was a religious Jew. The ability for all three men to consider the spiritual weight of AIDS certainly provided them with some additional cooperative affinities. Cohen, Mahler, and Mann would frequently talk late into the evening in Mahler's and Cohen's offices.

[52] Jonathan Mann, "WHO Control Programme on AIDS—informal update," no. 1, 1 October 1986.

[53] Thomas W. Netter, "AIDS Cases Are Said To Rise Sharply Worldwide," *The New York Times*, October 5, 1986, 1:9.

While Mann spoke cautiously about prospective therapeutic breakthroughs, he attacked aggressively what he considered the apathy and ambivalence that many global leaders were showing towards the disease. Providers had few weapons with which to fight AIDS beyond education and prevention; after all, effective AIDS prevention efforts required substantive national commitments. In October 1986, in conjunction with the release of CPA's new global AIDS estimates, Mann called on world leaders not to ignore a disease that had already resulted in 31,000 reported deaths in 74 countries. This was just the "tip of the iceberg," he maintained: "An epidemic that affects all continents is by definition a pandemic."[54] Still, he considered the fact that countries were reporting any numbers, rather than denying the disease's existence, to be a positive sign:

> AIDS cases reported to WHO give a limited reflection of the scope of the AIDS problem in the world. However, given the emotional and political climate which tends to characterize AIDS issues, we consider the reporting of even a fraction of known cases by national health authorities to be an expression of national willingness to deal constructively with the problem.[55]

Along with his battle against apathy and denial, Mann also attacked the symbolic actions that were more about political posturing than public health. His main target in this regard was the AIDS travel bans that some countries were starting to install.[56] "[Screening foreign visitors would be] senseless and ineffective," he told European health officials in early November 1986.

> At least a million people in the United States and an estimate of between 30,000 and 50,000 people in the United Kingdom are infected with the AIDS virus. For countries like these to consider screening selectively people from different parts of the world in order to try to protect their own home populations from infection does not make any sense and WHO is strongly opposed to it. This of course does not mean that some national health authorities will not take matters into their own hands and promulgate regulations that have no justification in terms of disease prevention. We have to assume that when this is done, it is done for a more political or symbolic purpose. It does not work to prevent transmission of this international disease.[57]

Countries should aggressively confront AIDS argued Mann, but not through powerless public policies and discriminatory actions.

Mann's increased prominence and activism around AIDS signaled something of a shift in the roles Mann and Assaad were now taking. They were still working together, of course, as perhaps is best exemplified by the publication, in early November 1986, of their jointly authored revision to the Global AIDS Strategy, entitled "AIDS: An International Perspective." The content largely reproduced much

---

[54] Jonathan Mann, "WHO Control Programme on AIDS – informal update," no. 1, 1 October 1986.

[55] Thomas W. Netter, "AIDS Cases Are Said To Rise Sharply Worldwide," *The New York Times*, October 5, 1986, 1:9. See also "AIDS Cases Doubling Yearly, Says Blewett," *Courier-Mail*, November 1, 1986.

[56] Chris Thomas, "Developing World Faces Devastation: WHO Expert," *Sydney Morning Herald*, November 3, 1986, p.7.

[57] Thomson Prentice, "Screening visitors for AIDS 'useless'" *The Times*, November 7 1986.

of the perspective and strategy that Assaad had championed for the previous 2 years, but the style had now changed, adopting Mann's more fervent and eloquent framing of the pandemic's import:

> HIV infection has created a serious challenge to medical and public health practice and even to the fabric of society. ... We cannot imagine a more difficult, serious or complex set of challenges. Yet we can afford complacency even less ... We are working together on AIDS during one of those rare historical moments, at the beginning, really, of a major new global public health challenge. Our responsibility is accordingly heavy, our opportunity to make a difference similarly great. In actions we take, or fail to accomplish during the next few years, we will indeed be judged by future generations.[58]

Still, by the fall of 1986, the transition of responsibilities for the global fight against AIDS had passed from Assaad to Mann. Assaad's delegation to Mann of this expanding leadership role certainly proved Assaad's confidence in him, though it also raised questions about Assaad's future role in AIDS. "I think [Assaad] was somewhat disappointed that he was being shunted aside a little bit," Walt Dowdle later told us.[59] Assaad had, after all, been WHO's point person on AIDS for the previous 2 years. What role would he now play? And if it were a diminished role, how would he move on to tackle seemingly more mundane public health questions after he has thrown himself into the battle against a disease like AIDS? Assaad was not the only one who would have to answer such questions in this story.

Whatever future shape Assaad's career was going to take, Mann's ascendance and the success of Mann and Assaad's leadership would have been impossible were it not for Mahler's decision finally to make AIDS one of WHO's priorities. This evolution had taken time. As we mentioned earlier, Mahler had not considered AIDS a top concern for WHO even as late as mid-1985. External pressure caused Mahler to rethink this, however. Beginning in late 1985, some governments began calling on Mahler to have WHO take a more active role in AIDS.[60] Then, in early 1986, politicians in Mahler's home country of Denmark began suffering political fallout for their own inaction on AIDS, and the diplomatic ramifications of ignoring AIDS were not lost on him.[61] Moreover, as we have mentioned, Mahler realized the flexibility that establishing the AIDS program as an extrabudgetary program would afford WHO, Assaad, and Mann.[62]

These other influences notwithstanding, the real source of Mahler's shift to giving AIDS greater priority was his increasing exposure to its ravages across the globe during 1986. Much of this exposure came from Assaad and Mann. Mann, who had seen AIDS's devastation up close, proved particularly persuasive. In the summer and fall of 1986, Mahler visited some hard-hit countries and truly began to grasp the

[58] Fakhry Assaad and Jonathan Mann, "AIDS: An International Perspective," Geneva: World Health Organization Media Service, November 1986, p.4.

[59] Walt Dowdle, Interview by Michael Merson, New Haven, CT, August, 2002.

[60] James Curran, Interview with Mike Merson, 2002.

[61] Ibid.

[62] Fiona Godlee, "The World Health Organisation: WHO in crisis," BMJ 26 November 1994;309:1424–1428.

extent to which AIDS had penetrated Africa and threatened Asia. WHO reports indicated that known cases had doubled from 15,000 in mid-1985 to 30,000 by mid-1986, and CPA staff estimated that between 1.5 and 3 million people were already infected with the virus, with projections topping 10 million infected. "Clearly it is an epidemic and it is everywhere," Mahler told reporters in mid-September after speaking to country delegates attending the Regional Committee for the Western Pacific region. "[AIDS] is knocking at the door of Asia. India has it now, Australia has quite a lot of it... No country is being spared."[63] Soon thereafter, Mahler met with the Ugandan Minister of Health, Ruhakana Rugunda, at the African Regional Committee Meeting in Brazzaville, who shared with Mahler the alarming AIDS situation in his country. Delegates from other African countries echoed his concerns.[64] After these trips to Asia and Africa and a number of discussions with Mann thereafter about the potentially grave and devastating consequences of the pandemic, Mahler appears to have reached a much deeper realization about what WHO was confronting with AIDS. He now stood ready to throw his full support behind Assaad's and Mann's efforts. Finally, they could count on WHO's full institutional support to run their program and hopefully obtain the needed funding that, heretofore, had not been there.

It was at precisely this point that Mann, Assaad, and Mahler ran into an unexpected obstacle to the full roll-out of the global AIDS program: Assaad became ill. Deathly ill. In fact, Assaad may actually have started showing signs of his illness in late 1985 and early 1986. You will recall it had been in December of 1985 that Assaad spent considerable time traveling back and forth to India to help the Indian Health Ministry establish its AIDS surveillance program. As we noted, Assaad found himself gripped with profound fatigue at the end of that process, "He came back completely worn out, exhausted," his wife Fawsia Assaad told us,

> ... [I noticed it] when he went back and forth to India. ... The confusion came from the fact that he was a medical doctor who knew about lots of things, and he was blocking the diagnosis himself. I think that he knew that it was leukemia, but he wanted to hope that it was something else. He suggested that it could be brucellosis so they had to go for analysis, and he hoped it would be tuberculosis.[65]

Over the next 6 months, as AIDS exploded onto the public stage, Assaad traveled extensively. During this period, he grew increasingly drained. Assaad attributed the weariness to his relentless schedule, and both he and his wife had hoped that the hiring of Mann would assuage some of the burgeoning AIDS workload. But the work kept coming, and Mann's appointment did little to diminish these demands. "He got Jonathan Mann to help," Fawsia explained. "... he felt very happy with [Mann], but I was not feeling happy, because he had said that when [Mann] came, he would travel less, but this didn't happen. He kept on traveling,

---

[63] "'No Country Is Spared,'" *Sydney Morning Herald*, September 17, 1986, 11.

[64] Daniel Tarantola, "Grande et petite histoire des programmes sida," *La Journal du Sida,* 1996, 86–8:109–116.

[65] Fawsia Assaad, Interview by Michael Merson, New Haven, CT, July, 2002.

even with [Mann], saying that [Mann] was too young ... he had to be guided—so it was no better. He kept on working and traveling everywhere."[66] By the summer of 1986, Assaad was so exhausted that he mentioned it to his doctor during his annual check-up. His doctor found nothing unusual and attributed the exhaustion to his long hours at work.[67]

In early September 1986, things appeared to worsen: Assaad's weariness became compounded with pneumonia-like symptoms and other disturbing signs.[68] Bill Parra, who was now assisting both Assaad and Mann, remembered the situation vividly: "Jonathan and I were in the room with him, briefing him on something that was going on in CPA," Parra recalled. "And I remember him saying to Jonathan after the end of the meeting. 'Jonathan, I wonder if you could stay because I want to ask you some questions about some symptoms'…when I went back to my office, Jonathan appeared there 15–20 min later. And he said, 'Bill, it is not good.'"[69] Over the next 2 months, Assaad endured numerous medical tests and several presumptive diagnoses before doctors finally determined, in late October following Assaad's daughter's wedding, that Assaad had developed a severe form of leukemia.[70] "A month before he died ... our doctor found two awkward cells and sent him immediately to hospital," his wife would later recall. "It was one of these very special cases: 'good for research' as the doctors said."[71]

Knowing he was going to die, Assaad began considering the fate of the AIDS program—whether it should remain within his division or be launched as its own special program—as well as the fate of his Communicable Diseases Division. Mahler tried to be optimistic with Assaad. "Mahler came and told him, 'Now you stop all this business and you get out of hospital,'" Fawsia reflected.[72] Still, some sort of transition needed to happen, and over the next month, Assaad and Mahler held long conversations about the AIDS program, in which Mahler recommended the AIDS program be separated from Assaad's division.[73] The program, Mahler explained, needed the visibility and bureaucratic freedom that the division was unable to provide.[74] Ultimately, Assaad agreed: "Fakhry felt that the program needed a global leader," explained Parra.

---

[66] Ibid.

[67] Ibid.

[68] Ibid; Fawsia Assaad, Interview by Stephen Inrig, Dallas, TX, October 5, 2010; William Parra, Interview by Stephen Inrig, Dallas, TX, October 14, 2010.

[69] William Parra, Interview by Stephen Inrig, Dallas, TX, October 14, 2010.

[70] Fawsia Assaad, Interview by Michael Merson, New Haven, CT, July, 2002; Fawsia Assaad, Interview by Stephen Inrig, Dallas, TX, October, 2010; William Parra, Interview by Author, October, 2010.

[71] Fawsia Assaad, Interview by Michael Merson, New Haven, CT, July, 2002.

[72] Ibid.

[73] Ibid.

[74] William Parra, Interview by Stephen Inrig, October, 2010.

He saw that [AIDS] was going to be big ... He envisioned that GPA someday could be 100 people – that was bigger than all the people in his division at the time. ... Even though he loved the idea of working on AIDS he recognized that his division couldn't handle it.[75]

Consequently, Mahler scheduled a press conference towards the end of November to announce the relocation and reprioritization of the AIDS program out of the Division of Communicable Diseases and into his office.

With Assaad sidelined by his illness, Mann took on greater responsibilities trying to raise awareness about AIDS's grave potential. In early November 1986, Mann met with "representatives from 37 Member States of the African Region" and 50 international scientists at WHO's 3-day African Regional Conference on AIDS held in Brazzaville.[76] The meeting explored a full range of issues related to the AIDS pandemic in Africa and, as Mann would later write, "the exchanges were open and friendly; many [country representatives] commented for the first time, AIDS was being openly discussed in a manner typical of meetings on diarrheal diseases or immunization."[77] The meeting differed profoundly from the one held the previous year in Bangui, where "it was difficult to talk about AIDS in Africa and to openly share information about it."[78] The 1986 meeting evinced only "a minimum of defensive behavior," Mann told the *New York Times*.

Along with the WHO regional office for Africa (AFRO) staff, Mann met individually with representatives from 15 African nations, all of whom requested WHO visit them to develop a CPA-sponsored AIDS program: "We said 'if this is something you want to do, then we will help by first sending an expert on AIDS to assess and devise a plan.'" By the end of 1986, Mann hoped to "send consultants to about eight countries with the expectation that programs will promptly be undertaken."[79] Mann's team decided to help the Ugandan government launch a national plan by December, with visits to Zaire and Zambia to follow immediately thereafter. Following the meeting, Mann returned to Geneva more completely aware of the pandemic's rapidly expanding pace in sub-Saharan Africa and cognizant of the demands countries in the region and elsewhere would soon place on WHO.

On November 19, 1 week after his return from Brazzaville, Mann and Mahler boarded a plane to New York to hold a press conference about the prioritization of

---

[75] Ibid.

[76] WHO Executive Board, "WHO Activities for the Prevention and Control of Acquired Immunodeficiency Syndrome, Seventy-ninth Session, Provisional agenda item 7.2," World Health Organization, November 25, 1986, EB79/12, p. 9.

[77] Jonathan Mann, "WHO Control Programme—informal update," no. 2, 1 December 1986. The purposes of the meeting were to conduct "a scientific review and update of the global aspects of the biology, immunopathogenesis, clinical features, laboratory aspects and epidemiology of HIV infection and AIDS; a scientific review and update of the clinical, laboratory and epidemiological features of HIV and related retroviruses in Africa; and a review of the practical experiences and activities to date in Africa." WHO Executive Board, "WHO Activities for the Prevention and Control of Acquired Immunodeficiency Syndrome, Seventy-ninth Session, Provisional agenda item 7.2," World Health Organization, November 25, 1986, EB79/12, p. 9.

[78] Lawrence K. Altman, "Africa Opening Door To More AIDS Research," *The New York Times*, November 17, 1986, A1.

[79] Ibid.

the WHO AIDS program. Mahler had finally become convinced of WHO's need to act on AIDS, particularly in light of his African trip in September, and he now expressed great confidence in Mann's ability to lead this effort. Assaad, who originally hoped to join the trip, was too ill to travel. In his absence, Mann and Mahler worked out on the plane the last details of their announcement, which included the level of funding they felt the program required.

And so, as we related earlier, it was on November 20, 1986, that Mahler announced to the world at UN headquarters in New York that he, and WHO, had underestimated AIDS. "One stands bewildered of the movement of AIDS," he told the gathered press. "[It presents] a developing health disaster of very great pandemic portions."[80] Thereafter, he explained, WHO would use its "international platform for coordinating and directing...AIDS prevention, control, research, [and] policy making" by establishing "a Special Programme on AIDS." The organization would seek "$200 million for AIDS over the next several years," he concluded, building ultimately to a projected $1.5 billion per year by the beginning of the 1990s.[81]

The global battle against AIDS had truly begun under WHO's leadership. It took far longer than it should have, but the agency primarily responsible for health matters within the UN system had finally stepped up to meet the challenge of what had all the makings of being the most serious global threat to health in centuries...a sexually transmitted disease, presumed to be fatal, with a long incubation period, and associated with marginalized and stigmatized behaviors and population groups.

On December 28, a little more than a month after Mahler's press conference, Assaad succumbed to his leukemia. In the years to come, Mann's leadership in global AIDS would eclipse the role Assaad had played in the early stages of the pandemic. This is as it should be: Mann would play a pivotal role in the global response to AIDS. But Assaad's efforts should not be forgotten. For 2 years, while still leading WHO's entire Communicable Disease Division, Assaad devoted himself tirelessly to the establishment of a global program on AIDS. To him went the thankless task of motivating country after to country to admit the presence of AIDS and the behaviors facilitating its spread. With very modest institutional support, he established a global disease reporting system, put mechanisms in place for the sharing of up-to-date information about the disease, and asserted scientific leadership for WHO in areas such as virology, laboratory diagnosis, and blood safety. Perhaps symbolically, as he was at heart a virologist, the last two activities he organized were WHO's first meeting on AIDS Vaccines held on December 15 and 16, 1986 and a meeting held in February 1987 to discuss new retroviruses that had recently been isolated in West Africa (eventually shown to be HIV-2). Assaad, of course, was unable to see either of these events take place. But it is important to remember the role he played in launching what would eventually be called the Global Programme on AIDS, and to reflect upon the countless unheralded individuals, like him, who have devoted themselves to the pursuit of health for the good of mankind.

---

[80] Halfdan Mahler, "Press Briefing on AIDS," 1877F/Med.CPA, 20 November 1986.
[81] Ibid.

Chapter 4
Assuming Global Leadership

Director-General Halfdan Mahler's announcement in November 1986 not only signaled the launch of the World Health Organization (WHO)'s high-priority AIDS program; it also denoted a change in the direction of the program. Fakhry Assaad had designed a program centered on stopping viral transmission, stressing disease surveillance and protecting the blood supply. With the advent of Jonathan Mann's leadership, WHO's program began to view AIDS in a much broader framework. In fact, over the next several years, Mann himself would go through several "conceptual prisms" before settling on what would become his trademark model in the fight against AIDS[1], the health and human rights framework. The global program's priorities and activities evolved with him. The next two chapters describe the evolution of Jonathan Mann and the WHO program he led, the Global Programme on AIDS (GPA).

Mahler's admission that he had underestimated the enormity of AIDS, and his bold decision that WHO should now take leadership in this area, guaranteed Mann would have substantial resources to build the AIDS program. As he took over from the ailing Assaad, the new resources available to Mann allowed him to push the program beyond Assaad's basic virological control approach towards a more robust public health program. To do this, in the latter part of 1986, Mann recruited a diverse set of public health specialists to shape the new program. One of his most important hires was Daniel Tarantola, a French nephrologist with a background in emergency humanitarian assistance, who boasted a 12-year career working primarily at the regional level in several WHO disease control programs (including smallpox eradication, immunizations, diarrheal diseases, and acute respiratory infections). I personally had worked closely with Tarantola during the first part of the 1980s, where he was the point person for the Diarrheal Diseases Control Programme (CDD) in

Within this chapter the singular pronouns *I* and *my* refer to Michael Merson alone, whereas the plural pronouns *we* and *us* generally refer to Michael Merson and Stephen Inrig jointly. Where *we* or *us* refers to Michael Merson and his colleagues at WHO, the object of the pronoun is clarified by context.

[1] For the purposes of this text, we will use the term AIDS to encompass both AIDS and HIV unless otherwise specified.

© Springer International Publishing AG 2018
M. Merson, S. Inrig, *The AIDS Pandemic*, DOI 10.1007/978-3-319-47133-4_4

the Southeast Asia and the Western Pacific regional offices; he had done outstanding work stimulating development of these programs in many Asian countries. In 1986, Tarantola was considering moving from WHO to the United Nations Children's Emergency Fund (UNICEF) when Mahler asked him to join the AIDS program. Mahler wanted him to guide the formation of country AIDS programs across the globe. Tarantola agreed.

Another key figure Mann and Mahler recruited was Manuel Carballo, a sociologist from Gibraltar who had worked for years in WHO's maternal and child health program. Carballo interested Mann, in part, because he had been responsible for leading WHO's international collaborative study on breastfeeding and the impact of breast milk substitutes on infant and maternal health. Carballo's initial role with the AIDS program was to direct the overall research component (before focusing more specifically on social and behavioral research).[2] Mann also reached out to Harvard University legal scholar Larry Gostin in December 1986 to conduct "a worldwide survey of legislative strategies to combat AIDS."[3] Other important staff included Jeff Harris, Jock Copland, Tony Meyer, Bob Hogan, and a few others, many of whom had strong connections to the Centers for Disease Control and Prevention (CDC) or the United States Agency for International Development (USAID).[4]

Bob Hogan's potential role had particular salience for me. Hogan was a long-time public health adviser who had worked in both smallpox eradication and immunizations in Africa and whom the CDC had seconded to WHO in the early 1980s to work with me as Program Management Officer for CDD. I had recruited Hogan for his unsurpassed excellence in implementing, managing, and evaluating public health programs, and he had proved invaluable in developing management training courses in CDD. Moreover, I was expecting to rely even more heavily on him because Mahler had just asked me to also lead WHO's Acute Respiratory Infections (ARI) Programme. Hogan's role with Mann's team began with informal consultations in late 1986, but in January 1987—during WHO's Executive Board meeting—Mahler formally requested that I lend Hogan to Mann's group for about one-third of his time, to which I very reluctantly agreed.[5] Still, Hogan's participation, along with

---

[2] Manuel Carballo, Interview by Michael Merson, 2002.

[3] Larry Gostin, "Society Tomorrow: Learning to live with Aids/Lessons for Britain of US action on disease," *The Guardian*, December 3, 1986; Larry Gostin, Interview by Stephen Inrig, June, 2010.

[4] Daniel Tarantola, Interview by Michael Merson, New Haven, CT, October, 2001.

[5] Ultimately, Hogan and Mann had different views of how one should run a global health program and Hogan returned to help me with CDD and ARI. "I didn't work there very long at all. We had half a dozen meetings and what Jock Copland and I and Bill [Parra] in particular were trying to do—Manuel [Carballo] was supportive of it and Daniel [Tarantola] was not—was to get Jonathan to be gradual, to develop operational intervention research. On the scale of research in CDD. To do that rapidly. We also urged him to establish close relations with the regional offices to get people recommended by regional offices to be stationed in countries to do this research, and as soon as the research had plausible results, to begin an implementation service-based program. Jonathan didn't want to do that, so we met as a group four or five times—then Jon and I met a few times and he asked me if I would become a GPA staff member and serve as his right-hand administrative person. I had no trouble in telling him that I was just not comfortable with the approach he was taking.... He first offered me that job in January—I turned it down. ...Jon came back to me—I remember a long lunch in some place in Chambesy and I said, Jonathan I am always available to you to talk,

the others previously named, suggested to me that Mahler and Mann were putting together a strong team. With pledges and contributions from donor nations totaling about $5 million by the end of 1986, Mahler and Mann began working with this team to craft a more comprehensive and multisectoral AIDS strategy.[6]

At this point, Mann made some important decisions about the direction of the AIDS program that would shape the global response. As we have mentioned, the Control Programme on AIDS (CPA) was no longer going to be housed in the Communicable Disease Division and instead would be moved directly into Mahler's office. Moreover, Mann and Mahler chose to rename CPA the "Special Programme on AIDS (SPA)" to have its name in line with the two other large extrabudgetary programs within WHO (the Special Programme of Research, Development and Research Training in Human Reproduction (HRP) and the Special Programme for Training in Tropical Diseases (TDR) programs). Mann, Mahler, and the growing SPA team decided upon three objectives for the program's focus: (1) to prevent HIV transmission; (2) to reduce the personal and social impact of AIDS; and (3) to unify national and global efforts against AIDS.[7] These objectives became the basic foundation for what would become SPA's Global AIDS Strategy.

The strategy that Mann, with the support of Mahler and Joe Cohen, Mahler's Senior Health Policy Advisor, envisaged was an iterative framework that would evolve "from a few key policies and limited guidelines to an extensive and complex instrument" as the pandemic became more multifaceted.[8] According to Kathleen Kay, a trained nurse and outstanding science writer from Australia whom Mann had hired as his technical writer and special assistant, the strategy's premier objective was to "unite the world." "It was at a time when no one had any direction, no one knew what to do," Kay explained to us. "It was a totally living thing."[9] Mann and his team envisaged this instrument as the embodiment of various codified elements ("policies, consensus statements, guidelines, and other materials") and strategic programs ("national and international programs, research, and intervention development") that unfolded in an organic fashion ("monitoring of progress and evaluation of effectiveness").[10] "It was a major political commitment," Kay further explained. "The global strategy evolved and was added to all the time, so that each World Health Assembly (WHA) resolution was all part of it, built on it. We were

---

but I think we have very different approaches to the development of a global program and I don't think I would serve well with the approach that you have." Robert Hogan, Interview by Michael Merson, New Haven, CT, August, 2002.

[6] Lawrence K. Altman, "Global Program Aims To Combat AIDS 'Disaster'" *The New York Times*, November 21, 1986, A:1. The new program had received the $5 million from Sweden, Norway, England, and the United States, as well as pledges from Denmark and Switzerland.

[7] Global Programme on AIDS, *Progress Report Number 6, May 1990*. Geneva: World Health Organization, WHO/GPA/DIR/90.4, 1990, 6.

[8] Kathleen Kay, Interview by Michael Merson, New Haven, CT, 2002.

[9] Ibid.

[10] Global Programme on AIDS, *Progress Report Number 6, May 1990*. Geneva: World Health Organization, WHO/GPA/DIR/90.4, 1990, 6.

very strategic in working out what was the resolution we wanted for next year."[11] The Global AIDS Strategy, under Mann, never became a finalized document or strategy; it was always evolving, always in motion.

Construing a global strategy in this way brought particular tradeoffs. On the one hand, it drew on many of the best traditions from WHO's battle for global health. For example, it drew on the social capital of WHO's successful effort against smallpox. Mahler, Cohen, and Tarantola had all participated in that effort and sought to muster the same spirit of global unity for the battle against AIDS. Mahler began making analogies between AIDS and smallpox during his November 1986 press conference, and he continued them over the next months and years.[12] Not only was the magnitude of AIDS comparable to smallpox for Mahler, so too was the opportunity:

> I think we certainly are going to have the same spirit in this one and the same kind of optimism, because smallpox eradication was held back throughout the first 30 years of WHO's existence, because everybody could find a reason why the job couldn't be done, in spite of having a vaccine. Now, here we need a good deal more optimism, and a lot of people will call us romantics, utopian and whatever. So be it. The problem is too serious.[13]

Their effort also drew on the precedent set by the Global Strategy for Health for all by the Year 2000, which meeting participants had adopted at the International Conference on Primary Health Care convened by WHO and UNICEF in Alma Ata, USSR in September, 1978. In contrast to many global plans of action crafted at international conferences, the Global Strategy for Health for All started with countries, and built models "up through regions to the global level," and then completed the cycle "by focusing on support to countries."[14] Mahler and WHO leadership had construed the Health for All strategy not as "a separate 'WHO strategy', but rather as an expression of individual and collective national responsibility, fully supported by WHO."[15] Conceiving the Global AIDS Strategy in this more fluid sense proved very attractive to Mahler and Mann in light of the complex and variable nature of the AIDS pandemic.

On the other hand, approaching AIDS in this way had some potential drawbacks. AIDS was a much more complex disease than smallpox. Smallpox was easily identifiable and had a short interval from infection to illness. Moreover, scientists understood smallpox's modes of transmission and natural history, and they had a relatively

---

[11] Kathleen Kay, Interview by Michael Merson, New Haven, CT, 2002.

[12] Robert MacNeil, "Convincing Performance?" *The MacNeil/Lehrer NewsHour*, November 20, 1986, Thursday. Transcript #2909; Nick Ludington, "WHO Says AIDS Could Claim 3 Million Victims in 5 Years," *The Associated Press*, November 20, 1986; Lawrence K. Altman, "Global Program Aims To Combat AIDS 'Disaster,'" *The New York Times*, November 21, 1986, A:1.

[13] Elizabeth Brackett, "AIDS Assault," *The MacNeil/Lehrer NewsHour*, November 21, 1986, Transcript #2910.

[14] *Global Strategy for Health for All by the Year 2000*. Geneva: World Health Organization, 1981, 11.

[15] Ibid.

inexpensive and highly effective vaccine available.[16] AIDS was bereft of almost all of these characteristics: it was difficult to identify until a patient was severely ill, had a long interval between infection and illness, lacked effective therapeutics, and faced considerable obstacles in development of a vaccine. In 1987, scientists had largely come to understand HIV's modes of transmission, but they were still ascertaining its natural history. The complexity of AIDS meant that the Global AIDS Strategy approach could be a risky one if program officers failed to formulate national, regional, and global strategies "with well-defined objectives and targets."[17] Recognizing that AIDS lacked "interventions that were undeniably effective," some on Mann's early team called for "a very vigorous research agenda" that could generate "interventions that were plausible" and could be incorporated into the management training programs already in place in WHO's network.[18] In the end, however, Mann and his team decided to adopt the vertical structure of the smallpox eradication effort and employ the flexible nature of the Health for All Strategy. "As the political and social response to HIV becomes increasingly complex," his team later explained, "and biomedical research brings not only new tools, but also new complexities to HIV/AIDS prevention and control, WHO must respond to new challenges as it seeks to further the three objectives of the Global AIDS Strategy."[19]

Launching this type of program within WHO required careful political maneuvering. Replicating a smallpox-style program required more than merely establishing an AIDS program—Assaad had already done that. Rather, to address the magnitude of AIDS properly, Mahler and Mann knew that the program needed the special prominence and extra flexibility that could only come by running it directly out of the Director-General's office. This decision proved strategically important to the shape of the global response to AIDS. WHO had, in times past, seen mixed success from its "operational activities" related to specific diseases. Observers viewed malaria eradication as something of a failure, for example, whereas most considered smallpox eradication a success.[20] Assaad had always worked through the WHO infrastructure and he had originally hoped to keep the AIDS program under the Division of Communicable Diseases.[21] But some of Mahler's team, particularly

[16] Richard A. Knox, "Scourge of AIDS Spreads Worldwide," *Boston Globe*, June 22, 1986, 3:1.

[17] WHO Executive Board, *Formulating Strategies for Health for All by the Year 2000: Guiding Principles and Essential Issues. Geneva: World Health Organization, Health for all series; no. 2, 1979.*

[18] Robert Hogan, Interview by Michael Merson, New Haven, CT, August, 2002; Ralph Henderson, Interview by Michael Merson, NH, February, 2003.

[19] Global Programme on AIDS, *Progress Report Number 6, May 1990.* Geneva: World Health Organization, WHO/GPA/DIR/90.4, 1990, 6.

[20] Daniel Tarantola, "Grande et petite histoire des programmes sida," *La Journal du Sida*, 1996, 86–8:109–116.] and Michael H. Merson, Robert E. Black, Anne Mills "Introduction," in Michael H. Merson, Robert E. Black, Anne Mills, eds,.*International Public Health: Diseases, Programs, Systems, and Policies.*Burlington, MA: Jones and Bartlett Publishers, June 2004, xxiv.

[21] On Assaad's bias towards working within the WHO structure, see Fawsia Assaad, Interview by Stephen Inrig, Dallas, TX, October 5, 2010 and Joshua Cohen, Interviewed by Michael Merson, New Haven, CT, August, 2002.

Cohen, had grown disenchanted with the ability of the regional offices to implement the Primary Health Care model. For this reason, and since AIDS represented a particularly "unusual" problem, Mahler, Mann, and Cohen chose to operate SPA directly from the Director-General's office and outside WHO's traditional infrastructure.[22] This choice provided the program with a high profile and maximum flexibility, but also opened it to substantial scrutiny and criticism from both inside and outside the agency.

Establishing the program on this footing, however, required getting support for the program and its Global AIDS Strategy from several official WHO bodies. The first step was obtaining the endorsement of WHO's Executive Board. This was especially important because the prospective budget Mahler had suggested the program needed in his November press conference dwarfed that of any previous program in the history of the organization. To put it in perspective, WHO's most acclaimed effort, the smallpox eradication program, had cost a total of only $300 million; Mann and Mahler were projecting that AIDS would cost $1.5 billion per year.

On January 19, 1987, the Executive Board took up the global AIDS situation. In what must surely have been a positive sign, several members expressed concerns about the state of the pandemic and WHO's response. Mahler described to Board members the current commitment WHO had made to the effort, which included $300,000 in devoted funds from WHO's regular budget and 15 staff drawn from other programs. He also detailed the pledges and donations, which now topped $10 million, from Finland, Sweden, Norway, Denmark, Netherlands, the United States, and the United Kingdom. "The main pressure on the program would be lack of time available for action," Mahler concluded, and while the requested budget was steep, it was also necessary because "there was no alternative to considering AIDS as a global crisis."[23] Mann followed Mahler's presentation to the Board with a summary of the proposed Global AIDS Strategy he and his staff had prepared.[24] The new program would report directly to the Director-General, recruit at least 32 professional staff, and require an annual budget of $43.7 million (with 60% of the funds devoted to national programs and 40% to global activities). A Global Commission on AIDS (GCA) would serve as a scientific, advisory, and assessment group to establish long-term priorities for the wide-ranging program, while a Committee of Participating Parties (CPP) would assist in mobilizing resources and coordinating communications between its members. After his own presentation, Mann, in an unusual step, invited Robert Gallo, then Chief of the Laboratory of Tumor Cell Biology at the United States National Institutes of Health, to provide an overview of recent advances in retrovirology. (In retrospect, Mann's choice of the controversial Gallo—at that time battling with French researchers over patents, taxonomy, and

---

[22] On some of the high-ranking disenchantment with Primary Health Care Model, see Daniel Tarantola, "Grande et petite histoire des programmes sida," *La Journal du Sida,* 1996, 86–8:109–116 and Daniel Tarantola, Interview by Michael Merson, New Haven, CT, October 2001.

[23] WHO Executive Board, "Provisional Summary Record of the Thirteenth Meeting," EB79/SR/13, 19 January 1987.

[24] WHO, *Programme on AIDS,* January 1987.

use of HIV samples—was curious, since scientific experts rarely participated in meetings of WHO's Executive Board).[25]

Having heard from Mahler, Mann, and Gallo, the Board "agreed with the broad outline of the program presented by the Director-General" and gave its approval.[26] On February 1, 1987, WHO officially launched the Special Programme on AIDS (SPA) under the leadership of Mann.

While Mann played a key role in defining the shape and trajectory of SPA, we should stress the critical role Cohen had in setting the program on its initial course. A Scotsman, Cohen had studied in the United Kingdom and the United States before working, in 1947, as a doctor in camps for holocaust survivors in Southern France. That same year, Cohen served as doctor-in-charge of the famous Haganah-ship EXODUS that transported Jewish emigrants from France to British Mandatory Palestine. In 1949, he formally emigrated to Israel where he eventually served in the Israeli Ministry of Health and developed a master plan for Israeli hospitals. In 1963, he began consulting for WHO in the area of health systems development, and in 1969 he joined WHO headquarters formally, working as the key architect of the WHO's Health for All by the Year 2000 initiative. There was no one whom Mahler relied on more for strategic thinking and direction than Cohen.

Cohen knew all too well the limitations of WHO's regional structure, and it was he, more than any other, who encouraged Mann to operate the AIDS program outside it.[27] "Jonathan was a very independent person," recalled Cohen, "and we saw no reason to hamper him because we knew nothing about the disease."[28] Admittedly, such a move proved controversial among WHO insiders, particularly the directors of the regional offices, but Mahler and his staff felt the nature of the pandemic called for it: "It was a big decision but I think events proved we were right," Cohen explained. "I admit that at the beginning it was done in a very partisan manner. Again because the thing was so strange."[29]

Cohen's push to run SPA outside WHO's traditional structure was no doubt a risky choice. As an agency, WHO has traditionally promoted health by financing health ministry programs in Member States and providing them with guidance on "health policy decisions."[30] WHO rarely provides direct health care or prevention services, and it seldom benefits individuals' health directly. Instead, WHO depends

---

[25] Since at least December 12, 1985, relations between Gallo and Luc Montagnier had been tense when the Pasteur Institute had filed a complaint "before the US Claims Court, arguing that Gallo and the National Cancer Institute had infringed an agreement not to use samples of LAV for commercial purposes." In May 1986, "a subcommittee of the International Committee on the Taxonomy of viruses decided … that the AIDS virus does not belong to the HTLV family. Instead, the committee said, the virus should be called Human Immunodeficiency Virus or HIV." "The Virus Reveals the Naked Truth," *New Scientist,* February 12, 1987, pp. 55–58.

[26] WHO Executive Board, "Provisional Summary Record of the Thirteenth Meeting," EB79/SR/13, 19 January 1987.

[27] Ingar Brueggeman, "In memoriam: Dr. Joshua Cohen." *Association of Former WHO Staff Quarterly News,* October 2010, QNT81:19.

[28] Joshua Cohen, Interviewed by Michael Merson, New Haven, CT, August, 2002.

[29] Ibid.

[30] World Health Organisation. Basic documents. 39th edition. Geneva: WHO, 1992.

Fig. 4.1 WHO Regular
Budget, 1976–1994.
Source: Printed with
permission from BMJ
Publishing Group Limited.
Fiona Godlee, "The World
Health Organisation: WHO
in crisis," *British Medical
Journal*, 309:1424–1428,
1994

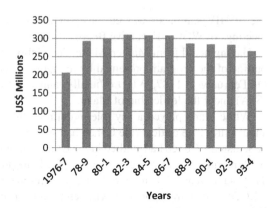

Years

on collaborative alliances between itself and national governments or intergovernmental agencies and its general operating budget goes towards this mission.[31] This
mandate renders WHO dependent on a health ministry's interests, priorities, and
institutional strength to accomplish its tasks, often making it difficult to ensure swift
action. In countries lacking substantive health infrastructure, WHO can have a difficult time affecting change.[32] Moreover, even where ministries are more effective
and WHO staff have considerable competence, WHO's bureaucratic structures can
hamper the staff's ability to provide timely and effective service.[33] Also, since the
election of the Regional Directors depends on votes from countries in the region
(see Appendix 1), regional offices can become encumbered with a political patron-
age system. This results in many WHO regional and country office appointees often
being political choices, some of whom struggle to provide adequate technical
assistance.[34]

SPA was going to be an extrabudgetary program from the beginning. Extrabudgetary
programs gave donor countries two points of strategic leverage. First, as we have
mentioned, they gave donor nations a measure of flexibility and autonomy to work
directly on a problem outside WHO's cumbersome structures. Second, by funneling
money into these extrabudgetary programs, donor countries are able to exert substantial control over WHO priorities. Thus, by the mid-1980s, Member States had
frozen the level of their contributions to WHO's regular budget (Fig. 4.1) and had
begun increasing their support to extrabudgetary programs they deemed more

---

[31] Fiona Godlee, "The World Health Organisation: WHO in crisis," *BMJ* 26 November 1994;
309:1424–1428.

[32] Fiona Godlee, "The World Health Organisation: WHO at country level -- a little impact, no strategy," *BMJ* 1994; (17 December) 309:1636–1639.

[33] Lee K, Walt G. *What role for WHO in the 1990s? Health Policy and Planning* 1992;7:387–90,
cited in Fiona Godlee, "The World Health Organisation: WHO at country level -- a little impact, no
strategy," *BMJ* (17 December) 1994;309:1636–1639.

[34] Ibid.; Charles Clift, "What's the World Health Organization for?" Chatham House Report,
Chatham House, London, May 2014.

effective and more responsive to their desires.[35] This shift made sense because these programs had distinct goals, comprehensible strategies, measurable outcomes, financial accountability, and programmatic autonomy. The upside, for donors, was that it gave them more say in WHO operations than their single vote in the World Health Assembly otherwise allowed. The downside, for WHO regional offices, was that it diminished some of their authority, incentivized vertical (i.e., disease-specific) programs in countries, and compromised the implementation of a larger, coherent region-wide approach like the horizontal approach embodied in Mahler and Cohen's Health For All strategy.[36]

No doubt, Cohen must have been aware that establishing SPA as an extrabudgetary program run out of the Director-General's office placed it at the intersection of competing WHO demands. It also raised the potential for intra-agency tensions. Mahler and Cohen were making an obvious tradeoff: SPA would more effectively address the AIDS pandemic, but risked creating a siloed infrastructure in countries around AIDS that could do little to reform or strengthen a nation's overall health system.[37] Its flexibility to promote a rapid response limited the likelihood that it would be part of a strategic distribution of resources in a given country.[38]

Part of Mahler and Cohen's calculus also appears to have been their view that establishing SPA as an extrabudgetary program, housed in Mahler's office, would allow the program to tap into the new and emerging multisectoral conception of health to which WHO was belatedly but slowly responding. WHO was, and is, an agency led largely by physicians. Physicians have a reputation for viewing disease through a medical lens and at times being condescending towards other approaches or perspectives. "A lot of us who are more traditional medical quacks, as I am, also have become so accustomed to manipulating people," Mahler explained to reporters in November 1986. "Make them addicted to your own kind of superior knowledge – at the very most you are paternalistic in your condescending sympathy – rather than … trying to mobilize that much more expensive empathy and look through their eyes."[39]

Instead of this rather paternalistic approach, the new multisectoral conception of health drew on disciplines and fields like sociology, education, and economics and focused on women's health, social development, and human rights. It promoted the

---

[35] Fiona Godlee "The World Health Organisation: WHO in crisis," *BMJ*, 1994, 309:1424–1428.

[36] Fiona Godlee, "The World Health Organization: WHO's special programmes: undermining from above," *BMJ* 1995; (21 January) 310:178–182.

[37] Cassels A, Janovsky K. A time of change: health policy, planning and organisation in Ghana. *Health Policy and Planning* 1992;7:144–54; Fiona Godlee, "The World Health Organization: WHO's special programmes: undermining from above," *BMJ* 1995; (21 January) 310:178–182.

[38] Danida. Effectiveness of multilateral agencies at country level: WHO in Kenya, Nepal, Sudan and Thailand. Copenhagen: Ministry of Foreign Affairs, 1991, cited in Fiona Godlee, "The World Health Organisation: WHO in crisis," *BMJ* 1994; (26 November) 309:1424–1428.

[39] "Dr Halfdan Mahler on Health Promotion," World Health Organization Europe, 1986. http://vimeo.com/51714332; accessed on December 27, 2012.

empowerment of communities to own and control their own health by setting their own priorities; making their own decisions; and planning and implementing their own strategies to attain better health.[40] It held the promise of multiple United Nations (UN) agencies working together on a problem of global importance.

Perhaps the best embodiment of this "new public health" was a conference that took place contemporaneously with Mahler's announcement about WHO's plan to launch SPA. Held in Ottawa, Canada, in late November 1986, WHO convened the International Conference on Health Promotion to address "growing expectations for a new public health movement around the world."[41] The concept of "health promotion" was distinct both from the concept of "disease prevention" and the more traditional "cure and rehabilitation." It focused instead on "enabling people to increase control over, and to improve, their health" by leveraging "healthy public policy, supportive environments, building healthy alliances, and bridging the equity gap." This meant viewing health as "a resource for everyday life" that draws on "social and personal resources, as well as physical capacities" to move "beyond healthy life-styles to well-being."[42]

WHO's reluctant engagement with these perspectives heretofore had created something of a leadership vacuum at both the international and national level, a vacuum that other UN agencies and intergovernmental organizations were willing to fill.[43] Unlike many at WHO, Mann and his team were interested in these concerns, and placing SPA in the Director-General's office provided Mahler and WHO with a high profile opportunity to move in this direction. In reality, as Mahler noted in an interview he gave in conjunction with the Ottawa conference, there was considerable skepticism within WHO about this new vision of public health and interagency cooperation. "I believe it took us a number of years after Alma Ata where most people were sneering cynics," Mahler explained:

So quite a number of years after Alma Ata … the old reflexes kept on manifesting themselves. … so I believe that gradually we have had some very strong internal conflictory debates in WHO and I think this has reflected what went on at national levels, that when people would say health promotion, people would say 'this is some very very hot air. It is absolutely nothing but one monumental illusion, just another kind of rebaptizing of the classical health education. So for me the real significance is that slowly but consistently, we have been trying to build up a body of conviction that it is not bluff when we are speaking about a new era in health … and that health promotion might just conceivably become *the* important lever for making a radical change in the way everybody is looking at health as you move towards the end of the century. So I see [the Ottawa conference] as an important milestone.[44]

---

[40] The Ottawa Charter for Health Promotion; First International Conference on Health Promotion, Ottawa, 21 November 1986; http://www.who.int/healthpromotion/conferences/previous/ottawa/en/index1.html; accessed on December 27, 2012.

[41] Ibid.

[42] Ibid., and "Dr Halfdan Mahler on Health Promotion," World Health Organization Europe, 1986. http://vimeo.com/51714332; accessed on December 27, 2012.

[43] Fiona Godlee,"The World Health Organisation: WHO in crisis," *BMJ* (26 November) 1994; 309:1424–1428.

[44] "Dr Halfdan Mahler on Health Promotion," World Health Organization Europe, 1986. http://vimeo.com/51714332; accessed on December 27, 2012.

Positioning SPA as they had gave Mahler and Cohen a large mechanism at WHO through which to develop these ideas. Accordingly they provided Mann and his team with maximum programmatic freedom. Considerable risk accompanied these decisions, as we said, because Mahler and Cohen would set Mann and his team up for substantial institutional push back both inside and outside WHO if SPA's results were slow to achieve or diplomatically damaging in their implementation. In hindsight, one could argue that a disease other than AIDS might have been better suited to the task.

Having embarked on this grand and urgent initiative, Mann and his team felt that operationally integrating SPA within WHO's larger infrastructure "was not possible nor even desirable."[45] "The [AIDS program] needed to respond rapidly to the pressing demand ...[that] 'something' needed to be done in order to stop the pandemic," Tarantola would later explain. According to Tarantola, Mann and his team believed that integrating AIDS programs into national health systems would be inefficient, ineffective, or actively resisted. "It was thus necessary," Tarantola concluded, "to mount administrative mechanisms, techniques, and financiers who would permit a program to start up within deadlines of a few weeks at the most."[46] Establishing a largely independent SPA appeared to be the best way to accomplish this goal.

With SPA approved by the Executive Board, Mann set several goals for his team: to alert "the world to the realities and dangers of AIDS;" to articulate "a conceptual framework for thought and action;" to link the "concern about AIDS to ... concrete actions;" and to implement aggressively an "active worldwide program."[47] The first step was raising awareness about the pandemic's severity, which Mann began to do immediately following Mahler's New York press conference by visiting several developing nations in late 1986 and early 1987.[48] "We are at a historic moment," he told the United States Senate's Labor and Human Resources Committee in mid-January, "[we are] at the beginning of a global epidemic whose ultimate magnitude cannot be predicted. It is clear that action now will have greater impact than action later."[49] "We essentially believe that all countries are involved to some extent in the AIDS pandemic," he reiterated in late March. "The really important thing is for

---

[45] Daniel Tarantola, "Grande et petite histoire des programmes sida," *La Journal du Sida,* 1996, 86–8:109–116.

[46] Ibid.

[47] Jonathan M. Mann, and Kathleen Kay, "Confronting the pandemic: the World Health Organization's Global Programme on AIDS, 1986-1989," *AIDS* 5 (suppl 2): s221–2229, 1991.

[48] Philip J. Hilts, "AIDS Rises in Latin America and Asia," *The Washington Post,* December 5, 1986, A13; "Science Watch: AIDS in the Third World," *The New York Times,* December 9, 1986, C:15.

[49] Jonathan Mann, "The World Health Organization's Perspective on AIDS: Global Dimensions and Prospects for Prevention and Control," Presentation to United States Congress, 15 January 1987.

Fig. 4.2 Special
Programme on AIDS
Poster 1987. Source: WHO

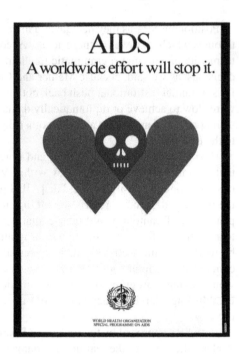

people to realize that this is a global problem and that it's a matter of degree, not its presence or absence."[50]

Mahler himself accelerated this awareness-raising effort upon receiving the Executive Board's blessing. "We are facing a situation of planetary urgency," Mahler explained at the 40th WHA in May 1987. "[It] requires immediate action."[51] Subsequently, Mann unveiled a global information campaign aimed at publicizing the epidemic's severity. A new image—two red hearts converging in a harrowing blue skull—symbolized the fight against AIDS (Fig. 4.2).[52] [Note—in general, this image was poorly received and SPA soon stopped using it]. Mahler and Mann also attacked the problem from a variety of angles. AIDS was an equal-opportunity disease, they argued, "there are no geographic 'safe zones' and no racial exemptions."[53] Other regions were not immune from the conditions present in Africa: "if you allow

[50] Thomas W. Netter, "Countries Moving In Battle On AIDS," *The New York Times,* March 22, 1987, 1:32.

[51] "AIDS threatens to spread across the planet, WHO director warns," *The Xinhua General Overseas News Service,* May 7, 1987, Item No: 0507126.

[52] "World Health Organization begins AIDS information campaign," *The Xinhua General Overseas News Service,* May 27, 1987.

[53] Sandra G. Boodman and Susan Okie, "Aggressive Prevention Efforts Proliferate: WHO Official Calls for World Cooperation, Warning There Are No Geographic 'Safe Zones'," *The Washington Post,* June 5, 1987, D1.

AIDS to get into the powder keg of Asia, then we really are going to have a problem," Mahler warned in June; "You have a potential here for an AIDS epidemic like Central Africa's," Mann told Brazilian officials in July.[54] AIDS posed dire economic and political consequences to nations if left unaddressed: "how many young movers and shakers can you lose before the net effect becomes a dampening of social progress?" Mann asked African leaders at the end of May;[55] "[The impact of AIDS on the middle class] has the potential for economic and political destabilization of some of the countries involved," Mann argued in the fall.[56] AIDS could also have long-term consequences for development: "The projected gains in infant mortality through the massive programs of recent decades may be cancelled by the exponential rise of AIDS among children in some African countries," Mann told participants attending the Second International Symposium on AIDS and Associated Cancer in Naples in October.[57]

Tying AIDS awareness to "an identifiable sequence and range of concrete actions" proved the next step for Mann and his team. Key to this process was the establishment of national AIDS programs that both addressed AIDS at a national level and aided global control efforts. "AIDS cannot be stopped in any country until it is stopped in all countries," Mann and his team concluded.[58] Assaad and Mann had already articulated the rudimentary shape of these programs in 1986, but Mann and his team gave them more structure in the ensuing months.[59] The process followed a set progression to be used in all countries (Fig. 4.3). Member States had to indicate their willingness to address AIDS and establish a national AIDS committee (or its equivalent) under their health ministry. WHO would then help conduct "an initial epidemiological and resource assessment" to determine AIDS prevalence in selected areas and across the country and to ascertain "the ability of the existing health system to support epidemiological, laboratory, clinical, and prevention components of the national AIDS program."[60] SPA advisors would then help the national AIDS committee improve their response capabilities in each of those areas in three phases: an "emergency" phase that addressed baseline concerns through a set of "urgent

---

[54] Barton Reppert, "Spread of AIDS to Asia a Potential 'Major Catastrophe,' WHO Chief Says," *The Associated Press,* June 24, 1987; Sam Seibert, Alma Guillermoprieto, and Ruth Marshall, "'An Epidemic Like Africa's': Brazil's doctors wonder how bad AIDS will get," *Newsweek,* July 27, 1987, Pg. 38.

[55] Blaine Harden, "AIDS Seen as Threat To Africa's Future: AIDS Hits African Urban Elites, Is Broad Threat to Development," *The Washington Post,* May 31, 1987, A1.

[56] Thomas Prentice, "AIDS ravages the elite of African cities," *The London Times,* October 9 1987, Issue 62895.

[57] Philip J. Hilts, "AIDS Takes Heavy Toll of African Children: Illness Could Wipe Out Recent Gains in Infant Mortality, Conference Told," *The Washington Post,* October 10, 1987, A1.

[58] WHO Special Programme on AIDS, "Progress Report Number 1," April 1987.

[59] Control Program on AIDS, "Global WHO Strategy for the Prevention and Control of Acquired Immunodeficiency Syndrome: Projected pp. 7–9, 18–20.

[60] Ibid., p. 8.

Fig. 4.3 Special Programme on AIDS: National AIDS program action course. Source: Control Programme on AIDS, "Global WHO Strategy for the Prevention and Control of AIDS: Projected Needs for 1986–1987," AIDS/CPA/86.2, June 1986

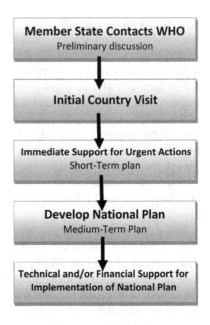

actions"; a short-term plan (STP) that addressed the essential steps the national AIDS program had to take in the first year to strengthen its AIDS response; and a medium-term plan (MTP) that guided planning and support for the following 3–5 years.[61]

As Chief of National Programme Support in SPA, Tarantola's responsibility was to provide Member States with technical and financial support to plan, design, implement, evaluate, strengthen, and monitor all the components of a national AIDS prevention and control program.[62] In March 1987, Mann and Tarantola set a goal of having 50 Member States establish their STPs by years end.[63] They had already visited several countries by this time, including Uganda and Haiti, but many doubted SPA could accomplish this.[64] In fact, Tarantola and his team were able to complete their goal by July of that year, and by year's end, SPA had visited almost 80 countries, over 60 of which had developed STPs and almost 30 of which had developed MTPs.[65] The pace continued thereafter such that in the 1988–1989 biennium GPA

[61] Special Programme on AIDS, "Strategies and Structure Projected Needs," WHO/SPP/GEN/87.1, World Health Organization, p. 10.

[62] Ibid, p. 5.

[63] Ibid, p. 11.

[64] Special Programme on AIDS, "Progress Report, Number 1; April 1987," World Health Organization, WHO/SPA/GEN/87.2, p. 12, 17.

[65] Jonathan Mann, "Status of Collaboration with Member States as of 28 July 1987," WHO Special Programme on AIDS, A20/370/2; Susan Okie, "Planning the Global Strategy on AIDS: World Health Officials Must Outrace the Epidemic's Ravages," *The Washington Post,* November 17, 1987, Z12.

organized more than 1300 missions to countries and, by 1990, 120 countries had developed national AIDS programs, 40 had developed MTPs, and 15 had already conducted some form of program review.[66] In his office, Tarantola kept a chart on the wall that tracked program progress and proudly displayed this impressive accomplishment.

SPA intended countries to develop national control plans that would work together as an interdependent network that would exchange AIDS information and provide mutual support.[67] Mann and his team used the ever-evolving Global AIDS Strategy as a framework for "common policies, guidelines and materials": its malleability responded to the needs of the unfolding pandemic while its prominence fostered global solidarity and global cooperation.[68] Mann and his team strategically worked WHO's system to this end: they convened WHO consultative meetings in Geneva to address critical and often controversial issues surrounding the pandemic faced by Member States and to lay the groundwork for new WHA resolutions. "Policy is only made by the Assembly or by the Director-General," explained Kathleen Kay,

> and we developed this way of using WHO consultations. ... We would then release the statements out of these consultations and it would be very clear that the WHO consultation was what WHO said. These statements helped change the climate and laid the groundwork for being able to get through resolutions the next year within the global strategy.[69]

This meant, of course, that SPA could use consultations to frame issues and advance policy perspectives they themselves supported. Some WHO colleagues considered this vision somewhat unrealistic ("One's not going to change the sexual habits of everybody in the world," an unidentified WHO official told a reporter), but Mann and his team felt it was essential: "we believe we will be able to dominate the disease instead of letting the disease continue to dominate us," he told reporters that October.[70]

The most prominent example of SPA's operational approach to the development of national programs was its efforts in Uganda. As we mentioned earlier, in the WHA in May 1986, Uganda was the first African nation to acknowledge the presence of AIDS in its own country. Ugandan health professionals first recognized AIDS as early as 1983, and by 1987 the nation was reporting 1100 cases, with high infection rates among sex workers, blood donors, truck drivers, and urban antenatal clinic attendees.[71] Fidel Castro, who had implemented a strict

---

[66] Gary Slutkin, Sam Okware, Warren Naamara, Don Sutherland, Donna Flanagan, Michel Carael, Erik Blas, Paul Delay, and Daniel Tarantola, "How Uganda Reversed Its HIV Epidemic," *AIDS Behav.* 2006 July; 10(4): 351–360.

[67] Kathleen Kay, "Overview of the First Global AIDS Strategy," UNAIDS, January 22, 1999.

[68] Jonathan M. Mann, and Kathleen Kay, "Confronting the pandemic: the World Health Organization's Global Programme on AIDS, 1986–1989," *AIDS* 5 (suppl 2): s221–229, 1991.

[69] Kathleen Kay, Interview by Michael Merson, New Haven, CT, 2002.

[70] R. Palmer, "For WHO, a battle won just means another war," *Herald,* October 27, 1987.

[71] Gary Slutkin, Sam Okware, Warren Naamara, Don Sutherland, Donna Flanagan, Michel Carael, Erik Blas, Paul Delay, and Daniel Tarantola, "How Uganda Reversed Its HIV Epidemic," *AIDS*

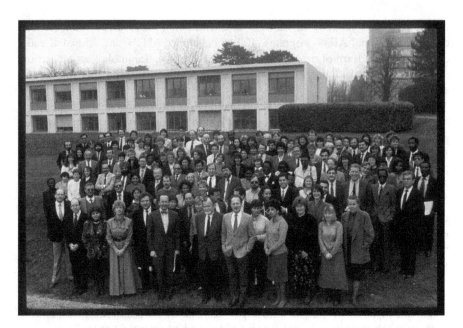

Picture 4.1 Jonathan Mann and the Special Programme on AIDS Staff, 1987 (Source: © World Health Organization/Erling Mandelmann)

AIDS control program in Cuba and whose health staff were working in Uganda during this time, pressured Uganda's leaders to act. In light of these alarming figures, and with Castro's prodding, Uganda launched its National Committee for the Prevention of AIDS and, in January 1987, asked WHO to help it craft a national emergency plan. The emergency plan included blood screening in urban areas, a health education program, and a sentinel surveillance program. Then, over the next 4 months, in collaboration with WHO, Uganda was able to secure $6 million in international pledges for the planning and implementation of its STPs and MTPs.[72] Uganda's STP initiated a public educational campaign, a blood safety

Behav. 2006 July; 10(4): 352; Thomas W. Netter, "Uganda Receives $6 Million To Combat AIDS," *The New York Times,* May 26, 1987, C4.

[72] Thomas W. Netter, "Uganda Receives $6 Million To Combat AIDS," *The New York Times,* May 26, 1987, C4; Blaine Harden, "AIDS Seen as Threat To Africa's Future: AIDS Hits African Urban Elites, Is Broad Threat to Development," *The Washington Post,* May 31, 1987, A1. The United States, Britain, Denmark, West Germany, Italy, Norway, Sweden, the European Community, the Geneva-based League of Red Cross and Red Crescent Societies, and the WHO all pledged to support the program. The WHO provided $400,000 for the emergency plan. Donors gave $1 million for the STP in $1987–1988, and an additional $4 million for 1988–1989. See Gary Slutkin, Sam Okware, Warren Naamara, Don Sutherland, Donna Flanagan, Michel Carael, Erik Blas, Paul Delay, and Daniel Tarantola, "How Uganda Reversed Its HIV Epidemic," *AIDS Behav.* 2006 July; 10(4): 352.

initiative, a hospital sterilization program, and a national prevalence survey. The health education campaign (known formally as the Information, Education, and Communication [IEC] Campaign and informally as the "Zero Grazing/Love Faithfully/Love Carefully" Campaign) served as the central component of its national AIDS program. The Ugandan Health Ministry led the IEC campaign in conjunction with WHO, UNICEF, and several international non-government organizations (NGOs) and Ugandan civil society groups. The program also involved multisectoral training, district mobilization (The District AIDS Mobilization Project [DAMP]), country-wide messaging, and media mobilization. By 1990, Uganda's AIDS budget had climbed to $18 million per year, with over 35 full-time Ugandan staff and six full-time WHO staff involved.[73] These efforts, along with several other factors, produced changes in Ugandan sexual behavior between 1989 and 1995, and while there was much subsequent debate over the reasons for this, prevalence rates dropped by half during that time (see Chapter 10).[74]

The Ugandan experience appeared to confirm that one of the most important factors in the Global AIDS Strategy was assessing and publicizing the scope of the pandemic. Some observers even considered this the key to Uganda's success: "The declining prevalence in Uganda ...it clearly was education," maintained Seth Berkley, a charismatic American medical epidemiologist who, while working for the CDC, helped establish and manage the Ugandan surveillance system for AIDS (and who would later go on to start and direct the International AIDS Vaccine Initiative [IAVI] and then become the CEO of the Global Alliance for Vaccines and Immunization [GAVI]), "but I think the education was driven by the panic across the country ... what [President] Museveni did was very brave and he really wanted the data out, wanted to push it, wanted to get it out there. That was what was important."[75] Mann, of course, had become painfully aware while working in Zaire that ignorance about the presence of AIDS (much less its extent) impeded action against it. The legacies of racism and colonialism and their associated impact on national reputations and economies were difficult to ignore. Still, any effective response to AIDS depended on an adequate understanding of its scope: "[It is] very important to develop an epidemiological base," Mann told reporters and health officials in mid-1987, "...such a base is essential for the planning of health care services and to monitor the success or otherwise of prevention

[73] Gary Slutkin, "Global AIDS 1981–1999: the response," *The International Journal of Tuberculosis and Lung Disease*, S28–29.

[74] Gary Slutkin, Sam Okware, Warren Naamara, Don Sutherland, Donna Flanagan, Michel Carael, Erik Blas, Paul Delay, and Daniel Tarantola, "How Uganda Reversed Its HIV Epidemic," *AIDS Behav.* 2006 July; 10(4): 357.

[75] Seth Berkley, Interview by Michael Merson, New Haven, CT, August 21, 2002.

programs."[76] Consequently, Mann and his team began working with WHO Member States to estimate the extent of infection within their borders. By mid-1987, 120 countries had already reported over 50,000 cases of AIDS, but Mann and his team felt confident the number was far higher, and began calling on Member States to obtain accurate projections.

To accomplish this, Mann recruited Jim Chin in March 1987 to head SPA's Surveillance, Forecasting and Impact Assessment Unit (SFI). Chin, who had been Chief of California State's Infectious Disease Section within the Bureau of Communicable Diseases Control, immediately began developing forecasting models using blood test results "to determine the frequency of infection with the virus in large populations" and to predict the existing scope and to project the future trajectory of the AIDS pandemic.[77] Since researchers knew so little about AIDS's natural history at this stage, it was difficult to determine how widespread the problem was or what long-term impact the disease might have. In 1987, Chin estimated between 5 million and 10 million people were infected worldwide: "A million here, a million there," Chin told reporters in 1987. "All we know is, we're talking, at least in terms of infected people, in millions."[78] Mann frequently set the number far higher in public forums: "the number of people infected … [would] reach at least 50 million to 100 million worldwide," he told audiences in July 1987.[79] The regional and global threat posed by a pandemic of that magnitude was truly alarming: "AIDS is the archetypal communicable disease," explained Manuel Carballo who lead Social and Behavioral Research, "We're all at risk."[80] In later years, some observers would criticize claims like this as alarmist, "glorious" myths employed to generate attention and money when less inflammatory numbers could have been employed.[81] For his part, Mann acknowledged the risk of using numbers carelessly: "The problem is so serious that overstating it doesn't help … If you think everybody is going to be infected, you can easily say it is hopeless. Why even bother?"[82] Still, discussing the potential scope of the pandemic had important awareness-raising value: "In Africa, AIDS could have widespread economic, social and political consequences," Mann explained. "What exactly they will be, it is too early to say … This is not a campaign that will be won or lost in a year or two. It

---

[76] John O'Neill, "Disease Outstrips Control Efforts," *Sydney Morning Herald,* July 21, 1987, Pg. 6.

[77] Jonathan M. Mann, and Kathleen Kay, "Confronting the pandemic: the World Health Organization's Global Programme on AIDS, 1986–1989," *AIDS* 5 (suppl 2): s221–229, 1991.

[78] Susan Okie, "Planning the Global Strategy on AIDS: World Health Officials Must Outrace the Epidemic's Ravages," *The Washington Post,* November 17, 1987, Z12.

[79] "AIDS Cases Increase in 122 countries," *The Xinhua General Overseas News Service,* July 30, 1987, In: 0730038.

[80] Susan Okie, "Planning the Global Strategy on AIDS: World Health Officials Must Outrace the Epidemic's Ravages," *The Washington Post,* November 17, 1987, Z12.

[81] See James Chin, *The AIDS Pandemic: The Collision of Epidemiology with Political Correctness.* Seattle, WA: Radcliffe Publishing, 2007, 200.

[82] Blaine Harden, "AIDS Seen as Threat To Africa's Future: AIDS Hits African Urban Elites, Is Broad Threat to Development," *The Washington Post,* May 31, 1987, A1.

will take a sustained effort. It will have to be built into the health systems of these countries."[83]

Particularly key in this endeavor, then, was SPA's ability to convince more African nations to test their populations and to expand the number of testing sites they had in place. "It's such a critical issue," Mann told reporters. "If you don't know how many people are being infected, you cannot know whether your program is having any impact and whether the investment is good or not." Most important for understanding the pandemic was to extend testing into rural parts of Africa, since most sentinel sites were being established in cities, while most Africans lived in rural areas. Admittedly, Mann acknowledged, this led to "an oversampling of the higher-risk population."[84] The answer, Mann's team was certain, was increased surveillance and improved projection models.

Along with its surveillance efforts, SPA explored the various behaviors putting people at risk for HIV transmission in various countries. Carballo led efforts to ascertain the main routes of viral transmission in various countries and tie that information to the observed epidemiological patterns. Nations differed in sexual behaviors and in the prevalence and frequency of tattooing, decorative scarring, intravenous drug use, and folk medicine injections. "There is no reason to believe that sexual behavior follows the same patterns in all societies, in all cultures, and in all age groups," Carballo told the media in 1987. "We need to know who [those using needles] are, where they work, whom they cater to, what they understand about sterilization and [AIDS] transmission." Carballo's unit therefore worked closely with SPA's surveillance team, as he developed questionnaires and other mechanisms to gain reliable information on risk behaviors and the best ways to reach high-risk groups. Up to 1987, limited work had been conducted in these areas: "most people working in the area of AIDS control and prevention strategy have realized early on that they are really working in the dark," Carballo explained.[85] His contributions included the undertaking of Knowledge, Attitude, Behavior, and Practices (KAPB) studies in countless countries, more focused studies of sexual behavior in a number of African countries, and the launching, with the technical assistance of Don DesJarlais and Sam Friedman from Beth Israel Medical Center in New York, of a 10-country, 13-city project to look at global patterns of injecting use.[86]

SPA also began deploying health, social, and educational programs in affected countries to "stimulate, support, and sustain individual behavioral change."[87] To aid

[83] Ibid.

[84] Lawrence K. Altman, "AIDS' Global Peril Is High On Agenda At Summit Meeting," *The New York Times*, May 31, 1987, 1:1.

[85] Ibid.

[86] Donald Des Jarlais, "Sexual Behavior and AIDS in the Developing World," in John Cleland and Benoit Ferry, eds, Taylor and Francis published on behalf of the World Health Organization, 1995. As for the substance abuse study, while it was never published, a copy of the fact sheet can be found on the WHO web site. http://www.who.int/substance_abuse/publications/en/IDUFactSheet. pdf?ua=1

[87] Jonathan Mann, "Human Rights and AIDS: The Future of the Pandemic," in *Health and Human Rights: A Reader.* Jonathan M. Mann, Sofia Gruskin, Michael A. Grodin, and George J. Annas,

in this effort, in April 1987 SPA convened a consultation on counseling those with AIDS that brought together a global group of clinicians, social workers, psychiatrists, activists, and sociologists from six countries to develop generic guidelines.[88] Soon this field expanded to include voluntary HIV testing and counseling.

Providing education and health services to individuals at risk "became the central mission of national AIDS programs."[89] High-income nations had the wherewithal to launch rapid and effective response programs, and most had done so by the time WHO launched SPA. Mann and his colleagues particularly held up as exemplary the United Kingdom's anti-AIDS effort: "The campaign in the United Kingdom is one of the first, one of the largest and, therefore, one of the most important public information activities for the general public regarding AIDS in the world," Mann told reporters in April 1987.[90] Switzerland's effort likewise gained SPA's approval.[91] Low- and middle-income countries had not moved as quickly in launching their AIDS control and prevention efforts, but Carballo noted that by 1987 SPA was even "beginning to see this in developing countries."[92] Uganda, as described above, clearly stood out as the benchmark in this regard.[93]

Several key assumptions reinforced SPA's education and prevention programs. First, as Mann would later explain, SPA "programs were designed with a view, either explicitly or implicitly, of HIV-related behavior as fundamentally individualistic and rational."[94] In later years, observers—including Mann himself—would denigrate these strategies as "the biomedical approach" or the "traditional public health approach" and insufficient to the task at hand.[95] Second, SPA imagined that they could implement efficacious small-scale prevention programs on a larger scale with relative ease. Roy Widdus helped lead some of this effort. Widdus, an expert in epidemiology and biochemistry, joined SPA as the de facto Deputy Director in the late 1980s after a decade working at the Institute of Medicine (IOM) of the United States National Academy of Sciences. At the IOM, he had overseen numerous projects on vaccine development and policy and served as Director of the Division of International Health. Widdus had been project director for the IOM's groundbreak-

eds., New York, Routledge, 1999, pp. 217–218.

[88] Special Programme on AIDS, "Progress Report, Number 1; April 1987," World Health Organization, WHO/SPA/GEN/87.2, p. 28.

[89] Jonathan Mann, "Human Rights and AIDS: The Future of the Pandemic," in *Health and Human Rights: A Reader.* Jonathan M. Mann, Sofia Gruskin, Michael A. Grodin, and George J. Annas, eds., New York, Routledge, 1999, pp. 217–218.

[90] Claudia Rader, "AIDS campaign alerts, and alarms, British," *The Advertiser,* April 7, 1987.

[91] Jim Lehrer, "AIDS: Dr. Jonathan Mann," *The MacNeil/Lehrer NewsHour,* June 3, 1987.

[92] Robert P. Hey, "Countries unite to fight spread of AIDS," *Christian Science Monitor*, March 19, 1987, p. 1.

[93] Jim Lehrer, "AIDS: Dr. Jonathan Mann," *The MacNeil/Lehrer NewsHour,* June 3, 1987.

[94] Jonathan Mann, "Human Rights and AIDS: The Future of the Pandemic," in *Health and Human Rights: A Reader.* Jonathan M. Mann, Sofia Gruskin, Michael A. Grodin, and George J. Annas, eds., New York, Routledge, 1999, pp. 217–218.

[95] Ibid.

ing 1986 analysis of the United States' response to the AIDS epidemic.[96] Some of the content of the report focused on Mann's work in *Projet SIDA*, and it was in conjunction with this that, in 1986 and 1987, Widdus and Mann grew to know each other. In 1987, Mann recruited Widdus to join SPA to structure new activities and broaden the program's research capacity. "I think we had faith that we would be able to figure out how to take those behavioral interventions at least to scale for the highest risk populations," Widdus recalled. "The thing we didn't realize at that time was that taking a small experimental research behavioral-change study to national scale could be totally thwarted by the cultural issues."[97] This common public health challenge—translating efficacious trial results into effective public health interventions—would dog WHO's AIDS program throughout its existence. Still, despite these challenges and rapidly expanding pandemic, just about all SPA staff imbued their role in the battle against the disease with passion and optimism.

The *esprit de corps* of this first generation of SPA staff facilitated this optimism and bonded the group to its mission. "I have never worked with such dedicated public health officials," Chin would later attest.[98] SPA staffer Gary Slutkin, an infectious disease physician who had run anti-tuberculosis programs in San Francisco and worked for the Ministry of Health's primary health care programs in Somalia before Mann hired him to help countries build AIDS programs in Africa (Slutkin is at the time of this writing the Executive Director of the heralded NGO Cure Violence in Chicago), agreed:

> I've never seen anything like it in my life. … I understand [smallpox] had this kind of a feeling, but it was the most exciting time of my life. … I've never been involved in anything like it - except when I worked in San Francisco General Hospital - in terms of commitment. But in terms of excitement and enthusiasm and the feeling that we were getting on top of this and we were on our way - everything was building, everything was going in the right direction … And I am not the only one who feels that way. We all felt that we were getting there - we all did. We all felt inspired, that the direction was right. We always came back from the field with something positive that had happened.[99]

Mann himself helped generate this energy. "I'm not sure he can survive these 16-hour days [but] so far he seems to be thriving on it," Chin told reporters in 1987. "If something is in the way, Jonathan says, 'Don't go around it, go through it.' … If we can clone Jonathan, if we can get a dozen Jonathan Manns, we might survive this year."[100]

While SPA generated considerable acclaim for its work, it was not without its critics. One issue was SPA's relationship with the traditional WHO infrastructure.

---

[96] Institutes of Medicine, *Confronting AIDS: Directions for Public Health, Health Care, and Research*. Washington, DC: National Academy Press. 1986.

[97] Roy Widdus, Interview by Michael Merson, New Haven, CT, October, 2001.

[98] James Chin, *The AIDS Pandemic: The Collision of Epidemiology with Political Correctness*. Seattle, WA: Radcliffe Publishing, 2007, 200.

[99] Gary Slutkin, Interview by Michael Merson, New Haven, CT, February 3, 2003.

[100] Susan Okie, "Planning the Global Strategy on AIDS: World Health Officials Must Outrace the Epidemic's Ravages," *The Washington Post*, November 17, 1987, Z12.

As we've mentioned, SPA's special status allowed it to operate outside WHO's standard organizational structure, particularly the regional offices, and many inside and outside WHO believed SPA intentionally did just that. "There was no doubt that there was an attitude within [SPA] that [WHO's regional structure] would slow us down," Slutkin later recalled. "There was a rebellious modality among all of us that we were going to do what was needed, no matter what … we intentionally avoided the regional offices."[101] While this strategy gave SPA considerable flexibility to respond quickly to the pandemic and support countries, the antagonistic relationship it built up between SPA and WHO's regional and country staff would have long-term consequences for the program.

An additional concern was whether SPA's approach to the national programs would ever enable countries to take responsibility and ownership of their anti-AIDS effort.[102] Mann and his team were able to mobilize a considerable amount of resources for countries, but it was not clear at this early stage whether countries truly understood the severity of AIDS within their borders and if they would provide funding for AIDS prevention efforts. The response from some nations, like Uganda, suggested that SPA could generate considerable buy-in from national authorities, as some of the initial funding for AIDS there had come from the Ministry of Health before SPA began its support to the national program. But other nations had not prioritized AIDS to the same extent as Uganda, and it was by no means clear that they would provide such local funding. The inescapably rapid start-up of SPA only fed these concerns. That is, while staffers in SPA considered themselves invited guests to provide concerned national health officials with needed resources to prevent and control AIDS in their country, some observers considered them little more than outsiders who imposed culturally inappropriate and prescribed approaches that would make little lasting change.[103]

However true this last criticism may have been, SPA played an essential role in helping many nations buttress their health systems. "It was really important, the support that SPA/GPA gave to Uganda," Seth Berkeley explained, countering this criticism:

> When I was there it was … the only working fax machine, and I just can't tell you how important those little logistics were – cars, vehicles. We set up the national surveillance system … Absolutely [SPA distorted the Ugandan health care system by putting in so much effort]!– but there was **no** health care system! It was a good thing.[104]

This meant that SPA helped some countries pursue larger health system goals, including the goals articulated in the Alma Ata declaration, through the resources it provided. Admittedly, SPA's efforts were imperfect. There were times when SPA staff insisted on using their standard approach to programming over locally developed ones, or would put systems in place which then lacked "the technical assis-

---

[101] Gary Slutkin, Interview by Michael Merson, New Haven, CT, February 3, 2003.

[102] Peter Piot, Interview by Michael Merson, New Haven, CT, October 26, 2002.

[103] Ibid.

[104] Seth Berkley, Interview by Michael Merson, New Haven, CT, August 21, 2002.

tance to keep [them] up" (e.g., surveillance). Sustainability of the activities promoted by SPA remained an open and important question, but at this early stage, most SPA staffers were more concerned about launching programs than worrying about the programs' long-term integration into the larger national infrastructure. To them, the impact of SPA's support to programs was quite positive.[105]

While Mann and his team set out to construct and implement the Global AIDS Strategy, he and Mahler recognized that their endeavor to lead the global AIDS fight depended entirely on the "continued, strong commitment by all its Member States to the principle of global leadership."[106] To this end, throughout 1987 and early 1988, Mahler and Mann went about ensuring broad support for the role of WHO's SPA using sequential resolutions to establish and ensure SPA's preeminence in the global fight against AIDS. In April 1987, Mann secured a consensus statement from the Third Meeting of Participating Parties For the Prevention and Control of AIDS that

> strongly recommend[ed] that the World Health Organization assume a global leadership role and responsibility for mobilizing and coordinating international initiatives and resources for global AIDS prevention, control and research and acknowledges the WHO Special Programme on AIDS as the focal point for international action in support of these activities.[107]

One month later, Mahler and Mann secured a resolution from the 40th WHA (Resolution WHA 40.26) that confirmed WHO's "role of directing and coordinating the global, urgent and energetic fight against AIDS," and called on bilateral, multi-lateral, and NGOs to "support the worldwide struggle against AIDS in conformity with WHO's global strategy."[108] Then, in June 1987, they gained support from the declaration adopted by the Group of Seven (G7) at its 13th Summit held in Venice,[109] which stated that "the World Health Organization (WHO) is the best forum for drawing together global efforts on a worldwide level to combat AIDS, and all countries should be encouraged fully to cooperate with the WHO and support its special program of AIDS-related activities."[110] In July 1987, at the 35th plenary meeting of

---

[105] Ibid.

[106] WHO Special Programme On AIDS, "Comprehensive Coordination Of Global And National AIDS Activities," WHO DOC 4951F 30 September 1987, 10.

[107] WHO "Consensus Statement," Third Meeting Of Participating Parties For The Prevention And Control of AIDS, Geneva, 27 and 28 April 1987 SPA/1NF/87.3.

[108] WHO Special Programme On AIDS, "Comprehensive Coordination Of Global And National AIDS Activities," WHO DOC 4951F 30 September 1987, 10; Fortieth World Health Assembly, Geneva, 4–15 May 1987, WHA40.26, Global strategy for the prevention and control of AIDS Hbk Res., Vol. III (1st ed.), 1.16.13 (Twelfth plenary meeting, 15 May 1987—Committee A, third report).

[109] Lawrence K. Altman, "AIDS' Global Peril Is High On Agenda At Summit Meeting," The New York Times, May 31, 1987, 1:1.

[110] G7 Chairman, "Chairman's Statement on AIDS, June 10, 1987," G7 Summit, Venice, Italy, June 10, 1987; See also "International News," The Associated Press, June 10, 1987; Venice Summit Statement on AIDS: WHO 'Best Forum' For Action," WHO Press, Press Release WHO/19, 11 June 1987; See also Lawrence K. Altman, "AIDS' Global Peril Is High On Agenda At Summit Meeting," The New York Times, May 31, 1987, 1:1 and WHO Special Programme On AIDS, "Comprehensive Coordination Of Global And National AIDS Activities," WHO DOC 4951F 30 September 1987, 10; "International News," The Associated Press, June 10, 1987.

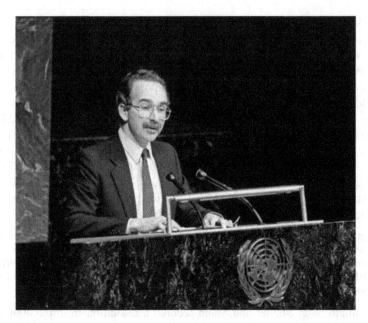

Picture 4.2 Jonathan Mann speaks at United Nations General Assembly, 1987 (Source: UN Photo/Saw Lwin)

the UN Economic and Social Council (ECOSOC) (held in New York), Mann and Mahler were able to secure Resolution E/1987/76, which "urge[d] all appropriate organizations of the United Nations system, including the specialized agencies as well as bilateral and multilateral agencies and non-governmental and voluntary organizations, to support the world-wide struggle against AIDS in close co-opera-tion with the World Health Organization in its role of directing and co-ordinating the urgent fight against AIDS and in conformity with the global strategy."[111] Finally, in October 1987, the 42nd session of the UN General Assembly unanimously adopted resolution 42/8, which confirmed that "the World Health Organization should direct and coordinate the urgent global battle against AIDS" and urged "all appropriate organizations of the United Nations system … in conformity with the [WHO's] Global Strategy, to support the worldwide struggle against AIDS."[112] The ECOSOC and UN General Assembly resolutions affirmed the clear leadership the UN was entrusting to WHO in the global fight against AIDS.

To reflect the scope of the global pandemic and WHO's now well acknowledged leadership role in the response to it, in January 1988, WHO's Executive Board chose

---

[111] ECOSOC, "Prevention and Control of AIDS, 1987/75," July 8, 1987; WHO Special Programme On AIDS, "Comprehensive Coordination Of Global And National AIDS Activities," WHO DOC 4951F 30 September 1987, 10.

[112] WHO, *Global Strategy for the Prevention and Control of AIDS: Report by the Director-General, A41/5*. Geneva: World health Organization, March 21, 1988, p. 3.

to rename the program the Global Programme on AIDS (GPA). At each stage in this iterative process, Mahler used his prominent global standing to ensure that AIDS made its way onto the agenda and that WHO's leadership in the global response was unchallenged. Initially, Mann was unaccustomed to WHO and the UN framework, but Mahler and his chief advisor Joe Cohen helped position Mann so he could best navigate the system.[113] Mahler and Mann then ensured the statements of each global body built off its predecessor to ensure support for WHO's "directing and coordinating role" at each level. The preeminence of WHO in the global fight against AIDS would remain a prevailing theme into the Director-General Hiroshi Nakajima era though, as we will see, it would soon be seriously challenged.[114]

---

[113] Joshua Cohen, Interviewed by Michael Merson, New Haven, CT, August, 2002.

[114] "World Leaders Call for Intensified Efforts Against AIDS," *The Xinhua General Overseas News Service,* December 1, 1988.

Chapter 5
Building and Coordinating a Multisectoral Response

Being recognized as the lead agency for national and global AIDS[1] control sounded good, but Jonathan Mann and Halfdan Mahler knew such formal statements were insufficient.[2] While the World Health Organization (WHO) was optimally positioned "to mobilize and coordinate" many of the health-related components of an AIDS campaign, the social, cultural, political, and economic facets of the pandemic demanded robust collaboration with other sectors at national, regional and global levels. Ensuring WHO's preeminence in the global fight against AIDS thus required Mann and Mahler to mobilize the necessary expertise and support from several sectors beyond the field of health.[3] This demanded extensive collaboration with numerous entities within WHO, the United Nations (UN), and the larger global community.

During its early years, the Global Programme on AIDS (GPA)[4] committed itself to "undertake joint programmes of cooperation, wherever appropriate and feasible, with other technical and development assistance agencies." These joint programs aimed at reducing duplication by utilizing "the relevant personnel skills and resources of other agencies in an agreed and appropriate fashion," and by placing GPA resources "at the

---

Within this chapter the singular pronouns *I* and *my* refer to Michael Merson alone, whereas the plural pronouns *we* and *us* generally refer to Michael Merson and Stephen Inrig jointly. Where *we* or *us* refers to Michael Merson and his colleagues at WHO, the object of the pronoun is clarified by context.

[1] For the purposes of this text, we will use the term AIDS to encompass both AIDS and HIV unless otherwise specified.

[2] Report of the Fifth Meeting of Participating Parties, Geneva, 27–28 April 1988. Geneva: World Health Organization, 1988, WHO/GPA/GEN/88.2, p. 2.

[3] Report of the Fourth Meeting of Participating Parties, Geneva, 12–13 November 1987, WHO/SPA/Gen.87.5, 3.

[4] Henceforth, in the text, Global Programme on AIDS (GPA) includes the periods the program was titled Control Programme on AIDS, (CPA), Special Programme on AIDS (SPA), and Global Programme on AIDS.

© Springer International Publishing AG 2018
M. Merson, S. Inrig, *The AIDS Pandemic*, DOI 10.1007/978-3-319-47133-4_5

disposal of other agencies for whatever support it can provide to maintain or enhance the coherence of their programmes within the Global Strategy on AIDS."[5]

The most immediate move Mann and his team made to leverage support was to collaborate with programs within WHO itself. Accordingly, over the next 3 years, GPA established numerous collaborative and consultative relationships with a host of WHO programs, initiatives, and divisions, including: the Global Blood Safety Initiative; Biologicals[6]; the sexually transmitted diseases program within the Division of Communicable Diseases[7]; the Expanded Programme on Immunization (EPI), (this included the convening of a joint consultation on HIV and routine childhood immunization[8]); the Family Health Division (this involved the organization of joint consultations on breastfeeding, perinatal infections, and virucide strategies[9]); and several jointly-sponsored conferences and consultations with Nursing[10], Oral Health[11], Occupational Health[12], the Special Programme for Research and Training in Tropical Diseases (TDR)[13], and the Special Programme for Research, Development and Research Training in Human Reproduction (HRP).[14]

---

[5] WHO Special Programme On AIDS, "Comprehensive Coordination Of Global And National AIDS Activities," WHO DOC 4951F 30 September 1987, p. 4; see also, Global Programme on AIDS. "Guiding Objectives and Principles for the Comprehensive Coordination of Global and National AIDS Activities. Fifth Meeting of Participating Parties, Geneva, 27-28 April 1988, GPA/ER/88.2 Rev.1.

[6] Special Programme on AIDS, "Progress Report Number 2," Geneva: World Health Organization, WHO/SPA/GEN/87.4, p. 10; "Global Strategy for the Prevention and Control of AIDS: Report by the Director-General," Geneva: World Health Organization, 1988, A41/5, p. 13; Global Programme on AIDS, "Progress Report Number 5, May 1989," Geneva: World Health Organization, 1989, WHO/GPA/DIR/89.4, p. 23.

[7] Special Programme on AIDS, "Progress Report Number 2," Geneva: World Health Organization, WHO/SPA/GEN/87.4, p. 10; "Global Strategy for the Prevention and Control of AIDS: Report by the Director-General," Geneva: World Health Organization, November 1988, p. 16; Global Programme on AIDS and Programme on STD, "Consensus Statement From Consultation on Sexually Transmitted Diseases as a Risk Factor for HIV Transmission, Geneva, 4–6 January 1989," Geneva: World Health Organization, 1989, WHO/GPA/INF/89.1, p. 1.

[8] Special Programme on AIDS, "Progress Report Number 2," Geneva: World Health Organization, WHO/SPA/GEN/87.4, p. 10; "WHO Consultation on HIV and Routine Childhood Immunization," Geneva: World Health Organization, August 1987, WHO/SPA/GL0/87.3.

[9] Special Programme on AIDS, "Statement on Breast-Feeding/Breast Milk and Human Immunodeficiency Virus (HIV)," World Health Organization, 1987, WHO/SPA/INF/87.8; Global Programme on AIDS, "Progress Report Number 5, May 1989," Geneva: World Health Organization, 1989, WHO/GPA/DIR/89.4, p. 24.

[10] "Global Strategy for the Prevention and Control of AIDS: Report by the Director-General," Geneva: World Health Organization, 1988, A41/5, p. 13.

[11] Special Programme on AIDS, "Progress Report Number 2," Geneva: World Health Organization, WHO/SPA/GEN/87.4, p. 11.

[12] Global Programme on AIDS, "Global Strategy for the Prevention and Control of AIDS: Report by the Director-General," Geneva: World Health Organization, November 1988, EB83/26, p. 17.

[13] Special Programme on AIDS, "Progress Report Number 2," Geneva: World Health Organization, WHO/SPA/GEN/87.4, p. 11.

[14] Special Programme on AIDS and Special Programme of Research, Development and Research Training in Human Reproduction, "Joint Statement: Contraceptive Methods and Human Immunodeficiency Virus (HIV)," World Health Organization, 1987, WHO/SPA/INF/87.9.

Member States and other groups also frequently asked GPA to address various technical questions related to the discovery of the new virus and concerns about its mode of transmission in different settings. These requests often led GPA to organize expert consultations with individual programs in WHO or to issue consensus statements on a number of topics, such as: the neuropsychiatric consequences of AIDS (of particular importance to the airline industry, which was concerned about the potential problems HIV-infected pilots might pose in-flight); HIV in the workplace; HIV in the military; and HIV transmission in sporting events.[15] The consensus statement on the latter called for immediate cleansing of skin lesions incurred in sporting events, and the removal of an athlete with a bleeding wound from an event until the bleeding stopped and the wound properly cleaned and covered. Many sports today continue to follow this protocol.

In addition to collaborating with other programs at WHO headquarters, GPA began using WHO's regional structure to implement sections of its program. For example, GPA asked the regional offices to prepare regional programs that GPA would, upon approval, fund, including: travel to GPA regional or inter-country activities; organization of GPA-related regional workshops; region-appropriate adaptation of GPA informational and educational materials; and GPA-related staff training.[16] Between 1987 and 1990, Mann and his team held numerous conferences, training courses, and planning meetings in all six WHO regions.[17] "Regional offices have a large and active role in the Global Programme on AIDS through support to prevention programs and adaptation of global materials to regional needs," Mann and his team explained in 1988.[18]

While GPA could claim, on paper, to have "established close working relationships with the regional offices," the actual relationship between them and GPA was more complicated.[19] As we explained in Chapter 4, to enable Mann to implement the program in the most effective and efficient manner, Mahler enabled Mann to direct GPA from his office, invested him with all program formulation, management, and directional authority, and had Mann report directly to him. Mann, therefore, had the power to determine "whether global and/or regional activities are consistent with and supportive of the Global Plan of Action on AIDS."[20] Mahler, as historians Elizabeth Fee and Manon Parry contend, "allowed Mann to bypass WHO's usual chain of command as head of the new GPA."[21] Accordingly, as GPA epidemiologist Jim Chin

---

[15] Consensus Statement from consultation on AIDS and Sports, GPA, Geneva, January 16, 1989.

[16] Global Programme on AIDS, "Report of the Fifth Meeting of Participating Parties, Geneva, 27–28 April 1988," Geneva: World Health Organization, 1988, WHO/GPA/GEN/88.2, p. 12.

[17] Special Programme on AIDS, "Progress Report Number 2," Geneva: World Health Organization, WHO/SPA/GEN/87.4, pp. 24–26.

[18] Global Programme on AIDS, "Global Strategy for the Prevention and Control of AIDS: Report by the Director-General," Geneva: World Health Organization, November 1988, EB83/26, p. 27.

[19] Special Programme on AIDS, "Progress Report Number 1, April 1987, WHO Special Programme on AIDS, WHO/SPA/GEN/87.2,,24 http://apps.who.int/iris/bitstream/10665/164060/1/WHA40_Inf.Doc-4_eng.pdf

[20] WHO Special Programme On AIDS, "Comprehensive Coordination Of Global And National AIDS Activities," WHO DOC 4951F 30 September 1987, p. 3.

[21] Elizabeth Fee and Manon Parry, "Jonathan Mann, HIV/AIDS, and Human Rights," *Journal of Public Health Policy,* 29(1): 59–60.

explains, Mann and his team "did not adhere to WHO's bureaucratic rules."[22] While most WHO programs in Geneva routed their communications to WHO country offices through the regional offices, GPA country staff uniquely reported directly to GPA in Geneva—indeed in many cases they even had their own offices outside the WHO country office—largely circumventing the regional office structure in their interactions with GPA in Geneva, and only afterwards sending copies of these communications to the regional offices to keep them informed of their activities.[23] "This was an operational routine that, to say the least, rankled all of the Regional Directors," concluded Chin.[24] According to Chin, Mann and his team had a particular aversion to sending correspondence, staff support, and program funds through the regional office for Africa (AFRO) in Brazzaville, Congo: "Jon[athan] …knew first hand of the inefficiency and outright corruption in the African Regional Office … He vowed that no GPA staff or country funds /support would be provided through AFRO."[25] In retrospect, one could argue that Mann should have paid more due deference to the hierarchical authority that prevailed in UN agencies like WHO.[26] As political scientist Christer Jönsson has noted, Mann's "readiness to depart from narrow organizational roles and to base initiatives on a conception of collective goals" may have threatened his standing within WHO because he was neglecting "the internal functions pertaining to his constituent organization."[27]

Mann, of course, believed the urgency of AIDS trumped whatever intra-agency squabbling GPA might have generated. When asked whether there was a danger in countries devoting too much attention to AIDS at the expense of other health issues, Mann replied that:

> AIDS is not the only priority at WHO, it is one of the major health priorities. If we do our AIDS prevention work well, we will actually strengthen the systems that are dealing with all those other important problems as well. … It's very narrow to take the view that health people should fight among themselves about which is a more important problem -- X or AIDS. It's actually pathetic to think that we health people might scrabble over the small crumbs of the budgets around the world that are available for health.[28]

Lacking a cure, vaccine or any other simple technological solution, Mann and his team also recognized that GPA needed to address the social and economic contexts and costs of AIDS by drawing on resources that other UN agencies could provide. Beginning in early 1987, Mahler and Mann began exploring potential partnerships and collaborations with several UN agencies—including the United

[22] James Chin *The AIDS Pandemic: The Collision of Epidemiology with Political Correctness.* Oxon, UK: Radcliffe Publishing, Inc., 2007, 200.

[23] Ibid.

[24] Ibid.

[25] Ibid.

[26] Christer Jönsson, "From 'Lead Agency' to 'Integrated Programming': The Global Response to AIDS in the Third World," *Green Globe Yearbook* 1996, p. 70.

[27] Christer Jönsson and Peter Söderholm, "IGO-NGO relations and HIV/AIDS: innovation or stalemate?" *Third World Quarterly,* 1995, 16(3): 473.

[28] Abigail Trafford and Susan Okie, "The Uphill Battle Against AIDS Worldwide," *The Washington Post,* August 25, 1987, Z6.

Nations Development Programme (UNDP), the United Nations Educational, Scientific and Cultural Organization (UNESCO), the United Nations Children's Emergency Fund (UNICEF), the United Nations National Population Fund (UNFPA), and the World Bank—to address the multisectoral causes, determinants, and consequences of the disease.[29] Some component of the AIDS pandemic and its response touched on the mission of these various agencies, and the challenge for Mahler and Mann was to draw upon their strengths without ceding strategic control and leadership over the global response to them.

This was a very real threat because, in response to the UN General Assembly's request for a coordinated UN response to AIDS, Secretary-General Javier Pérez de Cuéllar in 1987 had designated the Department of International, Economic, and Social Affairs (DIESA) in the UN as the coordinating authority for UN-associated AIDS programming. In response to this mandate, DIESA established a Steering Committee on AIDS and a Standing Committee on AIDS to coordinate AIDS efforts among UN agencies. While UNICEF, UNFPA, UNDP, and major UN departments belonged to this latter committee, WHO as a UN-specialized agency did not (though a liaison eventually began attending meetings).[30]

In response to DIESA's potential challenge to WHO's jurisdictional authority, Mahler in 1988 established the Interagency Advisory Group (IAAG) to coordinate activities of all agencies in the UN system (UN agencies and UN-specialized agencies) under the mandate of WHO's Global AIDS Strategy.[31] The IAAG included a broader swath of UN agencies (it included the World Bank, for example, which DIESA had not). GPA provided strong leadership in the organization, implementation, and agenda-setting of these meetings.[32] In addition, GPA began restructuring its Participating Parties meetings into what it eventually called the GPA Management Committee (GMC). The GMC included donor and recipient nations, participating UN agencies and other intergovernmental organizations, and (ultimately) various non-governmental organizations (NGOs). The Committee served GPA as a review and advising body that addressed funding, strategies, implementation, and global coordination. This entity would later play a key role in creation of the Joint United Nations Programme on HIV/AIDS (UNAIDS).[32] For our purposes, it is only important to note at this stage that, from the very beginning of GPA, WHO's authority in coordinating the global response was—at least on paper—complicated, contradictory, and open to contestation.[33]

[29] Special Programme on AIDS, "Progress Report Number 1, APRIL 1987," Geneva: WHO, 1987, WHO/SPA/GEN/87.2, p. 2.

[30] Christer Jönsson, "From 'Lead Agency' to 'Integrated Programming': The Global Response to AIDS in the Third World," *Green Globe Yearbook*, 1996, 66; Global Programme on AIDS, "Progress Report Number 5, May 1989," Geneva: World Health Organization, WHO/GPA/DIR/89.4, p. 18–19. The reader may find a full list of the other UN agencies at http://www.unsceb.org/directory#fp

[31] Global Programme on AIDS, "Progress Report Number 5, May 1989," Geneva: World Health Organization, WHO/GPA/DIR/89.4, p. 18–19.

[32] Christer Jönsson, "From 'Lead Agency' to 'Integrated Programming': The Global Response to AIDS in the Third World," *Green Globe Yearbook*, 1996, 66.

[33] Ibid.

These bodies, along with endorsements from the Group of Seven (G7), United Nations Economic and Social Council (ECOSOC), and the UN General Assembly gave GPA the leverage it needed to position itself between potential donors and national programs in such a way that it became "the 'gatekeeper' for participation … [in] national AIDS programs."[34] Centralizing oversight in this way, Mann argued, would reduce the potential for redundancies and free up national officials from a heavy load of bureaucratic reporting to focus on combating AIDS in their countries.[35] It also ensured that WHO retained control over the direction and content of the global AIDS response.

There were inherent institutional tradeoffs in having WHO as the coordinating agency in the global AIDS effort. For example, prior to the formation of GPA, "WHO officials had little experience in leading coordination of the UN system" beyond "specific public health projects."[36] Moreover, as we noted earlier, WHO rarely intervened directly in the provision of health care or disease prevention activities, working instead through Member States ("advising their governments on technical matters, financing the training of local health professionals, and trying to influence health policy decisions").[37] But since many health ministries and health systems in developing nations, particularly in sub-Saharan Africa, had serious weaknesses in leadership, manpower and management, WHO/GPA faced considerable limitations to its effectiveness "on the ground."

Health ministries also often lacked the mandate or ability to work outside the health sector. Consequently, Mahler and Mann decided to turn to UNDP for help in this regard. In most countries, the UNDP Resident Representative–who was responsible for executing UNDP activities–also served as the coordinator of all UN operational activities related to development, and UNDP staff possessed considerable expertise addressing socioeconomic issues in developing nations.[38] UNDP thus seemed the most obvious agency with which to collaborate to ensure coordinated efforts among UN agencies at the country level, and the development of programs that addressed the socioeconomic aspects of AIDS. From the outset, then, GPA collaborated with UNDP "to ensure linkages at the national level," including involvement in national program support activities and regional collaboration on support and planning.[39]

---

[34] James Chin *The AIDS Pandemic: The Collision of Epidemiology with Political Correctness.* Oxon, UK: Radcliffe Publishing, Inc., 2007, 201.

[35] Lawrence K. Altman, "AIDS' Global Peril Is High On Agenda At Summit Meeting," *The New York Times,* May 31, 1987, 1:1.

[36] Christer Jönsson, "From 'Lead Agency' to 'Integrated Programming': The Global Response to AIDS in the Third World," *Green Globe Yearbook,* 1996, 66; Leon Gordenker, "The World Health Organization: Sectoral Leader or Occasional Benefactor?" in Roger A. Coate, ed., *US Policy and the Future of the United Nations* (New York: Twentieth Century Fund Press, 1994, 179.

[37] Fiona Godlee, "The World Health Organisation: WHO in crisis," *BMJ* November 26 1994;309:1424–1428

[38] Christer Jönsson, "From 'Lead Agency' to 'Integrated Programming': The Global Response to AIDS in the Third World," *Green Globe Yearbook,* 1996, 66. Mike Merson interview. "WHO/UNDP Alliance to Combat AIDS: Policy Framework," in A41/5, p. 49.

[39] Special Programme on AIDS, "Progress Report Number 2, November 1987," Geneva: World Health Organization, WHO/SPA/GEN/87.4, p. 11.

It is within this context that, beginning in mid-1987, GPA (still SPA at the time) and UNDP staff began meeting to formalize a "WHO/UNDP Alliance to Combat AIDS." After the UN General Assembly called for the UN Secretary-General to ensure a coordinated response to AIDS in October 1987, WHO and UNDP leadership agreed to combine forces in support of national AIDS programs.[40] On 19 January, 1988, the WHO Executive Board endorsed the policy framework of the Alliance.[41] Initially, this Alliance was little more than a general framework of collaboration and lacked substantive details. It was drawn up to ensure that nations treated AIDS as more than merely a "health problem" and consequently incorporated AIDS activities into all their development plans and allocations.[42] In the Alliance agreement, UNDP pledged to support WHO in the formulation, coordination, implementation, and evaluation of national plans; ensure coordinated external support of those plans in light of each country's national priorities; and provide bridge funds of up to $2 million to ensure national programs had funding while awaiting the receipt of pledged donations. WHO retained hierarchical priority in the implementation of the Global AIDS Strategy and sole responsibility for technical and policy inputs in each participating nation. UNDP's Division for Global and Interregional Programs, led by Tim Rothermel, a savvy and highly trusted UNDP official who had worked closely with WHO in setting up TDR and the Diarrheal Diseases Control Programme (CDD), became the key coordination liaison between UNDP and WHO.[43] WHO and UNDP officials hammered out the details of the Alliance framework by February 1988, and at the end of March, Mahler and UNDP Administrator William Draper signed the agreement at a press conference at UN headquarters.[44] In the ensuing months, WHO and UNDP representatives would meet with governments to work out procedures for the Alliance's implementation.[45]

Not surprisingly, the WHO/UNDP Alliance to Combat AIDS raised concerns within UNDP. Some UNDP staff felt that many practical aspects of its framework

---

[40] "WHO/UNDP Alliance to Combat AIDS: Policy Framework," in A41/5, p. 49; "Co-operation against AIDS: Report of the Administrator" UNDP Special session, February 16–18 1988, DP/1988/I/Add.I. Item 2; World Health Organization, "Executive board, Eighty-first Session, Provisional Agenda Item 19: WHO/UNDP Alliance to Combat AIDS," Geneva: World Health Organization, 1987, EB81/INF.Doc./3.

[41] "Program Matters: Co-operation against AIDS, Addendum; DP/1988/1/Add.1" Governing Council of the United Nations Development Programme, 16–18 February 1988, pp. 1–2.

[42] "United Nations: WHO and UNDP form Alliance to Combat AIDS," IPS Inter Press Service, March 30, 1988.

[43] UNDP Governing Council, "Programme Matters: Co-operation against AIDS, Report of the Administrator," Geneva, 1988, DP/1988/1/Add. 1, pp. 1–3.

[44] Draper had previously served as President and Chairman of the Export–import Bank. "United Nations: WHO and UNDP form Alliance to Combat AIDS," IPS Inter Press Service, March 30, 1988.

[45] Global Programme on AIDS, "Progress Report Number 5, May 1989," Geneva: World Health Organization, WHO/GPA/DIR/89.4, p. 19.

lacked specifics, particularly in the area of administration, resource mobilization, distribution of responsibilities, and the future structure of the relationship.[46] Others supported the program but were cautiously aware of how difficult joint actions were among UN agencies.[47] Conversely, others saw the alliance as a model for collaboration among other UN agencies, particularly in an era of UN reform, and they called for the alliance to expand to include both other issues beyond AIDS and additional agencies beyond WHO and UNDP.[48] All in all, most observers inside and outside UNDP agreed with Mahler and Draper that the "unprecedented alliance" held great promise for "a well-coordinated, multilateral approach to the global struggle against AIDS."[49]

GPA also developed a relationship with UNICEF, an agency which at that time had been working closely with WHO in a number of areas, in particular child survival. This included immunization, oral rehydration therapy, breastfeeding, and use of growth charts, interventions that were top priorities for UNICEF's then Executive Director, Jim Grant. The collaborative relationship developed rapidly on several fronts. In February 1987, WHO and UNICEF issued a joint statement on immunization and AIDS with recommended sterilization practices for reusable needles and syringes during immunizations.[50] UNICEF also participated in a GPA consultation on breastfeeding/breast milk and HIV infection, partook in national donor meetings in countries, and appointed a consultant to liaise with GPA over UNICEF's role in the Global AIDS Plan.[51] Interagency collaboration continued in 1988 when GPA representatives met with UNICEF's Regional Directors to brief them on national program activities, and culminated in UNICEF's announcement, in May 1988, that it would launch a comprehensive AIDS prevention program, in conjunction with WHO, that included "health education, training of maternal and child care workers,...[safe] immunization programs, and country-by-country studies on the impact of AIDS on children."[52]

GPA launched collaborative ventures with other UN agencies as well. WHO and UNESCO held several joint consultations on the integration of AIDS information into educational settings throughout 1987 and 1988, and also collaborated on ways

---

[46] Governing Council of UNDP, "Special session: Co-operation with the World Health Organization and other agencies against AIDS; Summary Record of the 2nd Meeting, 17 February 1988," Geneva: UNDP, 1988, DP/1988/SR.2, 8, 10, 11.

[47] Ibid, p. 7.

[48] Ibid., pp, 7–8, 10–11.

[49] "United Nations: WHO and UNDP form Alliance to Combat AIDS," IPS Inter Press Service, March 30, 1988.

[50] WHO, "WHO Special Programme on AIDS, Report by the Director-General to the World Health Assembly, 27 March 1987," Geneva: World Health Organization, 1987, A40/5, p. 7.

[51] Special Programme on AIDS, "Progress Report Number 2, November 1987," Geneva: World Health Organization, WHO/SPA/GEN/87.4, p. 12.

[52] "Africa: UNICEF Plans to Combat AIDS in Women and Children," IPS-Inter Press Service, May 25, 1988.

to bring UNESCO-affiliated NGOs into global AIDS education efforts.[53] In 1987, GPA began collaborating with the World Bank on a study of the economic and demographic impact of AIDS and the cost of its care on developing countries.[54] That year marked the first time that the World Bank had invested in national health infrastructures with the intent of addressing specific health problems like AIDS, though over the next few years the World Bank would become an important donor to national AIDS programs' Medium Term Plans (MTPs) in countries like Brazil, Zaire, Uganda, Burundi, Tanzania, and Indonesia.[55] GPA also collaborated with UNFPA on bringing family planning and maternal and child health programs into the AIDS effort.[56] In addition, GPA worked with the International Labour Organization (ILO) in 1987 and 1988 to craft recommendations regarding AIDS in the workplace and the treatment of HIV-positive workers, and with the Food and Agriculture Organization (FAO) to study the impact a severe AIDS pandemic would have on agricultural supply and policy in developing nations.[57]

Beyond UN agencies, Mann and his team also had to maintain relationships with donor nations and international NGOs. Fakhry Assaad had already laid the foundation for this by establishing WHO's AIDS Collaborating Centers and the Committee of Participating Parties. But in the Cold War environment of the mid-1980s, many donor nations were far from convinced that multilateralism offered them greater benefits than bilateral programs. As political scientists Barry Hughes and Christer Jönsson have noted, bilateralism gives states greater control over their development funds, and "about three-quarters of all government aid flows remained bilateral by the late 1980s."[58] Nevertheless, several factors made it more attractive in the late 1980s for donors to fund multilateral, rather than bilateral, AIDS programs. First of all, "all Western governments were under enormous pressure to spend money on

---

[53] Special Programme on AIDS, "Progress Report Number 2, November 1987," Geneva: World Health Organization, WHO/SPA/GEN/87.4, p. 11; Global Programme on AIDS, "Progress Report Number 5, May 1989," Geneva: World Health Organization, WHO/GPA/DIR/89.4, p. 19.

[54] Special Programme on AIDS, "Progress Report Number 2, November 1987," Geneva: World Health Organization, WHO/SPA/GEN/87.4, p. 12; Jonathan Mann, "Trip Report for New York, Washington, Atlanta, 15–20 February 1988," World Health Organization, A20/372/7, etc.

[55] Thomas Land, "World Bank getting into fight against AIDS," *The Financial Post,* August 26, 1988, 1:13, National Council for International Health, "Press Briefing on Global AIDS Issues," *Federal News Service,* December 1, 1988; Global Programme on AIDS, "Progress Report Number 5, May 1989," Geneva: World Health Organization, WHO/GPA/DIR/89.4, p. 20.

[56] Special Programme on AIDS, "Progress Report Number 2, November 1987," Geneva: World Health Organization, WHO/SPA/GEN/87.4, p. 11; Jonathan Mann, "Trip Report for New York, Washington, Atlanta, 15–20 February 1988," World Health Organization, A20/372/7; Global Programme on AIDS, "Progress Report Number 5, May 1989," Geneva: World Health Organization, WHO/GPA/DIR/89.4, p. 20.

[57] Special Programme on AIDS, "Progress Report Number 2, November 1987," Geneva: World Health Organization, WHO/SPA/GEN/87.4, p. 12; Global Programme on AIDS, "Progress Report Number 5, May 1989," Geneva: World Health Organization, WHO/GPA/DIR/89.4, p. 21.

[58] Barry B. Hughes, *Continuity and Change in World Politics.* Englewood Cliffs, NJ: Prentice Hall, 1991, 104, cited in Christer Jönsson, "From 'Lead Agency' to 'Integrated Programming': The Global Response to AIDS in the Third World," p. 65.

AIDS ... So there is the domestic lobby that says 'you have to do something for AIDS,'" remembered Joe Decosas, a physician with expertise in sexually transmitted disease (STD)[59] who, at that time, was working for the Canadian International Development Agency (CIDA) and who would later become Chair of the GMC.[60] "Donors in this instance were giving to a problem, not to a solution," my former program management officer in the CDD program, Bob Hogan, recalled. "It was frustrating [for other WHO programs] because we had a problem, we had a solution, and we had an approach which had proven itself. Jonathan merely had a problem—but donors were wanting primarily to address their own domestic clients."[61] And so the money flowed. Part of this impetus also sprang from a second factor: that AIDS had arisen so rapidly, most nations felt they lacked the "knowledge, expertise, experience and financial and human resources" to run a successful bilateral AIDS program. "You know how long it takes to develop a bilateral project? 2 to 3 years ..." explained Decosas. "So there is ... this frantic trial to put something together like a bilateral program and in the meanwhile ..."we have GPA, let them deal with it.[62] On top of this, AIDS remained a profoundly sensitive issue for many nations in the late 1980s: "A number of major bilateral donors have stated clearly that their bilateral efforts to combat AIDS have been constrained by political sensitivities," Mahler explained at an AIDS meeting during the 1987 World Health Assembly, "... That is why [they] have decided to complement WHO's Programme and centrally funded activities."[63]

Member countries invested heavily in GPA over the next few years.[64] "Money was virtually pushed onto this program," explained Decosas.[65] The United States, which had been particularly parsimonious with WHO in the mid- to late-1980s, became one of the largest donors to the program; it gave approximately $15 million to GPA a year, beginning in 1988, coordinating this multilateral funding with its burgeoning bilateral investments (particularly its AIDS Technical Support [AIDSTECH] and the AIDS Health Communication Project [AIDSCOM] programs).[66] Mann had done

---

[59] For the purposes of this text, we use the term sexually transmitted disease(s) and the abbreviation STD rather than the other term sexually transmitted infection(s) or STIs.

[60] Joe Decosas, Interview by Michael Merson, New Haven, CT, October, 2001.

[61] Robert Hogan, Interview by Michael Merson, New Haven, CT, August, 2002.

[62] Joe Decosas, Interview by Michael Merson, New Haven, CT, October, 2001.

[63] WHO GPA (1992), *Report of the External Review of the World Health Organization Global Programme on AIDS*, GPA/GMC(8)/92.4 (Geneva: WHO GPA, Jan.) P. 4.

[64] Ibid.

[65] Joe Decosas, Interview by Michael Merson, New Haven, CT, October, 2001.

[66] "Panel, Earmarks Foreign Aid for AIDS Fight," *The Associated Press,* March 31, 1987; Halfdan Mahler, "Funding request letter to USAID, April 21, 1987." HRM-B12/372/2; Robert Meehan, "Project Implementation Order, 5/27/87,"; Joyce E. Frame, "Grant No. DPE-5965-G-IC-6059-00, Global AIDS Prevention and Control Program, Amendment No. 1, June 25, 1987," US AID; Barton Reppert, "U.S. Health Groups Seek To Restore WHO Funds," *The Associated Press,* June 29, 1987; Celia Hooper, "[United States has sacrificed its leadership]" *United Press International,* April 18, 1988; "Zambia: Intensifies Action Against AIDS," *IPS-Inter Press Service,* August 19, 1988; Jeffrey Harris, "Participation of AIDSCOM and AIDSTECH staff at Africa AIDS Donor Meetings," Washington, DC: USAID, June 9, 1988, 1–2; National Council for International Health, "Press Briefing on Global AIDS Issues," *Federal News Service,* December 1, 1988.

outstanding work convincing the United States Congress to divide its support for global AIDS between WHO and USAID's bilateral programs. He also requested to have the WHO appropriation earmarked in the federal budget so USAID leadership could not appropriate these funds otherwise. He had been able to do this in great part by gaining the support of then Republican Congressman John Porter from Illinois, who was a member of the United States House of Representative Appropriations Committee and Vice-Chair of its Foreign Operations Subcommittee (Porter would eventually leave Congress and go on to serve as one of the strongest champions for federally supported health research as chair of Research America). Canada, the United Kingdom, Japan, and the Scandinavian countries also donated considerable sums of money to GPA over the next few years.[67]

Donors were comfortable giving contributions to GPA as the structure of the program allowed them to exert influence through their position among the Participating Parties and subsequently as members of the GMC. Indeed, initially, all the donors to GPA were high-income nations, though by late 1987 several other non-donor countries took their place among the Participating Parties.[68] Initially, donor nations exercised little direct influence on the implementation of specific programs and strategies, focusing more attention on issues related to coordination of national and global activities and the funding of national programs.[69] One key concern they did have from the onset, however, was that GPA maintain proper and consistent communication and information exchange between itself, donor nations, national programs, and the WHO Collaborating Centers.[70] Mann tried to alleviate these concerns by communicating directly with national health ministers in a series of international conferences. The most prominent example of this came on January 28,

---

[67] "Britain to donate 3.6 million sterling pounds for aids control in east Africa," *The Xinhua General Overseas News Service*, March 12, 1988; Joan Breckenridge, "AIDS called a threat to health-care gains," *The Globe and Mail*, April 1, 1987; "Canada contributes to WHO's program on AIDS," *The Xinhua General Overseas News Service*, April 15, 1987, Item No: 0415088; "Canada's contribution to WHO," *The Xinhua General Overseas News Service*, February 12, 1988, Item No: 0212073; "World Health Organization (WHO) Asks Japan to Support International AIDS Strategy," *Japan Economic Newswire*, October 6, 1987.

[68] The nations at the fourth meeting of Participating Parties was Argentina, Australia, Belgium, Brazil, Canada, China, Denmark, Ethiopia, Finland, France, Federal Republic of Germany, Haiti, India, Indonesia, Italy, Japan, Jordan, Kenya, Mexico, the Netherlands, Norway, Philippines, Rwanda, Sweden, Switzerland, Thailand, the United Kingdom, Tanzania, the United States , the Union of Soviet Socialist Republics, Zaire, Zambia; cf. Special Programme on AIDS, "Report of the Fourth Meeting of Participating Parties, Geneva, 12–13 November 1987," Geneva: World Health Organization, 1987, WHO.SPA/GEN/87.5, pp. 14–17.

[69] WHO Special Programme on AIDS: Report by the Director-General," Geneva: World Health Organization, March 27, 1987, A40/5, p. 7; Special Programme on AIDS, "WHO Special Programme on AIDS, Provisional Agenda Item, 18.2; May 5, 1987," World Health Organization, A4C/Inf.DOC./8; Special Programme on AIDS, "Third Meeting of Participating Parties for the Prevention and Control of AIDS: Consensus Statement, Geneva, 27 and 28 April 1987," Geneva: World Health Organization, 1987, SPA/1NF/87.3, pp. 1–2.

[70] Special Programme on AIDS, "Third Meeting of the WHO Collaborating Centres on AIDS, Washington, D.C., 6 June 1987," Geneva: World Health Organizationi, June 1987, WHO/SPA/RDV/87.1, p. 4.

1988, when GPA and the Government of the United Kingdom jointly organized the World Summit of Ministers of Health on Programmes for AIDS Prevention in London. This was the largest conference to date sponsored by GPA with participants from close to 150 countries, including over 100 ministers of health. The conference reviewed the global AIDS situation and the role of information and education in AIDS prevention and control. A leading theme throughout the conference was a strong plea to fight bigotry and prejudice against persons with AIDS.[71] At the end of the conference, the ministers adopted the "London Declaration on AIDS Prevention" and designated December 1, 1988, as the world's day of dialogue on AIDS. That day (December 1, 1988) would go on to be the first World AIDS Day, a day that is still marked annually around the world.[72] Another important WHO-sponsored international conference was the First International Symposium on Education and Communication about AIDS, held in Mexico in October 1988 and attended by participants from 18 countries.[73]

We should note that, while the London Summit went a great way towards building confidence about WHO's commitment to consistent communication exchange with health ministers, it also had a diplomatic downside. In organizing the event, Mann had given Mahler and himself prominent places on the agenda. He had not invited any of WHO's Regional Directors to speak though they were in attendance. This oversight, we learned in our interviews, highly offended Hiroshi Nakajima, then Regional Director of the Western Pacific Region. This slight, whether intentional or not, would have important implications for the future of GPA because WHO's Executive Board had just nominated Nakajima as the next Director-General of WHO.[74]

To facilitate better oversight and communication, GPA and the Participating Parties moved to establish the aforementioned GMC composed of donor and recipient nations. GPA faced several obstacles to implementing national AIDS programs and the Global AIDS Strategy—including recruiting staff, delivering country support, linking with other organizations, and developing research priorities—and the GMC provided GPA with substantial opportunity to explore solutions to these problems, while also encouraging the program to pay due regard to local conditions and cultural contexts in its integration of AIDS prevention and control efforts into national health programs.[75] The new management committee would pose some tradeoffs though. With donors providing a growing pool of funds, as we shall see, they

---

[71] Trip report of Joe Asvall, Regional Director, EURO, dated March 23 1988.

[72] World Health Organization, "Global Strategy for the Prevention and Control of AIDS: Report by the Director-General, 22 November 1988," Geneva: World Health Organization, Executive Board, 1988, 9–10.

[73] World Health Organization, "Global Strategy for the Prevention and Control of AIDS: Report by the Director-General, A41/5, 21 March 1988," Geneva: World Health Organization, 1988, 12; Richard Herzfelder, "Media Losing Interest in AIDS, Delegates Told," *The Associated Press,* October 21, 1988.

[74] Hiroshi Nakajima, Interview by Michael Merson, Poitiers, October 13, 2002.

[75] Global Programme on AIDS, "Report of the Meeting of the Global Programme on AIDS Management Committee, 7–9 November 1988," Geneva: World Health Organization, 1988, GPA/GMC(1)/88.1, 3–4, 7.

began demanding greater accountability from GPA for program implementation and effectiveness.[76]

Alongside relations with donor nations, Mann and his team included various NGOs as program stakeholders.[77] The first steps came in early 1987, when GPA's leadership invited several international NGOs to participate in the larger Participating Parties group. By the end of 1987, GPA had expanded that group of NGOs to include organizations like the Christian Medical Commission, International Planned Parenthood Federation, and League of Red Cross and Red Crescent Societies. Though not NGOs in the conventional sense, GPA also included the Ford Foundation and the Rockefeller Foundation.[78] To facilitate the growing relationship with these entities, in 1988, Mann hired Robert Grose, an NGO-relations specialist from the Overseas Development Administration in the United Kingdom, as the GPA/NGO liaison officer.[79] Initially, Grose focused his efforts on the NGOs in "official relations" with WHO (mentioned above), but Mann and Grose quickly recognized the expanding role that local and regional NGOs were going to play in national AIDS programs and began establishing informal connections with them.[80] In a short time they came to view NGOs as integral to national AIDS programs and pushed to include trustworthy NGOs in the larger policy process.[81]

[76] Ibid, 38.

[77] Christer Jönsson and Peter Söderholm, "IGO-NGO relations and HIV/AIDS: innovation or stalemate?" *Third World Quarterly*, 1995, 16(3):466–469; Elizabeth Fee and Manon Parry, "Jonathan Mann, HIV/AIDS, and Human Rights," *Journal of Public Health Policy*, 29(1): 63.

[78] Special Programme on AIDS, "Meetings of Interested Parties for the Support of the National AIDS Prevention and Control Programmes," Geneva: World Health Organization, SPA/NPS/9.10.87, 3; The initial list of non-governmental groups included: CARE, CARITAS, Catholic Fund for Overseas Development, Catholic Relief Service, Christian Medical Commission (CMC), International Council of Nurses, International Planned Parenthood Federation (IPPF), International Union for Health Education, International Union against Tuberculosis and Lung Disease, International Union against the Venereal Diseases and the Treponematoses, League of Red Cross and Red Crescent Societies, Lutheran World Federation, Save the Children Fund (UK), Save the Children Fund (USA), and the World Federation of Hemophilia. Foundations included: African Medical and Research Foundation (AMREF), American Foundation for AIDS Research, Ford Foundation, The Rockefeller Foundation, and Project Hope. Special Programme on AIDS, "Report of the Fourth Meeting of Participating Parties, Geneva, 12–13 November 1987," Geneva: World Health Organization, 1987, WHO.SPA/GEN/87.5, pp. 18–20.

[79] US Department of State, "WHO Global Program on AIDS Management Committee Meeting," Geneva: US Mission Geneva, Nov. 8, 1988; Christer Jönsson and Peter Söderholm, "IGO-NGO relations and HIV/AIDS: innovation or stalemate?" *Third World Quarterly*, 1995, 16(3):466–469; Jeff O'Malley, Interview by Michael Merson, New Haven, CT, September, 2002.

[80] World Health Organization, "Global Strategy for the Prevention and Control of AIDS: Report by the Director-General, EB83/26, 22 November 1988," Geneva: World Health Organization, 1988, 8, 15; *Opportunities for Solidarity*, final report of the Montreal Meeting of NGOs involved in community AIDS service, Montreal 2–4 June 1989, p 6, cited in Christer Jönsson and Peter Söderholm "IGO-NGO relations and HIV/AIDS: innovation or stalemate?" *Third World Quarterly*, 1995, 16(3):466–7.

[81] WHO/GPA, Memorandum from Terry Mooney to Jonathan Mann, 7 March 1988, cited in Christer Jönsson and Peter Söderholm, "IGO-NGO relations and HIV/AIDS: innovation or stalemate?" *Third World Quarterly*, 1995, 16(3):466.

Encouraged by these initial efforts, AIDS activists in Canada, Brazil, and the United States sought support from WHO to establish a global forum for AIDS-related NGOs.[82] Soon after the 4th International Conference on AIDS in Stockholm in 1988, with several proposals in place and Grose now on board, GPA began to support the efforts of these groups. This gave them the "bureaucratic tidiness" inherent to WHO. GPA also hired Jeff O'Malley as a liaison officer to cultivate relations between WHO and AIDS-related NGOs. O'Malley was an experienced AIDS activist from Canada and would later go on to have a distinguished career in the UN, including working in UNDP and UNICEF.[83] Grose and Mann's ultimate goal, co-opting the vision of AIDS activists like O'Malley, was to create a "GPA-centered network ... [of] people in regular contact with each other" who could "strategize and map out a framework" of NGO engagement in local and global AIDS policy.[84] By 1988, GPA was working with over 35 international NGOs and 100 national NGOs in some form or function; and that number promised only to grow further in the years to come with the birth of the International Council of AIDS Service Organization at the 5th International Conference on AIDS in Montreal in June 1989. [85]

With this move—recognizing, collaborating with, and eventually financially supporting NGOs—Mann took a very groundbreaking step. International NGOs like the Red Cross had worked with WHO for many years, but Mann and his team truly pioneered the idea of incorporating a much wider range of NGOs—regional groups, activist groups, local AIDS service organizations—into GPA's plans. In later years, organizations like UNAIDS would take Mann's efforts even further by incorporating NGOs into the governance of international bodies.

Despite all these efforts, AIDS numbers continued climbing. By the fall of 1988, 80% of WHO member countries were reporting cases, with cumulative numbers of AIDS cases now surpassing 120,000, a 15-fold increase in 4 years.[86] This rapid climb skewed long-term projections even further.[87] Still, Mann and his team were seeing

---

[82] *Opportunities for Solidarity*, final report of the Montreal Meeting of NGOs involved in community AIDS service, Montreal 2–4 June 1989, p 6, cited in Christer Jönsson and Peter Söderholm, "IGO-NGO relations and HIV/AIDS: innovation or stalemate?" *Third World Quarterly*, 1995, 16(3):467.

[83] Christer Jönsson and Peter Söderholm, "IGO-NGO relations and HIV/AIDS: innovation or stalemate?" *Third World Quarterly*, 1995, 16(3):466–469; Jeff O'Malley, Interview by Michael Merson, New Haven, CT, September, 2002.

[84] Christer Jönsson and Peter Söderholm, "IGO-NGO relations and HIV/AIDS: innovation or stalemate?" *Third World Quarterly*, 1995, 16(3):467, and WHO/GPA, Memorandum from Terry Mooney to Jonathan Mann, 7 March 1988.

[85] World Health Organization, "Global Strategy for the Prevention and Control of AIDS: Report by the Director-General, A41/5, 21 March 1988," Geneva: World Health Organization, 1988, 12;World Health Organization, "Global Strategy for the Prevention and Control of AIDS: Report by the Director-General, EB83/26, 22 November 1988," Geneva: World Health Organization, 1988, 8, 15.

[86] Global Programme on AIDS, "Global Strategy for the Prevention and Control of AIDS: Report by the Director-General," Geneva: World Health Organization, November 1988, EB83/26, 3, 6; "Iran in Brief: Health Minister says AIDS cases discovered," *BBC Summary of World Broadcasts,* December 3, 1988.

[87] "No AIDS vaccine for 5–10 years, says WHO," *Herald,* December 1, 1988; "WHO official stresses need for AIDS education," *The Xinhua General Overseas News Service,* December 1, 1988.

some countries take positive steps. For example, 52 of 59 sub-Saharan African countries reported changes in sexual behaviors, particularly a reduction in the number of sexual partners and an increase in condom use.[88] In San Francisco, new infections among men who have sex with men (MSM) had started to decline.[89] In Amsterdam, infection rates among MSM had fallen from 10% in 1983 to less than 1% in 1988.[90] In other places, however, the trends were disconcerting: in Bangkok, infection rates among injection drug users (IDUs) went from zero to 15–20% in 2 years.[91] Mann was under no illusions about the dire nature of the situation: "the danger is widespread and is continuing to spread," he told reporters in November.[92]

In the 2 years since the launch of the program, GPA had seen considerable accomplishments in their awareness-raising campaign. "It is an unprecedented phenomenon in the history of world public health," Mann told reporters in December 1988, "There has never before been anything quite like the global fight against AIDS."[93] Indeed, GPA had established itself as the preeminent institution in developing, coordinating, and directing implementation of the global AIDS response. It had recruited a considerable number of program staff at headquarters, regional, and country levels and increased its budget to over $60 million annually. These resources enabled it to support collaborative efforts against AIDS with departments in WHO, agencies within the UN System, and organizations in the global health community[94] Mann and his team also tried to position WHO to coordinate activities in social and behavioral research under the leadership of Manuel Carballo and biomedical research under the leadership of David Heymann (Heymann was a Center for Disease Control and Prevention (CDC) epidemiologist who had been working in Africa for the previous 12 years whom Mann had recruited). These moves established GPA as the key agency for monitoring, forecasting, and evaluating the effects of the pandemic, as well as the chief entity orchestrating a global control and prevention strategy.[95]

---

[88] "WHO official stresses need for AIDS education," *The Xinhua General Overseas News Service,* December 1, 1988.

[89] Ibid.

[90] Brenda Watson, "World Health Group Lowers Worldwide AIDS Projection," *The Associated Press,* November 29, 1988.

[91] "WHO official stresses need for AIDS education," *The Xinhua General Overseas News Service,* December 1, 1988.

[92] Brenda Watson, "World Health Group Lowers Worldwide AIDS Projection," *The Associated Press,* November 29, 1988.

[93] Essma ben Hamida, "Heath: World Uniting To Fight AIDS," *IPS-Inter Press Service,* November 29, 1988.

[94] UNDP, "Co-operation With The World Health Organization and Other Agencies Against AIDS (DP/1988/I and Add.l and DP/1988/PROJECTS/REC/27 and DP/1988/PROJECTS/REC/28)," Geneva: United Nations Development Program, DP/1988/SR.2, 3–4; Global Programme on AIDS, "Global Strategy for the Prevention and Control of AIDS: Report by the Director-General," Geneva: World Health Organization, November 1988, EB83/26, 3, 6.

[95] UNDP, "Co-operation With The World Health Organization and Other Agencies Against AIDS (DP/1988/I and Add.l and DP/1988/PROJECTS/REC/27 and DP/1988/PROJECTS/REC/28)," Geneva: United Nations Development Program, DP/1988/SR.2, 3–4.

By the end of 1988, the program was "planning, implementing, monitoring and evaluating" national AIDS programs in over 140 countries.[96]

No one could deny that GPA had undergone a rapid and unprecedented expansion,
but Mann was not ignorant of the challenges ahead. The virus was still spreading
faster than the national programs could respond, and Mann believed the global
response still depended on the successful implementation of his three-pronged program: "education and information to change peoples' behavior; health care; and a
reversal of the stigmatization of AIDS sufferers."[97] One of Mann's key concerns was
how easily HIV spread in contexts of poverty, apathy, ignorance, and discrimination. Education and awareness alone would not slow the pandemic; nations needed
to invest in health access and health infrastructure: "it is pointless to talk of condoms without making them available to people," Mann explained. "Health care
must be improved if the battle against AIDS is to be effective."[98] As time went on,
Mann increasingly focused on these social determinants of health and vulnerability—the combination of information and education, health and social services provision, and human rights protection—as the comprehensive means by which the
world would slow the spread of AIDS.[99] This focus on health and human rights
would come to be a key though somewhat controversial weapon in Mann's
armamentarium against AIDS in the ensuing years, and to that we now turn.[100]

---

[96] Global Programme on AIDS, "Global Strategy for the Prevention and Control of AIDS: Report
by the Director-General," Geneva: World Health Organization, November 1988, EB83/26, 3, 6;
UNDP, "Co-operation With The World Health Organization and Other Agencies Against AIDS
(DP/1988/I and Add.1 and DP/1988/PROJECTS/REC/27 and DP/1988/PROJECTS/REC/28),"
Geneva: United Nations Development Program, DP/1988/SR.2, 3–4.

[97] Essma ben Hamida, "Heath: World Uniting To Fight AIDS," *IPS-Inter Press Service,* November
29, 1988.

[98] Ibid.

[99] "WHO official stresses need for AIDS education," *The Xinhua General Overseas News Service,*
December 1, 1988.

[100] Essma ben Hamida, "Heath: World Uniting To Fight AIDS," *IPS-Inter Press Service,* November
29, 1988

Chapter 6
Health, Human Rights, and the Global Programme on AIDS

By 1988, Jonathan Mann had come to conceive of AIDS[1] differently than when he had first arrived in Geneva 2 years earlier. Increasingly, he had come to understand AIDS as the interdigitation of biology, individual experience, and culture. This more robust comprehension of the pandemic pushed him, relentlessly, towards a broader interpretive framework for AIDS and public health, a position now frequently referred to as the health and human rights framework. Mann's evolving perspective would resonate with many others in global health and development. "It very much corresponded to my own views and feelings but which were not that well expressed," Peter Piot told us. "Jonathan was able to capture that in … a clear vision. I really think from a historic perspective that is his real contribution … the positioning of AIDS and the interpretation of AIDS in these terms … that it is not just a viral illness. That was I think an enormous contribution. Not only for AIDS but I think afterwards for many other health programs."[2] Not everyone was convinced that Mann's perspective was the correct or best one, of course, and Mann's innovative position on health and human rights could not shield him from Member States' demands for tangible results against the pandemic. Mann would ultimately interrupt his own efforts to operationalize this framework at the Global Programme on AIDS (GPA) with his abrupt resignation from the World Health Organization (WHO), but his time at WHO would steer the field in new and important directions. This chapter describes both the evolution of Mann's views on health and human rights and the pathway that led to his resignation as Director of GPA.

In the years after World War II, the integration of health and human rights moved forward on a number of fronts. Between the 1960s and 1980s, several non-govern-

Within this chapter the singular pronouns *I* and *my* refer to Michael Merson alone, whereas the plural pronouns *we* and *us* generally refer to Michael Merson and Stephen Inrig jointly. Where *we* or *us* refers to Michael Merson and his colleagues at WHO, the object of the pronoun is clarified by context.

[1] For the purposes of this text, we will use the term AIDS to encompass both AIDS and HIV unless otherwise specified.

[2] Peter Piot, Interview by Stephen Inrig, February, 2011.

© Springer International Publishing AG 2018
M. Merson, S. Inrig, *The AIDS Pandemic*, DOI 10.1007/978-3-319-47133-4_6

mental organizations (NGOs)—including Amnesty International, Physicians for Human Rights, and the International Federation of Health and Human Rights Organizations (IFHHRO)—mobilized "to conduct research and generate action to prevent and end grave abuses of human rights," including the health-related issues of incarceration, torture and mass violence, and "to demand justice for those whose rights have been violated."[3] At the same time, other NGOs—ranging from historical groups like the International Committee of the Red Cross to newer groups like *Medecins Sans Frontieres* and *Medecins Du Monde*—stepped up their efforts to deliver health care impartially to combatants on both sides during a conflict.[4] A burgeoning group of people were very interested in the linkages between health needs and human rights concerns at the precise moment that AIDS and its associated discrimination emerged on the global stage in the early 1980s.

From very early in the pandemic, people framed AIDS as more than a biomedical phenomenon.[5] Many politicians, policy-makers, public figures, and the public in general approached AIDS from a "social, moral, or spiritual" vantage point. Fear of AIDS and disapproval of groups associated with HIV transmission elicited blame, stigmatization, and numerous exclusionary actions. Partly in response to this conceptualization, and partly as a preemptive move, certain groups began asking questions about the human rights and civil liberties issues raised by various AIDS policies. Gay men in Europe and the United States were among the first to ask, largely because they were among the first groups significantly affected by AIDS and at a key point in their social identity. Many within these communities belonged to social networks that had formed during the gay rights freedom struggle of the 1960s and 1970s. They drew on these networks to launch AIDS service organizations and public advocacy groups.[6]

It was out of this context that groups began linking AIDS and human rights. Perhaps the first explicit mention came in 1983, when the Council of Europe—which had both a special committee on blood product safety and public proclamations against gay discrimination—issued several resolutions highlighting "the human rights aspects of the epidemic."[7] Between 1983 and 1985, the Council called for "[blood] donations by persons in risk groups without inappropriate discrimination

---

[3] Amnesty International, "About Amnesty International," London: Amnesty International Limited, 2010. http://www.amnesty.org/en/who-we-are/about-amnesty-international accessed on March 17, 2011. See also Physicians for Human Rights, "About PHR: PHR History," Cambridge, MA: Physicians for Human Rights, 2009; http://physiciansforhumanrights.org/about/founding.html accessed on March 17, 2011, and The International Federation of Health and Human Rights Organizations, "About Us," Utrrecht: IFHHRO, 2016 http://www.ifhhro.org/main.php?op=text&id=11

[4] Doctors of the World, "Notre Organisation," Paris: Medecins du Monde, http://www.mdm-international.org/spip.php?article78

[5] These next two paragraphs adapted from Christer Jönsson and Peter Söderholm, "IGO-NGO relations and HIV/AIDS: innovation or stalemate?" *Third World Quarterly*, 1995, 16(3): 464.

[6] Stephen Inrig. *North Carolina and the Problem of AIDS*. Chapel Hill, NC: University of North Carolina Press, 2011.

[7] Christer Jönsson and Peter Söderholm, "IGO-NGO relations and HIV/AIDS: innovation or stalemate?" *Third World Quarterly*, 1995, 16(3):467.

and emotive over-reaction amongst recipients," denounced "the use of this disease as a pretext for campaigns against homosexuals," and called on its members to "confront and, as far as possible, resolve the wider ethical, social and medical issues raised by the screening of donors."[8] As WHO took up the global problem of AIDS, it could not escape these larger social considerations.

Human rights protections in the fight against global AIDS did not play a central role in Fakhry Assaad's initial AIDS strategy at WHO. Once he took up the issue, Assaad considered AIDS to be a compelling and alarming public health problem that required an evidence-based response. Approaching AIDS as primarily a human rights issue would have been foreign to him, however, although Assaad and his wife, Fawsia Assaad, both had a strong commitment to human rights.[9] Nonetheless, human rights concerns—primarily the issue of AIDS-related discrimination—quickly forced their way onto Assaad's agenda. Few modern diseases carried as much potential for discrimination as AIDS—from subtle concerns about "AIDS carriers" to national policies restricting the rights of populations associated with AIDS. However, such widespread fears were relatively unique for WHO and the Centers for Disease Control and Prevention (CDC), so Assaad and his assistant Bill Parra may not have anticipated it when, in the early months of the program (before Mann joined WHO), they found themselves deluged with press and diplomatic interest and public hysteria over transmission risks associated with the disease. Frequently, concerned health officials would corner Assaad at international conferences and grill him on the safest standards for shipping AIDS-related materials or the most appropriate restrictions countries should place on infected travelers. The requests and concerns took on a life of their own, Parra recalled: "I think [Assaad] realized that this was something that was bigger than his division could do."[10] This additional aspect of AIDS was part of the reason for bringing Mann on board, and ultimately for setting up GPA as an entity outside the WHO Division of Communicable Diseases.

What might have happened to the focus on human rights and discrimination had the program remained with Assaad in the Communicable Disease division? "He would have made it a part; an essential part [of the program]," maintained Fawsia Assaad. "He would have made it a part of its normal [functioning], but he would have [focused] more on research and on [finding] medication."[11] Had Assaad lived longer, would he have liked the path Mann took the program? "I don't have any doubts that Fakhry would have supported Jonathan," Parra maintained.[12] As it turns out, Mann would push the concept of health and human rights in directions that were new, exciting, and controversial for WHO and the global health community.

---

[8] Leon Gordenker, Christer Jönsson, Roger A. Coate, and Peter Söderholm, *International cooperation in response to AIDS*. New York: Pinter, 1995, 38–39.

[9] Fawsia Assaad, Interview with Stephen Inrig, Dallas, TX, October, 2010.

[10] William Parra, Interview with Stephen Inrig, Dallas, TX, October 14, 2010.

[11] Fawsia Assaad, Interview with Stephen Inrig, Dallas, TX, October, 2010.

[12] William Parra, Interview with Stephen Inrig, Dallas, TX, October 14, 2010.

Mann's arrival at WHO did not immediately transform WHO's approach to health and human rights, largely because Mann himself had only begun his evolution on these topics. According to those who worked with Mann in Africa at *Projet SIDA*, other concerns consumed his time and attention. "He didn't get into any of the human rights issues, he didn't get into the stigma, none of that stuff," Tom Quinn recalled. "He was a pure breed epidemiologist investigating an outbreak of a disease. And that is what he did."[13]

Still, several things predisposed Mann to develop an interest in the human rights aspects of AIDS. First, his academic pursuits at college had attuned him to these considerations: he had majored in history at Harvard and had expressed considerable interest in "the history of diseases and how they influenced society and culture, especially in Europe."[14] Second, his family background surely influenced him: his father was a psychiatrist who worked with holocaust survivors and Mann's brother was a rabbi.[15] Finally, while he may have acted like a "pure breed epidemiologist" in Zaire, Mann's experience in Africa appears to have awakened in him some concerns about rights and discrimination. During his time there, for example, Mann grew close to *Projet SIDA's* lab coordinator Frieda Behets, and the two were known to spend considerable time engaged in "long, intellectual chats about those kinds of things."[16] In fact, towards the end of Mann's time with *Projet SIDA*, Quinn noticed an evolution in Mann's perspective on the pandemic. "I could not believe it—he was saying this is going to be the worst epidemic of all times, of our times .... He was making predictions," Quinn later recalled. "I think when he saw that he wasn't getting anywhere [convincing the United States Agency for International Development (USAID) and CDC of AIDS' magnitude] ...he had to take this to a different level. I think he thought WHO was the place to go."[17] So while it is unlikely that Mann arrived at WHO with a fully formed health and human rights framework, he was certainly positioned to look beyond more traditional public health frameworks in the battle against AIDS.

One of the most pressing issues facing the global community, as Mann took leadership of WHO's AIDS program, was whether nations could protect themselves from AIDS by screening travelers and foreign residents. These concerns had developed rapidly early in the emerging pandemic. In 1985, a global survey of AIDS legislation found no "immigration and travel restrictions for people with the HIV virus," but by 1987 several countries throughout the world had instituted such restrictions.[18] Indeed, by 1988, a WHO report found that at least 24 countries had

---

[13] Thomas Quinn, Interview with Stephen Inrig, Dallas, TX, February 3, 2011.

[14] Brenda Watson, "Top AIDS Official Has Busy Schedule, Momentous Task," *The Associated Press*, August 14, 1987.

[15] Manuel Carballo, Interview by Michael Merson, New Haven, CT, November, 2002; Michael Grodin, Interview with Stephen Inrig, Dallas, TX, 2010.

[16] Robin Ryder, Interview by Michael Merson, New Haven, CT, August, 2002.

[17] Thomas Quinn, Interview by Michael Merson, New Haven, CT, August, 2002.

[18] Dana Kennedy, "Seventy-Seven Countries Respond to AIDS Survey," *The Associated Press*, July 26, 1988.

introduced some sort of restriction on travelers living with AIDS, including (but not limited to) Belgium, Canada, China, Cuba, India, Iraq, Japan, Libya, Saudi Arabia, South Korea, the Soviet Union, Thailand, United States, and West Germany.[19]

The ramifications of these restrictions were apparent to Assaad and Halfdan Mahler even before Mann joined the program in the spring of 1986. The large-scale fear and discrimination actually caught them somewhat by surprise: "That was something that we had actually never experienced at WHO or CDC," remembered Parra. "That kind of concern that people would have about transmission and the kind of restrictions that people would place on people that had AIDS. That kind of discrimination never occurred."[20] Mahler himself (likely influenced by Assaad's experience and Mann's interest) brought up travel restrictions in a speech he delivered at the 2nd International Conference on AIDS in Paris in the summer of 1986: "AIDS has brought to the surface hidden fears, irrational suspicions and, consequently, irresponsible actions," Mahler explained. For example, "witness the attempts to restrict travel among countries."[21] In February 1987, Mann and Mahler chose actively and publicly to oppose such travel restrictions as counterproductive to the global fight against AIDS.[22]

Mann adopted a four part strategy to address the situation. First, GPA brought WHO's policy and moral weight to bear on these issues by hosting strategic consultations aimed at guiding the response and preventing missteps.[23] In early March 1987, GPA held a consultation in Geneva on global travel and AIDS.[24] The group concluded that such screening could only slow the epidemic briefly, at the expense of other more effective efforts; that barring HIV-infected individuals from means of transport made little sense in light of HIV's transmission mode; and that AIDS education was essential to resident and traveler alike.[25] "At best, and at great cost," Mann explained to reporters, "HIV screening of international travelers would retard only

---

[19] Ibid.; Sandra G. Boodman and Susan Okie, "Aggressive Prevention Efforts Proliferate: WHO Official Calls for World Cooperation, Warning There Are No Geographic 'Safe Zones,'" *The Washington Post,* June 5, 1987, D1; Hanns Neuerbourg, "Pressure Grows Around World for Drastic Steps against AIDS," *The Associated Press,* June 6, 1987; Jocelyn Ford, "Fear Of AIDS Sparks Stringent Gov't Reaction," *Japan Economic Newswire,* February 25, 1987; "Japan's Health Ministry Finalize Draft of AIDS Prevention Law," *Japan Economic Newswire,* March 6, 1987; Joan Breckenridge, "AIDS called a threat to health-care gains," *The Globe and Mail,* April 1, 1987; Robert Glass, "High-Risk Groups Targeted for AIDS Screening in Europe," *The Associated Press,* March 25, 1987.

[20] William Parra, Interview by Stephen Inrig, Dallas, TX, October 14, 2010.

[21] Halfdan Mahler, "Opening Speech, International Conference on AIDS, Paris, 23–25 June 1986" Geneva: World Health Organization, 1986.

[22] Jocelyn Ford, "Fear Of AIDS Sparks Stringent Gov't Reaction," *Japan Economic Newswire,* February 25, 1987.

[23] Kathleen Kay, Interview by Michael Merson, New Haven, CT, 2002.

[24] Halfdan Mahler, "WHO Special Programme on AIDS, Assembly Item 18.2, A40/5," World Health Organization, March 27, 1987, p. 1.

[25] World Health Organization, "WHO Special Programme on AIDS: Report by the Director-General," Geneva: World Health Organization, 1987, A40/5, p. 7.

briefly the spread of HIV... [so] the diversion of resources to HIV screening of international travelers and away from educational programs and measures to protect the blood supply is not justified."[26] Unfortunately, and contrary to what was desired, the consultation did not harness human rights law as a public health tool in this regard, and many countries went on to add, rather than drop, such travel restrictions.[27]

Second, perhaps recognizing the limited power WHO's consultations had on actual behavior of countries with a growing fear of AIDS, Mann sought to compile a list of relevant AIDS-related laws from WHO Member States. As we mentioned in Chapter 4, Mann hired United States legal scholar Larry Gostin to conduct this work. Gostin had received his bachelor's degree in psychology in New York during the early 1970s, began exploring the rights of mental health patients in North Carolina during his time at Duke University School of Law, and then, after graduating in 1974, spent much of the 1970s and early 1980s working on patient rights and civil liberties in the United Kingdom. By the mid-1980s, Gostin returned to the United States to teach at Harvard University, and he began transitioning from mental health law to the emerging field of AIDS and AIDS-related legal, regulatory, and policy issues surrounding AIDS.[28] In late 1986, Mann asked Gostin to expand his United States-based analysis to encompass the international community as well. Gostin agreed and began amassing examples of best and worst regulatory practices, from an ethical–legal standpoint, for dealing with AIDS. Ultimately completed in the summer of 1988, Gostin explained that the 150-page study was aimed at providing Member States with "the best and worst examples of how AIDS [was] being handled around the world."[29] These examples suggested ways that countries could structure legislation to deal effectively with AIDS while still complying with international laws related to health and well-being.[30]

The third tool Mann employed was a media based education campaign that drew attention to the ineffectiveness of bans on HIV-infected travelers. Mann took advantage of the opportunity afforded to him by the aforementioned March 1987

---

[26] "WHO rejects AIDS screening for travelers," *United Press International*, March 4, 1987; Hanns Neuerbourg, "Health Experts Advise Against Screening Travelers For AIDS, *The Associated Press*, March 4, 1987; "Testing of travelers not answer, panel says," *The Globe and Mail*, March 5, 1987.

[27] *Contra* Elizabeth Fee and Manon Parry, "Jonathan Mann, HIV/AIDS, and Human Rights," *Journal of Public Health Policy,* 29(1):63.

[28] Lawrence O. Gostin,, William J. Curran, and Mary E. Clark, *Acquired Immunodeficiency Syndrome: Legal, Regulatory, and Policy Analysis* (University Publishing Group) (1988) (First published U.S. Department of Health and Human Services); Harold M. Ginzburg & Lawrence O. Gostin, "Legal and Ethical Issues Associated with HTLV-III Diseases," *Psychiatric Annals* 16(3):180–185 (1987); Lawrence O. Gostin, "Acquired Immunodeficiency Syndrome: A Review of Science, Health Policy, and Law," *Health* Matrix: J. Of Law-Med. IV(2):3–13 (1986); Lawrence O. Gostin, "The Limits of Compulsion in Controlling AIDS," *Hastings Center Report* Dec. 24–29 (1986); Lawrence O. Gostin, "AIDS Policies Raise Civil Liberties Concerns," *J. of the National Prison Project* 10:10–11 (1986).

[29] Dana Kennedy, "Seventy-Seven Countries Respond to AIDS Survey," *The Associated Press,* July 26, 1988.

[30] Larry Gostin at the time of this writing is director of the O'Neill Institute for National and Global Health Law, the foremost institute of its kind in the world.

consultation, and also used various global forums and press conferences throughout the summer and fall of 1987 to reiterate WHO's position with medical professionals, health officials, and medical journalists.[31]

Fourth, and perhaps most importantly, Mann positioned himself and GPA as gatekeepers in global AIDS policy oversight: serving as arbiters of programs that could receive funding and host WHO conferences. Leveraging its influence and legitimacy into a "power of the purse," for example, WHO secured approval from the European Economic Community that it would not provide AIDS funds to countries unless they had their AIDS plan approved by WHO.[32] This leverage only increased as various global agencies acknowledged WHO's role in directing and coordinating the Global AIDS Strategy.[33] Likewise, as Mann explained to reporters at a July 1987 news conference, WHO would refuse to hold AIDS meetings "in a country which requires screening of participants for AIDS."[34] These leveraging tools became key mechanisms for encouraging countries to comply with WHO guidance on its consultation topics, though it would not be until 1989 and 1990 that the potential force of these inducements, particularly the one related to the convening of AIDS meetings, became obvious.

Mann moved rather quickly from concerns over bans on HIV-positive travelers to concerns about HIV screening in general. He was not alone in this, of course; by February 1987, health agencies like the CDC came out in favor of voluntary anonymous or confidential testing policies.[35] WHO was initially reluctant to take an official position on screening programs, but rather, in May 1987, it organized a consultation to provide guidelines for countries planning to implement screening programs. Inadequately designed programs, Mann argued, would be "intrusive, may threaten human rights, and are very likely to be both expensive and ineffective." Like the screening of travelers, Mann argued, generalized screening programs might divert "human, material and financial resources away from education programs and other vital human immunodeficiency virus prevention activities."[36] To avoid poorly planned screening programs, GPA published a set of guidelines that gave guidance on their rationale, potential candidates, counseling and implementation practices, data

---

[31] "Testing of travelers not answer, panel says," *The Globe and Mail*, March 5, 1987; Sandra G. Boodman and Susan Okie, "Aggressive Prevention Efforts Proliferate: WHO Official Calls for World Cooperation, Warning There Are No Geographic 'Safe Zones,'" *The Washington Post*, June 5, 1987, D1; Abigail Trafford and Susan Okie, "The Uphill Battle Against AIDS Worldwide," *The Washington Post*, August 25, 1987, Z6; Jennifer Parmelee, "Need For AIDS-Testing Foreign Visitors Disputed," *The Associated Press*, October 9, 1987.

[32] Lawrence K. Altman, "AIDS' Global Peril Is High On Agenda At Summit Meeting," *The New York Times*, May 31, 1987, 1:1.

[33] Ibid.; See also the discussion in the previous chapter.

[34] "AIDS Cases Increase in 122 countries," *The Xinhua General Overseas News Service*, July 30, 1987, IN: 0730038; "WHO Reports 55,396 AIDS Cases, Opposes Screening," *The Associated Press*, July 30, 1987.

[35] Carol Gentry, "AIDS tests not solution, officials say," *St. Petersburg Times*, February 25, 1987, 1A.

[36] Thomas W. Netter, "Uganda Receives $6 Million to Combat AIDS," *The New York Times*, May 26, 1987, C4.

utilization, and ethical–legal matters.[37] These guidelines provided a baseline from which GPA went on, in the following years, to make recommendations for testing programs among injection drug users, employees, sex workers, foreign diplomats, public safety officers, and airline pilots.[38]

At this stage, Mann had made some subtle shifts in his perspective. Perhaps the most obvious example was his heightened sensitivity to concerns about HIV screening. Back in 1986, when Mann coauthored an article on African AIDS epidemiology with Tom Quinn, Jim Curran, and Peter Piot, he and his coauthors had concluded that, while consideration needed to be "given to patient confidentiality, counseling, and ethical issues," nonetheless "the screening of women of child-bearing age and counseling regarding contraception for HIV-seropositive women [was] necessary in order to interrupt perinatal HIV transmission."[39] Moreover, in that paper Mann and his colleagues coupled AIDS education and testing together as part of a larger, proposed AIDS prevention and control strategy. By March 1987, however, Mann was retreating from these positions. First, he stated that he and other experts had become "highly skeptical about the value of screening" owing to its costs and social complications.[40] Additionally, Mann came to juxtapose AIDS education and HIV testing, arguing (as we have seen) that screening directed resources away from vital prevention activities.[41]

As Mann evolved on these policy and strategic considerations, he came increasingly to appreciate the concept of "human rights" and "human rights protections."

---

[37] Special Programme on AIDS, "Special Programme on AIDS Statement: Criteria for Screening Programmes For Human Immunodeficiency Virus (HIV)." Geneva: World Health Organization, May 198, 7SPA/INF/87.4, 1–2; Special Programme on AIDS, "Report of the WHO Meeting on Criteria for HIV Screening Programmes, Geneva, 20–21 May 1987," Geneva: World Health Organization, WHO/SPA/GLP/87.2, 9, 10. See also Thomas W. Netter, "Uganda Receives $6 Million to Combat AIDS," *The New York Times,* May 26, 1987, C4; "Mass-testing questions raised by health body," *The Globe and Mail,* May 26, 1987; Andrew Veitch, "Doctors to test for Aids in secret: Health Department questions legality of new BMA practice," *The London Guardian,* July 3, 1987; John O'Neill, "Disease Outstrips Control Efforts," *Sydney Morning Herald,* July 21, 1987, 6.

[38] Global Programme on AIDS, "Report of the Meeting on HIV Infection and Drug Injecting Intervention Strategies, Geneva, 18–20 January 1988," Geneva: World Health Organization, WHO/GPA/SBR/89.1, 9; Global Programme on AIDS, "Report of the Consultation on the Neuropsychiatric Aspects of HIV Infection, Geneva, 14–17 March 1988," Geneva: World Health Organization, 1988, WHO/GPA/DIR/88.1, 17; Global Programme on AIDS, "Statement from the Consultation on AIDS and the Workplace, Geneva, 27–29 June 1988," Geneva: World Health Organization and International Labour Office, WHO/GPA/INF/88.7, 2,3; Global Programme on AIDS, "Unlinked Anonymous Screening for the Public Health Surveillance of HIV Infections Proposed International Guidelines, Geneva, June 1989," Geneva: World Health Organization, GPA/SFI/89.3, 1–2; "Prejudice new AIDS peril," *Hobart Mercury,* March 12, 1988; Dana Kennedy, "Seventy-Seven Countries Respond to AIDS Survey," *The Associated Press,* July 26, 1988; Craig R. Whitney, "Soviets Say Foreigners Will Need AIDS Certificates," *The New York Times,* January 12, 1989, A13.

[39] Thomas C. Quinn, Jonathan M. Mann, James W. Curran, Peter Piot, "AIDS in Africa: An Epidemiologic Paradigm," *Science,* November 21, 1986, 234:962.

[40] Hanns Neuerbourg, "Health Experts Advise Against Screening Travelers For AIDS, *The Associated Press*, March 4, 1987.

[41] Thomas W. Netter, "Uganda Receives $6 Million to Combat AIDS," *The New York Times,* May 26, 1987, C4.

When he first joined WHO, Mann does not seem to have believed that mandatory screenings of residents and immigrants unilaterally violated human rights, feeling that it depended on what sanctions nations put in place for noncompliance, what quality-control measures nations established, and what confidentiality assurance mechanisms they put in place.[42] But he gained valuable political and rhetorical knowledge on this subject at the Group of Seven (G7) Venice Summit in June 1987. Coming out of the conference, the G7 called for all nations to conduct testing programs in accordance with human rights protocols and recommended that the group help establish "an international committee on the ethical issues raised by AIDS."[43] Mann had helped craft the rhetoric for the public proclamations eminating from this event, and it became clear through AIDS-related speeches and proposals at the G7 that he had also tapped into some resonant but as of yet inchoate "views and feelings" held by civil libertarians in both Europe and the United States.[44] This affirmation reinforced Mann's progression towards the health and human rights framework that he and GPA eventually developed and embraced.[45]

Mann's understanding of AIDS expanded further as he considered the socioeconomic impact of the disease. He and his colleagues had mentioned some of these infrastructural issues in their 1986 *Science* paper ("One cannot hope to prevent reuse of disposable injection equipment [in many African countries]," they wrote, "when many hospital budgets are insufficient for the purchase of antibiotics"), so Mann was already attuned to some of these concerns. But by 1987, Mann had become aware of the more complex consequences of the disease. In late March of that year, Mann participated in a conference on the socioeconomic impact of AIDS. "Health gains around the world are threatened," Mann explained to reporters at the conference. "There is a threat to the whole socioeconomic base of some countries."[46] Not only did AIDS rob countries of their most productive citizens, Mann explained, but evidence suggested that women could spread HIV to their children through breast milk, negating the child survival gains Africa had only just started to witness.[47] AIDS not only could threaten the major health advances that WHO had seen in developing countries,

[42] Ibid. Mass-testing questions raised by health body," *The Globe and Mail,* May 26, 1987; Lawrence K. Altman, "AIDS' Global Peril is High on Agenda at Summit Meeting," *The New York Times,* May 31, 1987, 1:1; Richard Pyle, "Statement Stresses Urgency, Human Rights, on AIDS Problem," *The Associated Press,* June 10, 1987; "Leaders back anti-AIDS, anti-drug efforts," *United Press International,* June 10, 1987; Tom Raum, "Low-Key Summit Ends With Human Rights Plea in AIDS Battle," *The Associated Press,* June 10, 1987.

[43] G7 Chairman, "Chairman's Statement on AIDS, June 10, 1987," G7 Summit, Venice, Italy, June 10, 1987; See also "International News," *The Associated Press,* June 10, 1987.

[44] Peter Piot, Interview by Stephen Inrig, Dallas, TX, February 2, 2011.

[45] Kathleen Kay, Interview by Michael Merson, New Haven, CT, 2002.

[46] Warren E. Leary, "AIDS Epidemic Threatens Third World Health Gains," *The Associated Press,* March 25, 1987.

[47] Celia Hooper, "AIDS could reverse world health gains," *United Press International,* March 25, 1987.

but it could severely damage their fragile economies, cripple fledgling democracies, and destabilize potentially volatile political situations.[48]

It was in light of these more structurally relevant consequences that Mann started speaking of "another epidemic" or "third epidemic": the "epidemic of social reaction and response—to the economic costs, the social impact, the cultural impact, and the political impact."[49] Mann would develop this imagery in greater detail as the pandemic wound on, but by mid-1987, Mann understood the first epidemic to be "the epidemic of the virus itself … a silent epidemic that … spread worldwide in the mid- to late-1970s," and the second epidemic to be "the disease of AIDS, which comes several years after the epidemic of infection."[50] The third epidemic, Mann posited, included the enormous social, cultural, economic, and political dimensions of the pandemic. These were of such magnitude, argued Mann, that they demanded global solidarity and globalized solutions. This was one of the reasons that in the fall of 1987, Mahler and Mann brought the issue of AIDS to the United Nations (UN) General Assembly and called on that body "to mobilize the entire UN system in the worldwide struggle against" the disease.[51]

One of the most important aspects of this "third epidemic" was the epidemic of fear and stigmatization of particular "minority" groups in a given population. "The depth and extent of personal and public reaction to AIDS throughout the world has been considerable," Mann and his team noted in the catalogue of projected needs that GPA published in March 1987.[52] "We are witnessing a rising wave of stigmatization: against Westerners in Asia, against Africans in Europe, against homosexuals, prostitutes, hemophiliacs, and recipients of blood transfusions," Mann told participants of the 3rd International Conference on AIDS in Washington, DC that summer.[53] Here too, Mann was tapping into a larger social movement over AIDS-related stigma and discrimination. In the United States, for example, the Supreme Court had just ruled that people with contagious diseases, including HIV, were protected against job discrimination; at the same time, advocates in New York had just launched the activist

---

[48] Ibid; Joan Breckenridge, "AIDS called a threat to health-care gains," *The Globe and Mail*, April 1, 1987; Lawrence K. Altman, "AIDS' Global Peril is High on Agenda at Summit Meeting," *The New York Times*, May 31, 1987, 1:1; John Schmitt, "Health: Predictions Gloomy at Chaotic World AIDS Conference," *IPS-Inter Press Service*, June 3, 1987; Jim Lehrer, "AIDS: Dr. Jonathan Mann," *The MacNeil/Lehrer NewsHour*, June 3, 1987.

[49] Celia Hooper, "AIDS could reverse world health gains," *United Press International*, March 25, 1987; Jim Lehrer, "AIDS: Dr. Jonathan Mann," *The MacNeil/Lehrer NewsHour*, June 3, 1987; John Schmitt, "Health: Predictions Gloomy at Chaotic World AIDS Conference," *IPS-Inter Press Service*, June 3, 1987.

[50] Jim Lehrer, "AIDS: Dr. Jonathan Mann," *The MacNeil/Lehrer NewsHour*, June 3, 1987.

[51] Jonathan Mann, "IV International Conference on AIDS: The Global Picture of AIDS," Geneva: World Health Organization, 12 June 1988.

[52] Special Programme on AIDS, "Strategies and Structure; Projected Needs," Geneva: World Health Organization, March 1987, WHO/SPA/GEN/87.1, 1–5.

[53] Lawrence K. Altman, "Key World Health Official Warns of Epidemic of Prejudice on AIDS," *The New York Times*, June 3, 1987, A1.

group called the AIDS Coalition to Unleash Power (ACT UP).[54] Not just the United States was affected, however. "The early hypotheses about the origins of the disease and the stigmatization of Africans that has occurred, particularly in Europe," Mann explained in the summer of 1987, "... has led to a reaction against that, and a defensiveness."[55] Discriminatory and accusatory discourse about African promiscuity and culpability in AIDS had grown so common that it infuriated African leaders and created such a sensitive international situation that United States State Department officials debated whether they should even consider supporting bilateral AIDS prevention programs in Africa.[56] "Everybody want[ed] to test," remembered Mann's special assistant Kathleen Kay, "many people wanted a quarantine."[57]

Mann refused to see this fear and discrimination as a series of discrete and unfortunate acts; rather he considered them as symptomatic of "dimly disguised" racial, religious, sexual, national, and socioeconomic prejudices.[58] "In every society facing AIDS," Mann explained to United States health officials in the fall of 1987, "certain complex, pre-existing issues have been highlighted and certain imbalances, deficiencies, and inequities in existing health and social systems have become evident."[59] To respond properly to AIDS, then, societies had to determine whether the status quo in health, education, and human rights was sufficient to the task. WHO's AIDS program could, Mann realized, play an important role in this social reassessment.

It is important here to stress a point made by political scientist Christer Jönsson.[60] Mann's theme of "the third epidemic" highlights the fact that there are numerous ways to frame a pandemic besides simply the biomedical image of a microorganism maximizing its reproductive potential owing to the particular structure of sociosexual interactions in the human species. By the time Mann took the helm of the AIDS program, several alternative conceptualizations—including moral, political, and theological ones—had emerged around AIDS. The calls for quarantine and other exclusionary or coercive public health strategies were often inseparable from value-laden judgments about those who had become sick and those assumed to be at higher risk for potential infection. There would be talk in later years about whether Mann should have "medicalized" the problem more, or whether others were

---

[54] Malcolm Ritter, "Court Decision On Job Discrimination Called Victory For AIDS Victims," *The Associated Press*, March 3, 1987; Larry Kramer, Interview with Sarah Schulman and Jim Hubbard. ACTUP Oral History Project, February 16, 2005. MIX: The New York Lesbian & Gay Experimental Film Festival. December 11, 2005, Actuporalhistory.org accessed on June 25, 2011.

[55] Jim Lehrer, "AIDS: Dr. Jonathan Mann," *The MacNeil/Lehrer NewsHour,* June 3, 1987.

[56] Blaine Harden, "AIDS Seen as Threat To Africa's Future: AIDS Hits African Urban Elites, Is Broad Threat to Development," *The Washington Post,* May 31, 1987, A1.

[57] Kathleen Kay, Interview by Michael Merson, New Haven, CT, 2002.

[58] Jonathan M. Mann, "Statement at an Informal Briefing on AID to the 42nd Session of the United Nations General Assembly, on Tuesday 20th October 1987." Geneva: World Health Organization, WHO/SPA/INF/87.12, 3.

[59] Jonathan Mann, "Statement to the U.S. National AIDS Commission," Geneva: World Health Organization, 2 November 1989, 3, 4, 5.

[60] Christer Jönsson and Peter Söderholm, "IGO-NGO relations and HIV/AIDS: innovation or stalemate?" *Third World Quarterly,* 1995, 16(3):46.

attempting to remedicalize the problem, but to his credit, Mann understood that it was difficult if not impossible to make these distinctions. Testing high risk groups depended on defining those groups, and it also implied one would have to take a position on patient autonomy vis-a-vis testing based on relative and imperfect assessment of risk levels. Surveillance of the disease begged questions about personal privacy and confidentiality. None of these things had "simple" medical or even public health (in the classical sense) answers.

It was in the summer of 1987, then, that Mann and Kay hit upon their public health rationale for preventing AIDS-related discrimination. It was not new or unique to them, of course, but they were the first ones to package the perspective in this way at WHO. Put simply, they maintained that discriminating against people with AIDS would drive those with AIDS or at risk for HIV infection to avoid detection and avoid contact with health and social services.[61] Threatening someone's job or denying them housing, Mann and Kay argued, would serve as a disincentive for someone to take actions beneficial to public health. A punitive strategy would likewise discourage "those most needing information, education, counseling, or other support services" from seeking or obtaining them.[62] With so many people calling for testing and exclusionary tactics like quarantine, Mann and Kay turned that rationale on its head: "If [people with AIDS] were fearful of being isolated as in quarantine, but also excluded from society—we had to come up with this public health rationale of why not to do the traditional things," Kay explained. "Instead of excluding people who were HIV-infected, we had to include them, because it was only by including them and by getting their cooperation, and their feeling of being supported by society—that HIV prevention would be effective."[63]

This public health rationale was the first formal step towards the eventual formation of Mann's health and human rights framework. At this stage, it did little more than highlight the instrumental role for human rights in public health. By "instrumental" here we mean something similar to what economist Amartya Sen intends when he describes the relationship between freedom and development. Sen argues that there are very good reasons to believe freedom and human rights effectively contribute to economic progress.[64] Similarly, with their public health rationale, Mann and Kay had come to see nondiscrimination and the protection of human rights as an effective means of contributing to public health in general and the fight against AIDS in particular. Mann and Kay not only felt the human rights of people with AIDS should be protected in their own right, but they felt that effective prevention campaigns would fail to reach their targets if countries and communities discriminated against AIDS.[65]

---

[61] Jonathan Mann, "IV International Conference on AIDS: The Global Picture of AIDS," Geneva: World Health Organization, 12 June 1988.

[62] Ibid.

[63] Kathleen Kay, Interview by Michael Merson, New Haven, CT, 2002.

[64] Amartya Sen, *Development as Freedom.* New York: Knopf, 1999, 36–37.

[65] Christer Jönsson and Peter Söderholm, "IGO-NGO relations and HIV/AIDS: innovation or stalemate?" *Third World Quarterly,* 1995, 16(3):464.

Again, Mann and Kay were not developing these thoughts from whole cloth. While Mann's interaction with human rights activists and theorists was only beginning, he had been discussing ways that human rights thinking applied to AIDS with Larry Gostin and Michael Kirby from early in his time at GPA. Along with Gostin, whom we introduced earlier, Kirby was an important figure in the emerging linkages between AIDS advocacy and human rights activism. Kirby was an Australian lawyer who served as Deputy President of the Australian Conciliation and Arbitration Commission from 1975 to 1983, and beginning in 1983, served as a judge on the Federal Court of Australia. An eloquent speaker, Kirby belonged to the International Commission of Jurists and, in 1988, was tapped by Mann to serve as Chair of GPA's Global Commission on AIDS. Together with Gostin, Kirby greatly influenced Mann on the role human rights protections could play in AIDS prevention efforts.

Gostin and Kirby were in good company thinking in this direction. As we mentioned earlier, these issues were beginning to percolate in Europe around the time that Mann arrived at WHO. About 3 years before his arrival, a group of international law experts had met in Siracusa, Italy, to "consider the limitation and derogation provisions of the International Covenant on Civil and Political Rights."[66] As it pertained to health matters like AIDS, a subcommittee at Siracusa determined that certain rights could be limited on public health grounds if a State was dealing with a serious threat to individual or population health. However, they argued, those rights curtailments were only legitimate if they were specifically aimed at preventing disease or injury, or at providing care for the sick and injured.[67] It was in this context, then, that Mann and Kay frequently stressed "that HIV is transmitted mainly through behaviors … which are private, secret, hidden … and illegal in some societies." Consequently, "exclusion of these persons [through loss of employment, forced separation from family, loss of education or housing] would be unjustified in public health terms" since the latter curtailments of rights and freedoms did nothing to stem the pandemic.[68]

Mann and Kay's public health rationale also grew up along emerging "harm reduction" public health models. Harm reduction involves an array of policies and interventions aimed at reducing the harmful consequences of high risk behaviors, like injection drug use or multiple sex partners. Harm reduction programs stress "low-threshold' intervention[s]" and emphasize choice "in keeping with the tenets of reasoned action theories" that view risk takers as "'health conscious' citizen[s]

---

[66] Urban Morgan Institute for Human Rights, "The Siracusa principles on the limitation and derogation provisions in the International Covenant on Civil and Political Rights," *Human Rights Quarterly*, 1985, 7(1): 3–14. See also Elizabeth Fee and Manon Parry, "Jonathan Mann, HIV/ AIDS, and Human Rights," *Journal of Public Health Policy*, 29(1):62–63.

[67] UN Commission on Human Rights, *The Siracusa Principles on the Limitation and Derogation Provisions in the International Covenant on Civil and Political Rights*, 28 September 1984, E/ CN.4/1985/4, 4–5. Available at: http://www.unhcr.org/refworld/docid/4672bc122.html [accessed 28 June 2011].

[68] Jonathan Mann and Kathleen Kay, "IV International Conference on AIDS, Stockholm, Sweden; AIDS: Discrimination and Public Health," Geneva: World Health Organization, WHO/GPA/ DIR/88.3, 1–3.

capable of 'rational decision-making' in keeping with publicly recommended 'risk avoidance.'"[69] Since GPA's national programs promoted many of these strategies, as Mann later explained, nondiscrimination efforts served to facilitate them: "field experience had demonstrated that the fear of profound personal and social consequences ... led those most likely to be infected to avoid participating in HIV prevention programs ... Thus, for the first time in history, preventing discrimination against infected people became an integral part of a strategy to control a pandemic of infectious disease."[70]

Even here, these views evolved. In some of his earliest speeches, Mann employed the idea of "not to exclude but include" more frequently than the term "human rights," in part because he and Kay worried that the term "'human rights' would be a bit of a red flag to the World Health Assembly (WHA)." Instead, he and Kay opted to talk about "nondiscrimination." Throughout the last half of 1987 and the first half of 1988, Mann and Kay worked to have the WHA adopt a nondiscrimination resolution. "That was a long process," Kay remembered. "First, starting with earlier speeches ... at the 3rd International Conference on AIDS (it was wording I remember that I had on my wall), Jonathan stated ...'There was a bigger epidemic of discrimination than of HIV'—that was the message."[71] Over the ensuing months, Kay and Mann approached the theme from a variety of angles, stressing the idea to include, rather than exclude.[72] At this stage, they were not in extensive dialogue with human rights experts about these issues, rather their ideas developed through interaction within GPA's senior leadership team. "In the early days of developing these ideas we talked together about the speeches and ideas," Kay recalled. "We talked through ideas a lot. They evolved."[73]

To obtain a WHA resolution on nondiscrimination, Mann, Kay, and Mahler again relied on the iterative strategy they had been using in other contexts. In the ensuing months, after raising the importance of nondiscrimination from the floor of the UN General Assembly in 1987 ("[The fight against AIDS] is also a fight against fear, against prejudice, and against irrational action born of ignorance."[74]), Mann worked with the Council of Europe to recommend that Member States devise AIDS policies that were "scientifically justified" and did "not interfere unnecessarily with [citizens'] individual rights to objective information, freedom and private life."[75]

[69] Tim Rhodes, "The 'risk environment': a framework for understanding and reducing drug-related harm," *International Journal of Drug Policy* 13 (2002) 85–94.

[70] "The History of Discovery and Response," in Jonathan Mann and Daniel Tarantola, eds. *AIDS in the World II,* New York: Oxford University Press, 1996, 433.

[71] Kathleen Kay, Interview by Michael Merson, New Haven, CT, 2002.

[72] Ibid.

[73] Ibid.

[74] Statement by the Secretary-General of the United Nations before the General Assembly. Press release SG/SM/816/GA/334 (October 20, 1987):3.

[75] Council of Europe, Committee of Ministers, Recommendation No. R (83) 25 Concerning Common European Public Health Policy to Fight the Acquired Immunodeficiency Syndrome (AIDS) (Nov. 26, 1987). From http://www1.umn.edu/humanrts/instree/europolicy.html accessed on June 28, 2011.

On December 1, 1987, GPA's consultation on the Social Aspects of AIDS Prevention and Control Programmes issued a statement indicating that AIDS prevention should respect and protect human rights and that exclusionary and discriminatory policies were unnecessary and counterproductive.[76] Mann then crafted documents focusing on inclusion rather than exclusion as background for the Summit of Ministers of Health in London in January, 1988.[77] He worked hard to ensure that the London declaration stated that AIDS prevention programs needed to protect "human rights and human dignity" and avoid "discrimination against, and stigmatization of HIV-infected people and people with AIDS and population groups," and that the Summit declare 1988 to be a Year of Communication and Cooperation about AIDS. He meant this "to forge a spirit of social tolerance among countries."[78] Several international meetings over the course of the following spring (including a Middle East conference on AIDS, a United Nations Development Programme (UNDP) meeting on AIDS, an Australian meeting on AIDS, and a WHO consultation on the neuropsychiatric implications of AIDS) reinforced the emphasis on human rights coming out of the Health Minister's meeting.[79] Particularly formative would be an international meeting in London in March, which connected Mann and Kay with members of the global human rights network.[80] At the conference, Mann stressed the need for global human rights organizations to help prevent discrimination against people with AIDS. Influence from these groups helped push Mann beyond the "instrumental" understanding of the relationship between AIDS and human rights that he and Kay had developed earlier.[81]

In May of 1988, the objective that Mann and Kay had been working on for a year finally came to fruition: the WHA passed a resolution against AIDS discrimination. Resolution WHA41.24 requested that WHO "take all measures necessary to advocate the need to protect the human rights and dignity of HIV-infected people and people with AIDS, and of members of population groups." The resolution also asked WHO's Director-General "to stress to Member States and to all others concerned the dangers to the health of everyone of discriminatory action against and stigmatization of HIV-infected people and people with AIDS and members of population

---

[76] Special Programme on AIDS, *Social Aspects of AIDS Prevention and Control Programs*, Geneva: World Health Organization, December 1, 1987, WHO/SPA/GLO/87.2.

[77] Kathleen Kay, Interview by Michael Merson, New Haven, CT, 2002.

[78] Global Programme on AIDS, "World Summit of Ministers of Health: London Declaration on AIDS Prevention, 28 January 1988," Geneva: World Health Organization, 1988, WHO/GPA/INF/88.6, 2–3.

[79] "Recommendation of mideast conference on AIDS," *The Xinhua General Overseas News Service* February 12, 1988, Item No: 0212010; UNDP, "Governing Council Special Session: Summary Record of the 2nd Meeting, 17 February 1988," Geneva: United Nations Development Programme, DP/1988/SR.2, 25 February 1988, 10; Paul Lewis, "AIDS Virus Seen Unlikely to Cause Mental Illness," *The New York Times,* March 19, 1988, 1:32.

[80] Jonathan Mann and Kathleen Kay, "IV International Conference on AIDS, Stockholm, Sweden; AIDS: Discrimination and Public Health," Geneva: World Health Organization, WHO/GPA/DIR/88.3, 1–3.

[81] Ibid.

groups, by continuing to provide accurate information on AIDS and guidance on its prevention and control."[82] WHO had officially adopted a nondiscrimination policy with regard to AIDS, and it further pressed GPA, as a part of its Global AIDS Strategy, to develop these ideas further and put them into concrete action.[83] This was no small feat.

Throughout the fall of 1988, Mann and Kay continued promoting their nondiscrimination public health rationale, and obtaining the WHO resolution enabled them to push forward in two different directions.[84] First, they continued operationalizing nondiscrimination policies in national AIDS programs. "This is an extraordinary consensus," Mann said in early 1988 about global support for nondiscrimination, "Now it is a matter of translating that consensus into reality."[85] In some countries, for example, previous government campaigns back in the 1970s had driven sex workers underground, which made it very difficult in the 1980s for national AIDS programs to reach this population with AIDS prevention messages, condoms, and other support. Other countries had rules related to premarital testing, mandatory testing, and even deportation or quarantine of individuals testing positive.[86] GPA had been working on these issues since the spring of 1987, but WHA 41.24 gave them greater authority to encourage adoption of nondiscriminatory policies and a greater mandate to penalize countries that utilized discriminatory policies.

Second, the WHA resolution gave Mann and his team license to develop the health and human rights framework further. Having used nondiscrimination as a more palatable concept to gain acceptance at the WHA level, Mann and Kay now began pushing beyond the inherent limitations of the public health rationale towards an expanded view of the relationship between AIDS and human rights. This ability to go beyond the public health rationale was important because its limitations were becoming quite clear to them. First, their focus on discrimination against people with HIV infection left unaddressed the fact that, in many societies, those who were not HIV infected but at heightened risk for HIV infection frequently faced AIDS-related discrimination. For example, regardless of an individual's serostatus, Africans bore the brunt of AIDS restrictions in Europe, while gays and Haitians endured AIDS-related discrimination in the United States. Second, they came to understand that the public health rationale had been heavily hampered by barriers to individual behavior change. Healthy behavior happened not merely in the absence

---

[82] "Global Strategy for the Prevention and Control of AIDS," World Health Organization, November 22, 1988, p. 14.

[83] Kathleen Kay, Interview by Michael Merson, New Haven, CT, 2002; Elizabeth Fee and Manon Parry, "Jonathan Mann, HIV/AIDS, and Human Rights," *Journal of Public Health Policy,* 29(1): 63.

[84] WHO Executive Board, "Executive Board, Eighty-third Session, Provisional agenda item 11: Global Strategy for the Prevention and Control of AIDS, Report by the Director-General," Geneva: World health Organization, EB83/26, 22 November 1988, 15.

[85] Andrew Veitch, "Fine words: The health minister's Aids summit in London," *The London Guardian,* January 29, 1988.

[86] Jonathan Mann, "IV International Conference on AIDS: The Global Picture of AIDS," Geneva: World Health Organization, 12 June 1988.

of fear, but also in the presence of support.[87] Third, Mann recognized that creating these positive environments required far more than nondiscrimination regulations and laws; it required adequate health and social systems.

It was with this new commitment to health and human rights that Mann began meeting with various members of human rights groups and NGOs. Initially, Mann thought the best way to collaborate with human rights groups on AIDS would be to establish a global system for monitoring AIDS-related human rights violations. "We need to know when and how discrimination occurs," he explained to an audience in March 1988.[88] While Mann proposed such a system, he never elaborated on how it would work and, perhaps realizing it might prove unfeasible, he subsequently dropped it from his policy considerations.[89] Instead, Mann began concentrating on the positive role "an informed and alerted human rights network can [play] through information and education about [human rights] and AIDS and through promotion of the human rights and dignity of all persons."[90] In anticipation that the WHA would issue its resolution on AIDS discrimination, Mann wrote to Mahler in April 1988 shortly before his departure from WHO seeking formal permission to begin meeting with human rights groups. "I believe the time has come for us to bring together the various organizations … involved with human rights, to discuss the relationship between AIDS, discrimination and human rights," he explained to Mahler.[91]

On May 27, 1988, having received Mahler's approval, GPA took the bold step of organizing an "informal consultation with representatives from UN agencies and 28 NGOs interested in development, human rights, and discrimination against people with HIV/AIDS."[92] At the meeting, Mann proposed that members of these three communities move forward in a collaborative, multidisciplinary approach to nondiscrimination.[93] Obtaining the WHA nondiscrimination resolution and now launching collaborative relationships with human rights NGOs appears to have pushed Mann considerably further along in his thinking about health and human rights. By the spring of 1988, it seems fair to say that Mann considered the issue of discrimination to be the focal point at which health and human rights intersected; they were "inseparably intertwined" in his mind.[94] "In thinking about AIDS, some

---

[87] Ibid.

[88] Robert Glass, "WHO Official Calls Masters & Johnson Study 'Irresponsible,'" *The Associated Press,* March 8, 1988.

[89] Ibid.

[90] Jonathan Mann and Kathleen Kay, "IV International Conference on AIDS, Stockholm, Sweden; AIDS: Discrimination and Public Health," Geneva: World Health Organization, WHO/GPA/DIR/88.3, 1–3.

[91] Jonathan Mann, "AIDS and Human Rights; Letter to Dr. H. Mahler, April 11, 1988," Unpublished document, April 11, 1988.

[92] "Global Strategy for the Prevention and Control of AIDS," World Health Organization, November 22, 1988, p. 15.

[93] Ibid.

[94] A.M. Rosenthal, "The Admiral on His Watch," *The New York Times,* June 10, 1988, A31.

seek to oppose the 'right of the many' to remain uninfected against the 'rights of the few' who are already HIV-infected," Mann explained at the 4th International Conference on AIDS in Stockholm that summer. "This is a false dilemma, for the protection of the uninfected majority depends precisely upon and is inextricably bound with protection of the rights and dignity of infected persons."[95] Now, having arrived at this point, Mann began exploring the relationship between the two and the extent to which they depended upon each other.

Mann also began considering what impact the WHO resolution would have on AIDS nationally and globally. First of all, it meant recognizing that discrimination fell on populations, and not merely individuals. This led him not only to talk about "HIV-infected persons [and] persons with AIDS" when discussing discrimination, but also to include a larger category of "stigmatized population groups."[96] Second, it meant bolstering support systems because nondiscrimination was similar to "negative" freedom: it might free people with HIV from having intentional obstacles to access placed in their way, but it was not the same as access itself. "Avoidance of discrimination," as the WHA resolution had been subtitled, was not the same as supporting access to care. And so, in the spring and summer of 1988, Mann began placing great emphasis on creating "a supportive social environment" within which prevention activities could take place.[97] This emphasis on "supportive social environments" echoed the message coming out of the "new public health movement" championed as goals in the Ottawa Charter.[98] "Public support must be firmly marshaled behind rational and humane AIDS prevention and control programs," Mann explained to the audience in Stockholm.[99]

Finally, and most importantly, Mann concluded that AIDS-related support would remain inadequate in a given country if the larger system of health inequities and inequalities remained. "We recognize that in doing this work we must inevitably confront the inadequacies of our health and social systems," he told the audience in Stockholm. "For if effective health information and education delivery systems already existed; if intravenous drug use was already effectively prevented or treated; if integrated blood transfusion services already existed in the developing world; if we already possessed useful information on sexual practices in each society—then the challenge of AIDS prevention would be correspondingly less. But AIDS remorselessly highlights and exposes the weaknesses, the inadequacies and inequities of our existing health and social systems and the gaps in our knowledge of

---

[95] Jonathan Mann, "IV International Conference on AIDS: The Global Picture of AIDS," Geneva: World Health Organization, 12 June 1988.

[96] Jonathan Mann and Kathleen Kay, "IV International Conference on AIDS, Stockholm, Sweden; AIDS: Discrimination and Public Health," Geneva: World Health Organization, WHO/GPA/DIR/88.3, 1–3.

[97] Jonathan Mann, "IV International Conference on AIDS: The Global Picture of AIDS," Geneva: World Health Organization, 12 June 1988.

[98] Ottawa Working Group on Health Promotion in Developing Countries, "Health promotion in developing countries. The report of a workgroup," *Health Promotion*, 1994; 15:259–275.

[99] Jonathan Mann, "IV International Conference on AIDS: The Global Picture of AIDS," Geneva: World Health Organization, 12 June 1988.

others and ourselves. In this way, the fight against AIDS has become part—a key element—in a broader fight for 'Health for All.'"[100] Thus, Mann explained to conference participants, "in addition to information and education, specific health and social services will be required to support risk-reducing behavior changes."[101]

This was not a completely new vision, of course: public health practitioners had focused on health systems and health inequalities at least since the publication of Rudolf Virchow's Report on the Typhus Epidemic in Upper Silesia in 1848.[102] Also, health equity formed the basis for Mahler's emphasis on the Health for All by the Year 2000 strategy that WHO adopted at the Alma-Ata conference in 1978. But what was new, for Mann, was the consideration of AIDS as symptomatic of much larger structural issues in societies across the globe.

Thus, at least two factors appear to have played a significant role in Mann's evolution on this point. The first was his realization that countries needed to have large infrastructural capacities in place to provide prevention services to their citizenry. For example, in response to questions about harm reduction efforts from a Soviet Union representative during a March 1988 meeting on UN agency collaboration against AIDS, Mann noted that while public health practitioners must use information and education to influence behavior, information and education alone were insufficient. "It was also necessary" Mann cautioned, "to provide social and health services in order to support the desired behavior."[103] Pushing the point further, Mann explained that "information on how to use condoms was of no use if condoms were not available, of poor quality, or too expensive. Telling intravenous drug users about the risks of contracting AIDS was of no use unless there was a drug treatment program."[104] National AIDS programs needed not only to attend to their blood supply and prevention policies, but they must also consider ways that their lack of health infrastructure might inhibit healthy behaviors. For Mann, in 1988 and 1989, this meant, for example, encouraging countries to expand their number of drug treatment programs.[105]

Along with considering the needs for greater prevention infrastructure within health systems, Mann focused on reforming care delivery. This new line of thought stemmed in part from the fact that, by the first months of 1987, the United States Food and Drug Administration (FDA) had approved the first drug showing promise against HIV, azidothymidine (AZT). AZT was a nucleoside analog reverse-transcrip-

---

[100] Ibid.

[101] Jonathan Mann and Kathleen Kay, "IV International Conference on AIDS, Stockholm, Sweden; AIDS: Discrimination and Public Health," Geneva: World Health Organization, WHO/GPA/DIR/88.3, 1–3.

[102] R.C. Virchow. *Archiv für pathologische Anatomie und Physiologie und für klinische Medicin.* Vol 2. Berlin, Germany: George Reimer; 1848;143–332.

[103] UNDP Governing Council, "Special session, Summary Record of the 2nd Meeting: Co-operation with the World Health Organization and other agencies against AIDS, 17 February 1988," New York: UNDP, 1988, DP/1988/SR.2, p. 13.

[104] Ibid.

[105] Jean Seligmann with Ruth Marshall, "Checking Up on a Killer," *Newsweek,* June 12, 1989, Pg. 59.

tase inhibitor (NRTI) that a United States cancer researcher, Jerome Horwitz, had synthesized in 1964 as an anti-cancer drug. While it had not worked against cancer, David Barry and his team at Burroughs Wellcome (and Duke University) had been able in the mid-1980s to show that it was active against HIV.[106] Consequently, the FDA had approved the drug to much fanfare.

Such a development seemed surely a potential breakthrough in the battle against AIDS. However, as Mann and his GPA team turned their attention to the drug, they recognized that it came with considerable trade-offs that made it impractical to supply across the globe. For one thing, the drug was cost-prohibitive. Moreover, some believed the drug to be relatively toxic at its prescribed dosage. Also, researchers had not been able to follow patients taking the drug long enough to ascertain the duration of its efficacy. Still, the drug held considerable promise, and Mann and his team expected that countries would demand global distribution. Mann recognized the challenge this posed to many health systems, which often did not have the infrastructure to provide long-term treatment. "The assumption in the United States is that those on AZT will remain on it until they die or until something else comes along that is shown to be more effective," Mann explained to reporters in late June 1988. "You have to be in a system that can assure lifetime commitments." "Political instability, poverty, and the frailty of medical institutions make that unrealistic in many countries," noted *New York Times* reporter Lawrence K Altman.[107] With the possibility of chronic AIDS care on the horizon for many affected countries, Mann and other practitioners began exploring the role WHO would play in helping resource-poor nations bolster their health infrastructure.

Consequently, Mann began talking to faculty at the Harvard School of Public Health about the burden WHO would have "organizing AIDS treatment and prevention for these countries."[108] As 1988 wound on, Mann paid increasing attention to the inequities that existed in health systems and across societies. He began talking about a system that could ensure "equitable global distribution of future treatment drugs and vaccines" across the globe.[109] He never articulated how such a system would work or how GPA could induce pharmaceutical companies to participate in such a system, but the idea itself and the principles that inspired it—rather than its feasibility or the logistics involved—were what grabbed Mann's attention. Here again, Mann was not operating in a vacuum. Many of these questions were prompted by HIV-positive gay men and their allies in the United States and elsewhere. HIV-activist groups, like the Lavender Hill Gang and ACT UP, were beginning to ask hard questions about the structure of health care delivery in the United States as it related to access to care and distributive justice among sexual, gender, and racial

---

[106] Stephen Inrig, "In a place so ordinary: North Carolina and the problem of AIDS, 1981—1997," by Duke University, 2007, 474 pages; 3321835.

[107] Lawrence K Altman, "Poor Nations Plagued With AIDS Pose Haunting Ethical Questions," *The New York Times,* June 28, 1988, C3.

[108] Ibid.

[109] Elizabeth Fee and Manon Parry, "Jonathan Mann, HIV/AIDS, and Human Rights," *Journal of Public Health Policy,* 29(1):62–63.

minorities (it would be a number of years before AIDS activists in low- and middle-income countries took up the issue with fervor).[110]

This new focus on the structure of health systems and the problem of access pushed Mann and GPA further along the continuum of health and human rights. We should note that it was not uncommon for WHO staff to focus on the economic disparities between and within health systems. In 1988, for example, WHO's new Director-General, Hiroshi Nakajima—who would come to play an important role in the story of global AIDS—noted that the gap in access to medical and preventive services between high-income countries and low- and middle- income countries had widened since the 1970s. Nakajima argued that debt-ridden developing countries could not afford these services, and that even those committed to making sound health policies found themselves unable to implement them owing to a lack of resources. AIDS was one example Nakajima gave: "The spread of knowledge on AIDS depended on increasing literacy among women in developing countries," he had told reporters shortly after he took office in October 1988, "[but] the number of illiterate women in the third world ha[d] increased in the previous years."[111] What differed in Mann's approach was that he came to see such inequitable distribution within and between countries as violations of justice and human rights.

How did he propose to tackle the problem? Initially, he thought the best approach would be through activism: as noted above, he advocated establishing a global net-work to monitor human rights abuses of people with AIDS. To this end, among others, in 1988 he set up "a human rights office within GPA … specifically empha-sizing nondiscrimination and equitable access to health care."[112] Mann hired Katarina Tomaševski to head the office. Tomaševski was a Yugoslavian professor of international law and political science who had worked for the Danish Centre for Human Rights, the Research and Information Centre on Censorship in London, and the Netherlands Institute of Human Rights. She had experience on an array of human rights projects ranging from the right to food, freedom of information, and a "policy-framework for integrating human rights into development policies, pro-grammes, and projects."[113] (Tomaševski would go on to serve as the first United Nations Special Rapporteur on the Right to Education of the United Nations Commission on Human Rights from 1998 to 2004).

In her position, Tomaševski began "initiating, commissioning and supervising research and coordinating policy development concerning legal, ethical and human rights aspects of HIV/AIDS prevention and control."[114] Over a period of several

[110] Susan Chambre, *Fighting for Our Lives: New York's AIDS Community and the Politics of Disease* (New Brunswick, NJ: Rutgers University Press, 2006).

[111] "WHO Chief Urges More Aid For Hygiene in 3rd World," *Japan Economic Newswire,* October 25, 1989.

[112] Elizabeth Fee and Manon Parry, "Jonathan Mann, HIV/AIDS, and Human Rights," *Journal of Public Health Policy,* 29(1):61.

[113] Katarina Tomaševski, "Curriculum Vitae"; Sophia Gruskin, Interview by Stephen Inrig, July 28, 2010.

[114] Katarina Tomaševski, "Curriculum Vitae."

months, working with a young law student named Sophia Gruskin and the NGO liaison Jeff O'Malley, Tomaševski briefed and trained GPA staff and consultants about the integration of human rights into national AIDS programs, organized global and regional meetings on AIDS and human rights, and collaborated with the relevant UN bodies and NGOs on the intersection of AIDS and human rights.[115]

It is probably fair to say that Tomaševski helped Mann evolve further in his understanding of human rights. Whereas he initially viewed human rights primarily through the lens of AIDS, Tomaševski helped him to view AIDS—and other health issues—through the lens of human rights. As Joe Cohen, Mahler's senior policy adviser remembered, Mann began pushing this conceptualization further than anyone at WHO had done before: "by focusing on the rights of people who otherwise would be an easy prey for AIDS. This was this peculiar combination of the specificity which has an effect on the generality. Using AIDS as an example of the importance of protecting human rights."[116] For example, Mann differed from Nakajima on female illiteracy. Nakajima would support finding creative ways of "providing basic [AIDS] knowledge to women and mothers unable to read," while Mann would ask what prevented women from being able to learn to read in the first place.[117]

Of all the issues Mann sought to address, AIDS and the rights of women appears to have been the concern that formally pushed him to his pioneering view on health and human rights. This new understanding was the outgrowth of Mann's recognition of two overlapping issues: that socioeconomic context played a role in the status of peoples' health, and that women generally occupied a disproportionately vulnerable position with regard to their social and economic status in most societies. Mahler had clearly articulated a position on the first issue: "In WHO," Mahler had told the UN General Assembly in 1987, "we never forget that the broad social impacts are as much a part of the pathology of AIDS as the virus itself."[118] Those concerned about the broader issue of women's health at WHO had unambiguously communicated a position on the second issue: "The report of [the Conference on Safe Motherhood, in Nairobi in March 1987], cited evidence of broad discrimination against women and girls," Mann recalled in 1989, "[they] have higher death rates, higher likelihood of being malnourished, and less access to education than boys."[119]

Finding that the human rights perspective was acutely embodied in the issue of women's health, Mann began in 1989 to work closely with Angele Petros-Barvazian Director of WHO's Family Health Division and the focal point for WHO'S

---

[115] Katarina Tomaševski, "Curriculum Vitae"; Sophia Gruskin, Interview by Stephen Inrig, July 28, 2010.

[116] Joshua Cohen, Interviewed by Michael Merson, New Haven, CT, August, 2002.

[117] Gene Kramer, "WHO Chief: Sex Discrimination, Youth Alienation Threaten World Health," *The Associated Press,* December 16, 1988.

[118] Halfdan Mahler, "Statement by Dr. H. Mahler, Director-General at an Informal Briefing on AIDS to the 42nd Session of the United Nations General Assembly on Tuesday 20th October 1987," Geneva: World Health Organization, WHO/SPA/ZNF/87.13, p. 2.

[119] Jonathan Mann, "Women, Children, and the Global AIDS Strategy," Geneva: World Health Organization, November 27, 1989, 1.

Programme on Women, Health and Development. An Iranian woman, Petros-Barvazian and others had worked hard over the years to promote the advancement of women and raise their overall health and social status. At WHO and the UN, this had manifested itself in a host of conferences and consultations on the position of women, including the United Nations Conference on the Advancement of Women (Mexico, 1975), the Primary Health Care Conference (Alma-Ata, 1978), the End of Decade United Nations Conference (Nairobi, 1985), the Safe Motherhood Conference (Nairobi, 1987), and the Conference on Better Health for Women and Children through Family Planning (Nairobi, 1987).[120]

Several outcomes grew out of this new emphasis on AIDS and the rights of women. First, Mann and his team started calling attention to the growing burden that AIDS was placing on women throughout the world, as well as the disproportionate obligations of care, treatment, and social support that women shouldered in the wake of the pandemic's devastation. In light of the heavy burden of AIDS on women, GPA (particularly Gunilla Ernberg, a lawyer from Sweden who had joined GPA in 1988 and served as one of Mann's regional program officers) began pushing "to involve women at all levels within [national AIDS programs] and to strengthen and support the role of Women's NGOs in AIDS."[121] While these ideas were in their incipient form, towards the end of 1989, Mann came to recognize that, up until that time, GPA had given insufficient attention to women in HIV prevention. AIDS campaigns, Ernberg noted, had targeted "barmaids, pregnant women, and prostitutes," but had been inadequately focused on women in general. This meant that GPA lacked materials specifically targeted towards women's organizations, and its condom education material did an insufficient job helping equip women to negotiate condom use with reluctant or resistant partners.[122]

This change in perspective helped Mann specifically, and GPA more generally, better understand sexual behavior and risk within the context of broader social factors. Factors like "labor migration, the separation of household members, and gender/patriarchal relations, particularly women's economic dependence on men and the cultural imperative to have children."[123] The move beyond the public health rationale was palpable. As Susan Timberlake, the lawyer whom I would later hire to run GPA's health and human rights efforts, explained, "Basically what we were saying was, 'women shouldn't get raped because they'll catch HIV' … We were trying to get people to care about women and rape and HIV by putting the three together." It became clear, however, that this public health rationale risked glossing over the most important point: that women should not be raped. "The fundamental human

---

[120] Global Programme on AIDS, "Report on the Consultation with International Women's NGO's on AIDS Prevention and Care; Geneva, 21–22 December 1989," Geneva: World Health Organization, GPA/DIR/91.3, 1, 3–6, 8.

[121] Ibid.

[122] Ibid.

[123] Colleen O'Manique, "Global Neoliberalism and AIDS Policy: International Responses to Sub-Saharan Africa's Pandemic," *Studies in Political Economy,* Spring/Summer 2004, 73: 61–62.

rights issue," Timberlake explained, "... was the treatment of women."[124] It was this perspective that Mann ultimately understood in the fall of 1989 and began to champion.

To this end, in November, 1989, GPA and the government of France organized a conference on the Implications of AIDS for Women and Children, with cosponsorship of the United Nations Children's Emergency Fund (UNICEF), United Nations Educational, Scientific and Cultural Organization (UNESCO), United Nations Development Programme (UNDP), International Labour Organization (ILO), World Bank, and the Council of Europe.[125] "It is highly symbolic," Mann said as he opened the conference, "that this International Conference on the implications of AIDS for mothers and children is the last major international AIDS meeting of this decade." The fact that it was the last meeting of the decade reflected the "relatively lower priority which AIDS in mothers and children has thus far received," Mann acknowledged.[126]

The conference reflects well the next stage in Mann's evolution on health and human rights. The next month GPA hosted a consultation with international women's NGO's on AIDS prevention and care. The discussions at the consultation exhibited Mann and GPA's new perspective, centering not only on educating women about AIDS, but about providing them with basic literacy and nutrition. Thereafter, GPA started exploring interventions that addressed the economic autonomy of women and income-generation to confront both the economic impact of AIDS as well as the economic vulnerability that exposed women to AIDS at higher rates in the first place.[127] Many of these projects would not emerge until the early 1990s, but Mann and GPA began designing them towards the end of 1989. As a next step, however, on February 13, Mann and his team announced that the theme of World AIDS Day for 1990 would be Women and AIDS.[128]

We believe concerns about the rights of women crystallized for Mann and others in GPA leadership an "expanded" view of human rights, one that looked not at AIDS specifically, but at health more generally. "[If one] is not blinded by the term 'human rights' and looks into how you can transform your action inspired by the human rights principles ...," Daniel Tarantola explained, "[then] rather than my deciding who is going to attend [sexually transmitted disease (STD)[129]] clinics, let us look at who gets higher rates of STDs and why it is that they don't get the appropriate treatment." The role of women in the AIDS pandemic led Mann to begin

---

[124] Susan Timberlake, Interview by Michael Merson, New Haven, CT, August, 2002.

[125] Jonathan Mann, "Women, Children, and the Global AIDS Strategy," Geneva: World Health Organization, November 27, 1989, 1.

[126] Ibid.

[127] Colleen O'Manique, "Global Neoliberalism and AIDS Policy: International Responses to Sub-Saharan Africa's Pandemic," *Studies in Political Economy,* Spring/Summer 2004, *73:* 61–62.

[128] "1990 world AIDS day to focus on aids in women," *Xinhua General News Service,* February 14, 1990, Item No: 0214218.

[129] For the purposes of this text, we use the term sexually transmitted disease(s) and the abbreviation STD rather than the other term sexually transmitted infection(s) or STIs.

asking larger questions within the world of public health. Tarantola explained, questions like "'is there any group that is subjected to more discrimination than others?' ... In the French context ... people from the Magreb—they don't have more sex than the others, but they are discriminated against in France and therefore have less access to diagnostics and treatment. ... then you say, 'We need to do something about those people from the Magreb. We need to create clinics where they will be comfortable culturally, feel equal and well served'. ... That's basically what we call a human rights approach."[130] The vulnerability of women allowed Mann to concretize this perspective, and grappling with these issues in 1988 and 1989, transformed his perspective. Consequently, he entered the 1990s intending strongly to advocate for this more expanded view. He would be unable to operationalize these visions at GPA, however, because his time there was about to come to an abrupt and surprising halt.

---

[130] Daniel Tarantola, Interview by Michael Merson, New Haven, CT, October, 2001.

Chapter 7
The Resignation of Jonathan Mann

On Friday morning, March 16, 1990, Jonathan Mann delivered a letter announcing his resignation to the office of World Health Organization (WHO) Director-General Hiroshi Nakajima. Fed up with the way he felt Nakajima was impeding the global AIDS[1] effort, Mann declared that he could no longer serve as the head of WHO's Global Programme on AIDS (GPA). By noon, Mann had told his key staff about his decision, and then sat down to pound out a memo to the entire GPA staff and send news of his resignation to donors and reporters.[2] "On the basis of my experience during the last 2 years," Mann explained in his letter to Nakajima, "I have now come to the conclusion that there is a great variance between our positions on a series of issues which I consider critical for the Global AIDS Strategy and the WHO GPA. Under these circumstances, I have decided to resign as Director of the Global Programme on AIDS, effective as of the end of my current contract, in June 1990."[3]

The news would come as a shock to many inside and outside the field of AIDS; to many, Mann stood atop the world of public health. It was not a secret that the relationship between Mann and Nakajima had deteriorated quickly. This decision of Mann's was not an impulsive act, however: best we can tell, Mann appeared to have been considering the move for some time, and his decision was a product of a number of factors, the conflict with Nakajima being the most frustrating and pre-cipitating one. Whatever the reasons, Mann's move would leave GPA in a state of great uncertainty and disarray. His departure also revealed that, along with the

---

Within this chapter the singular pronouns *I* and *my* refer to Michael Merson alone, whereas the plural pronouns *we* and *us* generally refer to Michael Merson and Stephen Inrig jointly. Where *we* or *us* refers to Michael Merson and his colleagues at WHO, the object of the pronoun is clarified by context.

[1] For the purposes of this text, we will use the term AIDS to encompass both AIDS and HIV unless otherwise specified.

[2] Daniel Tarantola, Interview by Michael Merson, New Haven, CT, October, 2001; Jonathan Mann, "Letter to Jeff Harris, March 16, 1990." Manuel Carballo, Interview by Michael Merson, New Haven, CT, November, 2002.

[3] Jonathan Mann, "Letter to Dr. Hiroshi Nakajima, March 16, 1990".

© Springer International Publishing AG 2018
M. Merson, S. Inrig, *The AIDS Pandemic*, DOI 10.1007/978-3-319-47133-4_7

acclaim he had rightly received for his efforts against AIDS, his program and his leadership were not without its critics both within and outside WHO.

We believe that the path towards Mann's resignation actually began on the evening of January 29, 1988, when WHO's Executive Board nominated Japan's Hiroshi Nakajima to serve as the next Director-General. The election was very close, and it took four rounds of voting before Nakajima was able to secure the necessary majority of votes. Indeed, Nakajima had trailed Carlyle Guerra de Macedo from Brazil, the Regional Director of the Pan American Health Organization [PAHO] (and outgoing Director-General Halfdan Mahler's choice for successor), in the first three rounds of voting. In the end, Japanese staff member Yuji Kawaguchi, Director of Planning, Coordination, and Cooperation in WHO headquarters, masterminded a brilliant strategy that increased Nakajima's vote total each round and eventually secured his election (see Chapter 10). The news greatly pleased the Japanese government, who had worked hard to support Nakajima's candidacy as it very much desired to have one of its nationals become, for the first time, an elected director of an agency in the United Nations (UN) system. But while the news pleased Japan and many of Nakajima's supporters, it would create considerable disruption inside and outside WHO, and eventually spell the end of Mann's time at GPA.

Having received his medical degree from Tokyo Medical University, Nakajima joined WHO in 1974 as a scientist in its Drug Evaluation and Monitoring program. In 1976, he became Chief of WHO's Drug Policies and Management Unit, and 2 years later he became Regional Director of WHO's regional office for the Western Pacific (WPRO). It was from that position that Nakajima successfully ran and received the nomination for Director-General in 1988. While it was not certain at the time of his election, most observers felt that Nakajima represented "the traditional medical model of health" that some criticized WHO for embodying. As Fiona Godlee, who eventually became Editor in Chief of the British Medical Journal explained, WHO had failed to embrace institutionally the concept of "health as a broad social issue," despite the expansive multisectorial vision exemplified in Mahler's Health for All by the Year 2000 vision. Nakajima seemed to favor filling most of WHO's professional posts with physicians, rather than other health professionals and technical experts. He was also deeply committed to WHO's established regional structure, which meant he not only felt comfortable housing most of WHO's supported endeavors in national health ministries, but he looked askance at efforts to operate outside WHO's traditional infrastructure and seemed largely uninterested in inter-UN agency collaboration.[4] All these ways of working contrasted markedly with Mann's modus operandi for GPA.

This misalignment between Nakajima and Mann might not have caused serious problems, had it not been for the fact that Nakajima held a markedly different appreciation of and approach to AIDS than Mann. As something of an "old school" public health professional, Nakajima felt that the best approach to AIDS was the one he claimed to have practiced successfully in WPRO: the sexually transmitted

---

[4] Fiona Godlee, "WHO in retreat: is it losing its influence?" *BMJ* 3 December 1994;309:1491–1495.

disease (STD)[5] approach. As Nakajima told us in an interview at his farm in France, "When the HIV/AIDS issue started, my approach, WPRO's approach, was STDs... [For example] the Singapore government, which was a strong government, immediately asked [WPRO] for supplies, equipment, and experts. All sex workers were registered in Singapore, with weekly checking and so on."[6] Nakajima felt this model to be the most appropriate to address AIDS, and he disagreed with Mann's approach, which he thought framed AIDS as "more of a behavioral problem, a cultural problem." Nakajima's attachment to what many called "the biomedical model" clearly clashed with Mann's more social and economic "human rights" approach, which Mann was just starting to develop around the time that Nakajima ascended to the position of Director-General.[7]

An example of the differences between Nakajima's and Mann's way of thinking could be seen in their approach to human rights. Nakajima felt Mann's stress on human rights lacked rigor. "Human rights is important," Nakajima admitted, "but in my observation ... nobody understands human rights. We understand gays' rights, women's rights (that women should not be infected by HIV by force), child rights (without knowing that they had been infected by their mothers), but what is human rights itself? ... The human rights charter from the UN is not clear – it's vague."[8] Even though Nakajima recognized a legitimate place for human rights in the fight against AIDS, he felt Mann's application of those ideas was both culturally insensitive and strategically narrow. Mann imposed a very "Western" concept of human rights on participating nations, Nakajima felt: "behavior change, condoms, and mass movement was Jon's approach, with a quilt and human rights!" Moreover, as Marjory Dam (WHO's Washington, DC-based External Relations Officer who had served since 1987 as the liaison between WHO and the United States government) explained to us, Nakajima felt "[Mann] was too fixated on ... this French idea about human rights, and that ... there was more to the epidemic than that."[9] For Nakajima, a more appropriate AIDS strategy would focus on "medical, biomedical, [and] scientific research."[10] "I discussed with Jon very much ...the issue of biomedical research," Nakajima explained to me. He and Mann discussed topics like "vaccines, drugs, other means like vaginal tablets," Nakajima explained, but Mann did little to pursue research on these, he felt.

Moreover, Nakajima believed Mahler, Mann, and Daniel Tarantola relied too heavily on the smallpox eradication model as a paradigm for the AIDS program, when to his mind AIDS was far more difficult to diagnose and prevent than smallpox.

---

[5] For the purposes of this text, we use the term sexually transmitted disease(s) and the abbreviation STD rather than the other term sexually transmitted infection(s) or STIs.

[6] Hiroshi Nakajima, Interview by Michael Merson, Poitiers, October 13, 2002.

[7] "World News Tonight—ABC," *ABC News Transcripts,* June 9, 1989; Michelle Lalonde and Andre Picard, "AIDS Montreal Conference: Minute of silence to honor dead gives rare unity to conference," *The Globe and Mail,* June 10, 1989.

[8] Hiroshi Nakajima, Interview by Michael Merson, Poitiers, October 13, 2002.

[9] Marjory Dam, Interview by Michael Merson, New Haven, CT, September 29, 2001.

[10] Hiroshi Nakajima, Interview by Michael Merson, Poitiers, October 13, 2002.

Nakajima knew, for example, about the large chart Tarantola had hung in his office listing all the country team visits GPA staff had made. Nakajima felt this was epidemiologically suspect, because at the local level it suggested that GPA had already determined its strategy for fighting AIDS in those countries without visiting regional representatives or health ministers or determining the specific features of the epidemic in a given country or region. Nakajima was deeply skeptical about Tarantola's approach.

Mann first got a glimpse of this difference in perspectives in the winter of 1988, not long after Nakajima had taken up his new position. That winter, Nakajima gave an interview with the French newspaper *Le Monde* wherein he expressed some discomfort with the nondiscrimination resolution that Mann had secured from the World Health Assembly (WHA) earlier that year. Mann was shocked when he read a prepublication version of the interview. According to Kathleen Kay, Mann threatened to resign from GPA unless Nakajima allowed him to "fix" the interview to better reflect WHO's stance on nondiscrimination.[11] Nakajima relented and Mann rewrote the piece, but the episode proved informative for both Mann and Nakajima. For Nakajima, it must clearly have sent the signal that Mann had little concern about hierarchy and was willing to confront an organizational superior who differed with him on a policy issue. For Mann, it plainly raised profound concerns about the support he felt he could expect from the new Director-General on GPA's approach to AIDS and human rights, as well as the extent to which Nakajima would be willing to contradict, publicly, the expressed position of his own organization and the WHA.

Beyond these professional or strategic qualms, both men seem not to have liked each other on a personal level. Some of this sprang from personal and cultural differences: Nakajima—as a senior Japanese man—felt Mann, a younger American, was flippant and showed inadequate respect towards authority.[12] Nakajima also seems to have felt that Mann was an attention seeker, and inappropriately so: If Mann had focused on "research and so on, his face was not in the newspaper," Nakajima explained to me, "but if he talked ... of these extremely controversial issues, his name was everywhere."[13] We think it is fair to speculate that Nakajima perceived that Mann's publicity-seeking behavior came at the expense of the attention that Nakajima felt he deserved as head of WHO. Much of this may have had little to do with Mann directly, of course: Nakajima was succeeding a very popular Director-General, Halfdan Mahler, a director whom few had wanted to step down from his post. Struggling as he may have been to define his own leadership in the shadow of Mahler's illustrious reputation, Nakajima must have viewed Mann—and perhaps any other similarly gifted individual—as a threat or distraction to his own public perception.

Mann, for his part, seems likewise to have had a strong personal dislike for Nakajima. Part of this must have stemmed from Mann's previous relationship with Mahler: Mann had been very close to Mahler, and (especially) his senior policy advisor Joe Cohen, and Nakajima's different personality, approach, and values

---

[11] Kathleen Kay, Interview by Michael Merson, New Haven, CT, 2002.

[12] Claire Chollat-Troquet, Interview by Michael Merson, New Haven, CT, August 12, 2002.

[13] Manuel Carballo, Interview by Michael Merson, New Haven, CT, November, 2002.

could not overcome that.[14] As Tarantola told us "…when Mahler left we cried, and when Jonathan left we cried."[15] Beyond this, however, Mann appears to have had a visceral and personal aversion to Nakajima.[16] As Bob Black (who served on GPA's External Review Committee and was Chair of the Department of International Health at the Bloomberg School of Public Health for 30 years) explained, Mann—like some others at WHO—"didn't respect Nakajima at all … [and] he just couldn't tolerate Nakajima telling him what to do, even over trivial things."[17] At one point during Mann's tenure, Dam remembers suggesting to Mann that he seek Nakajima's advice on something as a means of showing deference. Dam had learned personally, in working with Nakajima, that showing small amounts of deference to his positional authority went a long way to ensuring a healthy working relationship, "And Jonathan said 'I can't do that,…because I don't want to hear anything he has to say; I don't want or need any advice from him," Dam recalled.[18]

Perhaps the reality of Nakajima's relationship with Mann was that Mann represented a dramatic inversion of Nakajima's own strengths and weaknesses. Nakajima valued biomedical research because he was a highly knowledgeable biomedical technician, whereas Mann considered such research far less of a priority for GPA. Mann was an extraordinary communicator, a gifted and passionate writer, and an exceptional diplomat who exhibited unrivaled ease and charm, whereas Nakajima was at best a flawed communicator in English, French, or even his native Japanese. Truth be told, neither men have been praised as exceptional managers or administrators in the traditional sense, though Nakajima clearly excelled as a shrewd politician while Mann possessed the unique ability to captivate a team or audience with his vision of the world. It is easy, therefore, to understand why Nakajima found himself uncomfortably outshone by a younger and more dynamic individual.

The friction between Mann and Nakajima came at a particularly inopportune time for Mann, owing to a series of external pressures bearing down on GPA all at once. By the spring of 1989, research by GPA staffer Victor Agbessi indicated that the health infrastructure in many African nations would be insufficient to cope with the epidemiological burden of AIDS.[19] For Mann and his GPA team, it became depressingly clear that nations could expect a "massive rise in AIDS cases" if the world failed to respond very soon with a "solid, sustained, and coordinated" effort.[20] The numbers in May of that year suggested HIV infection was far more prevalent

[14] Ralph Henderson, Interview by Michael Merson, NH, February, 2003.

[15] Daniel Tarantola, Interview by Michael Merson, New Haven, CT, October, 2001.

[16] Larry Gostin, Interview by Michael Merson, New Haven, CT, September, 2002; Manuel Carballo, Interview by Michael Merson, New Haven, CT, November, 2002; Bob Black, Interview by Michael Merson, New Haven, CT, August, 2002.

[17] Bob Black, Interview by Michael Merson, New Haven, CT, August, 2002.

[18] Marjory Dam, Interview by Michael Merson, New Haven, CT, September 29, 2001.

[19] "Africa: insufficient funds to fight AIDS," The Xinhua General Overseas News Service, May 16, 1989, Item No: 0516077.

[20] "AIDS cases on the rise," The Xinhua General Overseas News Service, May 18, 1989, Item No: 0518042.

than originally thought and that the trajectory of the pandemic was worsening.[21] Rather than plateauing as many observers had hoped, the pandemic remained very dynamic (as Mann revealed in his May 1989 report to the WHA), continuing to worsen in places it already existed even as it spread into new regions.[22] As a worst case scenario, Mann warned, between 45 and 90 million people might acquire the virus by the year 2000.[23] But, by November, Mann and his team found themselves already revising these frightening estimates upward. They suspected that the number of infections in South Asia and Eastern Europe were going to increase markedly, even as new surveillance sites in sub-Saharan Africa suggested that Africa could still expect explosive growth, particularly in the Southern part of the continent.[24]

The problem was—for Mann, for GPA, and for people affected by AIDS—these numbers had failed to translate yet into sufficient and sustained global action. "A backlash of complacency … [was] threatening the success of international campaigns to prevent the spread of AIDS," Mann explained at the 2nd International Conference on Health, Law, and Ethics in London in the summer of 1989.[25] Part of Mann's case for this complacency came from the problem of "media fatigue" that researchers had chronicled: "The number of newspaper articles on AIDS had gone up eleven-fold between 1984 and 1987," Mann explained, "but had since dropped by 50%."[26] Equally frustrating for Mann was the fact that, at the Group of Seven (G7) Summit in Paris the week before, AIDS did not garner as much attention as rainforest depletion.[27] "It may be a lot easier to talk about rainforests in someone else's country than sexual relations and drugs in your own country," Mann complained.[28] Mann was particularly worried about Western nations like the United States or the United Kingdom, which seemed to be refocusing their AIDS resources inwards, with far less priority given to global AIDS.[29] "Dangerous complacency about AIDS

---

[21] "New Warning on AIDS Spreading Through the 1990's," *The Associated Press,* May 19, 1989; "A Tenfold Rise In AIDS Is Seen," *The New York Times,* May 19, 1989, D16; Daniel Q. Haney, "Health Official Predicts Nine Times More AIDS Infections In 1990s," *The Associated Press,* June 4, 1989.

[22] Daniel Q. Haney, "Health Official Predicts Nine Times More AIDS Infections In 1990s," *The Associated Press,* June 4, 1989.

[23] "Weekend News Sunday Late," *ABC News Transcripts,* June 4, 1989.

[24] Rebecca Kolberg, "AIDS battle threatened by complacency," *United Press International,* November 2, 1989; "India records maximum AIDS cases in southeast Asia," *Xinhua General News Service,* September 28, 1989, Item No: 0928152; Thomson Prentice, "Experts predict six million Aids victims by 2000; Africa," *The London Times,* October 19 1989, Issue 63529; Rebecca Kolberg, "AIDS battle threatened by complacency," *United Press International,* November 2, 1989; "AIDS Spreading Rapidly Among Drug Users In Europe, WHO Says," *The Associated Press,* February 3, 1990.

[25] Aileen Ballantyne, "AIDS drive 'beset by complacency': 'Media fatigue' and prejudice attacked at conference," *The London Guardian,* July 18, 1989.

[26] Ibid.

[27] Thomson Prentice, "AIDS chief claims casualties will soon reach one million; Health Law and Ethics conference," *The London Times,* July 18 1989, Issue 63449.

[28] Ibid.

[29] Thomson Prentice, "Fear over cuts in Aids campaigns," *The London Times,* November 25 1989,

is spreading," Mann warned then United States President H.W. Bush's AIDS Council in November 1989. "If indifference or denial lead to relaxation of current efforts or to a decrease in future commitment to AIDS, we will falter and fall further and further behind the pace of the worldwide epidemic," Mann concluded.[30]

However, Mann and his team could take some solace in the fact they were making some headway against the virus. Clinical trials of the drug azidothymidine (AZT) suggested some promise for helping asymptomatic people with HIV (we would only learn later how short-lived were the effects of this monotherapy), while evidence was mounting that condoms, clean needles, and behavioral interventions could slow viral transmission. Moreover, dozens of countries and countless non-governmental organizations (NGOs) by the end of the 1980s were taking up the fight against AIDS. Nevertheless, despite these promising signs, GPA observers recognized that the pandemic was outstripping these modest gains, particularly in resource-poor countries.

On top of these frustrating trends, or perhaps because of them, Mann started sensing a very real measure of donor dissatisfaction. Donor countries had rapidly poured considerable funds into GPA—indeed, GPA had raised in 3 years more funds than any WHO program in the agency's history—but the data compelled Mann to admit that the pandemic was still speeding up, rather than slowing down. This meant Mann needed to raise an ever larger pot of money to respond to the growing pandemic. For donor countries, however, this posed a problem, because despite these increasing budgetary requests (for the 1990 budget Mann "presented … an ambitious plan"), Mann had been unable to spend all the money he already had.

These issues came to a head during the 1989 year-end GPA Management Committee (GMC) meeting, when "many donors expressed concern about the large growth proposed," and asked "whether such an increase was realistic."[31] Moreover, the GMC wondered what activities Mann would be willing to cut if he proved unable to raise funds to meet the proposed budget. "Mann states that all elements of the budget were priorities," the meeting notes read. "He did not indicate where he would cut if this became necessary."[32] With the crushing reality of the expanding pandemic weighing on him, Mann must not have felt he could suggest that any parts of his program were expendable.

At some point in the GMC meeting, the donors expressed concern about the budgeting process and the methodology by which GPA was establishing its priorities each year, given the fluid nature of the pandemic. As they reviewed the budget,

Issue 63561.

[30] Rebecca Kolberg, "AIDS battle threatened by complacency," *United Press International,* November 2, 1989; Kenneth B. Noble, "Better Reporting Seen in Zaire's AIDS Case Count," *The New York Times,* December 22, 1989, A9.

[31] US Mission Geneva, "Meeting of Global Management Committee of the WHO Global Programme on AIDS," US Department of State, December 1989, p. 1.

[32] Ibid.

several items remained unclear to them, and so the GMC asked for clarification and requested a full review of the budget at its next meeting in April 1990.[33] Joe Decosas (see Chapter 5) feels that, at this point, Mann was caught in something of a catch-22 "… the people round the table were bureaucrats who were basically evaluating on their ability to spend their money [and] they had an agency in front of them which was only spending 60% of its budget. … Then afterwards, GPA rapidly cranked up its mechanisms to program money and people started to look and say, what are you spending it on?"[34] At the same time, Decosas recalled, Mann was "under pressure from the regional offices [who under Mahler had been] bypassed and suddenly under Nakajima had their power back and were retaliating. So Mann was squeezed between a bureaucratic apparatus that he could no longer manipulate and move and a group of donors who were becoming increasingly more hostile."[35] Perhaps, in an effort to gain control of what was becoming an increasingly intrusive oversight process—and highly cognizant of GPA's reputation and prominence— Mann raised the prospect of undertaking an external review of GPA at its 5-year mark (1992), and offered to provide a "draft scope of work … for discussion at the next GMC meeting."[36]

The donors, the meeting report suggests, had moved out of whatever honeymoon phase may have existed between themselves and GPA and were now much more vested in the budgeting process and outcomes of the program. This was not surprising, since most of them had given their initial contributions to GPA at a time when there was great concern about the rapid growth of the pandemic and GPA presented them the only viable and substantive response. By 1989, however, a number of donors had launched their own substantial bilateral assistance AIDS programs. As a consequence, many of them were now fielding requests for financial support from domestic organizations (particularly NGOs) who were undertaking activities in AIDS-affected countries. The donors therefore were increasingly scrutinizing their donations to GPA. This was partly because they had to rationalize giving contributions to GPA rather than to domestically-based organizations who might be more politically important to the government and capable of achieving similar outcomes. In addition, some donors were concerned about reports they had been receiving about the underperformance of some WHO regional and country offices, particularly those in the African region. If those reports were true, as many suspected, reapportioning their donations to bilateral programs made a lot more sense.

In light of this budget scrutiny and uncertainty, Mann must have been disappointed when, at the end of 1989, a few donor nations indicated they would not increase their budgetary contributions for fiscal year 1991. The Nordic countries and Canada indicated that they intended to keep their donations static, while the United States announced that it planned on trimming its GPA funding. In an effort

---

[33] Ibid.

[34] Joe Decosas, Interview by Michael Merson, New Haven, CT, October, 2001.

[35] Ibid.

[36] US Mission Geneva, "Meeting of Global Management Committee of the WHO Global Programme on AIDS," US Department of State, December 1989, p. 1.

to soften the blow, "the US stated that the level of US funding to GPA should not be seen as a diminution of support to GPA," read the GMC minutes, "because overall AIDS funding would increase due to increased funding through USAID bilateral channels."[37] The United States decision to increase funding to its bilateral programs gave little solace to Mann and his team, however, who still had an expanding pandemic on their hands and less funds than they needed.

The expanding pandemic and increased scrutiny and diminished support from donors came at the same time that Mann had been experiencing tightening oversight from Nakajima. For example, soon after he became Director-General in 1988, Nakajima instituted an internal management review of GPA. Ostensibly, Nakajima established the review to assess GPA's management performance at headquarters, regional level, and country level. Mann and his team, however, suspected that Nakajima's review was mere posturing to change the management structure of GPA. It was, we believe, another reason, a defensive or strategic counter-move, that Mann proposed that the GMC launch an external review. Our hunch is that he likely believed the external review could serve as a counterweight to Nakajima's presumably negative evaluation. The problem was—as Mann quickly discovered when the GMC budget discussion turned into a GMC budget review—that there was no guarantee he could maintain control over the process or its outcomes.

Mann therefore came to the end of 1989 with a measure of discouragement. "The world has come to a major fork in the public-policy road as it confronts the challenges posed by the disease AIDS," Mann told reporters in an interview towards the end of 1989. Depending on which route the world took, Mann explained, it was "in danger of losing the war against AIDS."[38] The world had made significant progress, Mann explained, and the world could continue down that path, but doing so "require[d] a long-term commitment to combating the disease ... a reversal of what he s[aw] as the smug contentment of some Western nations, ... [and] a recognition by the more-affluent nations, including the US, that they must increase the amount of money they are providing for the worldwide effort." The other path was easier, requiring no commitment, no increase of funds, and no demand for engagement. But taking it would "undo the past decade's progress in fighting AIDS."[39] It was by no means clear that leaders and nations would take that first path, however.

Within this context, the tension between Mann and Nakajima likely became toxic. At a fundamental level, Mann and Nakajima were clashing over matters of bureaucracy. In crafting so much of his program with little regard for the larger WHO infrastructure, Mann had used up whatever social capital he might have had with Nakajima. As a former Regional Director, Nakajima had felt snubbed by Mann and GPA's disregard for WHO's regional offices. For example, the regional offices

---

[37] Ibid.

[38] "World faces defeat in AIDS war warns expert," *Hobart Mercury,* November 3, 1989.

[39] Robert P. Hey, "Mann: AIDS Battle Needs US Commitment," *Christian Science Monitor,* November 9, 1989, p. 7.

frequently wanted to share in the largesse of GPA to help governments establish
AIDS testing facilities, but Mann had downplayed the importance of testing and
kept the funds largely out of the regional infrastructure. Indeed, Nakajima and
regional leaders frequently found themselves excluded from GPA activities in their
regions: "[GPA people] running around the region was OK," Nakajima later told us,
thinking back on his time as a Regional Director, "but I was the chief of WHO for
the region, and headquarters should at least have informed me that GPA people were
coming to the region." Recall that Nakajima had taken this omission as personal
disrespect, a fact best exemplified by his actions at the 1988 London Health
Ministers' meeting. At the meeting, Mann had not shown Nakajima the appropriate
level of respect Nakajima felt was his due, given his recent elevation to Director-
General-elect; nor had Mann invited him to speak at the meeting.[40]

These were more than personal and professional slights for Nakajima, but rather
were, in his view, symptoms of a dysfunctional approach to AIDS within WHO.
Nakajima felt that Mann had purposefully kept GPA centralized at headquarters
both to thwart the regional structure and to aggrandize himself. He was particularly
chafed by Mann's habit of frequently traveling to countries to address issues himself
rather than delegating them to WHO regional offices.[41] "If you do not decentralize,"
Nakajima told us, "you cannot solve the problem. ... if I accepted all Mann's
requests, half of WHO money [would be] gone!"[42] Consequently, Nakajima and his
surrogate, Yuri Kawaguchi, frequently blocked or delayed Mann's requests for
travel until it was too late for Mann to attend various events.[43] Indeed, Kawaguchi—
who had (as we mentioned) masterminded Nakajima's election (and later reelection) as Director-General—would serve as the main filter on Mann's activities.
Kawaguchi reviewed all of Mann's memorandums to Nakajima before they reached
the latter's desk and he played a key role in determining the scope of Mann's administrative relationship with the Director-General. Later, when I took over as Interim
GPA Director, I was surprised to find a large stack of memorandums from Mann to
Nakajima that Kawaguchi had apparently intercepted and which presumably had
never made it off Kawaguchi's desk.

On top of denying, delaying, or ignoring travel requests, Nakajima forced Mann
to adopt several administrative concessions. For example, Nakajima required Mann
to follow WHO protocol for "the preparation, approval, and organization of meetings," which included Director-General approval.[44] Mann had not previously had to

---

[40] Hiroshi Nakajima, Interview by Michael Merson, Poitiers, October 13, 2002.

[41] Ibid.

[42] Ibid; This statement was perhaps ironic given that the GPA budget did constitute about half the
WHO budget.

[43] James Curran, Interview by Michael Merson, New Haven, CT, March 9, 2002; Manuel Carballo,
Interview by Michael Merson, New Haven, CT, November, 2002; Kathleen Kay, Interview by
Michael Merson, New Haven, CT, 2002; Daniel Tarantola, Interview by Michael Merson, New
Haven, CT, October, 2001.

[44] Jonathan Mann, "Memorandum: WHO/GPA Meetings: Planning, Approval, and Organization,"
WHO Global Programme on AIDS, May 15, 1999.

adhere to these rules under Mahler. Nakajima also requested that Mann take on a Deputy Director, something that flew in the face of Mann's hands-on management style.[45] Mann had hoped to counter these bureaucratic interventions by setting up a Global Commission on AIDS and various Steering Committees to run in conjunction with the GMC.[46] These, he hoped, would serve as a buffer between Nakajima and himself. But he could not escape the push from within WHO to decentralize and regionalize his program, despite concerns both he and some donors raised about the African regional office. In the end, Mann was also unable to evade the growing administrative control Nakajima sought to impose on him and on GPA.[47]

Nakajima's bureaucratic moves to pull GPA back under WHO's formal structure, curtailing Mann's previous autonomy, were felt by GPA leadership to be highly detrimental to the program: "To watch what we had put so much energy into being stopped," Kathleen Kay later recalled. "It was soul destroying."[48] In December 1989, the process had grown so onerous and the team so demoralized that Mann and some of his key staff strongly considered resigning. After some reflection, though, the group decided to stay on at least until the summer (Mann was seconded to WHO by CDC and his contract was set to end in June 1990).[49] By February 1990, however, Mann again began strongly considering resignation: "from about 6 weeks before he actually resigned it just was getting harder and harder," Kay explained, "...they'd let ...off for a while—then they'd do it again. There was a couple of weeks before [Mann quit] when Jonathan thought he might resign, but he didn't."[50] During the last weeks of February and the first weeks of March, therefore, rumors began to fly across WHO headquarters that Mann would resign, though Mann remained tight lipped about the situation.[51] Mann may have also been under the impression that, even if Nakajima reappointed him, it would only be for 1 year.[52]

The tipping point appears to have been when Nakajima prevented Mann from attending a meeting in late February 1990. The occasion was the first major meeting of Eastern European national AIDS program managers and experts. The recent collapse of the Iron Curtain had brought a new openness between Eastern European countries that threatened to heighten the spread of AIDS, and Mann wanted to learn

[45] Jonathan Mann, "Memorandum: GPA Deputy Director," WHO Global Programme on AIDS, October 4, 1989.

[46] Global Programme on AIDS, "Terms of Reference of the Global Commission on AIDS, the Research Steering Committees and the Steering Committee on AIDS Prevention and Control Strategies (GPA/GMC(2)/89 INF.DOC.2)," WHO Global Programme on AIDS, December 5, 1989.

[47] US Mission Geneva, "Meeting of Global Management Committee of the WHO Global Programme on AIDS," US Department of State, December 1989, p. 1.

[48] Kathleen Kay, Interview by Michael Merson, New Haven, CT, 2002.

[49] Ibid.

[50] Ibid.

[51] "American Head of WHO AIDS Program Resigns," The Associated Press, March 16, 1990.

[52] James Curran, personal communication, April 11, 2016.

more about this first hand. It was therefore not an unimportant meeting. The previous year (1989), reporters had filed several stories from the Soviet Union revealing that nurses in some hospitals had reused syringes, infecting 70 babies and young children with HIV in the process.[53] That tragic news was quickly surpassed when medical teams determined that similarly reused syringes were responsible for the infection of over 700 children at hospitals and orphanages in Romania.[54] In light of these tragic events, WHO's regional office for Europe (EURO) organized "a meeting of health officials from all Eastern European nations in Copenhagen starting February 27."[55] "Several other European countries have asked for help from WHO since change began sweeping through Eastern Europe," Mann explained to reporters. "The meeting in Copenhagen [was] being held to decide how to determine the scope of the problem and how to strengthen the health care systems of the countries."[56] The meeting's main goal was to "put the finishing touches on our (AIDS) plan for Eastern Europe," Mann explained to reporters. "If they succeed, and find the funds to carry out the program, 'we'll be limiting the AIDS epidemic in the '90s.'"[57]

In accordance with the arbitrary 3-month in advance travel request policy Nakajima had imposed on him the previous December, Mann submitted the paperwork to attend the meeting. Nakajima refused Mann's request, telling him there was no reason for him to attend.[58] While Mann's requests had been denied or delayed before, because of the importance of the meeting, according to Tarantola, this denial proved to be the breaking point for his relationship with Nakajima. Mann now faced a decision: should he break the rules and attend, giving "ground to Nakajima to retaliate," or should he submit to Nakajima's decision and soldier on within an increasingly circumscribed range of activity. Mann opted not to attend the meeting, sending Tarantola in his stead, but it was this decision by Nakajima that seems to have reignited Mann's commitment to resign.

In mid-February, during a trip to Cuba, Mann appears to have concluded that Nakajima's team only planned to set more administrative obstacles in his way and limit his "freedom to travel and to speak on behalf of WHO on HIV/AIDS issues."[59] Mann was in Cuba to press the Cubans firmly on the human rights implications of their AIDS quarantine policies, but the Cubans were unwilling to consider changing them. He was "disturbed and sad," both about the failure of his trip to Cuba and the resistance he expected to face upon his return to Geneva. Fernando Zacarias, a staff

---

[53] Judy Foreman, "AIDS/Montreal '89: Soviet doctor recounts AIDS hospital tragedy," *The Boston Globe,* June 4, 1989, p. 12.

[54] "700 Romanian kids AIDS-infected," *The Toronto Star,* February 7, 1990, A16.

[55] Philip J. Hilts, "Upheaval In The East:: W.H.O. Emergency Team Is Sent To Romania to Assess AIDS Cases," *The New York Times,* February 8, 1990, A14.

[56] Ibid.

[57] Robert P. Hey, "East European Opening Prompts Warning on AIDS," *Christian Science Monitor,* March 1, 1990, p. 8.

[58] Fernando Zacarias, Interview by Michael Merson, New Haven, CT, January, 2002.

[59] Daniel Tarantola, Interview by Michael Merson, New Haven, CT, October, 2001.

member of PAHO who was responsible for AIDS activities in the region and was traveling with Mann on the trip, noted Mann's profound disquiet: "[Mann] said, 'How is it that I can't see my boss to discuss issues, I am not getting the support.' ... I think that [Mann] understood that his contribution as an initiator of [this global movement] was about to be over."[60] When Marjory Dam picked Mann up at the airport in Washington, DC on his way back from Cuba, she sensed the same thing: "I was there at the gate to meet him, and I almost didn't recognize him, he looked so ... pale and thin and terrible," Dam recalled. "That was when he told me in the car that he was worried about travel claims and things like that."[61] The administrative barriers being raised by Nakajima's staff were taking their toll on Mann's well-being.

These administrative obstacles created such frustration for Mann that, according to Nakajima, Mann came to him in early March with an ultimatum: promote him to the level of an Assistant Director-General (ADG) and reinstate the programmatic autonomy he had previously had under Mahler (limited rules on finances, administration, travel authorizations, and recruitment procedures) or Mann would resign.[62] Such a request for an ADG position and authority was not unprecedented: Ralph Henderson, who was also a CDC staffer seconded to WHO, had earlier asked for similar authority (which he did not receive) when he had lead WHO's Expanded Program on Immunization (EPI).[63] Even if Nakajima had wanted to grant Mann that authority, he could not. Henderson was now serving as an ADG, having stepped down from EPI and Nakajima was operating under an unwritten rule of governance that stated that WHO should have only five ADGs, one each from the five permanent members of the UN Security Council. Recalled Nakajima, "I said to Jon, 'I am sorry that I have this precedent and I cannot increase and have a second ADG from the USA. Jon was furious.'"[64]

And so, on the morning of Friday, March 16, 1990, with tensions growing over his program's budget and direction, and with the bureaucratic conflicts between himself and Nakajima at an impasse, Mann tendered his resignation as Director of GPA. March 16 happened to be the day that WHO planned to release a new UN stamp intended to support WHO's efforts against AIDS. That morning Nakajima, Mohammed Abdelmoumene (an Algerian and WHO Deputy Director-General), and Lars Kallings (a Scientific Advisor to the Swedish government who was then serving as chair of the Global Commission on AIDS) planned to join Mann in WHO's Executive Board Room to announce the stamp's release.[65] Before the presentation, Kallings rode with Mann on the elevator to the seventh floor, to pick up Nakajima

---

[60] Fernando Zacarias, Interview by Michael Merson, New Haven, CT, January 2002.

[61] Marjorie Dam, Interview by Michael Merson, New Haven, CT, September 29, 2001.

[62] Hiroshi Nakajima, Interview by Michael Merson, Poitiers, October 13, 2002.

[63] Ralph Henderson, Interview by Michael Merson, NH, February, 2003.

[64] Hiroshi Nakajima, Interview by Michael Merson, Poitiers, October 13, 2002.

[65] "UN stamps issues in support of 'Fight AIDS Worldwide.'" *Xinhua General News Service*, March 16, 1990, Item No: 0316223.

for the presentation. As the three rode down, according to Kallings, Mann asked Nakajima if he had received his resignation letter.[66] Since apparently Kawaguchi had the letter and had not yet shown it to the Director-General, Mann's question caught Nakajima by surprise.[67]

Meanwhile, the news of Mann's resignation had quickly spread among GPA staff. Consequently, about 100 of them gathered outside the Executive Board Room during the ceremony and, as Mann exited the room at the ceremony's end, they lined the hallways and cheered him.[68] Their outburst clearly demonstrated that the staff understood that Mann's resignation "was sending a message out that WHO could no longer fulfill its tasks by the way it was now managed by the new Director-General," as Tarantola explained, "...we completely understood that....we never felt that he was abandoning us. We felt in fact that he was giving such a powerful message to put WHO back on track"[69] Mann briefly addressed the crowd, saying that "the circumstances surrounding the program over the last few months ... had led him to the conclusion that this was the appropriate [action]."[70] Then, according to observers, Mann raised his clenched fist in a salute to his loyal staff.[71]

Mann's resignation was clearly a shocking turn of events, though he had not intended it to take immediate effect – Mann, a CDC employee seconded to WHO, had announced that he would resign at the end of his contract with WHO in June. Still, the announcement was momentous, and Mann, always a skilled communicator, had timed it to coincide with the meeting of the Global Commission on AIDS (GCA) being held early the following week (which was why Kallings happened to be at WHO at the time of Mann's resignation). Some GCA members had learned of Mann's resignation before that meeting started: Mann, for example, had informed Jim Curran of his resignation, when he picked him up at the Geneva airport that day. Curran was a GCA member and head of the HIV Division at CDC. Likewise, June Osborne, who was then Dean of the School of Public Health at the University of Michigan and one of Mann's closest friends, remembers learning about his resignation either through Mann himself or from the journalists who almost immediately began peppering her with questions once they had caught wind of the situation.[72]

The press quickly moved in to unpack the situation. Nakajima, who had attended the UN stamp ceremony before leaving that evening for Afghanistan, said little to reporters beyond releasing a statement noting he regretted Mann's announcement, "which happened, without previous consultation, at a time when the organization is confronted with new challenges concerning the fight against

---

[66] Lars Kallings, Interview by Michael Merson, New Haven, CT, September, 2002.

[67] Ibid.; Manuel Carballo, Interview by Michael Merson, New Haven, CT, November, 2002.

[68] Manuel Carballo, Interview by Michael Merson, New Haven, CT, November, 2002.

[69] Daniel Tarantola, Interview by Michael Merson, New Haven, CT, October, 2001.

[70] Manuel Carballo, Interview by Michael Merson, New Haven, CT, November, 2002.

[71] Philip J. Hilts, "Leader in U.N.'s Battle on AIDS Resigns in Dispute Over Strategy," *The New York Times*, March 17, 1990, 1:1.

[72] James Curran, Interview by Michael Merson, New Haven, CT, March 9, 2002; David Chandler, "Leader of global fight against AIDS resigns," *The Boston Globe,* March 17, 1990, 21.

AIDS."[73] One of Nakajima's aides indicated that Mann's resignation had surprised the Director-General.[74]

Mann, for his part, spent the weekend fielding questions and giving press interviews about his resignation. By this time, the story had gone global and most of the world's leading newspapers had reported Mann's resignation.[75] "When Jon resigned he made a big splash," Walt Dowdle remembered. "He didn't just say 'I am moving on to do other things of interest' and so on and so forth. When he resigned he made a big effort to make sure that he made as many points as he could about Nakajima's leadership."[76] It was during this time that Mann gave an interview with *Le Monde*, wherein he was quite critical of Nakajima.[77] "[That was] a sort of point of no return interview as far as his relationship with Nakajima was concerned," remembered Osborne.[78]

It is not clear the extent to which Mann's interview with *Le Monde* affected the situation, but by the Monday following Mann's resignation, Nakajima—in a move that appears to have surprised Mann—announced that he had accepted Mann's resignation, and that it would be effective immediately. Nakajima therefore removed Mann from his post and set out straight away to replace him. Mann had taken no steps to transition his position; he seems to have expected that Nakajima would let him remain as GPA Director during the final months of his contract to put things in order. "[Mann] hadn't thought of that possibility in his scenario," Nakajima's wife Martha later recalled about Nakajima's swift decision.[79] For his part, Nakajima apparently was prepared for such a scenario, so while the timing of the resignation caught him by surprise, the possibility—indeed likelihood—of it did not. "There was some rumor that he was preparing to resign," Nakajima remembered, "so I was already prepared to replace him."[80]

The rapidity with which Mann resigned and was removed created an immediate crisis both for the United States government and for GPA. Since Mann was a CDC employee seconded to WHO, the United States government had to address the political fallout that accompanied a very public tiff between one of its high-level employees and a prominent UN agency director. At the same time, it also had to address the immediate personal needs of Mann and his family. On March 19, the first day of the GCA meeting, Nakajima ordered Mann to vacate his GPA office and

---

[73] "American Head of WHO AIDS Program Resigns," *The Associated Press*, March 16, 1990; David Chandler, "Leader of global fight against AIDS resigns," *The Boston Globe*, March 17, 1990, 21.

[74] Kelly Toughill, "Top AIDS doctor quits over feud with boss," *The Toronto Star*, March 17, 1990, A6.

[75] Philip J. Hilts, "Leader in U.N.'s Battle on AIDS Resigns in Dispute Over Strategy," *The New York Times*, March 17, 1990, p. 5; http://www.nytimes.com/1990/03/17/us/leader-in-un-s-battle-on-aids-resigns-in-dispute-over-strategy.html.

[76] Walt Dowdle, Interview by Stephen Inrig, Dallas, TX, August 10, 2010.

[77] Kathleen Kay, Interview by Michael Merson, New Haven, CT, 2002.

[78] June Osborne, Interview by Michael Merson, New Haven, CT, October 26, 2002.

[79] Hiroshi Nakajima, Interview by Michael Merson, Poitiers, October 13, 2002.

[80] Ibid.

relocate to one in a relatively secluded office block far from the GPA offices while WHO and CDC worked out his future arrangements.[81] "Here I was, Jon's supervisor," Curran remembers, "… now that he didn't have a job and they wanted him out of the place."[82] Having resigned from his job at WHO, Mann was no longer covered by his visa from the Swiss government to remain in the country. Curran was able to secure an agreement that CDC could assign Mann to Nyon, where he lived, and Mann could work there and look for another position until his children finished their school term. Mann later returned to his GPA office and cleared out his desk.[83]

In four tumultuous days, Jonathan Mann ceased to be the leader of a program he had worked tirelessly to create over 4 years, a program that was leading the global response to a pandemic that was entering its tenth year, caused by a deadly virus, and whose course was unclear. This moment would go down as one of the most significant in the course of the global response to AIDS.

---

[81] Lars Kallings, Interview by Michael Merson, New Haven, CT, September, 2002; Kathleen Kay, Interview by Michael Merson, New Haven, CT, 2002.

[82] James Curran, Interview by Michael Merson, New Haven, CT, March 9, 2002.

[83] Ibid.

Part II
From Mobilization to Managing in a Pandemic

Chapter 8
The Transition

At 10:10 a.m. on Tuesday, March 20, 1990, my administrative assistant, Gillian Mignon, informed me that the World Health Organization (WHO)'s Deputy Director-General, Mohammed Abdelmoumene, was on the phone. At the time, I was serving as Director of WHO's Diarrheal Diseases Control Programme (CDD), a position I had held since 1980, and also as Director of WHO's Acute Respiratory Infections Programme (ARI), a position I had held since 1987. It was not uncommon for Abdelmoumene to call me about some aspect of these two programs, so I did not think his call unusual. However, I quickly noticed that the generally low-key Abdelmoumene sounded tense and spoke rapidly over the phone. "Meet me at 11:00 a.m. in the Director-General's office" Abdelmoumene said. "We want to talk to you about the Global Programme on AIDS."[1]

By this time, of course, I had heard that Jonathan Mann had resigned the previous Friday as Director of the Global Programme on AIDS (GPA), and about the accompanying scene on the first floor of the main WHO building. Beyond that, I knew little about what had happened. I do recall speaking with Bob Hogan, my Program Management Officer, about the situation that afternoon. We both had begun to speculate about potential candidates to replace Mann as GPA Director. There seemed, at that stage, no obvious successor. Jim Curran appeared the most likely candidate, since he headed the AIDS program at the Centers for Disease Control and Prevention (CDC), had a close relationship with Mann, and was well respected by the AIDS community in the United States and globally. I did not consider myself a prospective candidate. While my management experience and relationship with the donor community could be considered assets, I had no experience in the field of AIDS, knew very little about GPA and its history, and my French was embarrassingly poor.

Within this chapter the singular pronouns *I* and *my* refer to Michael Merson alone, whereas the plural pronouns *we* and *us* generally refer to Michael Merson and Stephen Inrig jointly. Where *we* or *us* refers to Michael Merson and his colleagues at WHO, the object of the pronoun is clarified by context.

[1] For the purposes of this text, we will use the term AIDS to encompass both AIDS and HIV unless otherwise specified.

© Springer International Publishing AG 2018
M. Merson, S. Inrig, *The AIDS Pandemic*, DOI 10.1007/978-3-319-47133-4_8

Even though I did not expect to be picked for the post, I found myself surprisingly anxious when, at 11:00 a.m. Nakajima's staff ushered me into his office. With Abdelmoumene at his side, Nakajima cut straight to the point: would I serve as Interim Director of GPA until he found Mann's replacement? I asked a few questions, requested a day to consider his proposal, and left the room. The next day, at 5:30 p.m., I agreed to the Director-General's request. Little did I realize the complexities that lay ahead.

How had I come to this point? My interest in medicine came from my paternal grandfather. A cardiologist, he had lived in Brooklyn, close to my family's apartment, and I spent many hours "hanging out" in his office as a young child, playing with his instruments and marveling at his x-ray machines. Both the proximity to his practice and my great respect for him made him an important figure in my upbringing and whetted my appetite for a career in medicine. My interest in public health emerged more gradually, during my medical training at State University of New York (SUNY) Downstate School of Medicine in Brooklyn. I came to medical school with an interest in infectious diseases, a subject that sensitized me to issues of poverty and health disparities, and did my clinical rotations at Kings County Hospital in the East Flatbush area of Brooklyn, which in those days was one of the most impoverished areas of the borough and the city of New York. Then, in the summer between my third and fourth year of medical school, I took the opportunity made available by the then Chairperson of Obstetrics and Gynecology, Louis Hellman, to travel to Nepal and work in the government's family planning program supported by a United States Agency for International Development (USAID) fellowship. It was this experience that first exposed me to the health challenges in low- and middle-income countries.

Those experiences guided my path into the world of public health and medicine. During my first year of medical residency at Johns Hopkins Hospital in Baltimore, Maryland, I was able to spend 3 months working on the hospital ship S.S. Hope (which at that time was docked for the year in Natal, in Northeastern Brazil). During those 3 months, I provided clinical care for patients hospitalized aboard the ship, served as an instructor for the Brazilian medical students onboard, and worked twice a week in clinics in the local hospital on shore. Even more so than my experience in Nepal, my time in Natal gave me enormous insight into the plight of the poor and solidified my commitment to a career in global health (we used the term "international health" in those days).

Right after my first year of residency I became eligible for the draft. I opted to enroll in the Commissioned Corp of the United States Public Health Service (USPHS) and join the Epidemic Intelligence Services at CDC, where I was assigned to the Enteric Diseases Branch in Atlanta for 2 years (I ended up remaining a third year to serve as head of the branch). This placement gave me the opportunity to work abroad. For example, I conducted research on the etiology of travelers' diarrhea in Mexico and investigated an outbreak of cholera on Guam in 1974.[2] It was because of these experiences that

---

[2] Michael Merson., et al. "Cholera on Guam, 1974 Epidemiologic Findings and Isolation of non-toxinogenic Strains." *American Journal of Epidemiology* 105.4 (1977): 349-361; and Michael Merson, et al. "Travelers' diarrhea in Mexico: a prospective study of physicians and family members attending a congress." *New England Journal of Medicine* 294.24 (1976): 1299-1305.

the CDC Director tapped me to lead a CDC team that was sent to Guam to provide quarantine clearance for about 110,000 Vietnamese refugees brought there by the United States military in the spring of 1975 at the end of the Vietnam War, under an inter-agency program called Operation New Life.[3] After these refugees were cleared, they were transferred to temporary housing at four United States military bases on mainland United States, from which they would be resettled by voluntary agencies.

When my 3 years at CDC ended, I split a 2-year fellowship between Boston (Beth Israel and Children's Hospitals) and Baltimore (Johns Hopkins and Baltimore City Hospitals) and planned to obtain board certification in infectious diseases. I never took that exam, however, because during the second year of my fellowship, my mentor at Johns Hopkins, Brad Sack, arranged for me to spend 3 months in Dhaka, Bangladesh, conducting a study on the treatment of enterotoxigenic E. coli diarrhea at the Cholera Research Laboratory (now called the International Centre for Diarrhoeal Diseases Research). This experience convinced me that I wanted to pursue a career in global health research and practice, rather than one as an academic infectious disease clinician. Since the USPHS had paid my salary during my 2 years of fellowship, I owed it 3 years of service. Hence, when my fellowship at Johns Hopkins ended in June 1977, I opted to return to the Cholera Research Laboratory as Chief Epidemiologist under the auspices of the USPHS detailed from CDC in Atlanta, where I participated in a host of exciting studies on diarrhea etiology and transmission.

I was living in Dhaka only a little over a year when Dhiman Barua, a famous cholera bacteriologist from Kolkata who worked in WHO, invited me to join him in starting a new global program on diarrheal diseases control. It was a difficult decision, but in 1978, I moved with my family to Geneva and joined WHO on secondment from CDC as a medical officer in the newly established CDD Program. I expected to work in WHO for only 2 years, fulfilling my 3-year commitment to the USPHS, but I remained there for the next 17 years. Two years after I joined CDD, to my great surprise, Barua told me that he had to retire. Though he was in the best of health, he had reached WHO's then mandatory retirement age of 60 years, and was no longer eligible to be employed by WHO. Since he and I were the two main staff members in the program, this meant that, if I returned home, the program would have no one to lead it who had been involved in its initial development. Consequently, in 1980, I agreed to remain on as Program Director of CDD.

Fortunately, the program performed well and grew considerably under my watch. We owed our success to several factors. First, we promoted a simple technology, oral rehydration therapy, that greatly reduced diarrhea mortality and which health programs in low- and middle-income countries could readily adapt and put to use. Second, oral rehydration aligned nicely with WHO's priorities, fitting particularly well with the primary health care approach recently championed in Alma Ata. Third, our program dealt with children, so it had widespread donor empathy and support. Finally, we collaborated closely and successfully with other United Nations (UN) agencies—like the United Nations Children's Emergency Fund (UNICEF) and the United Nations Development Programme (UNDP)—and with bilateral programs,

---

[3] Daniel Haulman. "Operation Babylife and New Life." Air Moblity Command Museum. Available at https://amcmuseum.org/history/operation-babylift-and-new-life.

like USAID. I am proud of my time with CDD and the contributions we made to the reduction of childhood mortality over the past three decades. Since the start of the program, global diarrhea deaths have declined considerably.[4]

Our accomplishments in CDD led WHO's Director-General, Halfdan Mahler, to ask me in 1987 to also direct the ARI Program. Mahler's rationale was that diarrhea and pneumonia were the two leading causes of death in children, and their case management approaches were similar in that they focused on recognition of a few, easily recognizable signs and symptoms and provision of treatment at the community and first-level facility level. I accepted the position, became Director of both programs, and was happily serving in that capacity when I received the phone call from Abdelmoumene on March 20th.

As mentioned above, the request from Nakajima to serve as Interim Director of GPA came as a surprise. After asking for time to consider it, I began weighing my options: I talked it over with Hogan and called several people in the United States for insight and advice. I wasn't sure what to do. The same reasons I had assumed I would not be a candidate for the position remained: I knew little about AIDS, I knew even less about the politics of AIDS, and my French was limited. I remember feeling very conflicted.[5] I was not concerned about leaving the day-to-day work of the CDD and ARI programs for a short period, as I had excellent senior staff and knew that, with the help of Hogan, I could continue to manage both programs.

Nakajima, on the other hand, apparently felt quite certain that I was the correct fit for GPA. As we described in Chapter 7, rumors of Mann's dissatisfaction and potential resignation had surfaced in the early months of 1990, which—when he heard them—gave Nakajima time to consider his options. "So ... even before Mann's resignation," Nakajima later explained, "I had screened [potential candidates] and thought about this."[6] It is unclear when Nakajima began considering me, but others had apparently suggested me as a potential replacement. On one occasion (according to Tony Piel, then Director of Program Development in the Director-General's Office), Nakajima and Mann once had a heated discussion over AIDS policy and Mann threatened to resign. During this interchange, Abdelmoumene, who was in the office with Mann and Nakajima at the time, penned a note to Piel, informing him that Mann was threatening to quit. Piel, familiar with my work as Director of CDD and ARI, sent a note back to Abdelmoumene recommending that "if Jonathan goes through with this, then call Michael Merson."[7] Not long thereafter, according to Piel, "Abdelmoumene sent me a [third] note out and he said 'we are taking your suggestion seriously.'"[8]

[4] Numbers taken, and extrapolated back to 1980s, from Danzhen You, Jin Rou New and Tessa Wardlaw on behalf of the United Nations Inter-agency Group for Child Mortality Estimation, "Levels & Trends in Child Mortality, Report 2012: Estimates Developed by the UN Inter-agency Group for Child Mortality Estimation," Geneva: UNICEF, 2012 http://www.apromiserenewed.org/wp-content/uploads/2015/03/UNICEF_2012_child_mortality_for_web_0904.pdf

[5] Robert Hogan, Interview by Michael Merson, New Haven, CT, August, 2002.

[6] Hiroshi Nakajima, Interview by Michael Merson, Poitiers, October 13, 2002.

[7] Anthony Piel, Interview by Michael Merson, Sharon, CT, December 22, 2001; Letter from Anthony Piel to Mike Merson, 22 December 2001.

[8] Ibid.

From a diplomatic perspective, choosing me made good political sense for Nakajima. "The way he was thinking," remembered Walt Dowdle, who was CDC Deputy Director at the time, "was that he had to have somebody as the Interim Director, and he thought that, in view of Jon[athan]'s resignation, he probably ought to have an American—but one he could trust."[9] Choosing a non-American, particularly someone from within GPA, might have appeared as a defeat for Nakajima, and so no one should have expected he would do that. I think this explains why, even before consulting with United States officials, Nakajima asked me to serve as Interim Director.[10] Nakajima would later tell me himself that "it had to be an American because they were the largest donor to the program."[11]

Nakajima's move also made sense to some high-level health officials. During the weekend immediately following Mann's resignation, Hogan had spoken with several other people within WHO, including Piel, Manual Carballo, and Warren Furth (who had recently stepped down as Assistant Director-General), about a potential replacement. According to Hogan, most of them considered me "the most plausible candidate for that job."[12] After Nakajima appointed me, Jim Grant, Executive Director of UNICEF, wrote to congratulate me on Nakajima's "good move," while United States officials voiced their support to me, to Nakajima, and to the press when they learned about my appointment.[13] Dowdle, whom CDC Director and Assistant Secretary for Health James Mason had immediately sent to Geneva upon hearing of Mann's resignation, considered my appointment fortuitous: "Before I got on the plane, we discovered that Nakajima had asked you to come on board as the Interim Director. That was not done in consultation with us … I think that was a pretty smart move. When we discovered this, in fact, we said 'Hey, why not—good idea!'"[14]

Within GPA, however, my selection was understandably much more controversial. Some felt it was merely a pretext for a more definitive move by Nakajima. "I think … once the resignation was there, and it was clear that they were going to appoint you as an interim," Roy Widdus remembered, "everyone in the program thought that there was a very strong probability that you would be named as the Director."[15] Whether it was Nakajima's initial intent or not, those within GPA saw my appointment as Nakajima's exertion of control over the program. Many felt that I would bring both personal and philosophical changes to the program. Michael Kirby, the first Chair of the GPA Global Commission on AIDS, for example, felt

---

[9] Walt Dowdle, Interview by Michael Merson, New Haven, CT, August, 2002; Nakajima confirmed, in our interview with him, that he felt he needed to hire an American. See Hiroshi Nakajima, Interview by Michael Merson, Poitiers, October 13, 2002.

[10] Walt Dowdle, Interview by Michael Merson, New Haven, CT, August, 2002.

[11] Hiroshi Nakajima, Interview by Michael Merson, Poitiers, October 13, 2002; Mohamed Abdelmoumene, Interview by Michael Merson, Geneva, October 28, 2014.

[12] Robert Hogan, Interview by Michael Merson, New Haven, CT, August, 2002.

[13] James P. Grant, "Letter to Michael Merson, March 22, 1990," New York: UNICEF, 1990; Louis Sullivan, "Letter to Hiroshi Nakajima, April 11, 1990," Geneva: United States Mission to International Organizations, 1990; "AIDS Program Gets Acting Head Following Resignation of Dr. Mann," *The Associated Press*, March 21, 1990.

[14] Walt Dowdle, Interview by Michael Merson, New Haven, CT, August, 2002.

[15] Roy Widdus, Interview by Michael Merson, New Haven, CT, October, 2001.

I lacked "the fire and *elan* of Jonathan Mann," and that my appointment signified Nakajima's desire to remedicalize AIDS, diminish the emphasis on human rights, and shift attention away from developing nations towards AIDS in the developed world.[16] Whether or not these fears were founded, the depth with which they were felt by GPA staff indicated just how much work I had to do to win them over if I hoped to be effective as an Interim Director.

Initially, as we described above, the Director-General appointed me on a short-term basis, primarily to "hold the fort" while I conducted a search for a permanent Director. To this end I wrote a letter to all the staff in the CDD and ARI programs informing them that I expected to return and how the programs would be run in my absence.[17] This would provide time to find a permanent replacement, someone with whom Nakajima and GPA staff could feel comfortable. There was, at this stage, no anger or bad feelings between the United States government and WHO about the way Nakajima had handled Mann's resignation; United States officials felt they "owed WHO and Nakajima a lot" and wanted to salvage the relationship by finding an acceptable replacement for Mann.[18] I felt that I was part of this immediate task, working primarily "to ensure a smooth transition."[19] However, as the relationship between Mann and Nakajima quickly deteriorated and Nakajima was determined to immediately remove Mann from his position, I was instead thrust into a situation that required me to bring some stability to GPA while finding Mann's replacement.

I took that task seriously: I had only agreed to take the interim position on the condition that I could help in the search for Mann's replacement. To my surprise, the pool of candidates turned out to be small: I received only ten resumes from interested candidates sent either by the candidates themselves or by governments from different countries. In my view, the strongest of these candidates was Michael Adler, a leading expert in sexually transmitted diseases[20] (STDs) from the United Kingdom and the founding editor of the journal *AIDS*, whom I would meet a few years later when visiting Diana, Princess of Wales, at Kensington Palace. None of the ten candidates seemed acceptable to Abdelmoumene and Nakajima, so I began calling around to gather resumes from more contenders.[21] This, too, proved frustrating, however, because several obstacles stood in the way of some very viable candidates. For example, some with whom I talked had the sense that Nakajima wanted an

---

[16] Michael Kirby, "Global Commission on AIDS, Third Meeting, Geneva, 22–23 March 1990: AIDS—Third Meeting of GCA." Unpublished Document.

[17] Marjorie Dam, Interview by Michael Merson, New Haven, CT, September 29, 2001.

[18] Walt Dowdle, Interview by Michael Merson, New Haven, CT, August, 2002.

[19] "U.N. body appoints new AIDS director," *The Toronto Star,* March 21, 1990, A22; "WHO appoints acting director of global AIDS program," *Xinhua General News Service*, March 21, 1990, Item No: 0321027; "Dr. Michael H. Merson Appointed Acting Director For Global AIDS Programme." *World Health Organization Press*, March 26, 1990.

[20] For the purposes of this text, we use the term sexually transmitted disease(s) and the abbreviation STD rather than the other term sexually transmitted infection(s) or STIs.

[21] Robert Hogan, Interview by Michael Merson, New Haven, CT, August, 2002.

American in the position and the United States government was eager to retain it; this discouraged applications. At the same time, none of the suitable American candidates were available. As mentioned earlier, Jim Curran was, to my mind, the best person for the position. "I didn't speak French," Curran explained to us in an interview, "[and] I didn't know international health that much, or Africa."[22] The truth is that the United States government greatly valued Curran domestically and believed his leadership of the HIV Division at CDC was too vital for him to leave to head up GPA. Tapping Curran for GPA would merely have shifted a search for leadership to the CDC and in the end the United States government would not release him. So Curran stayed in Atlanta.

As for me, I continued searching diligently for Mann's replacement. I do not feel I was being self-serving in this—though I recognize some might disagree— but three factors began to point, or perhaps had always pointed, to me as the leading candidate for the position. For one, Nakajima obviously felt comfortable with me. In fact, in mid-April, Nakajima formally offered me the job, but I turned him down.[23] Second, not only did I have Nakajima's approval, but I also had United States government support as well. Many American officials felt working effectively in WHO, much less working with Nakajima, was a special skill all its own; since I had thrived in that context, they were comfortable with me staying on.[24] United States officials made this plain to me in late April, when I flew to Washington, DC to discuss the search personally with Louis Sullivan, Secretary of Health and Human Services. Sullivan told me that I was his candidate for the job and would have his full support if I took it on. Third, in addition to the support from Nakajima and the United States government, several GPA donors, including Norway and the United Kingdom (and its representative and Chair of the GPA Management Committee, Barbara Kelly), encouraged me to take the job and implored Nakajima to "keep [me] on, and keep GPA moving."[25]

However, I remained very ambivalent. I was well aware of my limitations with respect to my knowledge of AIDS, AIDS politics, and the AIDS community.[26] Equally important, and unbeknownst to Nakajima or anyone else at WHO at the time, I had been informed that I was on the short list and the most likely candidate to replace D. A. Henderson as Dean of the Johns Hopkins (now Bloomberg) School of Public Health. Johns Hopkins consistently ranked as the top public health school in the United States, and it was an exciting and attractive opportunity for me. I had been at WHO for over a decade by this time, and had started thinking about the next stage of my career. Indeed, before Mann resigned, I had interviewed multiple times

---

[22] James Curran, Interview by Michael Merson, New Haven, CT, March 9, 2002.

[23] "AIDS: 6th Meeting of Global Management Committee of the WHO Global Programme on AIDS," Washington, DC: US Department of State, May 15, 1990.

[24] James Curran, Interview by Michael Merson, New Haven, CT, March 9, 2002.

[25] "AIDS: 6th Meeting of Global Management Committee of the WHO Global Programme on AIDS," Washington, DC: US Department of State, May 15, 1990.

[26] Robert Hogan, Interview by Michael Merson, New Haven, CT, August, 2002.

for the Johns Hopkins position.[27] I was therefore not expecting to take up a new challenge at WHO but instead, by the summer of 1990, to be moving back to Baltimore, where I had done much of my medical training. The interim position did little to interfere with that trajectory; becoming GPA Director certainly would.

While I contemplated my options, I did my best to keep GPA functioning on an even keel as its Interim Director. This meant I largely worked to maintain ongoing program activities and handle any acute problems as they arose. I avoided making decisions that would have a significant impact on the person who would occupy the permanent position. This being the case, I quickly came to realize just how momentous the AIDS pandemic was. Its magnitude caught me off guard. While smaller in scope to some diseases, it nonetheless posed a devastating threat to many countries, especially those with a high or potentially high HIV incidence.[28] The enormity of GPA's response was equally striking. "There has been nothing like it," I concluded in my presentation to the GPA Management Committee (GMC), which held its scheduled meeting as planned on April 26. "As someone who has been deeply involved in child survival efforts for the past 12 years, I can tell you that the worldwide efforts to reduce childhood mortality ... pale in comparison to the response to AIDS ... [and] much of the credit for this must be given to Dr. Jonathan Mann."[29] (Picture 8.1)

It was evident that the dispute between Mann and Nakajima, and Mann's subsequent tumultuous departure, threatened to derail the immense progress GPA had made and hamper the urgent and continued efforts that were required of the program to slow down the pandemic. GPA staff felt tremendous loyalty to Mann, and with him gone, they understandably viewed me and my potential intentions and influence quite skeptically.[30] Nakajima tried to smooth my way by reassuring GPA staff of their integral role in WHO, but few of them held Nakajima with high regard, and his assurances had little impact. Many leaders in the field outside GPA even expressed concern for it's future.[31]

It took me little time to grasp the devastating impact of Mann's resignation on staff morale. The day Nakajima announced me as Interim Director, GPA's staff gathered together to meet with him and me in the Executive Board Room. The room was filled to capacity, and on the faces of the staff I saw a mixture of fear, anger, and

[27] Ann Gibbons, "New Head for the WHO Global Program on AIDS: do changes at the World Health Organization signal a new direction for its international AIDS program?" *Science*, June 15, 1990, 248:1306–7.

[28] Michael Merson, "GPA Diagnosis, April 16, 1990;" Michael Merson, "Director's Report, GPA Management Committee, April 26, 1990;" Mike Merson, Interview with Stephen Inrig.

[29] Michael Merson, "Director's Report, GPA Management Committee, April 26, 1990."

[30] Michael Kirby, "Global Commission on AIDS, Third Meeting, Geneva, 22–23 March 1990: AIDS—Third Meeting of GCA." Unpublished Document.

[31] "U.N. body appoints new AIDS director," *The Toronto Star,* March 21, 1990, A22; Thomson Prentice "World AIDS specialists fall out over key programmes for action," *The London Times* March 21, 1990; Christie McLaren, "Canadian groups fear departure will hurt global fight against AIDS," *The Globe and Mail,* March 21, 1990; "WHO officials' departure worries Canadian AIDS groups," *Xinhua General News Service*, March 21, 1990; Item No: 0321203.

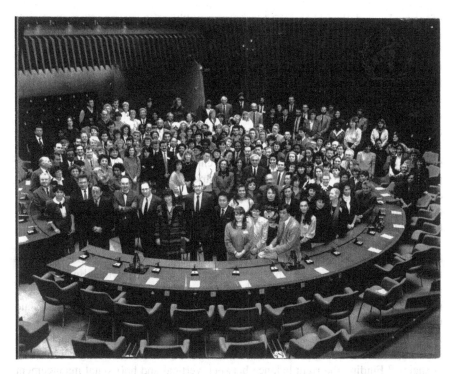

Picture 8.1 GPA Staff in WHO Executive Board Room, February 1990 (Source: © World Health Organization/Alain Gassmann)

incredulity. I imagined it was similar to what the staff of an explosive start-up company might have experienced after their well-regarded CEO resigned precipitously with no transition plan in place. People were astounded, demoralized, and frightened; no one knew what to make of what had happened.

Most seemed to think they knew what to make of me, however; to them my presence was not wholly innocent. Nakajima had long doubted GPA's efficiency and effectiveness with respect to its research, operations, management, and support to national AIDS programs. GPA staff must certainly have felt he had brought me in not only to stabilize the program, but also to improve and reform it to be more in line with his way of thinking.[32] Appointing me for such a task implied that GPA was somehow dysfunctional, a judgment that many believed Nakajima was in no position to make, and one that stood in contrast with GPA's external appearance of robust effectiveness and growth. Indeed, at the time Mann resigned, GPA had grown far more rapidly than program in WHO's history. By 1990, its staff numbered almost 400, its annual budget stood at almost $100 million, 123 countries had short-term plans (STPs), 95 countries were developing medium-term plans (MTPs), and

---

[32] Michael Merson, Personal notes, March 1990.

65 countries had already arranged "resource mobilization meetings" to fund their national efforts.[33]

Yet despite these remarkably rapid achievements, or perhaps because of them, I found that GPA harbored numerous organizational redundancies and inefficiencies. Soon after assuming the Interim Directorship, I sent a memo to Nakajima detailing some of these: there was considerable overlap in responsibility among different units; there were too many people reporting directly to the Director; and some staff carried excessive workloads. Moreover, it seemed that the proposed reorganization of GPA, which Mann and his colleagues had worked on since late 1989 and was scheduled to begin on April 1, portended even more redundancy and coordination problems. Under the valid pretext of the impending hiring of a new Director, I decided early on that it was best to postpone the reorganization process.[34] Also, about 1 month later, I sent Nakajima an alternative, simplified organizational structure that the new Director might wish to implement.[35]

GPA faced other issues as well. Since 1988, WHO's Executive Board had called on GPA to regionalize its operations, although both GPA's leadership and donors had very reluctantly agreed to this idea. When I came on board, the regionalization process was underway (i.e., shifting more of the responsibility from GPA in Geneva to WHO Regional offices), and so I set about determining how GPA could continue towards its regionalization goals.[36] At the same time, many national programs were in a state of flux over their MTPs, their relationship within their national health ministries, and their support from bilateral, multilateral, and non-governmental agencies.[37] Finding the right balance between vertical and horizontal management of these programs demanded considerable time and careful attention.[38]

I also needed to address GPA's budget, its research agenda, and the potential impact of the ongoing internal and proposed external evaluations. The 1990 and 1991 budgets were slated at about $100 million, but there was considerable uncertainty about the source of these funds. The global economic picture was darkening, donors were demanding more accountability, and GPA had some over-expenditures

---

[33] Global Programme on AIDS, *Report of the External Review of the World Health Organization, Global Programme on AIDS,* Geneva: World Health Organization, January 1992, 7.

[34] Michael Merson, "Director's Report, GPA Management Committee, April 26, 1990."

[35] Michael Merson, "Workplan request from Acting Directors, GPA; April 9, 1990"; Michael Merson, "GPA Diagnosis, April 16, 1990"; Michael Merson, "Confidential Memorandum to the Deputy Director-General on the Revised Structure for GPA, April 23, 1990."

[36] Michael Merson, "Director's Report, GPA Management Committee, April 26, 1990"; "AIDS: 6th Meeting of Global Management Committee of the WHO Global Programme on AIDS," Washington, DC: US Department of State, May 15, 1990.

[37] For more on the various issues and concerns related to the National Programs, decentralization, budget, internal and external reviews, see "AIDS: 6th Meeting of Global Management Committee of the WHO Global Programme on AIDS," Washington, DC: US Department of State, May 15, 1990; Michael Merson, "Director's Report, GPA Management Committee, April 26, 1990"; Michael Merson, "GPA Diagnosis, April 16, 1990."

[38] Michael Merson, "GPA Diagnosis, April 16, 1990," Michael Merson, "Director's Report, GPA Management Committee, April 26, 1990," Walt Dowdle, Confidential Memorandum to Michael Merson, April 26, 1990.

and under-expenditures in key budget areas. Some donors were calling for GPA to revise its budget targets downwards.[39] I had to digest all this in rapid fashion in order to present the GMC with a revised 1990 budget and budgetary projections for 1991 at its aforementioned meeting.[40] Each of the unit chiefs thankfully made my work easier by providing me a work plan for the period of April to June. On the research front, which was one of Nakajima's key concerns about GPA, I (and some of the donors) had the sense that GPA could do more to establish relevant policies and provide support to test new drug and vaccine candidates. I also felt GPA's behavioral research agenda needed strengthening, although I recognized such research was more difficult in many ways than biomedical research. One challenge was the lack of extensive behavioral research capacity in developing nations, particularly around sexual behavior, which Manuel Carballo and his team had recognized early on (see Chapter 11). Expansion of research infrastructures needed ideally to be done in collaboration with national programs in order to ensure the results of this research were relevant and could be implemented by these programs.[41]

The internal and external program evaluations also cast a shadow over GPA, and I needed to become fully acquainted with them. The internal review was in the second phase of its management evaluation, while the external review—called for by the GMC at its last meeting—was only in its early planning stages. Ross Noble, who at that time was Senior Program Officer, Multilateral Technical Cooperation for the Canadian International Development Agency (CIDA) and represented Canada on the GMC, reflected back on what the donors had in mind when they had called for an external evaluation at the same time that GPA's leadership was in such flux:

> "At the April [1990] meeting—Terry Mooney [a Canadian working as the external relations officer in GPA] came up to me and said, 'We need more money for programs,' and I said: 'Terry, this program has been drawing your annual budget now for something like 80 or 90 million. ... I have to be able to go back to my masters and justify why we should increase this program, to which we are already giving generously.' And he persisted ... and during the course of the meeting I thought, 'I'm just going to test things out with the other donors to see if they feel the same way.' Our [ie. Canada's] feeling was that, 'we're not going to give any more money to this program. If you're asking for more money, then you show us what you have been able to do with the money so far, going back to 86 '... So I compared notes with my Swedish and Dutch colleagues and I said: 'I think we had better go back on this, and ask the program to think about doing an evaluation, because if they are asking for more money, the only way they are going to get it from my government is if they can show results—and maybe it's time for a review.' They seemed to agree with that and that really was the genesis for the call for an evaluation.'"[42]

---

[39] "AIDS: 6th Meeting of Global Management Committee of the WHO Global Programme on AIDS," Washington, DC: US Department of State, May 15, 1990.

[40] Michael Merson, "Director's Report, GPA Management Committee, April 26, 1990," Global Programme on AIDS, "Progress Report Number 6, May 1990," Geneva: World Health Organization, WHO/GPA/DIR/90.4, 7.

[41] Michael Merson, "Director's Report, GPA Management Committee, April 26, 1990."

[42] Ross Noble, Interview by Michael Merson, Geneva, October, 2001.

---

1. To review GPA's basic strategies and modes of
   operation ...
2. To assess GPA's accomplishments and contributions to
   global and national AIDS prevention and control efforts.
3. To assess the process used by GPA for priority setting ...
4. To review progress towards meeting targets
5. To assess the effectiveness, cost effectiveness, and
   efficiency of GPA's operation.
6. To assess the relevance of GPA activities to national
   health care systems ...
7. To assess the suitability of GPA's management
   structure, procedures, and priorities to enhance
   national and international efforts for AIDS prevention.
8. To assess GPA's activities and interactions with other
   parts of WHO at all levels, the UN system, and other
   institutions and organizations ...
9. To consider the future role and priorities of GPA
10. To make recommendations relevant to the terms of
    reference.

Fig. 8.1 Terms of reference for external review, 1990. Source: Bernadette Olowo-Freers, Gill Walt, et al. Report of the External Review of the World Health Organization, Global Programme on AIDS, Geneva: World Health Organization, January 1992, pp. i – iii

In light of these considerations, I began talking with individual donors to better understand their intentions behind the external review, their preferences for the review's terms of reference (see Fig. 8.1), and the impact this additional scrutiny would have on GPA's ability to function effectively.[43] The overall goal of the external review was "to provide the Management Committee and the Director-General with an independent, formative evaluation of the relevance and, to the degree possible, impact of the first 5 years of the program's activity, including recommendations for enhancing GPA's contribution to global AIDS prevention and control."[44] At its meeting in April 1990 (my first meeting as Interim Director), the GMC created a working group to draw up the full terms of reference for the review and to select a committee to conduct the evaluation. It planned for the Committee to present "a summary report ... to the GMC in November 1991 and a full and final report at the GMC

---

[43] "AIDS: 6th Meeting of Global Management Committee of the WHO Global Programme on AIDS," Washington, DC: US Department of State, May 15, 1990.

[44] Global Programme on AIDS, *Report of the External Review of the World Health Organization, Global Programme on AIDS*, Geneva: World Health Organization, January 1992, pp. i–ii.

meeting in June 1992."[45] Gaining a grasp of the state of GPA would be no small task. Among other challenges, it meant recognizing how much scrutiny GPA had recently come under in terms of using their contributions to achieve program outcomes that met their expectations.

In addition, I had to be cognizant of two pressing issues. The first was the impending 6th International Conference on AIDS, scheduled to be held in San Francisco starting on June 20. An important complicating factor for the conference was that, in 1987, the United States Congress had added HIV to its list of dangerous contagious diseases that could be used to exclude entry of foreigners into the United States. This put WHO and GPA in a difficult position with respect to the conference, because we had publicly criticized nations that had enacted such regulations on travelers. Many in GPA and WHO had seriously considered whether to withdraw WHO's co-sponsorship of the conference. However, for reasons that were unclear, Mann had not reached a formal conclusion on what stance the organization should adopt on the conference before he resigned. With the gathering only 2 months away, a decision had to be made.

Negotiating WHO's response therefore fell to me, along with Nakajima and other senior WHO staff. No one expected a timely change in United States government policy, since that would require Congressional action (indeed, it would not be until January 2010 that Congress would formally remove HIV/AIDS from the list of communicable diseases for which entry was denied). I worked with United States health officials to come up with a compromise: HIV-positive foreigners would be able to request a waiver that would permit them to obtain a 10-day visa in order to attend international conferences in the United States. This solution still failed to please several global health and AIDS advocacy organizations and many of them would decide to boycott the conference for that reason. The solution's weaknesses aside, I felt that it enabled WHO to continue co-sponsoring the conference while maintaining our stance on nondiscrimination and upholding the human rights of persons living with HIV and AIDS.[46] We knew, however, we would have to find a better solution going forward (for much more on this, see Chapter 12).

The second, and even more pressing, issue I faced was the impending World Health Assembly (WHA), which was set to start on May 7. Nakajima had told me that he wanted to have a permanent replacement for Mann in place before the WHA began.[47] Since AIDS and GPA were on the Assembly's agenda, Nakajima felt having a permanent Director in place was essential to vindicate his decision to remove Mann from his position so swiftly after he resigned. As the WHA approached, Nakajima felt that my efforts as Interim Director of GPA had confirmed his initial support of me for the permanent position. He trusted me, and my success in the CDD and ARI programs fit his bias towards technical solutions to health problems.[48]

---

[45] Ibid.

[46] Deborah Mesce, "White House Hopes New Visa Policy Will End Boycott Threat," *The Associated Press*, April 14, 1990.

[47] Vitaly Makarchev, "World Health Assembly Session To Discuss Environment, AIDS," *TASS*, May 7, 1990.

[48] Lars Kallings, Interview by Michael Merson, New Haven, CT, September, 2002.

So, in the days immediately leading up to the WHA, Nakajima again asked me for-mally to take the position. This time, I accepted.

What convinced me to change my mind? As I reflected on it, I realized that my interest in the Johns Hopkins Deanship bespoke the fact that I was looking for an exciting new challenge; I now realized that there could be no greater challenge than the AIDS pandemic. I had strong support from Nakajima, the donors, and the United States government. Moreover, the more I thought about it, the more I came to real-ize that, while I might have another opportunity to lead a public health school (though maybe not of the caliber of Johns Hopkins), I may not have the chance to head another global program. And, of course, GPA was not just any global program. As Interim Director I had seen firsthand the impact the pandemic was having around the world, and playing a leadership role in the global response was a special oppor-tunity. Would it not be a remarkable achievement, I thought, if we could reverse the projections of up to 100 million persons infected with HIV through strong public health actions and find a cure or effective vaccine? I also thought that the manage-ment experience I had gained directing two WHO global programs and my good relationships with the WHO Regional Directors would allow me to better integrate GPA into WHO's infrastructure without compromising its delivery at regional and country levels.

Looking back, I realize that I approached this decision with a considerable amount of naiveté: I did not have AIDS expertise and had not met the experts in the field; I knew little about the history of the pandemic; and I did not appreciate the history and unique culture of GPA. I did not understand how much better it would have been if I had worked in the AIDS field before, and how valuable that background would be at times in building partnerships and making strategic decisions. As I had never even worked in the field of STDs, I underestimated how difficult it would be to change the behaviors that put persons at risk of HIV infection, and I was not fully aware of the depth that social determinants had on these behaviors. Moreover, I had no experience with the world of activism and, consequently, I did not realize how difficult it would be to gain the essential trust of AIDS activists (as Mann had) who were fighting hard for access to AIDS medicines and against intolerable AIDS discrimination practices. Additionally, I had little experience dealing with high media demands, and failed to appreciate the extent to which GPA required a strong media presence. Lastly, my managerial style at the time focused on performance and outcomes, and thus I could seem rather abrupt at times, particularly when compared to Mann's more personal approach. Mann and his team were very loyal to each other and I would be a culture shock for them.[49] Had I better understood some of these things, perhaps I would not have taken the position. But based on what I knew and felt at the time, I believe I would make the same decision again if presented with the same circumstances. Thus on May 4, 3 days before the WHA convened, I agreed to be the next Director of GPA and withdrew my candidature for the Deanship at Johns Hopkins School of Public Health. Johns Hopkins eventually selected Al Sommers for the position, and he served as an outstanding Dean for 15 years.

---

[49] Manuel Carballo, Interview by Michael Merson, New Haven, CT, November, 2002.

The response to my appointment was mixed. Outside GPA, in the professional public health community, many saw my appointment positively. "I think we feel bad about Jon[athan] Mann," Tom Quinn, Mann's close friend, *Projet SIDA* collaborator, and National Institutes for Health (NIH) infectious disease specialist, told reporters, "but I think Merson's a good choice ... No one's complaining about Merson."[50] D.A. Henderson, saw my appointment as a "strengthening move": "New institutions or programs often benefit from one type of individual to get them started," Henderson told reporters from the journal *Science*, "and they often require another type with another sort of orientation, management style, and skill to carry it on."[51]

Inside GPA and the larger AIDS community, however, my appointment generated considerable uncertainty. Some worried that I would "come in and decimate the behavioral side of things ... [that I] had no respect for the cultural or behavioral side."[52] Others felt that, as I knew nothing about AIDS, I had few legitimate claims to leading the program: "[Your appointment] was a surprise, because you were not one of 'us'—who had worked to build it up, in the AIDS world," remembered Lars Kallings. "... it would have been more natural to have a person who was in the HIV/AIDS field."[53] Even more critical, some understandably felt that I was aligned with Nakajima against Mann's human rights approach, favoring a more technical, biomedical strategy instead. "Nakajima was much more a technical person than a spiritual person," Kallings reflected. "He did not expect a cure, but [he envisioned] that some technical solution would be found ... a typical WHO solution. And you were the one who could help out, because you had that understanding of simple public health measures."[54]

Ultimately, then, many within GPA and the larger AIDS community viewed me as "Nakajima's man" who was going to change the direction of GPA, "and do draconian things."[55] I was largely unaware of the depth of these feelings, perhaps because I had implemented a strong behavioral component within the CDD program, and felt that I was being appointed by Nakajima largely on my merits as a successful program manager.[56] Only later on did it become clear how many would only see me through this "Nakajima's man" lens. This would pose particular problems for me going forward.

---

[50] Ann Gibbons, "New Head for the WHO Global Program on AIDS: do changes at the World Health Organization signal a new direction for its international AIDS program?" *Science*, June 15, 1990, 248:1306–7.

[51] Ibid.

[52] Thomas Coates, Interview by Michael Merson, New Haven, CT, February, 2002.

[53] Lars Kallings, Interview by Michael Merson, New Haven, CT, September, 2002.

[54] Ibid.

[55] Ibid.

[56] Thomas Coates, Interview by Michael Merson, New Haven, CT, February, 2002; Lars Kallings, Interview by Michael Merson, New Haven, CT, September, 2002.

Chapter 9
Enhancing Program Delivery

Monday, April 16, 1990, was Easter Monday, an official holiday at the World Health Organization (WHO) headquarters in Geneva. Still, I found myself working in my Global Programme on AIDS (GPA) office. The weather had been moderate and much of the building lay empty as WHO staff enjoyed a long weekend in the brisk Swiss air. The semi-solitude of the office gave me a chance to think, after what had been a whirlwind month as Interim Director of GPA. At my desk, with the reading light on against the cool gray sky in the window, I wrote a three-page memo to the Director-General, Hiroshi Nakajima, diagnosing GPA's present status and suggesting areas where I felt it required improvement.

Most of my thoughts seemed straightforward. I warned that the high incidence of AIDS[1] among certain populations portended disaster; AIDS demanded the unprecedented action WHO and its Member States had already taken and Nakajima could ill afford to expect otherwise. I also told him that GPA had developed strong alliances with the United Nations Development Programme (UNDP) and other United Nations (UN) agencies, and that these needed to continue for GPA to succeed. Furthermore, I cautioned him that he would have to be patient with GPA's regionalization process: the magnitude of AIDS and the limitations of the WHO regional and country offices meant that regionalization would need to proceed far more slowly than the Regional Directors preferred if GPA and WHO were to adequately address the pandemic and provide the necessary leadership.

GPA faced several obstacles to effectiveness, I informed Nakajima. National AIDS programs were so new that WHO had to be careful not to rush their integration into larger health programs. Most lacked managerial support, training, and guidelines for care, and many needed clearer targets and objectives towards which

---

Within this chapter the singular pronouns *I* and *my* refer to Michael Merson alone, whereas the plural pronouns *we* and *us* generally refer to Michael Merson and Stephen Inrig jointly. Where *we* or *us* refers to Michael Merson and his colleagues at WHO, the object of the pronoun is clarified by context.

[1] For the purposes of this text, we will use the term AIDS to encompass both AIDS and HIV unless otherwise specified.

© Springer International Publishing AG 2018

M. Merson, S. Inrig, *The AIDS Pandemic*, DOI 10.1007/978-3-319-47133-4_9

they could operate. GPA's organizational structure and reporting relationships within the larger WHO infrastructure were inefficient and needed improvement. I closed the letter with some suggestions for how to address these problems once someone was selected to take the helm of GPA.

I left the memo for my assistant to finalize (we did not have email in those days) and went away reflecting on what I had written. In its present iteration, I had some initial doubt as to whether GPA could effectively position itself to fight such a rapidly expanding pandemic; doing so effectively would require redirection and refinement. The question was whether GPA, WHO, and indeed the larger global health community, was up to the transformation that seemed necessary. I felt like there were five areas where our actions would be crucial: (1) containing the global spread of AIDS; (2) enhancing program delivery; (3) supporting research; (4) addressing human rights; and (5) improving coordination. As I made my way home, I pondered the fact that many of the issues I had mentioned in my memo to Nakajima had existed for some time. But I felt that if we made solid progress on these—while managing the unpredictable effect Mann's resignation might have on the program—GPA could really turn the tide on the pandemic. Now serving as the new Director of GPA, I was beginning to feel confident that I would be able to help make this happen.

To begin with, I was optimistic that I could navigate the internal politics of WHO, by which I mean the Regional Directors. Not long after Nakajima announced my appointment as Director of GPA, I found myself thinking about how to best work with them. I knew each very well, having collaborated closely with them when I led the Diarrheal Diseases Control (CDD) and Acute Respiratory Infections (ARI) programs. As we explained earlier, the Regional Directors (including Nakajima at the time) had found GPA's autonomy profoundly frustrating. With Mann's resignation—with new leadership atop GPA and a former Regional Director heading WHO—the Regional Directors saw an opportunity to reshape GPA more to their liking. This was a reminder—if not a realization—that GPA did not have the mandate to pursue whatever course it thought necessary to lead and coordinate the global response to the pandemic. It was clear that it would require more than epidemiological insight and evidence-based interventions. Delivering on AIDS at the global level would require navigating a host of obstacles standing in the way of effective program implementation.

I should add that the concerns of the Regional Directors were related to the key question on how WHO structured its operations and provided support to national AIDS programs. A long history lay behind these tension points: they stretched back at least to the 1976 World Health Assembly (WHA), when Director-General Halfdan Mahler had decentralized WHO's budgeting structure, radically shifting the percent of WHO's regular budget allocated to its regional and country offices from 30 to 70% and thereby enabling the regional offices to operate almost independently from WHO headquarters. Despite these changes, Mahler's strength of will, his leadership, and his "one WHO" philosophy kept WHO united. And, as we discussed in Chapter 4, Mahler and his senior policy advisor, Joe Cohen, were willing to situate programs, like GPA, in the Director-General's office and operate outside the WHO infrastructure. The Regional Directors did not view Mahler's decision on the placement of GPA and Mann's operational practices amicably, however, particularly in light of GPA's track record of providing little support to activities undertaken by regional and country offices.[2] They clearly supported the process of regionalization.[3]

As a former Regional Director, Nakajima certainly shared this desire for regionalization. Nakajima and the Regional Directors wanted GPA to complete the regionalization process to maintain organizational integrity: Nakajima argued that, if GPA continued operating outside the regional structure, it would inevitably balkanize WHO as a whole. Moreover, Nakajima's more restrained leadership style allowed the Regional Directors' push for autonomy to blossom.[4] Consequently, upon assuming his position, Nakajima began pressuring Mann to integrate GPA progressively back into the larger WHO infrastructure. In response, Mann and GPA had started integrating GPA's programs in five of WHO's six regions with some success (the exception being the African region).

This push for regionalization created considerable tension between WHO leadership and GPA staff and its donors.[5] GPA staffers, almost all of whom had been hired under Mann, worried that regionalization would hamper the global response to the pandemic and compromise progress in particularly hard-hit regions, especially in sub-Saharan Africa.[6]

Many of GPA's donors agreed with these concerns. With Mann gone, Nakajima in charge, and me at the helm of GPA, they felt regionalization would weaken the broad prevention perspective Mann had been able to implement directly from WHO headquarters.[7] Many held particular concerns about WHO's African regional office (AFRO): they doubted its capacity to support national AIDS programs effectively; they were concerned about the competence of its staff, since many had been appointed for political reasons; they suspected that regional and country WHO staff were spending GPA funds inappropriately; and they even worried that the regional office was rife with corruption. Unfortunately, Gottlieb Lobe Monekosso, AFRO's Regional Director, a Cameroonian physician, had done little to allay their fears when asked to address his region's performance in dealing with the AIDS pandemic at recent meetings of the GPA Management Committee (GMC), the Executive

---

[2] Michael Merson, "Report of the Director: Sixth meeting of the Management Committee, Geneva, 23–24 April 1991; Provisional agenda item 3," Geneva: Global Programme on AIDS, GPA/GMC(1)/91.3; 22 April 1991.

[3] Michael Merson, "Report of the Director, Fifth Meeting of the Management Committee, November 26, 1990" Geneva: World Health Organization GPA/GMC(2) 90.3, 1990.

[4] Fiona Godlee, "The World Health Organisation: The regions—too much power, too little effect." *BMJ* 1994, 10 December, 309:1566–1570; Fiona Godlee, "The World Health Organisation: WHO at country level—a little impact, no strategy," *BMJ* 17 December 1994; 309:1636–1639.

[5] Michael Merson, "Report of the Director, Sixth Meeting of the Management Committee, April 1991," Geneva: World Health Organization GPA/GMC; Gill Walt, Interview by Stephen Inrig, Dallas, TX, September 23, 2010.

[6] Gary Slutkin, "Global AIDS 1981–1999: The Response [The Pittsfield Lecture]," *The International Journal of Tuberculosis and Lung Disease* 4, no. 2 (February 1, 2000): S24–33.

[7] Gill Walt, Interview by Stephen Inrig, Dallas, TX, September 23, 2010.

Board, and WHA.[8] Moreover, AFRO's location in war-torn Brazzaville made it a difficult office with which to communicate, much less visit. Having broad experience supporting country programs in Africa through the regional office during my time with CDD, I knew that the regionalization process would be difficult to achieve, but at least initially I truly believed GPA could do it.

I had made it a priority in the first 6 months of my tenure with GPA to meet with representatives from almost all the donor nations to secure their ongoing support and raise, if possible, their overall contributions. This was not a difficult task, as I knew many of them from my time in CDD and ARI and our relationships for the most part were strong. Their intent to continue their ongoing support heartened me during those meetings, although a few indicated they did plan to scale back their contributions. As a whole, the donors were clear about what they desired from GPA: they wanted to see their funds driving HIV and AIDS rates down; they wanted GPA to ensure that the national program plans were effective, particularly in Africa; and they wanted a more coordinated global response to the pandemic.[9] This last desire had important implications for the regionalization process and how GPA worked within WHO, as well as with other UN agencies (as we shall see in Chapter 14). While we assured the donors that GPA shared these commitments, we soon learned that a few important donor nations had started thinking about alternative global governance structures for responding to the pandemic.

In the meantime, GPA continued pursuing regionalization. Some donors suggested GPA regionalize everywhere besides Africa, but we knew that regionalizing GPA *except* for AFRO would have been politically impossible. Monekosso would merely have protested the move in WHA and the 51 countries in his region would have supported him. What was unclear was whether GPA could create transparent and credible processes by which regionalization could be successfully achieved in Africa.

The first step in pursuing regionalization, while maintaining donor confidence, was to establish procedures preventing the misuse of donor funds. In the first 6 months of my tenure, then, I visited all the regional offices, including two trips to AFRO in Brazzaville. My goal was to understand the office better and assure myself about AFRO's capacity to operationally and financially manage GPA's collaboration in the region. I then arranged for a senior level administrative support team to visit AFRO to review its progress towards regionalization.[10] We also put in place, as requested by GMC, an interim review of progress in the African Region, the results of which we presented to the GMC in the spring of 1991. The review team was satisfied that no substantial or insurmountable problem existed in AFRO's financial management; supply management; technical staff; and staff management. It also

---

[8] Michael Merson, "Report of the Director: Sixth meeting of the Management Committee, Geneva, 23–24 April 1991; Provisional agenda item 3," Geneva: Global Programme on AIDS, GPA/GMC(1)/91.3; 22 April 1991, 16.

[9] Michael Merson, "Report of the Director, Fifth Meeting of the Management Committee, November 26, 1990" Geneva: World Health Organization GPA/GMC(2) 90.3, 1990.

[10] Ibid.

instructed us to continue the regionalization process using the criteria that the team had endorsed for transferring country responsibilities from Geneva to AFRO.[11]

To facilitate the transfer of country responsibilities from Geneva to AFRO, I tasked Gunilla Ernberg, (a Swedish lawyer who had served as one of Daniel Tarantola's administrative officers and had overseen GPA support to national programs in two regions) with monitoring AFRO's financial reports and records. AFRO's finances were particularly complicated during Mann's tenure because AFRO countries managed their accounts using a different format than GPA. This administrative inefficiency was worsened by frequent expenditure discrepancies between GPA and AFRO country reports.[12] Ernberg set out to rectify much of this.

Ernberg established a team that formally approved each African country for regionalization, which meant that it was ready to fall under the responsibility of AFRO. She developed a comprehensive and deliberate process, which was understandably time consuming. Once a country met her team's criteria, Ernberg or a member of her team would visit the country to confirm this was the case. I trusted Ernberg and her team fully. I had always admired her diligence and devotion to GPA, and felt that we had established a system that prevented corruption and misuse of funds. I realized that the process was not perfect, but we never found funds being deliberately mismanaged and never hesitated to withdraw funds from a project if we felt it was warranted. On one occasion, for example, we found that a small regional project that cost about $80,000 was being poorly managed and promptly halted payments.[13] Despite these measures, it was a tough sell convincing some of our donors we had met their standard of integrity. By September 1991, we had made significant progress, successfully regionalizing 25 countries in the African region; we still had to manage 19 countries from GPA headquarters because they had not yet fully met our criteria. Nevertheless the GMC began expressing "serious reservations about the capacity of the regional office to cope with the workload created by regionalization."[14] I think, however, that Ernberg accomplished as much as anyone could have done in this particular task.

Ernberg's assignment represented just one of the many ways I set about to reorganize GPA to improve its performance and management. As we mentioned, Mann had already initiated a reorganization of the headquarters staff a few months before he resigned, and, during my interim period as Director, I had drawn up for Nakajima

---

[11] Interim Review Team "Interim Review of Regionalization of GPA Technical Cooperation Activities in the African Region: Provisional agenda item 5; Sixth meeting of the Management Committee, Geneva. 23–24 April, 1991, Geneva: Global Programme on AIDS, GPA/GMC(1)/91.11, 21 March 1991.

[12] Global Programme on AIDS, *Report of the External Review of the World Health Organization, Global Programme on AIDS,* Geneva: World Health Organization, January 1992, p. 13.

[13] Mort Rosenblum, "U.N. AIDS-Fighting Agency Having Problems; With AIDS-Losing Battle." *The Associated Press,* July 5, 1992.

[14] Report of the Seventh Meeting of the Management Committee, 19–21 November, 1991, WHO; Global Programme on AIDS, *Report of the External Review of the World Health Organization, Global Programme on AIDS,* Geneva: World Health Organization, January 1992, p. 30.

a revised and simplified organizational structure.[15] That first summer as head of GPA, I asked Walt Dowdle from the Centers for Disease Control and Prevention (CDC) to return to Geneva (he had helped me tremendously in the days immediately following Mann's resignation) to give me his advice and assistance on this reorganization and other matters. Dowdle was indispensable in helping me streamline GPA's structure in ways that best met its objectives. The resulting plan created five divisions under the GPA Director: Programme Management; Policy Coordination; Epidemiological and Biomedical Research; Strategy and Intervention Development; and National Program Support (see Fig. 9.1).[16] I obtained approval for this revised reorganization plan from Nakajima and began the process of implementing it during the late summer and early fall of 1990.

Crucial in this regard—particularly with respect to learning about the staff at GPA and how it had operated over the previous 3 years—was Mann's closest colleague in GPA, Kathleen Kay. Kay as described in Chapter 4, was an Australian nurse who, soon after graduating from nursing school, had carved out a career for herself writing medical articles, disease treatment manuals, and public health curricula. By the mid-1980s, she had become consumed by the problem of AIDS and began researching and writing about the topic. In the fall of 1986, she set up a breakfast meeting between herself, then an aide to the Australian Health Minister, and Mann, when he was visiting the country to attend an AIDS conference. After their meeting, Mann invited her to join GPA and used money from Mahler's discretionary fund to bring her on as a technical writer. As we described earlier, she was his chief strategist in the development and articulation of the Global AIDS Strategy. Kay had initially stepped down 3 days after Mann's resignation in a show of solidarity with him and in protest of Nakajima, but she approached me very soon after I was appointed Interim Director and graciously offered to remain in the program for 3 months to help guide me during this difficult transition period. I think she did this out of loyalty to the staff and GPA. For her help and generosity of spirit I was, and I am to this day, extremely grateful.

The most important piece of advice that Kay gave me, besides graciously navigating me through the program staff, was to recommend removing Yugi Kawaguchi from my reporting hierarchy to the Director-General. Kawaguchi, as we mentioned in Chapter 7, had severely limited Mann's operational effectiveness and access to Nakajima. Kay's advice seemed so wise at the time that I made it a key condition for accepting the GPA Directorship, and I believe the fact that I reported directly to Nakajima—rather than through a surrogate—helped to give me much more programmatic freedom than Mann had under Nakajima.

---

[15] Note for the Record, Meeting held with GPA staff on 2 July 1990, GPA reorganization. I based the reorganization on three factors: (1) the priorities of the program as established in its formative documents and approved Global AIDS Strategy; (2) consultations with unit chiefs, regional directors, donor organizations, associated UN agency heads, collaborating researchers, Health Ministers, and other WHO leadership and staff; and (3) the style of management I preferred.

[16] Global Programme on AIDS, Proposed Organization Structure, n.d. unpublished document.

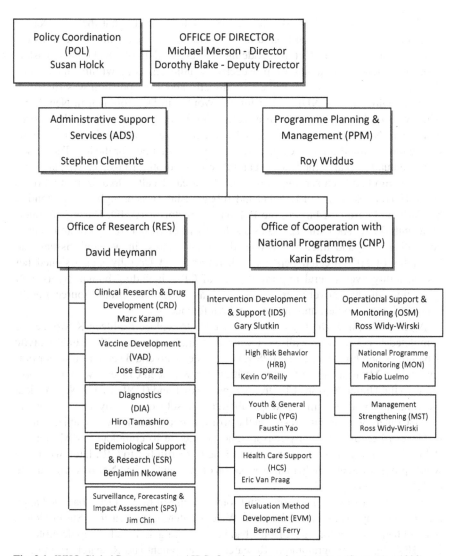

Fig. 9.1 WHO Global Programme on AIDS: Organization at headquarters (September 1990)

As I was receiving help from Kay, I was recruiting others to join me. One of my urgent needs was to find a Deputy Director to replace Hans Emblad. Emblad had also been very supportive during my transition to GPA, but had eventually decided to leave the program and become Director of WHO's Program on Substance Abuse. While this was a great opportunity for Emblad and a position for which he was highly suited, it gave me the difficult task of replacing a very important position early on in my term as Director.

The question was, whom should I choose? I felt, ideally, that the new Deputy Director should be a woman from a low- or middle-income country to serve as my counterbalance and to reflect the pandemic's future epidemiological course. I asked many colleagues for names of prospective candidates both within and outside WHO. One person who approached me directly about the position was Elizabeth Reid, the Director of UNDP's Division for Women in Development in New York, when we met for the first time at a welcoming reception for me at UNDP headquarters in New York. I did not know Reid, and since I was looking for someone from a low- or middle-income country, I did not consider her for the job. The person who eventually became the leading candidate was Dorothy Blake, a physician from Jamaica who had been serving as the Pan American Health Organization (PAHO) and WHO representative in Trinidad and Tobago. Blake was brought to my attention by Carlyle Guerra de Macedo, the Regional Director of PAHO. During my interview with Blake, she came across as a solid manager with a strong commitment to combating the pandemic. She also had a keen interest in women's issues and the rights of HIV-infected persons. I therefore hired Dorothy and assigned her responsibility over several important areas of GPA, including human rights, collaboration with non-governmental organizations (NGOs), external resource mobilization, advisory bodies, and international conferences.[17]

Along with a new Deputy Director, I needed to replace Kathleen Kay once she completed her 3 months with us. I wanted to find someone with strong analytic capabilities and knowledge of AIDS-related issues who could serve as a senior policy advisor. My first choice for this position was Kathleen Cravero, who was working with the United Nations Children's Emergency Fund (UNICEF) in New York at the time and with whom I had collaborated closely during my last 3 years in CDD. Cravero was very interested in the position, but in the end was unable to move to Geneva because of family reasons and her desire to complete her Masters of Public Health degree at Columbia. I was able to recruit her to GPA later, when she would prove invaluable help in the formation of the Joint United Nations Programme on HIV/AIDS (UNAIDS).

Now concerned whether I could find someone else of her caliber, I had the happy fortune one day, while eating lunch in WHO's cafeteria, to run into Susan Holck, whom I had not seen for years. Holck had been working as a medical epidemiologist in WHO's Special Programme of Research, Development and Research Training in Human Reproduction for a number of years, conducting research related to female contraceptive use, and, like myself, had previously worked at CDC in Atlanta. In the midst of our conversation, it struck me that she might be a perfect fit as a policy adviser and I spontaneously asked her if she might be interested in joining GPA. We met a few times after this to discuss the position and I became more and more convinced she would be the ideal person to lead our policy coordination office. However, she was not sure she was ready to give up her research. I must have worn her down because, after repeated requests on my part, she agreed to join GPA as our senior policy advisor. I soon learned that my instincts about her were correct. She worked

---

[17] Ibid.

tirelessly on the many critical policy questions that we faced, and I came to rely on her to develop sound policy guidelines through consensus and to ensure the accuracy of all our publications. There were few persons in GPA whose judgment I trusted more.

I also needed to replace Daniel Tarantola, who headed National Program Support. Unlike Mann, Kay, and Emblad, who resigned from GPA on their own volition, Tarantola's departure would be the only high-level change associated with my reorganization effort. It was one of the most difficult decisions I ever had to make. Tarantola, as we mention in Chapter 4, had a long history in WHO and I knew him well, our having worked together when I led the CDD program. Tarantola had been critical to GPA's support of the first national AIDS programs in many countries in late 1986 and early 1987, and had led this effort thereafter. Moreover, he was greatly admired and even revered by almost all GPA staff. But he also bore much responsibility—perhaps even more than Mann—for the sometimes tense relationship between GPA and the WHO regional and country office staff that GPA's operational autonomy had created. My dilemma was this: I felt I had to respond to the concerns expressed by the Regional Directors about the autonomous way GPA had been operating at the country level and to reintegrate the program into WHO's larger structure, and I had doubts we could achieve this if Tarantola remained as head of National Program Support.

Before making a final decision, however, I thought I should seek advice from the Deputy Director-General, Mohamed Abdelmoumene, since they knew each other well and I trusted Abdelmoumene's political judgment. We discussed it and his view was that it would be best to find an alternative leadership position for Tarantola. Since he was both a colleague of Tarantola and a fellow francophone, Abdelmoumene felt he was better suited than I to explain this decision to him. Also, and most importantly, as Deputy Director-General, he could offer Tarantola a new position as Chief of WHO'S Relief and Rehabilitation Unit within WHO's Emergency Response Program. This position would give Tarantola the opportunity to carry out assessment, planning, and other technical missions in the context of rehabilitation of health systems in countries affected by war, a position consistent with his pre-WHO experience serving in emergency humanitarian medical missions in Africa.

To this day, I do not know exactly what Abdelmoumene said to Tarantola. I only know, having spoken with Abdelmoumene many years later,[18] that he remembers telling him it would be "good for everyone" and "best for him in the long term" if Tarantola were to leave GPA and assume leadership of the Relief and Rehabilitation Unit, and that Tarantola seemed to welcome this opportunity. Moreover, if Tarantola would have objected to this plan, Abdelmoumene explained, he would have explored other possibilities for him.[19] It seems hard to imagine that Tarantola welcomed this decision, having given so much of his time and energy to GPA, but perhaps Nakajima's track record and the programmatic changes portended by my presence may have made him think otherwise. More likely than not, this move, like Mann's resignation, was deeply painful for Tarantola. It certainly provoked an outcry among

---

[18] Meetings with Mohamed Abdelmoumene (MA), October 28, 2014, Geneva, Switzerland.
[19] Ibid.

his supporters,[20] and the fact that Tarantola left WHO a year later (in 1991) to join Mann at Harvard University's School of Public Health leaves me to think that he received the decision to move out of GPA more poorly than Abdelmoumene would have had me believe.

Was this the right decision? On reflection, I realize how impactful a decision this was, one that influenced the entire program and many GPA staff less than 4 weeks into my Directorship. Could I have handled this differently? When Abdelmoumene told me, "let me do it," I knew that both he and Nakajima wanted it done, and that they were trying to take the heat off me. But in retrospect, I think I should have spoken face to face with Tarantola about my concerns and given him an opportunity to convince me that he could have stayed on. I do not know if my decision would have been any different, what with the Regional Directors being so firm in their views. But I believe the way we did it … I did it … made Tarantola resent me more than he might have if I had spoken with him myself. Certainly, it did nothing to improve my relationship with Mann, which was now—perhaps in part because of this—starting to deteriorate. This became quite clear when, soon after we had informed Tarantola of our decision, Mann left an angry message for me with Penny Ratcliff, my assistant, who had previously worked for Mann, informing me of his extreme disappointment at Tarantola's transfer out of GPA.[21]

Tarantola's departure from GPA was as great a loss, in operational terms, as the loss of Mann's leadership. To replace him as head of National Program Support, I recruited Karin Edstrom, a Swedish obstetrician, who had worked for more than a decade at WHO headquarters in the Maternal and Child Health and Family Planning Unit. She was an expert in adolescent reproductive health and had much experience working with WHO regional and country offices, including those in the Africa region. Edstrom led the reorganization process for National Program Support over the summer and early fall of 1990 and quickly found that she had her hands full trying to fill Tarantola's shoes. Anyone would have.

Another challenge I faced was to find a place for Lars Kallings. Kallings had expressed his desire to join the program soon after I became Director. He had been an early and persistent warrior in confronting the pandemic: he was serving at the time as Chair of the Global Commission on AIDS, was the founder and first President (1988–1990) of the International AIDS Society, had been Director-General of the Swedish National Institute for Infectious Disease Control (1982–1988), and had served as Vice Chairman of the WHO Executive Board (1988–1990). Indeed, I suspect he would have applied to be Director of GPA had he not felt that an American would be selected for the position. Kallings told me that he wanted more than a "ceremonial role" and preferred to "coordinate research development."[22] In the end, we agreed he would serve as my Scientific Advisor, a position for which I felt he was well suited, given his long-standing involvement in scientific and policy affairs related to AIDS.

---

[20] Jonathan Mann, "Message to Michael Merson," May 30 1990.

[21] Ibid.

[22] Letter for Lars Kallings to Michael Merson, May 30, 1990.

In addition to making these key hires, I asked Stephen Clemente and his administrative team to update the job descriptions of all our program staff. At the start of GPA, to accommodate rapid program growth, WHO had waived some of its recruitment and staffing rules in its hiring practices. This allowed GPA to respond rapidly to the pandemic, but it also created some confusion and overlap in scope of authority and responsibility. As part of the reorganization, we reviewed these job descriptions to ensure every position adequately spelt out its justification and responsibilities. I felt this reorganization helped GPA better implement our programmatic priorities while resolving some logistical issues. For example, it reduced programmatic fragmentation for those within and outside GPA and removed the job insecurity for those staff previously working under temporary contracts, leading I hoped to a more secure and productive workforce.[23]

Besides Tarantola, I did not ask any other GPA staff to leave the program. Some did, of course, leave of their own accord. But the state of affairs in which I found myself does beg the question of whether, in such a management situation, one should replace senior and mid-level managers on assuming the Directorship of an agency or institution. As Stef Bertozzi (whom I would later recruit to lead GPA's policy work and would replace me as GPA Director) reflected, GPA was built up as an "OXFAM within the UN system."[24] By this he meant it had been a program that had attracted staff fiercely committed to fighting the pandemic and intensely loyal to GPA and Jonathan Mann, with little interest in achieving managerial efficiency or measuring program effectiveness. They also, under Mann's leadership, had been told to consider themselves as distinct from WHO. As Jose Esparza recalled, "I remember that Jonathan didn't like us to refer to ourselves at WHO, but GPA...Very often when I wrote WHO, it was scratched and replaced by GPA."[25]

This school of managerial thought would have encouraged me to "clean house" when I arrived, to bring in new individuals to fill senior and mid-level management positions. I did not think this was a good idea then, and reflecting back I still believe that today. Such a move would have been too disruptive and would likely have crippled the program. Even if there are cases where such wholescale change might be in order, GPA was not one of them: the expertise of the GPA staff was unmatched in the world and having more of them leave would have needlessly fed the already growing perception that I was Nakajima's man and stood against all that Mann had established and achieved. My hope, rather, was that I could continue to build the program and in time gain the confidence of the staff. To that end, upon the advice of Walt Dowdle, I began convening daily morning meetings with GPA's senior management staff to build trust, foster teamwork, and gain organizational efficiency. The senior staff had not worked in that way before, and had been brought together only under extraordinary circumstances so I felt such an intentional, cohesion-building practice would benefit all of us. This practice, which we started in the

---

[23] Note for the Record, Meeting held with GPA staff on 2 July 1990, GPA reorganization.

[24] Stefano Bertozzi, Interview by Michael Merson, Cuernavaca, May 15, 2005.

[25] Jose Esparza, Interview by Michael Merson Seattle, WA, October, 2001.

Table 9.1 GPA technical assistance, 1988–1991

	Jan. 88	Jan. 89	Jan. 90	Jan. 91
Technical visits	111	152	159	169
STPs	75	118	123	130
MTPs	26	51	95	113
Resource mobilization meetings	5	29	65	87
Programme reviews		1	10	34

Source: Reprinted from "Report of the External Review of the World Health Organization Global Programme on AIDS, January 1992, page 9"

summer of 1990, allowed us to exchange information on a daily basis about the most urgent issues and challenges facing the program and to discuss how we would go about planning and strengthening our activities. I am not sure these meetings ever helped me build the trust that I had hoped for; earning that trust would prove difficult and time was short.

One of the most important areas I gave my full attention was the planning of national AIDS programs. GPA had helped countries launch their national programs through short-term plans (STPs) beginning in late 1986 and early 1987. Every country with a national program started with such a plan, followed soon thereafter by the development of 3-year medium-term plans (MTPs), and some of these were just coming up for review as I began my time at GPA (Table 9.1). The first MTP reviews were to be in countries such as Tanzania, Kenya, Ethiopia, Senegal, Zambia, Bhutan, Nepal, Sri Lanka, and Thailand.[26] With such an extensive list of countries due for review over the next several months and even more on the horizon, we began preparing ourselves to help these countries transition smoothly from their initial MTPs to new ones (which we termed second-generation MTPs) that were to be more efficient, targeted, sustainable, and multisectoral in their design.

National program planning had been one of GPA's strengths from the beginning. Tarantola and his team had, early on, created a standardized approach to planning to help countries get up and running. This was necessary given the number and speed at which new programs were being initiated. However, GPA had not updated this approach to take into account the latest knowledge about the epidemiology of AIDS and best practices on prevention and care (see Chapter 11).

Consequently, we developed a new approach for the planning process: one that was both simpler and more sophisticated; strengthened the public health focus of national programs; and could be used to formally train national program managers. As a first step, we crafted a public health framework for an ideal national AIDS program and provided program managers with a series of steps for implementing

---

[26] 1991 Progress Report, Global Programme on AIDS, WHO, Geneva; GPA Progress Reports; Global Programme on AIDS, *Report of the External Review of the World Health Organization, Global Programme on AIDS,* Geneva: World Health Organization, January 1992, p. 9.

its constituent parts.[27] For example, we prepared tools to determine prevalence rates in the general population. If these rates were high, we encouraged epidemiological surveillance, blood safety, and broad-based campaigns; if rates were low, we recommended interventions targeting high-risk groups. Then, we developed a menu of proven strategies and interventions from which program managers could select according to the needs of their country's epidemic. For countries with high sexual transmission prevalence, we stressed condom use and safer-sex promotion; for countries with high drug-related prevalence, we encouraged harm reduction strategies and the promotion of safe sex practices. We linked each of these interventions to the primary objectives of our idealized framework.[28] All this allowed countries greater flexibility and tailoring of their programs to meet their individual epidemiological situations. Finally, we offered a set of priority prevention indicators and simple evaluation methods that countries could employ to monitor their activities and assess the extent to which they were meeting their targets.[29] Our plan was to package these steps into a program planning process that enabled each national program manager to proceed through them in ways appropriate to their context.[30]

The revision in MTP preparation was thus coupled with plans to improve management of national programs. Personally, I viewed improved management as central to the success of national programs. National AIDS program managers and mid-level district supervisors needed more information on how to set program priorities, establish program targets, and evaluate progress towards those targets.[31] GPA needed to do a better job of providing national program managers with this type of guidance. Their STPs and MTPs were deficient in sound management practices, particularly around priority setting and budgeting. Many GPA staff and long-term consultants in countries were epidemiologists and often themselves lacked training and experience in planning, leading, and implementing large-scale programs, and many national AIDS program managers likewise did not have the requisite skills and experience.[32]

Our plan was to train our program managers on these basic management concepts following the framework described above (a principle that was followed later

---

[27] Michael Merson, "Report of the Director: Sixth meeting of the Management Committee, Geneva, 23–24 April 1991; Provisional agenda item 3," Geneva: Global Programme on AIDS, GPA/GMC(1)/91.3; 22 April 1991, 16.

[28] WHO/GPA Recommended Objectives, Strategies, Interventions and Activity Areas for National AIDS Programmes, 10 April 1991.

[29] Michael Merson, "Report of the Director: Sixth meeting of the Management Committee, Geneva, 23–24 April 1991; Provisional agenda item 3," Geneva: Global Programme on AIDS, GPA/GMC(1)/91.3; 22 April 1991, 16.

[30] Michael Merson, "Report of the Director, Fifth Meeting of the Management Committee, November 26, 1990" Geneva: World Health Organization GPA/GMC(2) 90.3, 1990.

[31] Michael Merson, "Director's Report, GPA Management Committee, April 26, 1990," Geneva: World Health Organization, 1990.

[32] Global Programme on AIDS, Report of the External Review of the World Health Organization, Global Programme on AIDS, Geneva: World Health Organization, January 1992, p. 14.

on by UNAIDS in its appeal to "know your epidemic"[33]). I knew from experience that it would take a couple of years to develop a suitable program management course. In the meantime, as a bridging step, we decided in early 1991 to strengthen our provision of technical and financial support to countries. This included the organization of several week-long workshops for GPA technical officers assigned to African, Asian, and Latin American countries that were aimed at simplifying the development, implementation, accountability, and evaluation of MTPs.[34]

Much of the impetus for such a management approach to planning came out of my experience in the CDD Program. There we had developed a course that taught national CDD program managers how to define their diarrheal diseases problem, select the most relevant interventions, decide on priorities, set targets for their program, monitor progress towards those targets, and evaluate the effectiveness of the program in reducing diarrheal mortality, hospitalization, and morbidity. Before I left the ARI program, a very similar course was under development for program managers of national ARI programs. I don't claim being innovative in using this approach: I learned about it from Ralph Henderson, the Director of the Expanded Programme on Immunization (EPI), shortly after I arrived at WHO in 1978 and I give him credit for introducing it to WHO. As I pushed the development of the course in GPA, I soon realized there were others who saw little value in this approach to planning. Some viewed it as too "American", which to some extent it may have been. Others felt AIDS was primarily a development issue, and that GPA should place priority on actions that reduced poverty and ensured gender equality rather than on public health approaches to reduce transmission. Still others felt the course did not sufficiently take into account the human rights framework they believed critical to AIDS prevention and care, though I was very open to including this content in the course if we received guidance on how to operationalize this framework in national programs.

Despite these concerns and objections, I moved forward with the preparation of the course as I believed it was essential to bring these solid management principles into national AIDS programs. Thus, during 1990 and 1991, I worked with Bob Hogan, Patsy Whitesell (a training specialist whom I had previously hired to write the CDD program managers training course), and others to develop a course that would bring management skills to high-level national and regional AIDS program staff, senior health ministry officials, directors of national NGOs, and leaders from key professional groups involved in implementing national AIDS programs. By the end of 1991 we had completed drafts for many of the instructional modules, but we were not ready to field test the course until mid-1992. I put much of my own time

---

[33] "UNAIDS Annual Report 2007"Geneva: Joint United Nations Programme on HIV/AIDS (UNAIDS) 2008 UNAIDS/08.21E / JC1535E www.unaids.org/en/media/unaids/contentassets/dataimport/pub/report/2008/jc1535_annual_report07_en.pdf

[34] Michael Merson, "Report of the Director: Sixth meeting of the Management Committee, Geneva, 23–24 April 1991; Provisional agenda item 3," Geneva: Global Programme on AIDS, GPA/GMC(1)/91.3; 22 April 1991, 16.

into this effort—even leading the field test of the course—because I wanted to emphasize the importance I placed on a serious approach to planning.[35]

We completed the course in early 1993, translated it into French and Spanish, and helped the regional offices organize courses for national AIDS program managers. We also started preparing a similar course for mid-level managers (as the CDD and EPI programs had successfully done). Unfortunately, because of all that transpired over the next 2 years, we never completed it. Nor did we ever fully overcome the resistance described above to these types of management courses. Nonetheless, we remained committed to using a sound public health approach within national AIDS programs, setting measurable and attainable targets, and providing appropriate approaches that low- and middle-income countries could implement to reach these targets in the short, medium, and long term.

While there was no hard evidence to prove this, we at GPA believed these efforts helped countries make significant progress in their planning efforts which, as illustrated in the next chapter, improved the outcomes of their programs. Beginning in 1991 with Tanzania, and often with the advice and assistance of GPA staff, countries began planning their second-generation MTPs, which as noted above were more multisectoral in orientation than the first plans. By December 1993, almost 60 countries had prepared such plans, often using the Facilitator's Guide from the GPA program management course. Near the end of 1993, Erik Blas, a hard working Danish national who directed this area of activity, convened a meeting of AIDS program managers from five African countries to review this planning process, the report of which laid out recommendations that provided important guidance for program planning.[36]

We also supported external reviews of many national AIDS programs. This process had been a priority for Tarantola and his team, and under his direction, GPA supported 14 such reviews by July 1990 (in 13 African countries and Thailand). By 1993, the program had supported 110 such reviews and another 55 were conducted over the next 2 years. A report issued in 1994 indicated that these reviews had provided "a useful management tool in the program cycle of first generation national AIDS programs."[37] In particular, they had "provided an official forum to raise concerns and criticisms, had directed public and private attention to the AIDS problem,…and had sharpened the focus of national AIDS programs on priority program areas, clarified roles and management issues, and sped up program implementation."[38] A key recommendation of the report was that national AIDS programs should

---

[35] Ibid.; Dr. M.H. Merson, "WHO European Regional Meeting on Psychosocial Aspects of HIV/AIDS and Evaluation of Prevention Strategies" LISBON, 1 JUNE 1990, mhml/l June 1990, 2; Michael Merson, "Report of the Director, Fifth Meeting of the Management Committee, November 26, 1990" Geneva: World Health Organization GPA/GMC(2) 90.3, 1990.

[36] Review of experiences in five countries in planning and managing multisectoral AIDS programmes, WHO/GPA GPA/CNP/OSM 10 December 1993.

[37] Report of the Study of the Process for NAP Reviews (1989–1993), Global Program on AIDS, Geneva, October 1994.

[38] Ibid.

conduct a single review rather than undertaking multiple reviews at the request of individual funding agencies,[39] a policy that was also later advocated strongly by UNAIDS.[40]

One area where I felt GPA could have an important early impact was blood safety. At the beginning of GPA, Mann and his team devoted considerable attention and resources in support of the Global Blood Safety Initiative (GBSI). GBSI was a cooperative endeavor to help countries develop safe and effective blood transfusion services. Its core participants included GPA, the WHO unit of Health Laboratory Technology, the United Nations Development Programme (UNDP), the League of Red Cross and Red Crescent Societies (now called the International Federation of Red Cross and Red Crescent Societies), and the International Society of Blood Transfusion. GBSI established several important programs, including the identification of several "accelerated strategies" for reducing transfusion-related HIV transmission and developed a checklist of "essential consumables and equipment necessary to collect, process, store and distribute blood and blood products safely."[41] Jean Emmanuel, a Zimbabwean physician, was working on these projects when I arrived, and he recognized early on that we needed to enhance our support at the national level in the area of blood safety. He developed training materials for use in national transfusion services, established blood safety review mechanisms at national level, and brought about great credibility for WHO and GPA in this area.

Ultimately, GBSI closed down in 1993 and this area of work was turned over to WHO's Blood Transfusion Safety Unit under Emmanuel's leadership. However, GPA continued to assist many countries in establishing national blood transfusion advisory committees and worked with this Unit to develop distance learning materials for program staff and managers at the national level responsible for prevention of blood-borne HIV transmission.[42] GPA also produced (often in conjunction with the League of Red Cross and Red Crescent Societies) several additional training materials to support blood and blood donor safety.[43] Though blood transfusion was responsible at the time for only 6–10 % of HIV infections globally, swift action to advance the safety of blood transfusions would turn out to be one of the major accomplishments of GPA's prevention and control efforts.

Also, and most importantly, with the number of reported AIDS cases increasing dramatically, particularly in sub-Saharan Africa, GPA began thinking more holistically about provision of care for people with HIV and AIDS. While in the

---

[39] Ibid.

[40] *"Three ONEs" Key Principles.* Geneva: UNAIDS, 2004, Conference Paper 1, Washington Consultation 25.04.04; http://data.unaids.org/UNA-docs/Three-Ones_KeyPrinciples_en.pdf

[41] World Health Organization, "WHO Global Programme on AIDS 1987–1995: Final Report with Emphasis on 1994–95 Biennium" (Geneva: World Health Organization, May 1997), 23.

[42] *Preventing HIV Transmission through blood and Blood Products (Including Nosocomial Transmission)* WHO/GPA/CNP/93.2 A-E.

[43] *Guidelines on Costing of Blood Transfusion Services* (WHO/GPA/BLS/95.2; *Guidelines for Blood Donor Counselling on HIV* (WHO/GPA/TCO/HCS/94.2); *Recruiting, Educating and Retaining Safe Blood Donors* (WHO/GPA/BLS/95.1), pp. 24–25.

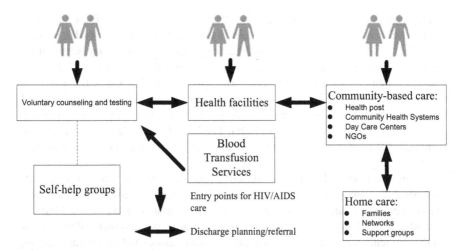

Fig. 9.2 The HIV/AIDS Continuum of Care. Source: Reprinted from Global Programme on AIDS 1987–1995. Final report with emphasis on 1994–1995 Biennium, page 32. WHO 1997. http://apps. who.int/iris/bitstream/10665/65955/1/WHO_ASD_97.1.pdf

early 1990s various antiretroviral drugs (ARVs) were emerging as possible treatment for HIV infection and AIDS, there was no evidence at that stage that effective treatment would soon be available. Consequently, GPA felt compelled to develop a care approach that was primarily supportive and palliative. In light of this, we articulated a "Comprehensive Care Across the Continuum" paradigm that examined the comprehensive care needs of people with AIDS and enunciated the "coordinat[ion] and pooling [of] medical and social services, and creat[ion] of care-giving linkages between conventional medical facilities and social services and NGOs" (Fig. 9.2).[44] Eric Van Praag, an energetic Dutch public health specialist with enormous overseas experience (he had worked for 8 years in Tanzania and Bangladesh before serving as the WHO Team Leader in Zambia from 1988 to 1991) lead this effort.[45] He and his team organized, in September 1994, an initial consultation of a wide range of experts, including persons living with AIDS (PLWAs), to identify and prioritize mechanisms for providing AIDS care across the continuum (i.e., from home to health facility). The conclusion of this meeting (*Provision of HIV/AIDS Care in Resource Constrained Settings*)[46] called on governments to include care for AIDS patients in their heath development plans, collaborate with NGOs in meeting the health needs of PLWAs, and encourage

---

[44] Michael Merson, "Report of the Director: Sixth meeting of the Management Committee, Geneva, 23–24 April 1991; Provisional agenda item 3," Geneva: Global Programme on AIDS, GPA/GMC(1)/91.3; 22 April 1991, 32–34.

[45] Eric van Praag now serves, at the time of this writing, as the Senior Regional Technical Adviser for FHI 360 living in Tanzania).

[46] *Provision of HIV/AIDS Care in Resource Constrained Settings* (WHO/GPA/TCO/HCS/95.14).

implementation research on continuum of care. Recognizing that there was enormous variation between national health systems, GPA also created a process whereby national AIDS programs could tailor general clinical management guidelines to the realities of local conditions. This "Nominal Group Process" approach brought together a nationally representative group of health professionals to provide comprehensive insight into care processes in an individual country.[47] GPA led workshops on the development and operationalization of this continuum of care model and launched studies in India, Thailand, Ghana, Zambia, Uganda, and Kenya to gauge the feasibility and sustainability of this approach in resource-limited settings.[48]

Having developed this framework, GPA provided various kinds of support to national AIDS programs as they articulated the numerous steps and transitions in the continuum of care. For example, we urged programs to encourage high-risk individuals, like female sex workers and injection drug users, to seek AIDS care and STD treatment and conducted studies on the factors associated with health-seeking behavior.[49] For AIDS counselors and their trainers, GPA developed a *Source Book for HIV/AIDS Counselling Training* to use as a reference for providing competent care.[50] We provided similar resources on counseling and its relative benefits to policy-makers and program managers.[51] For medical and paramedical providers delivering care at various stages of the continuum, GPA prepared a slide collection and booklet (*Clinical Aspects of HIV Infection in Adults*) with detailed information on clinical care of AIDS.[52] We also conducted studies and developed materials to aid the provision of care for PLWAs in home and community settings and explored ways to integrate home care with the larger continuum of care.[53] Looking back, GPA was clearly among the first to undertake efforts to ensure comprehensive care

[47] *Adapting WHO Guidelines for the Clinical Management of HIV Infection to Country Needs"* (WHO/GPA/TCO/HCS/94.8). This guideline was field tested in four countries and one subregion (involving 17 countries), representing a spectrum of different drug supply systems, HIV prevalence rates and health services systems; Michael Merson, "Report of the Director: Sixth meeting of the Management Committee, Geneva, 23–24 April 1991; Provisional agenda item 3," Geneva: Global Programme on AIDS, GPA/GMC(1)/91.3; 22 April 1991, 36.

[48] World Health Organization, "WHO Global Programme on AIDS 1987–1995: Final Report with Emphasis on 1994–95 Biennium" (Geneva: World Health Organization, May 1997), 32–34.

[49] Ibid., 21–22.

[50] The *Source Book for HIV/AIDS Counselling Training* (WHO/GPA/TCO/HCS/94.9).

[51] *Counselling for HIV/AIDS: A Key to Caring* (WHO/GPA/TCO/HCSI95.15); World Health Organization, "WHO Global Programme on AIDS 1987–1995: Final Report with Emphasis on 1994–95 Biennium" (Geneva: World Health Organization, May 1997), 37.

[52] *Clinical Aspects of HIV Infection in Adults* (GPA/IDS/HCS/93.4); World Health Organization, "WHO Global Programme on AIDS 1987–1995: Final Report with Emphasis on 1994–95 Biennium" (Geneva: World Health Organization, May 1997), 36.

[53] "Home and Community Care for Persons with HIV/AIDS" in Lyon (1993) and Montreal (1995); World Health Organization, "WHO Global Programme on AIDS 1987–1995: Final Report with Emphasis on 1994–95 Biennium" (Geneva: World Health Organization, May 1997), 32–34.

and support for PLWAs… one could argue that this was one of the most important contributions the program made during its history.

We also collaborated closely with AIDS Service Organizations, AIDS-related NGOs, and other country-level NGOs to improve national program outcomes. By 1990, largely through Mann's personal initiative and support, NGOs had come to constitute an important component in a number of national AIDS programs. This included organizations like The AIDS Support Organization (TASO) in Uganda (under Noerine Kaleeba), the Positive and Living Squad in Zambia (under Winston Zulu, who was the first Zambian to talk publicly about AIDS), and Empower in Thailand (under Chantawipa Apisuk), all of which contributed greatly to their nations' early efforts. Mann was truly a pioneer in this area, and quickly upon arriving at GPA I came to understand the critical role these groups played in the effective prevention and control of AIDS.

It was out of this recognition that, during my first year as Director, GPA established a 15% minimum allocation target for NGOs in national AIDS program budgets (we made this a formal allocation recommendation in 1991). This meant that national governments had to direct 15% of their GPA resources towards NGO-related activities. This had never been done before in WHO, and it ensured that governments would bring the multisectoral expertise of NGOs into their national activities. GPA also continued the Partnership Program, a program started by Mann in 1990 and directed by Bob Grose, which provided seed-grants to community-based NGOs to pursue innovative care and prevention efforts at the community level. During 1991, GPA awarded grants directly to 38 NGOs in 25 countries, totaling over $1 million.[54]

Also in the summer of 1990, GPA offered a contractual services agreement to an umbrella group of AIDS-related NGOs under the auspices of Richard Burzynski, Executive Director of the Canadian AIDS Society. This group was born out of the 5th International Conference on AIDS in Montreal where a number of these NGOs, whom GPA had sponsored to attend, put forth the idea of creating such an organization.[55] The funds GPA provided helped give them the capacity to organize and establish the International Council of AIDS Service Organizations (ICASO), which they did at the International Conference of NGOs Working on AIDS held in Paris in November 1990.[56] Formally launched in 1991, ICASO would come to play an important role in the fight against AIDS by mobilizing and supporting diverse community organizations with the shared goal of building an effective global response to AIDS. Burzynski served admirably as its Executive Director from 1993 to 2008.

---

[54] Michael Merson, "Report of the Director: Sixth meeting of the Management Committee, Geneva, 23–24 April 1991; Provisional agenda item 3," Geneva: Global Programme on AIDS, GPA/GMC(1)/91.3; 22 April 1991, 16.

[55] Jeff O'Malley, Interview by Michael Merson, New Haven, CT, September, 2002.

[56] Michael Merson, "Terms of Agreement for launching the International Council of AIDS Service Organizations," Geneva: World Health Organization, July 19, 1990.

In the same vein, GPA was also influential in creating and supporting the Global Network of People Living with HIV/AIDS (GNP+). Since the earliest years of the pandemic in the United States, PLWAs had shown a remarkable ability to advocate for themselves, and it was their actions that led to the formulation, in 1983, of the Denver Principles, which defined their basic rights as individuals.[57] Dietmar Bolle, a British national, had the idea to establish conferences to bring together PLWAs from around the world in 1986, and their first international conference was held in London in 1987. The conference met in several European cities until 1991, when it returned again to London for its 5th International Conference in September. GPA provided support towards this conference as well as for a regional conference for PLWAs in Latin America and for meetings of the GNP+ Steering Committee.[58]

Finally, GPA worked to update its Global AIDS Strategy and then went before WHO's Executive Board in early 1992 to obtain its approval for these revisions. GPA decided to revise the Strategy for three reasons. First, it required updating to reflect the changing demographics of the pandemic and the 5 years of accumulated experience in AIDS prevention. Second, it needed to include more information on technically and ethically sound approaches of known or presumed effectiveness for meeting some of the pandemic's new challenges. These included (a) treating STDs; (b) providing adequate and equitable health care to patients with AIDS; (c) reducing the risk of HIV infection by improving the status of women in developing countries; (d) planning for the various socioeconomic effects of the pandemic in low- and middle-income countries; and (e) effectively communicating the public health rationale for combating AIDS-related stigma and discrimination.[59] Lastly, we wanted to express the Strategy in more succinct and concrete terms—a sort of action statement for the global response—rather than through an evolving document like the one Mann and Kathleen Kay had produced earlier. Susan Holck and Suzanne Cherney (a long time WHO staff member whom Holck had recruited to GPA to prepare my presentations and other program documents) took the lead revising the Strategy, seeking input from many others in GPA. The hope was that expanding and revising the Global AIDS Strategy in this way would make it more useable and helpful to countries.

The reality, however, was that, despite all the efforts described in this chapter, it sometimes felt like we were running out of time. When I joined GPA, the program faced considerable obstacles implementing programs effectively: WHO regional

---

[57] Victoria A. Harden, *AIDS at 30: A History* (Kindle Edition). New York: Potomac Books. Kindle Edition., 2012, Kindle Locations 818–819.

[58] 1991 Progress Report, Global Programme on AIDS, page 14.

[59] WHO AIDS Series: "The Global AIDS Strategy," Geneva: World Health Organization, 1992. http://whqlibdoc.who.int/aids/WHO_AIDS_11.pdf; Alexander G. Higgins, "World Health Organization Revises Strategy to Meet AIDS Crisis Among Women," *The Associated Press*, January 28, 1992. http://www.apnewsarchive.com/1992/World-Health-Organization-Revises-Strategy-to-Meet-AIDS-Crisis-Among-Women/id-d3ce51e17b5544057bfb40e9fdd6f1ce

office uncertainties; organizational inefficiency; staffing challenges; national complacency; outmoded planning strategies; inexperienced program management at country level; and the need to better engage NGOs. GPA was trying its best to address these challenges, but we were facing a complex and relentless pandemic, and growing impatience among our donors.

Chapter 10
Containing the Global Spread of HIV

It was hard to know what motivated Theresa Kaijage most, but between 1985 and 1989, her life became consumed with the fight against AIDS[1] and for the lives it was destroying in her homeland of Tanzania. Perhaps it was the 28-year-old mother of four who, along with her children, had been violently driven into homelessness by her in-laws. They blamed her for the death of their son, an accountant, and her husband, from AIDS. Perhaps it was Dinah Mutalemwa, the 27-year-old widow of Wilbert Mutalemwa, who had recently tested positive for HIV after her husband's death from AIDS the previous year; Kaijage had encouraged Wilbert to overcome his fears of rejection and tell his wife and family about his diagnosis. Perhaps it was the month-old infant that residents found deserted by the side of the road, "barely alive and suffering from exposure and malnutrition," and whom doctors had confirmed had HIV, after police brought the baby to the nearest hospital.[2]

An American-trained social worker, in the late 1980s Kaijage became the defacto "chief counselor and friend" of HIV-positive people living in Dar es Salaam. "People didn't know what to do," Kaijage explained to reporters in 2001. "The medical community was paralyzed. People just didn't have the skills to deal with AIDS." And so, in 1989, Kaijage gathered together a group of HIV-positive Tanzanians, widows, widowers, former lovers, surviving parents, and surviving children to form the AIDS advocacy and counseling group WAMATA (in Swahili, WAMATA is an acronym meaning "people in the fight against AIDS"), which at the

---

Within this chapter the singular pronouns *I* and *my* refer to Michael Merson alone, whereas the plural pronouns *we* and *us* generally refer to Michael Merson and Stephen Inrig jointly. Where *we* or *us* refers to Michael Merson and his colleagues at WHO, the object of the pronoun is clarified by context.

[1] For the purposes of this text, we will use the term AIDS to encompass both AIDS and HIV unless otherwise specified.

[2] Adapted from Neil Henry, "Africans, Facing AIDS, Haltingly Talk of It; Tanzanian Counsel Service Struggles Against Despair, Official Apathy," *The Washington Post*, September 17, 1990, sec. A.

© Springer International Publishing AG 2018

M. Merson, S. Inrig, *The AIDS Pandemic*, DOI 10.1007/978-3-319-47133-4_10

time was Tanzania's only advocacy organization for people with AIDS.[3] With more than 13,000 Tanzanians testing positive for HIV and far more projected to be infected but untested, WAMATA's task was daunting. In the Northwestern corner of Tanzania—where the country borders Uganda, Rwanda, Burundi, and Lake Victoria—AIDS hit particularly hard, with many fathers and mothers dying, "leaving tens of thousands of impoverished orphans."[4]

Kaijage's story was hardly unique. In the early 1990s, in places as far apart as Dominican Republic and Burundi, AIDS raised its head and ravaged communities. Stopping or at least slowing its spread remained quite obviously the overriding goal as I took over leadership of the Global Programme on AIDS (GPA). But while this was easy to say, achieving it was another matter. By the time countries began reporting even a few cases of AIDS within their borders, we at GPA knew it was only the tip of the iceberg and that a much greater number of people had already been infected. Getting ahead of the epidemic in each country demanded that GPA understand just how far behind we were, and, as we entered the 1990s, it grew increasingly clear just how far that was.

This dilemma became real to me during my first year in GPA. HIV and AIDS case reports were notoriously imperfect at this early stage in the pandemic, particularly given the limited surveillance infrastructure of many low- and middle- income countries; nonetheless, the data we had were alarming. The World Health Organization (WHO) published global AIDS numbers as reported by countries in its *Weekly Epidemiological Record*. At the end of 1989, 203,599 cases of AIDS had been reported globally. A year later, those numbers had increased by 50%. Every region had seen an increase, with the highest reported increases occurring in Africa (up 112% to 81,019 cases), in Asia (up 77% to 872 cases), in Europe (up 47% to 41,947 cases), and in the Americas (up 40% to 188,211 cases). The prospects in particular countries were even more alarming: in South Africa, for example, the prevalence of HIV was doubling every 8.5 months. This meant that the number of HIV-positive South Africans between the ages of 15 and 49 years would rise to "between 317,000 and 446,000 by the end of 1991."[5] The explosion of HIV and AIDS was by no means unique to South Africa. Indeed all across sub-Saharan Africa, GPA saw the numbers and projections climb significantly, particularly when one looked at seroprevalence among pregnant women in capital cities across the African continent (Table 10.1).[6]

---

[3] Ervin Dyer, "Soldier in War against Disease Plaguing Africa Is Studying Here," *Pittsburgh Post Gazette*, December 1, 2001; Neil Henry, "Africans, Facing AIDS, Haltingly Talk of It; Tanzanian Counsel Service Struggles Against Despair, Official Apathy," *The Washington Post*, September 17, 1990, sec. A.

[4] Neil Henry, "Africans, Facing AIDS, Haltingly Talk of It; Tanzanian Counsel Service Struggles Against Despair, Official Apathy," *The Washington Post*, September 17, 1990, sec. A.

[5] G.N. Padayachee and R. Schall. "Short-term predictions of the prevalence of human immunodeficiency virus infection among the black population in South Africa." *S Afr Med J.* 1990 Apr 7;77(7):329–33.

[6] Anne Buvé, "The HIV Epidemics in Sub-Saharan Africa: Why So Severe? Why So Heterogeneous?" in Philippe Denis and Charles Becker, eds., *The HIV/AIDS Epidemic in Sub-Saharan Africa in a Historical Perspective*. Senegalese Network "Law, Ethics, Health" Online edition, 2006, pp. 41–56; http://www.dphu.org/uploads/attachements/books/books_1448_0.pdf

Table 10.1 Trends in HIV-1 seroprevalence (%) among pregnant women in selected cities and provinces in sub-Saharan Africa

Region	City	1989	1990	1991	1992
Central Africa					
	Kinshasa	6.5	4.8	6.6	10.8
	Yaoundé	0.2	1.3	1.6	1.7
West Africa					
	Abidjan	5.5	4.0–9.6	10.0	9.0–13.5
	Cotonou		0.4	0.4	0.0
	Maiduguri	0.1	0.2		
East Africa					
	Kampala	24.5	25.0	27.8	29.5
	Nairobi		5.8–17.5	7.6–15.8	8.5–15.0
	Dar es Salaam	8.9	9.0		11.0
Southern Africa					
	Lusaka		24.5		22.6
	Gaborone		6.0		14.9
	Gauteng Province		0.7	1.1	2.5

Source: Anne Buvé, "The HIV Epidemics in Sub-Saharan Africa: Why So Severe? Why So Heterogeneous?" in Philippe Denis and Charles Becker, eds., *The HIV/AIDS Epidemic in Sub-Saharan Africa in a Historical Perspective*. Senegalese Network "Law, Ethics, Health" Online edition, 2006, pp. 41–56

These were alarming numbers, no doubt. But I still believed we could make a demonstrable impact against the pandemic. I was confident that the public health management approaches which had worked with WHO's Expanded Programme on Immunization (EPI) (see Chapter 9) and that were starting to have an impact in the Diarrheal Diseases Control Programme (CDD), would also be effective here; and I believed strongly that WHO and the larger United Nations (UN) community could unite to make a difference. Certainly, there were challenges—and weakness inherent in health systems—but I believed we could eventually overcome them, gain the support of the donors, and slow down and perhaps even reverse the course of the pandemic.

With this confidence, I set out to draw on the strength of GPA's reorganization and all the support that GPA could provide to bolster national AIDS programs. As described in Chapter 4, few of the African countries affected by AIDS in the late 1980s and early 1990s were as severely stricken as Uganda. As we described in Chapter 3, Uganda had been the first African country to admit publicly at the World Health Assembly (WHA) that it was facing a rapidly emerging AIDS epidemic. Not surprisingly, Uganda had made an early commitment to fight its epidemic, and GPA had provided substantial support to this end. At the time I joined GPA, Ugandan President Yoweri Museveni had established a multisectoral program out of his office, which directed the national AIDS response and coordinated the efforts of several government offices (including the Ministry of Health) and members of civil society (e.g., political, religious, and community groups like The AIDS Support Organization [TASO] and the Islamic Medical Association of Uganda).

I became very aware of Uganda's situation in the first few months after becoming GPA Director. I was working in my office one afternoon when Noerine Kaleeba (TASO's founder) (Picture 10.1) walked in and introduced herself, and we spoke about the AIDS situation in Uganda for over an hour. For Kaleeba, AIDS was very personal. A physical therapist, she had nursed her husband before he died from a transfusion-related HIV infection in January 1987. Not long before his death, she and several of her colleagues began meeting informally in her husband's hospital room to care for and support one another. So many people with AIDS had been abandoned by their families. About 4 months after her husband's death, Kaleeba and 14 of her colleagues (seven of whom were living with HIV) formally launched TASO to provide home care and community support for people living with AIDS and their families in Uganda.[7] Under Kaleeba's leadership (she served as Executive Director from 1987 to 1995), TASO would go on to launch outreach clinic sites, AIDS service centers, and regional coordinating offices throughout the country. By 2012, TASO had cared for over 300,000 Ugandans living with AIDS, as well as their families.[8]

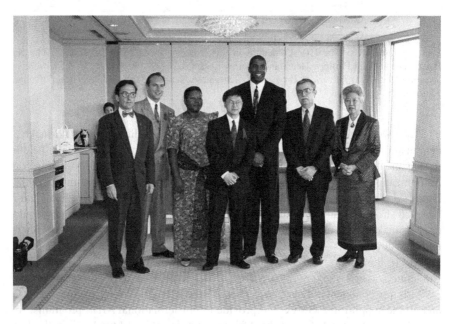

Picture 10.1 The International Symposium on AIDS'93 Conference, Tokyo. February 1993. Noerine Kaleeba (third from *left*) and Michael Merson (second from *right*). Also pictured are Earvin "Magic" Johnson (third from *right*) and David Ho (fourth from *right*). Photo courtesy of The Nippon Foundation

---

[7] Noerine Kaleeba, Frontline: The Age of AIDS, May 5, 2005, http://www.pbs.org/wgbh/pages/frontline/aids/interviews/kaleeba.html

[8] "The AIDS Service Organization: Celebrating 25 Years of Positive Living and Great HIV and AIDS Service," *New Vision*, September 24, 2012. http://www.newvision.co.ug/new_vision/news/1307287/aids-support-organisation#sthash.MFBoLV3r.dpuf

This effort by Kaleeba drew the attention of President Museveni, who in 1986 had launched a mass media campaign against AIDS and in the summer of 1987 was forming a national AIDS committee.[9] Subsequently, Museveni selected Kaleeba to serve on this committee, giving her work a national platform. By the time I met her, even though TASO was still a relatively new entity, it had already opened five clinics and its needs were acute.[10]

At the end of our meeting, Kaleeba implored me to come to Uganda for a brief trip, "I really would like you to come and visit some of the people I am working with," she said. I hesitated—there was much to do in assuming the leadership of GPA—but Kaleeba persisted. And so I went a few weeks later. Shortly after checking into my hotel, I squeezed into her one-door Suzuki and, in about 15 min, we were driving up a raggedy road to meet the TASO staff who were stuffed into a former polio clinic in the back corner of Mulago Hospital. It was TASO's first AIDS clinic, which had opened in 1987. It only had one doctor, and was the only clinic where AIDS patients could receive care.

I remember Kaleeba saying in the local language something like, "Here is our man! He's the man who is responsible for the global response; you ask him what you want." The patients immediately started asking me for medicine. I was overwhelmed by their feeling of desperation. When I asked what was bothering them the most, they told me they could not eat; that their mouths and throats were so painful they could not swallow. Assuming the problem was thrush caused by the fungus *Candida*, I asked why they weren't receiving treatment. Kaleeba replied that they did not have the necessary medicine. So remembering what I had learned in medical school, I suggested using "something simple" like gentian violet. Kaleeba explained the impact of my suggestion,

> after you left, everybody's mouth was painted with gentian violet. It helped tremendously.
> ... We didn't [think of that before]—even those of us who had been trained because this was
> a scary disease, it was a new disease. ... yet in terms of immediate relief, that was a big
> break-through. For people who were bedridden we continue even today to use ... [It was]
> important for you to say that, because simple things that we had always known about care,
> diarrhea for example... whatever they ate, they lost. But even the simple [therapies] that we
> have—we didn't at that time necessarily think about it, because the message we had in our
> ears was, this is a new disease, this requires new equipment.[11]

After visiting the TASO clinic, I visited the inpatient wards at Mulago Hospital. There, I was overwhelmed by the number of AIDS patients I saw. In fact, the entire medical and pediatrics wards were full with only AIDS patients. Joep Lange, a Dutch physician who was there the following year to help set up a research study on the drug Kemron (see Chapter 11) was able to capture so well what I had observed, "I was shocked to see the internal medicine wards almost entirely occupied by

---

[9] Noerine Kaleeba, Frontline: The Age of AIDS, May 5, 2005, http://www.pbs.org/wgbh/pages/frontline/aids/interviews/kaleeba.html

[10] These were TASO Mulago (November 1987), TASO Masaka (May 1988), TASO Tororo (November 1988), TASO Mbarara (January 1989), and TASO Mbale (March 1990). Peter Kitonsa Ssebbanja, *United against AIDS : The Story of TASO*, 1st ed. Oxford, UK : Strategies for Hope Trust; 2007.

[11] Noreen Kaleeba, Interview by Michael Merson, Geneva, October, 2001.

people with AIDS; two in each bed and many lying on mattresses on the floor. At regular intervals I saw people who had just died being carried away. Besides a lack of running water, there were virtually no diagnostic tools and little to no medications."[12]

My brief time in TASO's clinic and my visit to Mulago Hospital, perhaps more than any other single event, drove home to me that the greatest needs in this pandemic would not be solved by visiting foreigners with packaged lectures about protection and harm reduction; it would come only when we combined the very best clinical research to find effective treatment with the deepest levels of human compassion.

This first trip to Africa to see the AIDS pandemic was also where I learned the subtleties around prevention. After visiting the wards at Mulago Hospital, I asked the nurse who had been my host whether the hospital distributed condoms to their patients in light of the seriousness of the epidemic in the country. She replied that Mulago Hospital was a Catholic hospital and therefore could not give out condoms. I probed a little further and inquired whether this might be possible for HIV-infected persons. She hesitated a bit, then admitted that in fact the staff would give condoms to HIV-infected persons. Noting how barren the laboratories were in the hospital, and knowing they had no diagnostic tests for HIV, I then asked her how the staff knew if someone was HIV-infected. She calmly replied that "we assume that all our patients are HIV-positive," meaning of course that they in fact offered condoms to everyone. If only this had been a more common practice throughout Africa.

Indeed, this example of innovative prevention in Uganda was indicative of what was going on at a larger scale owing to President Museveni's commitment to fighting AIDS, and the support being provided by GPA and other multilateral and bilateral organizations. As Gary Slutkin, Chief of our Intervention Development and Support Unit, described in a later article, Uganda was the first country with whom WHO developed "a single national plan and budget ... [and] the first country to progress through all of the steps: a Short Term Plan (STP), Medium Term Plan (MTP), joint donor meeting, program review, and reprogramming processes."[13] Those in GPA who contributed most to this effort were Slutkin, Ross Widy-Wirski, a Polish epidemiologist, and Don Sutherland, a Canadian public health specialist. In the late 1980s and early 1990s, Uganda would receive $18 million in external financial support (compared to between $1 million and $4 million received by other countries in the region). In fact, external and national financial support for Uganda's AIDS effort was four to twenty times more than any other AIDS program in low- and middle-

[12] Joep Lange, Africa on the Rise, University of Amsterdam, Sept, 2014 http://www.pharmaccess. org/Images/Joep_Lange_-_Africa_%20on_the_Rise.pdf

[13] Gary Slutkin et al., "How Uganda Reversed Its HIV Epidemic," *AIDS and Behavior* 10, no. 4 (July 2006): 351–60, doi:10.1007/s10461-006-9118-2; Jonathan M. Mann and Daniel Tarantola, *AIDS in the World*. Cambridge, MA: Harvard University Press., 1991; World Health Organization, "WHO Global Programme on AIDS 1987–1995: Final Report with Emphasis on 1994–95 Biennium" Geneva: World Health Organization, May 1997.

income countries.[14] The prevention strategy and messaging "emphasized faithfulness and fidelity, … provided information on all forms of HIV transmission and all forms of protection, [including] information on delaying age of on-set of sexual activity and the protective value of condoms." While "overall condom distribution was … an amount that could not have influenced overall reductions in HIV prevalence as substantial[ly] as [would be] observed," knowledge about condoms "was high, and use increased substantially."[15]

Slutkin notes that the "Ugandan people, problem, or program" were not unique in Africa with respect to AIDS and their response to it. What was different was the "intensity, depth, breadth, and extensiveness" of Uganda's implementation "of its behavior change campaign, the level of involvement of all sectors, the pragmatism and extension of the district level work deep into communities," aided by significant financial, religious, and civil society support and enablement.[16] Slutkin remembers "returning from usual 'mission travel' to multiple countries in the region, including Rwanda, Burundi, Kenya, Tanzania, and sometimes Malawi or Zambia, and noting that there was no comparison between what was going on in Uganda and these other countries."[17]

Despite these promising efforts, AIDS was spreading rapidly and having a devastating effect in Uganda (by 1992, observers were calling Uganda "the AIDS capital of the world"[18]). It would take a few years before any positive impact of its prevention efforts would be evident. Between 1990 and 1993, for example, HIV prevalence rates among 15–24 year olds at antenatal sentinel surveillance sites remained startling high (Table 10.2).[19] The disease was wreaking such damage among Ugandan families and communities that Action Aid Uganda, a national AIDS Service Organization, predicted that the country would have at least 500,000 AIDS orphans by the mid-1990s.[20] In 1992, Warren Nyamugasira, a socio-economist working for World Vision International (Uganda), estimated that the number of AIDS orphans would end up much higher: "There are no national figures on the number of children orphaned by AIDS in Uganda but estimates put it at 1.5 million

[14] Jonathan M. Mann and Daniel Tarantola, *AIDS in the World*. (Cambridge, MA: Harvard University Press., 1991); "A Measure of Success in Uganda: The Value of Monitoring Both HIV Prevalence and Sexual Behaviour" (Geneva: The Joint United Nations Programme on HIV/AIDS (UNAIDS), May 1998), http://www.unaids.org/en/resources/documents/1998/19980530_value_monitoring_uganda_en.pdf

[15] Gary Slutkin et al., "How Uganda Reversed Its HIV Epidemic," *AIDS and Behavior* (July 2006) 10(4):351–60, doi:10.1007/s10461-006-9118-2.

[16] Ibid.

[17] Ibid.

[18] Moira Farrow, "AIDS & Africa; In Uganda, the Epidemic Is a Plague. The Country Has an Estimated 1.5 Million AIDS Orphans," *The Ottawa Citizen*, February 3, 1992.

[19] Gary Slutkin et al., "How Uganda Reversed Its HIV Epidemic," *AIDS and Behavior* (July 2006) 10(4):351–60, doi:10.1007/s10461-006-9118-2.

[20] Anthony Swift, "AIDS: Courage of a Country Where Thousands are Facing Death; Uganda/A Special Report," *The Guardian (London)*, April 23, 1992, p. 12.

Table 10.2 HIV prevalence (%) Antenatal Sentinel Surveillance Sites in Uganda for 15–24 years
old, 1990–1993

Antenatal sentinel surveillance sites in Uganda	1990–1993
Nsambya	30.6 (25–36)
Rubaga	24.0 (18–30)
Mbarara	30.7 (25–36)
Jinja	17.7 (14–22)
Mbale	15.0 (12–18)
Tororo	15.5 (11–20)

Source: Adapted from AIDS and Behavior, How Uganda Reversed Its HIV Epidemic, Volume 10,
2006, page 358, Gary Slutkin, Sam Okware, Warren Naamara et al. With permission of Springer

and I don't think that's far-fetched."[21] "Unless we can get help, unless we can
educate our people," journalist and former Ugandan Ambassador to West Germany,
Francis Odida, told reporters that same year, "we face the risk of being wiped from
the face of the earth. We already have whole villages which have been virtually
wiped out."[22] "It's a nightmare," Nyamugasira added, "there is such a feeling of
hopelessness about this disease."[23]

For Slutkin and his GPA team, there was no certainty that the "intense messaging" that was part of Uganda's AIDS effort would have any substantive effect on the
trajectory of Uganda's epidemic.[24] "It was not our impression at the time," Slutkin
recalls, "that this [intensive messaging] would necessarily translate into effective
change. The thinking at the time was that there needed to be a still more professionally designed [Ugandan health education] program with more of a strategic
basis, [responding to] findings and criticisms that were noted in the 1988 program
review… and a problem thought common to all programs in the region."[25] We will
return to Uganda later in the chapter.

Uganda was of course not alone. In the early 1990s, using predictive models for
HIV over the next 10 years, Jim Chin, GPA's senior epidemiologist, predicted that
HIV would kill up to 3 million women of child-bearing age, orphaning up to 11%

---

[21]"Life and Death in Africa: In the AIDS Capital of the World, the Dying Are Children and
Grandmothers and Everyone in between," *The Vancouver Sun (British Columbia)*, February 1,
1992,http://www.lexisnexis.com.msmc.idm.oclc.org/lnacui2api/api/version1/getDocCui?lni=3SR8-
V1X0-002F-R4CV&csi=270944,270077,11059,8411&hl=t&hv=t&hnsd=f&hns=t&hgn=t&oc=0
0240&perma=true

[22]Mark Douglas, "Ugandan AIDS Epidemic Warning," *The Advertiser*, May 11, 1992.

[23]"Life and Death in Africa: In the AIDS Capital of the World, the Dying Are Children and
Grandmothers and Everyone in between," *The Vancouver Sun (British Columbia)*, February 1,
1992,http://www.lexisnexis.com.msmc.idm.oclc.org/lnacui2api/api/version1/getDocCui?lni=3SR8-
V1X0-002F-R4CV&csi=270944,270077,11059,8411&hl=t&hv=t&hnsd=f&hns=t&hgn=t&oc=0
0240&perma=true

[24]Robert C. Hornik, *Public Health Communication: Evidence for Behavior Change* (L. Erlbaum
Associates, 2002).

[25]Gary Slutkin et al., "How Uganda Reversed Its HIV Epidemic," *AIDS and Behavior* 10, no. 4
(July 2006): 351–60, doi:10.1007/s10461-006-9118-2.

of all children under 15 in some parts of the African continent.[26] In Central and East Africa, as many as 20% of young adults in some urban centers were infected, and it was feared that the mortality rate for adults would at least double over the next decade.[27] By the early 1990s, in capital cities across the African continent, AIDS had become a leading cause of death among adults. In Abidjan, capital of Cote d'Ivoire, AIDS was the leading cause of death in men (in the late 1980s and early 1990s it accounted for almost one half of all adult male deaths in the city) and the second greatest cause of mortality among women.[28] By the early 1990s GPA estimated that 400,000 children had developed AIDS since the beginning of the pandemic, and nearly 90% of those lived in sub-Saharan Africa.[29] For all my efforts to strengthen GPA and my initial confidence that we could get on top of the pandemic, HIV was transmitting rapidly and extensively in sub-Saharan Africa, and it was not evident if or when we could slow it down.

While the burgeoning pandemic in Africa appeared to be insurmountable, there was no sense of our giving up. GPA continued prioritizing its efforts in Africa, while concurrently working diligently in other parts of the world where AIDS incidence was much lower and there was still a good chance of preventing an African-like pandemic. In particular, we gave much attention to Latin America and the Caribbean region (particularly Brazil) and to South and Southeast Asia (especially Thailand).

The AIDS pandemic in Latin America and the Caribbean region posed an interesting challenge because of its great variability. Each country faced a unique epidemic, and thus GPA had to approach each country in very individualized ways. Whereas in Brazil and Uruguay, AIDS was primarily a problem among injection drug users (IDUs), in Haiti, Guyana, and Honduras, transmission was mostly through unsafe sex, and in Argentina, both types of transmission were occurring.

Brazil had started its national AIDS program in May 1985, after the Ministry of Health finalized its national AIDS control plan (NACP), but by 1991 its response was far more tepid than the epidemic required. There was a need to forge a deeper commitment to AIDS prevention and care in the country. At that time, the number of recorded AIDS cases in Brazil was the third highest in the world, behind only the United States and Uganda. I first visited the country in 1991 to raise awareness about the problem, meeting with often recalcitrant activist communities (Picture 10.2) who more than anything else wanted access to azidothymidine (AZT) monotherapy for treatment of AIDS cases and felt that GPA and the government were not working hard enough to provide access to the drug (GPA's caution in providing the drug stemmed from concerns about AZT's efficacy, as we describe in Chapter 11).

One of our strongest allies in Brazil was the business community, which early on launched a broad social marketing campaign to educate Brazilians about AIDS.

---

[26] Frances Williams, "New chief for world anti-Aids campaign," *The Independent* (London), May 15, 1990, 3.

[27] Deborah Mesce, "WHO Predicts AIDS Will Increase in Developing Nations, Among Heterosexuals," *The Associated Press*, June 12, 1990.

[28] "AIDS Takes a Heavy Toll in Africa," *St. Louis Post-Dispatch*, August 21, 1990, 2B.

[29] "New Estimates on Child Victims Push Up Global Total," *The Associated Press*, September 25, 1990.

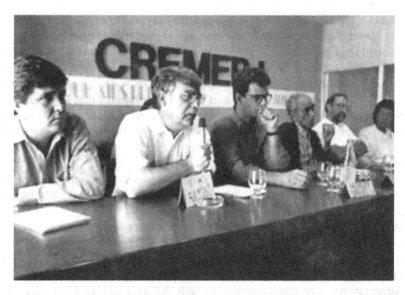

Picture 10.2 First National Meeting of People Living with HIV and AIDS, Rio de Janeiro, 1991. From left to right, Eduardo Côrtes, Director of the Brazilian National AIDS Program; Michael Merson, Director of the World Health Organization's Global Programme on AIDS, Richard Parker, ABIA; Herbert de Souza (Betinho), ABIA; Fernando Zacarías, Director of the Pan American Health Organization's Regional Program on AIDS; Álvaro Matida, Director of the State of Rio de Janeiro Program on AIDS. Source: Photo courtesy of Grupo Pela Vidda

Beginning in 1991, the Brazilian government reorganized its NACP to provide a more comprehensive commitment to HIV prevention and care. The program established special AIDS commissions throughout the country, and the Ministry of Health pledged $20 million for educational campaigns and public health endeavors[30] and established stronger links with civil society and other parts of the Brazilian government. Over the next 6 years, the federal government committed $90 million to its effort against the disease and secured a 6-year loan agreement with the World Bank, dubbed AIDS Project I, that topped $160 million. The project supported new payment systems for hospitalization of AIDS patients, an expanded network of trained hospitals and professionals equipped to care for people with AIDS, and the formation of multidisciplinary teams to care for patients and their families and connect them to services. This comprehensive program included "the promotion of HIV testing; promotion and education on condom use; the provision of disposable syringes; increasing the availability and provision of incentives for pre-natal testing, and the prevention of other sexually transmitted diseases[31] (STDs)."[32]

---

[30] "WHO warns of AIDS spread in Brazil," *Agence France Presse*, August 16, 1991.

[31] For the purposes of this text, we use the term sexually transmitted disease(s) and the abbreviation STD rather than the other term sexually transmitted infection(s) or STIs.

[32] Guido Carlos Levia and Marco Antonio A. Vitoria, "Fighting against AIDS: the Brazilian experience," *AIDS* 2002, 16:2373–2383.

This commitment that Brazilian leaders and activists made with the assistance of GPA and the World Bank was impressive, but it would ultimately be surpassed in December 1996, when the federal government decided (federal law 9313) to provide antiretroviral drugs (ARVs) free to all citizens through Brazil's public health system.[33] This resulted in a dramatic drop in AIDS-related hospitalizations and AIDS-related opportunistic infections and considerable savings in treatment costs. This was one of the first demonstrations of the impact of ARVs in a low- and middle-income country and a great stimulus to the eventual global movement for access to these drugs.[34] A few years later, Brazil, through negotiations with multinational pharmaceutical companies and exclusive manufacturers of certain medications, would be one of two countries (with India) to bring down the price of ARVs and increase their access in all low- and middle-income countries (see Chapter 18).

What about other countries in Central and South America during the first half of the 1990s? In some countries, we saw a fast rise in the number of infections followed by a leveling off and even a decrease in new infections; in other countries—like the Dominican Republic—we had cause for concern (Fig. 10.1). By 1993, sentinel surveillance of STD patients in some clinics showed HIV prevalence rates of 7.8%, up from 4.3% in 1991.[35] Similarly HIV prevalence among commercial sex workers had risen from less than 2% in 1986 to almost 12% by 1993.[36] Likewise, in Guyana, HIV

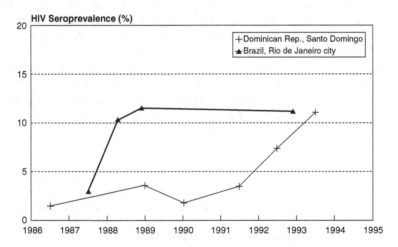

Fig. 10.1 HIV seroprevalence for commercial sex workers; Latin America: 1986–1993. Source: Jinkie Corbin, Anny Ross, Peggy Seybolt, Lisa Mayberry, and David Rudolph, Health Studies Branch, International Programs Center Population Division, "HIV/AIDS in Latin America and the Caribbean, Research Note No. 19," Washington, D.C.: US Census Bureau, November 1995, Figure 4

---

[33] Ibid.

[34] GC Levi et al., "Fighting Against AIDS: the Brazilian Experience," *AIDS* 2002 16:2373–2383.

[35] Jinkie Corbin et al., "HIV/AIDS in Latin America and the Caribbean" (Health Studies Branch, U.S. Bureau of the Census, November 1995).

[36] Ibid.

rates among commercial sex workers had been negligible in 1987 and 1988, but by 1993 rates had risen to around 25%.[37] Still, we had strong reason to be optimistic about the outcomes in Latin America and the Caribbean. We felt we had been able to get in front of the epidemic in many places and, in many countries there were enough resources and strong leadership to ensure the battle could be won.

In Southeast Asia GPA focused much of its early efforts on Thailand and had been involved there before I joined the program. Importantly, however, it was during the March 1990 program review—which occurred at about the time that I became Interim Director—that Thailand's Ministry of Health and our GPA review team realized that AIDS in Thailand "was no longer a principally homosexual and drug user problem," which at the time was the type of epidemic Thailand thought it had and consequently was directing its resources accordingly.[38]

The first reported case of HIV in Thailand was a Thai man, who had returned to Thailand in 1984 after being diagnosed in the United States. Since this first case and the ones immediately following involved men who have sex with men (MSM), Thai authorities had targeted high-risk populations for HIV testing as soon as HIV antibody tests became available in 1985. The government was mainly concerned with HIV among MSM in those early years, but eventually it expanded its effort to include IDUs, particularly after officials saw HIV prevalence rates jump from 16 to 44% in that population within a space of 9 months in 1988.[39] But the Ministry of Public Health in Thailand had also taken an innovative step, translating GPA's sentinel surveillance guidelines into national practice,[40] and then training public health teams on their use in every province. This gave it the ability to track the trajectory of the epidemic in the country and make appropriate and timely recommendations for prevention.[41]

What Thai officials were seeing in the surveillance reports at the end of the 1980s alarmed them. Whereas, in 1987, the country had only about 1000 reported cases, by 1990 that number had climbed to 50,000. Among commercial sex workers a 1% HIV prevalence rate in 1987 had increased to around 40% in some cities.[42]

---

[37] Ibid.

[38] Gary Slutkin, "Global AIDS 1981–1999: The Response [The Pittsfield Lecture]," *The International Journal of Tuberculosis and Lung Disease* 4, no. 2 (February 1, 2000): S24–33.

[39] The numbers came from 18 drug treatment centers across the country. Wiwat Rojanapithayakorn and Robert Hanenberg, "The 100% Condom Program in Thailand," *AIDS*, 1996, 10:1–7.

[40] Gary Slutkin et al., "Sentinel Surveillance for HIV Infection : A Method to Monitor HIV Infection Trends in Population Groups" (Geneva: World Health Organization, 1988), http://www. who.int/iris/handle/10665/61728; Gary Slutkin et al., "Use of HIV Surveillance Data in National AIDS Control Programmes : A Review of Current Data Use with Recommendations for Strengthening Future Use" (Geneva: World Health Organization, 1990), http://www.who.int/iris/ handle/10665/59785#sthash.gF0ZEhU0.dpuf; G. Slutkin, "Global AIDS 1981–1999: The Response [The Pittsfield Lecture]," *The International Journal of Tuberculosis and Lung Disease* (February 1, 2000) 4(2): S24–33.

[41] Gary Slutkin, "Global AIDS 1981–1999: The Response [The Pittsfield Lecture]," *The International Journal of Tuberculosis and Lung Disease* (February 1, 2000) 4(2): S24–33.

[42] Deborah Mesce, "WHO Predicts AIDS Will Increase in Developing Nations, Among Heterosexuals," *The Associated Press*, June 12, 1990.

Most concerning were HIV prevalence rates in Northern Thailand (especially Chiang Mai province), which had abruptly soared among new military recruits (to 13%) and pregnant women (to 5%). Thai officials recognized that these data portended a real crisis for the country, not only because of an AIDS threat to the general population, but also because of its potential effect on the tourist industry, which was at the heart of the national economy. "The rates of increase that we have seen in Asia in the past 2 years have been even sharper than those we saw earlier in Africa," I told Asian health leaders in the summer of 1990. "If the situation continues like this in Asia, we will have another problem there, like we do in Africa, within 10 years."[43] We encouraged them not to despair, however. "You have a warning that the United States and Europe did not have, that Africa did not have, and that Latin America did not have," I explained at a conference in August, "You will need to have the courage to speak about AIDS and about sexual behavior openly and to deal with these issues openly within the context of your social, cultural and religious norms."[44]

Fearing a generalized epidemic, in 1991, Thai officials dramatically shifted their national AIDS strategy and implemented an "intensive and extensive prevention program that focused on high risk populations, multi-channel messaging, social norm change, socioeconomic interventions, human rights protections, and rapid nationwide implementation."[45] This comprehensive, nationwide, prevention program concentrated particularly on Thailand's sex industry.[46] The main objectives of the campaign were to "raise awareness about the chances of AIDS; reduce high risk behavior; and provide care to people suffering from AIDS."[47] A broad spectrum of Thai society rallied to support this new strategy, including the Prime Minister, Parliament, the National Economic and Social Development Board, business leaders, and provincial governors. Prime Minister Anand Panyarachun formed and chaired the National AIDS Commission which led the program, and he played a key role in its success. I was impressed by his commitment and determination to stem the growing epidemic. What struck me at the time was that Thailand was the first country in Asia, and one of the first in the world (along with Uganda and a few others) to respond to AIDS at the "Head of State" level. Not surprisingly, 25 years later, due to continued strong national commitment and universal access to health care, Thailand also became the first country with a generalized HIV epidemic to eliminate mother to child transmission of HIV.[48]

---

[43] Malcolm Gladwell, "AIDS Spreading 'Dramatically' Worldwide; WHO Estimates Up to 10 Million Infected; Cases in Asia Surge," *The Washington Post*, August 1, 1990, A1.

[44] Michelle Hardy, "Help urged in AIDS fight," *The Advertiser*, August 6, 1990.

[45] Werasit Sittitrai, "HIV Prevention Needs and Successes: A Tale of Three Countries," Geneva: UNAIDS, 2001, 9–14.

[46] Ibid.

[47] Wiwat Rojanapithayakorn and Robert Hanenberg, "The 100% Condom Program in Thailand," *AIDS*, 1996, 10:1–7.

[48] What does it take to control an epidemic? Learning from Thailand's experience. Mastro, T, November 15, 2016. FHI 360. http://degrees.fhi360.org/2016/11/what-does-it-take-to-control-an-epidemic-learning-from-thailands-experience/; accessed February 10, 2017.

How had Thailand almost entirely restructured its national AIDS strategy? Much of the credit goes to Wiwat Rojanapithayakorn, who directed Thailand's AIDS Program in the late 1980s.[49] Rojanapithayakorn was a Thai physician who became aware of AIDS in 1983 when, while serving as an STD epidemiologist in the Thai Public Health Ministry's Department of Communicable Disease Control, he visited the Centers for Disease Control and Prevention (CDC) in Atlanta and heard about the disease. Upon returning to Thailand, Rojanapithayakorn launched a program to integrate AIDS into Thailand's STD education effort. He climbed quickly through the health system ranks, being appointed Thailand's first Director of its AIDS Program in 1987 and director of Ratchaburi's provincial CDC in 1989. It was in Ratchaburi province that same year that Rojanapithayakorn started the now famous 100% condom use program.

The 100% condom use program was born out of crisis: HIV had spread quickly through the country by the time Rojanapithayakorn arrived in Ratchaburi. He found condom use rates remarkably low both among sex workers and the men that frequented them. Sex workers frequently lacked the bargaining power to enforce condom use, he noted, and the only way he could see that changing was to instead target the owners of brothels and other commercial sex establishments. This recognition came at a time when his division was spending considerable resources on testing sex workers every 3 months to detect HIV infection. A lot of money was being spent without any resulting behavior change.

Rojanapithayakorn decided to deploy a "monopoly" approach that levied penalties on business owners who did not require sex workers in their establishments to use condoms. The proposal required some diplomacy, however, so Rojanapithayakorn sought support from the Ratchaburi Provincial Governor, Peera Boonjing, and other provincial authorities. Boonjing helped Rojanapithayakorn bring others on board, and in late 1989, Ratchaburi province began levying penalties on all commercial sex business owners and managers that refused to enforce 100% condom utilization ("no condom – no sex" was the mantra). When, after a few months, the project showed a considerable decrease in STD rates among sex workers, Rojanapithayakorn began expanding the program to nearby provinces. By 1991, Rojanapithayakorn was able to convince Uthai Sudsukh, then Permanent Secretary of Public Health for Thailand, to deploy the program nationally as part of the national AIDS committee strategy. In August 1991, Sudsukh convinced the national AIDS committee to issue a resolution requiring that all Thai provinces implement the 100% condom use program.

One of the key allies in the promotion of this endeavor was Mechai Viravaidya, who since 1973 had headed the non-governmental organization (NGO) Population and Community Development Association and would become known as the "condom king" of Thailand. Appointed by Prime Minister Panyarachun as Minister for Tourism, Information and AIDS, Viravaidya became the public face of—and one of GPA's key bridges to—a very large movement by Thai family planning and

---

[49] The following paragraphs on the 100% Condom Programme in Thailand adapted from Wiwat Rojanapithayakorn, "Description on the Development of the 100% Condom Programme in Thailand," unpublished document, n.d.

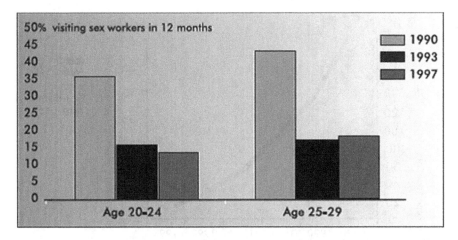

Fig. 10.2 Risk reduction in urban males visiting sex workers, 1990–1997. Source: Reprinted from HIV Prevention Needs and Successes: A Tale of Three Countries. An update on HIV prevention success in Senegal, Thailand, and Uganda, page 11. UNAIDS, 2001

population control NGOs to promote condom uptake in Thailand as part of the country's 100% condom use program. By April 1992, every province in Thailand had implemented the program.

The program's outcomes were impressive. The reported percentage of sex acts with commercial sex workers protected by condoms rose from 14% in 1989 to over 90% by December 1994.[50] At the same time, the number of men aged 20–29 years reporting visits with a sex worker dropped from 35–43% in 1990 to 17–18% by 1993 (Fig. 10.2).[51] Over the same period, the number of STDs reported among men declined markedly, as did the reports of condom non-use in urban males visiting sex workers (Fig. 10.3).[52] Eventually, there was a significant decrease in HIV prevalence in 21-year-old Thai military conscripts (Fig. 10.4). With a comprehensive and sustained commitment, including to the 100% condom use program among sex workers, Thailand was truly able to contain its epidemic.

While GPA contributed substantial resources to this effort (around $5 million per year), the GPA team in Thailand was relatively small compared to those we had in many African countries (such as Uganda). However the GPA Technical Officer, Steve Kraus, worked very closely with Thai national AIDS program staff, providing whatever technical support was needed. While a decade later HIV rates in Thailand would

[50] Wiwat Rojanapithayakorn and Robert Hanenberg, "The 100% Condom Program in Thailand," *AIDS*, 1996, 10:1–7.

[51] Werasit Sittitrai, "HIV Prevention Needs and Successes: A Tale of Three Countries," Geneva: UNAIDS, 2001, 9–14.

[52] Wiwat Rojanapithayakorn and Robert Hanenberg, "The 100% Condom Program in Thailand," *AIDS*, 1996, 10:1–7.

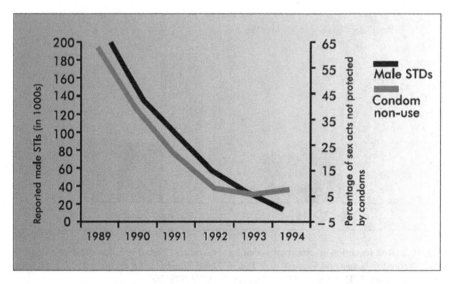

Fig. 10.3 Comparison of increase in condom use with decline in reported male STDs on a national scale, Thailand 1989–1994. Source: Reprinted from HIV Prevention Needs and Successes: A Tale of Three Countries. An update on HIV prevention success in Senegal, Thailand, and Uganda, page 13. UNAIDS, 2001 success in Senegal, Thailand and Uganda, page 11. UNAIDS, 2001

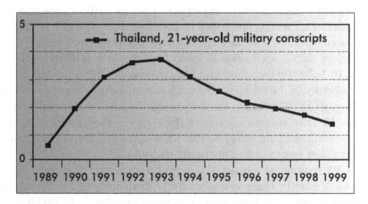

Fig. 10.4 Trend in prevalence in 21-year-old Thai military conscripts. Source: Reprinted from HIV Prevention Needs and Successes: A Tale of Three Countries. An update on HIV prevention success in Senegal, Thailand, and Uganda, page 14. UNAIDS 2001

climb again (though nowhere near the levels they had previously reached[53]), these early results in Thailand showed GPA that, with a concerted cooperative effort, it was possible to bring the pandemic under control, at least in situations where much of the

---

[53] Lawrence Altman, "Former Model of Success, Thailand's AIDS Efforts Falters, UN Reports," *The New York Times* July 9 2004.

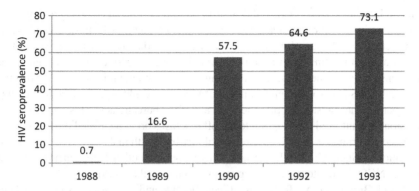

Fig. 10.5 HIV seroprevalence (%) in Manipur IV drug users. Source: R. C. Bollinger, S. P. Tripathy, and T. C. Quinn, "The Human Immunodeficiency Virus Epidemic in India. Current Magnitude and Future Projections," Medicine Volume 74, no. 2 (March 1995): 97–106

HIV transmission occurred in sex trade establishments. Rojanapithayakorn would later advocate this 100% condom use program in Cambodia, Vietnam, Laos, Philippines, and China and was awarded the Prince Mahidol award in Public Health in 2009 for his efforts.

The dramatic results in Thailand gave us hope for other South and Southeast Asian countries. One of our deepest concerns was the situation in India. The numbers of HIV infections there had climbed from "virtually nil" in the late 1980s to "at least 500,000" in 1990.[54] That summer there was evidence that "70% of the prostitutes in Bombay who came from Southern India were infected."[55] Over the next several years, rates among commercial sex workers and STD clinic patients continued climbing at alarming rates in a number of Indian cities.[56] Among IDUs in Manipur, HIV also spread very rapidly, from <1% seroprevalence in 1988 to over 73% by 1993 (Fig. 10.5).[57] But while these numbers were alarming, and we saw HIV rates climb in several additional South and Southeast Asian countries over the next several years, there was time to respond and, in most cases, to take preventative steps that kept HIV from reaching the levels we saw in many sub-Saharan African countries.[58]

While GPA and bilateral donors had provided support to the Indian government since Fakhry Assaad's early visit there in 1985 (see Chapter 2), the national response was initially modest at best. This all changed when the government, desiring more foreign currency to help spur its economy, decided to accept a soft loan from the World

---

[54] "WHO assessment of AIDS epidemic grows grimmer," *United Press International*, July 31, 1990.

[55] Malcolm Gladwell, "AIDS Spreading 'Dramatically' Worldwide; WHO Estimates Up to 10 Million Infected; Cases in Asia Surge," *The Washington Post*, August 1, 1990, A1.

[56] R. C. Bollinger, S. P. Tripathy, and T. C. Quinn, "The Human Immunodeficiency Virus Epidemic in India. Current Magnitude and Future Projections," *Medicine* (March 1995) 74(2): 97–106.

[57] Ibid.

[58] Rod Mickleburgh, "WHO reports million more AIDS-virus infections Figures since last April buttress grim predictions," *The Globe and Mail*, February 12, 1992.

Bank to launch a country-wide AIDS control program.[59] I recall receiving a phone call at home early one morning in late 1991 from Olavi Elo, a Finnish physician and WHO Representative to India, asking me to come there immediately to discuss plans for this program with the Ministry of Health. I traveled to India the following week and, after an intense series of meetings, reached an agreement with the ministry to establish the National AIDS Control Organization (NACO), which would be connected to the ministry but operate outside its often tedious and slow bureaucracy. This was a critical decision, as it allowed the program to get off to a fast start and ensured involvement of the State governments (which have responsibility for health in the country) through the formation of State AIDS cells. This, in turn, encouraged other UN agencies, bilateral donors, NGOs, and international corporations to join in these efforts.

Patrick Brenny, GPA's Technical Officer, did outstanding work assisting NACO in formulating HIV prevention and continuum of care policies and strategies, coordinating outside technical assistance, and mobilizing a multisectoral government response. While the program showed some early successes in improving knowledge about HIV and providing care and support to HIV patients, some States were slow in implementing their programs (including those with HIV prevalence rates of 3–5% in pregnant women). Additionally, these programs had limited impact on marginalized populations, particularly commercial sex workers and IDUs, owing to the severe stigma and discrimination associated with these behaviors (this situation would greatly improve with the initiation, in 2003, of the AVAHAN project, supported by the Bill & Melinda Gates Foundation [see Chapter 18]). The government would eventually integrate NACO back into the Ministry of Health, angering AIDS activists in the country.[60]

GPA also had concerns about China. China is, of course, a very large country steeped in traditions that made it difficult to openly address AIDS and its associated high-risk behaviors. This led, initially, to considerable denial in the country during the first years of the pandemic. China had all but abolished STDs and commercial sex work under Mao Zedong and thus officials in its Ministry of Health felt confident that the measures it had in place—laws against commercial sex work, homosexuality, and illicit drug use; mandatory blood screening of high-risk groups and of returning nationals from abroad; and banning of imported blood and blood products—were sufficient to prevent an epidemic from occurring. However, China's decision in 1992 to endorse a socialist market economy was quickly increasing wealth among its population, leading to a rapid rise in commercial sex work and consequently STD rates, and HIV began spreading rapidly. I visited Beijing often to meet with the national AIDS program leadership in the Ministry of Health and appealed to them to implement HIV education programs targeted towards young people and measures to destigmatize high risk groups. By 1994, some positive developments had occurred, including: the creation of a National Association of Sexually Transmitted Diseases; the formation of a national AIDS Prevention and Control Program (in cooperation with GPA); and the launch of an AIDS educational program for the public and for college students. In my final visit to China as GPA Director, in 1994, I

---

[59] Olavi Elo, Interview by Michael Merson, Geneva, September 21, 2001.
[60] Dimsa Sachan, "India's AIDS department merger angers activists." *The Lancet*, 384(9946):842, 6 September 2014.

recall that national authorities were particularly concerned about the risks of transmission from contaminated blood. This, in retrospect, makes me wonder if they were aware then of the illegal and dangerous blood collection practices that were going on among farmers in rural areas in Henan Province and elsewhere. We did not know about them at the time, but in 2000 the international press exposed these practices, which by then had resulted in many thousands of AIDS cases.[61]

As the 1990s wound on, some of the promising signs in the fight against AIDS that GPA was seeing in Asia and South America also emerged in Africa. In Uganda, the effect of the national effort began bearing fruit as data from most sentinel surveillance sites across the country (an imperfect but nonetheless valuable metric to assess HIV prevalence and program impact) suggested that HIV had reached its peak prevalence in 1992 and thereafter began a dramatic decline throughout the country (Figs. 10.6 and 10.7). Between 1990 and 1996, delayed onset of sexual intercourse and condom utilization also increased (Table 10.3).[62] While the natural course of the epidemic can explain some of this decline, much of it was no doubt a result of the efforts of the national AIDS program led by Sam Okware and Warren Naamara, the courageous leadership of President Museveni, the strong commitment of many Ugandans working in various sectors in and out of government, and the support and guidance of GPA, the World Bank, the United States Agency for International Development (USAID), and several other UN agencies and governments. Much has been debated and written about the reasons for the success in Uganda, but in my view Slutkin has said it the best: it was due to the "intensity, depth, breath, and extensiveness of programming of its behavior change campaign, the level of involvement of all sectors, including local churches and mosques, and the high level of financial support the program received".[63]

Uganda was not alone in its success: A few other African countries saw similar progress in slowing down their epidemic. For example, Senegal's leaders had made a bold commitment to act against AIDS early in the pandemic by forming a national AIDS Council in 1986. In 1992, GPA and other donors brought considerable funds together enabling Senegal to invest over $20 million during the next 4 years in AIDS prevention efforts.[64] Senegal's AIDS control program, led by Ibra Ndoye (see Picture 10.3), had several advantages: it was based on the foundation of a very strong, preexisting STD program, which included frequent screening of commercial sex workers; its male population had high circumcision rates; Muslim cultural norms reduced widespread sexual risk behaviors; and the program had high buy-in from faith communities who did not object to the promotion of condoms through

---

[61] Elizabeth Rosenthal, "In Rural China, a Steep Price of Poverty: Dying of AIDS," *New York Times*, Oct 28, 2000.

[62] Werasit Sittitrai, "HIV Prevention Needs and Successes: A Tale of Three Countries," Geneva: UNAIDS, 2001, 1–4; Gary Slutkin, Sam Okware, Warren Naamara et al., "How Uganda Reversed its HIV Epidemic," *AIDS Behav.* 10(4): 351–360 2008.

[63] Gary Slutkin, Sam Okware, Warren Naamara et al., How Uganda Reversed its HIV Epidemic, *AIDS Behav.* 10(4): 351–360 2008.

[64] Elizabeth Pisani, "Acting Early to Prevent AIDS: The Case of Senegal," Geneva: UNAIDS, 1999, 99.34E, 11.

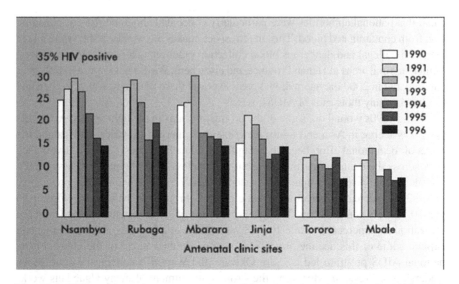

Fig. 10.6 HIV prevalence in pregnant women. Selected sentinel sites, Uganda, 1990–1996. Source: Reprinted from HIV Prevention Needs and Successes: A Tale of Three Countries. An update on HIV prevention success in Senegal, Thailand, and Uganda, page 1. UNAIDS, 2001

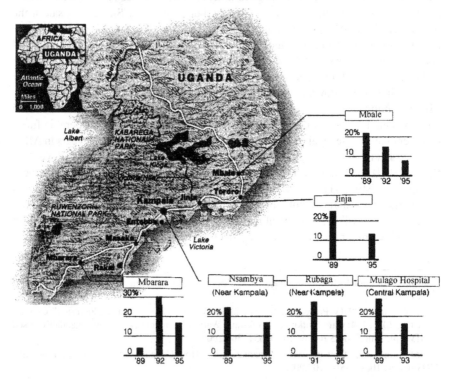

Fig. 10.7 Decreases in HIV infection rates among pregnant women in six cities in Uganda, as reported in the *New York Times*, 1996. Source: Reprinted with permission of the International Union Against Tuberculosis and Lung Disease. Copyright © "The Union." G. Slutkin, "Global AIDS 1981–1999: The Response [The Pittsfield Lecture]," *The International Journal of Tuberculosis and Lung Disease* 2000 Volume 4, no. 2, S24–33

Table 10.3 Decrease in HIV prevalence (%) in 15–24 year olds in Uganda between 1990–1993 and 1995–1996

Antenatal sentinel surveillance sites	1990–1993	1995–1996	P
Nsambya	30.6 (25–36)	14.7 (13–17)	<.001
Rubaga	24.0 (18–30)	17.5 (14–21)	<.05
Mbarara	30.7 (25–36)	14.0 (11–17)	<.001
Jinja	17.7 (14–22)	12.1 (9–15)	<.05
Mbale	15.0 (12–18)	7.4 (5–10)	<.001
Tororo	15.5 (11–20)	12.2 (9–15)	NS

Source: Adapted from AIDS and Behavior, How Uganda Reversed Its HIV Epidemic, Volume 10, 2006, page 358, Gary Slutkin, Sam Okware, Warren Naamara et al. With permission of Springer

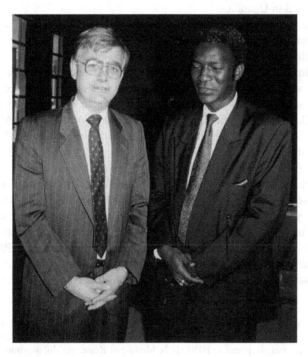

Picture 10.3 Michael Merson (*left*) and Ibra Ndoye (*right*) at the AIDS Programme Manager's Meeting in Mbour, Senegal 1991. Photo printed with permission from Ibra Ndoye

aggressive social marketing campaigns. Smaller programs, in places like Tanzania, likewise saw progress. There, under the leadership of David Nyamwaya, a GPA-supported project used trained peer-outreach workers to encourage partner reduction and condom utilization among truck-drivers and sex workers along the trans-African highway. Both groups reported increases in condom utilization, and GPA pushed to expand the project into several neighboring countries.[65]

---

[65] Clare Nullis, "Health Agency Urges More Promotion of Condoms," *The Associated Press*, June 22, 1992.

When such successful responses to AIDS occurred in sub-Saharan African countries, as international economist Jeff Gow observed, it was often due to a confluence of several factors. These included: extensive community engagement; intentional efforts to normalize, prioritize, and destigmatize AIDS; tangible adoption of risk reduction behaviors, particularly with regard to sexual behaviors; widespread promotion of national efforts against AIDS; designated program champions at each level in the leadership hierarchy; interagency and non-governmental partnerships at the local, regional, and national level; mobilization of resources, setting of priorities, adequate financial initiatives; and efficient use of "local institutions, communities, and the public and private sectors."[66] Researchers would not establish the evidence for this panoply of contributing factors until later, but at the time, all these factors certainly existed in Uganda.

Despite these promising signs of progress in a few countries, there were far more reports of countries struggling to slow down the rapid spread of HIV. Even as we saw dramatic declines in Uganda after 1992, in other countries in the region the epidemic continued almost unabated (Fig. 10.8).[67] In East Africa, as a whole, HIV/AIDS accounted "for more than 50% of adult medical admissions into some of the national and provincial hospitals as well as for 10–15% of pediatric admissions."[68] During this period, AIDS became the most common cause of death in East Africa among those aged 15–45 years, while rates of AIDS-related tuberculosis climbed threefold in many countries.[69] HIV infection rates among pregnant women in Francistown and Gaborone in Botswana reached a startling 40% (Fig. 10.9).[70]

South Africa is another country where GPA's early involvement is worthy of mention. There were a number of reasons in the early 1990s to imagine that the epidemic in that country would be as catastrophic as it turned out to be; we suspected that the most important one was the heavy in and out migration associated with the mining industry and the commercial sex industry that grew up alongside it.[71] GPA's ability to intervene was severely limited by the UN boycott of South Africa put in place in 1962 as a result of apartheid. Most significantly, this boycott meant GPA was unable

---

[66] Jeff Gow, "The HIV/AIDS Epidemic in Africa: Implications for U.S. Policy," *Health Affairs (Project Hope)* 21, no. 3 (June 2002): 57–69; see UNAIDS, Guide to the Strategic Planning Process for a National Response to HIV/AIDS, Module 4: Resource Mobilization, Best Practice Collection Geneva: UNAIDS, 2000.

[67] Jacques du Guerny, "AIDS and agriculture in Africa: can agricultural policy make a difference?" Food and Agriculture Organization of the United Nations, 1999, Rome, Italy. See also Rand L. Stoneburner and Daniel Low-Beer, "Population-Level HIV Declines and Behavioral Risk Avoidance in Uganda," *Science* (April 30, 2004) 304(5671): 714–18, doi:10.1126/science.1093166.

[68] F. S. Mhalu and E. Lyamuya, "Human Immunodeficiency Virus Infection and AIDS in East Africa: Challenges and Possibilities for Prevention and Control," *East African Medical Journal* (January 1996) 73(1): 13–19.

[69] Ibid.

[70] "HIV/AIDS epidemiological surveillance report for the WHO African Region: 2007 update." World Health Organization. Regional office for Africa, 2008, p. 25.

[71] Lucia Cornoa and Damien de Walqueb, "Mines, Migration and HIV/AIDS in Southern Africa," *J Afr Econ* (2012) 21(3): 465–498.

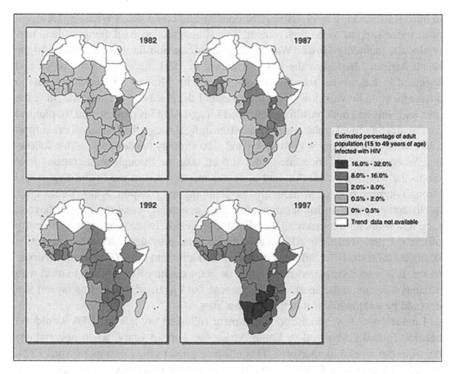

Fig. 10.8 HIV in sub-Saharan Africa. Source: Food and Agriculture Organization of the United Nations, 1999, Jacques du Guerny, "AIDS and agriculture in Africa: can agricultural policy make a difference?" Food, Nutrition, and Agriculture, Rome, Italy. Reproduced with Permission

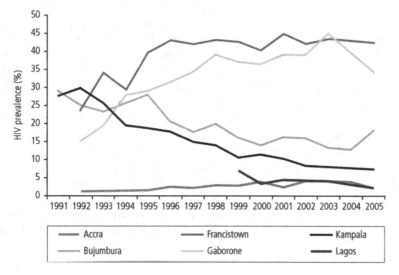

Fig. 10.9 Trends in median HIV prevalence among pregnant women aged 15–49 years attending ANCs in selected cities in the WHO African Region, 1991–2006. Source: The World Health Organization regional office for Africa. HIV/AIDS epidemiological surveillance report for the WHO African Region: 2007 update. 2008

to have staff working in or visiting the country and could not provide any technical or financial support to the government. This situation concerned many medical professionals, including Gustav Wolvaardt, a physician and the Health Attaché to the South African Mission to the UN in Geneva. In 1991, he came to my office and appealed to me to visit the country and meet with Ministry of Health officials to advise them on how to slow down the spread of the disease. Carefully weighing the pros and cons and not consulting with others, I agreed to his request, and we planned for the meeting to take place when I was transiting through the Johannesburg airport a few weeks later on my way to Swaziland. The strategy we devised was the following: Wolvaardt would meet me at the airport, take me through immigration, drive me to the Ministry of Health, and after our meeting return me to the airport and through immigration, all without anyone stamping my passport. A few weeks later, in November 1991, we implemented our plan, essentially breaking the UN boycott for a few hours for me to advise the Ministry of Health. In the meeting with Ministry officials, I reviewed their AIDS surveillance data, provided advice on prevention strategies most likely to curb their epidemic, and left them some GPA technical documents. It was an eerie experience both to be in the country illegally and to meet with officials working in the apartheid government, but I justified it by telling myself that it would be worthwhile if it helped to save lives.

I never knew how much the government followed my advice. GPA would not become formally involved in South Africa for 2 more years, when negotiations began to put an end to apartheid. This ultimately led to the election, in April 1994, of Nelson Mandela as President and to the formation of a unity government. Doris Schopper, a German public health physician who had recently joined GPA's Policy Unit after working for 8 years for *Medicine San Frontiers*, had a close colleague on South Africa's transition team who arranged for her to visit the country a number of times starting in October 1993 and to participate in the formulation of a national AIDS strategy and plan. Most of her visits focused on trying to improve prevention practices in the mining sector which she confirmed fueled the epidemic not only in South Africa, but in the entire region. Many of the miners, who were migrants from more than ten different countries, would frequently engage in commercial sex when they came out of the mines and lived in dormitories. They would then often spread HIV when they returned to their home countries.[72] When Mandela came to power, his African National Congress party was initially reluctant to make AIDS a priority. It had, of course, a host of other pressing issues to deal with, but it also feared that a focus on AIDS (very much a taboo subject) might damage its image at a time when it needed to project legitimacy and competence. Unfortunately, it made this political choice while South Africa fast became one of the countries with the highest rates of HIV in the pandemic, particularly in its black population. Mandela himself did not speak publicly about AIDS until 1997 (at the World Economic Forum in Davos). It would not in fact be until after his presidency had ended 2 years later that

---

[72] Ibid.

he would speak out forcefully against AIDS and its associated stigma, though by then the number of AIDS cases in South Africa had skyrocketed.[73]

The truth was that, by the mid-1990s and, despite our achievements in some countries, we in GPA still did not know whether we could sufficiently control the pandemic. When I took up the position at GPA, I had every hope that we could stem the tide. In some regions, like Asia and South America, we had seen some real gains. In some of the hardest-hit places in Africa, like Uganda, we had seen both terrible devastation and remarkable responses. But in other parts of sub-Saharan Africa, and in the newly liberated parts of Eastern Europe, the worst was still to come. The virus, of course, had arrived in many of these countries long before GPA had started, and as more countries awoke to the realities they faced, we saw our resources becoming more and more inadequate.

Most discouraging, for people like Gary Slutkin, was the belief that much of this could have been avoided. Reflecting back on the success of the Uganda program, Slutkin noted that there were differences in the "implementation of the program itself ... compared to all of the neighboring countries at the time."[74] Principally, this meant that the program was more intense, extensive, vigorous, and broadly based than those in neighboring countries. Slutkin felt that "the other countries in Africa were thought to be simply *'behind'* Uganda in planning, implementation and in their own movement toward enhanced support," but that "given the full support, proper planning, and strength of implementation," programs in other African countries could have met with similar success.[75] While we think to some degree this underestimates the essential leadership that President Museveni provided in the response to the epidemic in Uganda, there is much truth in this statement. For us, as for Slutkin, "there [was] no technical or program reason ... why all, or most other countries could not perform similar reversals."

Why did this not happen? As we mentioned in Chapter 9, changes at the international level—with GPA, with WHO, with the UN, and with the donors were all part of the reason.[76] "Beginning in the early and mid-1990s," Slutkin concludes, "serious interruptions in programming in neighboring countries began to occur as the WHO/GPA global effort began to be less globally coordinated, more bilaterally fragmented, and less prevention focused."[77] In addition, there was no other entity able to fill in the gaps left behind by GPA's regionalization, particularly in the provision of technical support. This was particularly important because, by 1992, African nations began to realize what was required to address their epidemic and demands for assistance

---

[73] Stephanie Nolen, "Mandela arrived late to the fight against HIV-AIDS," *The Globe and Mail,* December 4, 2013. http://www.theglobeandmail.com/news/world/nelson-mandela/mandela-arrived-late-to-the-fight-against-hiv-aids/article548193/

[74] Gary Slutkin et al., "How Uganda Reversed Its HIV Epidemic," *AIDS and Behavior* (July 2006) 10(4): 351–60, doi:10.1007/s10461-006-9118-2.

[75] Ibid.

[76] Ibid.

[77] Ibid; See also G. Slutkin, "Global AIDS 1981–1999: The Response [The Pittsfield Lecture]," *The International Journal of Tuberculosis and Lung Disease* (February 1, 2000) 4(2): S24–33.

outstripped our ability to meet them. This forced us to shift some of our funds from countries with promising programs to nations with more urgent needs, thereby undermining the progress made. In Uganda, for example, we decreased our funding by about one-third in 1992 to shift money to other countries.[78] This placed considerable limitations on Uganda's AIDS program, though they were eventually able to find resources elsewhere, including from USAID and the World Bank. A few years later, when the Joint United Nations Programme on HIV/AIDS (UNAIDS) started and donor funds provided directly to African countries declined, Helene Gayle (who at the time was responsible for AIDS at USAID) would note that the support GPA provided national AIDS programs, however imperfect it had been at times, had been essential in helping countries develop programs.[79] In countries that lacked funding and had inadequate leadership, or who awoke to the pandemic only after GPA's country allocated funds diminished, the absence of such support would be severely felt, a theme we will pick up later in Chapter 14.

---

[78] Mort Rosenblum, "U.N. AIDS-Fighting Agency Having Problems; With AIDS-Losing Battle." *The Associated Press,* July 5, 1992.

[79] Gary Slutkin, Interview by Michael Merson, New Haven, CT, February 3, 2003; Helene Gayle, Interview by Michael Merson, New Haven, CT, February, 2002.

Chapter 11
Supporting Research

We described in Chapter 10 how, in the fall of 1990, I made my first trip to Uganda to see the African AIDS[1] pandemic firsthand. As I walked around the overcrowded AIDS Support Organization (TASO) clinic with its Director, Noerine Kaleeba, I heard a few patients ask about Kemron. "Kemron," I thought, "never heard of it." I soon learned that Kemron was a low dose (150 IU/day) of oral interferon alpha. A compound developed by the Kenya Medical Research Institute (KEMRI), Kemron allegedly completely alleviated the symptoms associated with AIDS (and AIDS-related complex) and effectively treated the opportunistic infections associated with the disease. KEMRI, referring to the treatment as "A Miracle Drug Against AIDS," had released the drug for sale to the public on July 27th, 1990.[2] Moreover, it reported that about 10% of those treated with the drug had achieved a complete cure (that is the "loss of HIV antibody seropositivity").[3]

These claims were phenomenal, of course, and soon several media reports added to the hype by touting the drug as a cure for AIDS and emphasizing that Africans

---

Within this chapter the singular pronouns *I* and *my* refer to Michael Merson alone, whereas the plural pronouns *we* and *us* generally refer to Michael Merson and Stephen Inrig jointly. Where *we* or *us* refers to Michael Merson and his colleagues at WHO, the object of the pronoun is clarified by context.

[1] For the purposes of this text, we will use the term AIDS to encompass both AIDS and HIV unless otherwise specified.

[2] Jane Perlez, "In Kenya, a New AIDS Drug Gets Mired in Politics and Financial Disputes," *The New York Times*, October 3, 1990, sec. World, http://www.nytimes.com/1990/10/03/world/in-kenya-a-new-aids-drug-gets-mired-in-politics-and-financial-disputes.html

[3] D. K. Koech, A. O. Obel. "Efficacy of KEMRON (low dose oral natural human interferon alpha) in the management of HIV-1 infection and acquired immunodeficiency syndrome (AIDS)." *E Afr Med J* 1990;67:SS64–70; E. T. Katabira, N. K. Sewankambo, R. D. Mugerwa, E. M. Belsey, F. X. Mubiru, C. Othieno, P. Kataaha, M. Karam, M. Youle, J. H. Perriens, and J. M. Lange, "Lack of efficacy of low dose oral interferon alfa in symptomatic HIV-1 infection: a randomised, double blind, placebo controlled trial," *Sex Transm Infect.* 1998; 74(4): 265–270.

© Springer International Publishing AG 2018
M. Merson, S. Inrig, *The AIDS Pandemic*, DOI 10.1007/978-3-319-47133-4_11

working in Africa had developed it. The news had already reached AIDS support groups in Uganda, Kaleeba explained to me, and patients in the TASO clinic had started pooling funds and were planning to send people to buy the drug. After my return from Uganda, I began hearing from health officials in other countries asking whether the Global Programme on AIDS (GPA) could help authenticate claims about Kemron. These urgent questions about Kemron, coupled with my firsthand exposure to AIDS in Africa, drove home the realization that GPA needed to scale up its care and treatment research activities. Donors and other observers were beginning to question GPA's leadership in the global fight against AIDS, and I felt we could strengthen our legitimacy and primacy by helping guide and support AIDS research at the global level. This was also important to Director-General Hiroshi Nakajima, as he had made clear to me on many occasions.

As the donors provided more money each year to GPA, it was understandable that they were increasing their scrutiny over the types of activities we were supporting. Earning the donors' trust and slowing down the pandemic meant implementing evidence-based interventions, and research was required to decide which interventions best influenced outcomes. GPA had supported and even conducted some research since the launch of the program, but one of Walt Dowdle's concerns—when he reviewed the program with me in the days just after Jonathan Mann resigned, and again when he returned to Geneva in the summer of 1990 to advise on program goals and reorganization strategies—was that GPA make available data on outcomes of intervention studies on AIDS prevention. He urged me to do so swiftly if GPA was to address the pandemic most efficiently, effectively, and comprehensively.[4] Particularly concerning to Dowdle was his impression that GPA had adapted very little from the World Health Organization (WHO)'s experience on the control of other sexually transmitted diseases (STDs).[5] It was with Dowdle's appeal in mind that I sought to improve the staffing, structure, and management of our research to better position GPA to identify effective interventions and promote evidence-based programs.

Under the leadership of Manuel Carballo, GPA had supported a considerable number of observational studies on high risk sexual behavior (using national Knowledge, Attitude, Belief and Practice and Partner Relations or KABP/PR surveys) and drug injecting behavior (through collaborative research studies) in countries where GPA had helped establish national AIDS programs. We wanted to build off this research and made plans to establish a Steering Committee on Social and Behavioral Research to guide future research in this area. Also, David Heymann (our head of research) and Hiko Tamashiro had supported important biomedical research in key areas, such as establishing an AIDS case definition, elucidating WHO's staging system for clinical AIDS, and developing reliable commercial HIV diagnostic tests. This work had to be expanded. Additionally, GPA needed to bolster its clinical research profile and, as noted above, expand our intervention research efforts to better identify practical

---

[4] "Media Reaction: W.H.O. AIDS Expert Interviewed," October 31, 1990, 1.

[5] For the purposes of this text, we use the term sexually transmitted disease(s) and the abbreviation STD rather than the other term sexually transmitted infection(s) or STIs.

behavior-change strategies[6] and understand factors driving risk behaviors.[7] Finally, it was important for us to expand the efforts that Jose Esparza had initiated in the area of vaccine development. Esparza, a highly respected Venezuelan virologist who had originally been recruited to WHO to work on a rotavirus vaccine (see Introduction), had launched a GPA Network for HIV Isolation and Characterization, which brought together 15 laboratories across the globe to provide insight into the "genetic, antigenic, and biological variability of HIV." We anticipated that the results coming from this network would help identify strains for possible HIV vaccines.

We put together a team to strengthen the program's research capacity.[8] My strategy, which was based on my experience in the Diarrheal Diseases Control Programme (CDD), was to identify those areas where GPA could best increase its support of research while concurrently advocating that other agencies and institutions support basic, clinical, and behavioral HIV-related research.[9] This, I felt, would prevent us from spreading ourselves too thin and thereby having too little impact. With regard to potential therapies, I was particularly keen to have Heymann and his unit chiefs develop clear policies and plans for testing new drug and vaccine candidates, improve GPA's technical support to local investigators, support comparative effectiveness research, and enhance the ethical and technical quality of our research.[10,11] This involved revising the 1982 international ethical guidelines for research involving human subjects to better apply to AIDS research.[12]

By mid-1991, we had convened five global research steering committees, each consisting of eight to ten international experts, and tasked them to review, prioritize, and support research activities in the areas of vaccine development; clinical research and drug development; diagnostics; epidemiological research, surveillance, and forecasting; and social and behavioral research.[13] These were chaired by leaders in their field: Hans Wigsell, from Sweden (vaccine development); David Cooper from Australia (clinical research and drug development); Mike O'Shaughnessy from Canada (diagnostics); Peter Piot from Belgium (epidemiological research, surveillance, and forecasting); and Tom Coates from the United States (social and

---

[6] Michael Merson, "Director's Report, GPA Management Committee, April 26, 1990," Geneva: World Health Organization, 1990.

[7] Global Programme on AIDS, "The Problem, WHO Activities, and Financial Needs, June 1990," Geneva: World Health Organization, 1990, 2.14.1, 22.

[8] "Media Reaction: W.H.O. AIDS Expert Interviewed," October 31, 1990, 1.

[9] Ann Gibbons, "New Head for the WHO Global Program on AIDS," Science, June 15, 1990; 248:1306–1307.

[10] Michael Merson, "Director's Report, GPA Management Committee, April 26, 1990," Geneva: World Health Organization, 1990.

[11] Ibid.

[12] Michael Merson, "Report of the Director, Fifth Meeting of the Management Committee, November 26, 1990" Geneva: World Health Organization GPA/GMC(2) 90.3, 1990, 9–10.

[13] Michael Merson, "Report of the Director: Sixth meeting of the Management Committee, Geneva, 23–24 April 1991; Provisional agenda item 3," Geneva: Global Programme on AIDS, GPA/GMC(1)/91.3; 22 April 1991, 10–12.

behavioral research). All these committees were supported by their respective administrative units within GPA. This was merely a jumping-off point; while GPA had some distance to go before fulfilling its potential in the research domain, I felt like we were beginning to instill a sense of technical excellence in our research programs.[14]

While GPA pursued technical excellence in these five areas, Heymann and I understood that at times GPA would best be suited to play a more facilitating role in the global AIDS research agenda. For example, other more suitable funding agencies could support basic research to develop drugs or vaccines and conduct phase I and II clinical trials of new products, while GPA could help establish sites where later, phase III trials of promising candidates could occur in low- and middle-income countries. GPA could also hold such international trials to the highest technical and ethical standards, and collaborate with research institutions and pharmaceutical companies to ensure that poorer countries could obtain afford-able safe and effective products.

This latter responsibility sometimes meant making difficult decisions. One of our tasks, for instance, was addressing false leads about cures and treatments. As an example, not long after I began with GPA, international observers asked us to weigh in on claims about a potential AIDS therapy in Romania. Researchers there were testing an alleged anti-HIV drug developed by British oil engineer David Hughes—dubbed FLV23-A—on 83 children in Bucharest's Colentina Hospital with support from funders in the United States and United Kingdom. This trial had started, even though the United States National Cancer Institute had reported that the drug was "totally inactive," and the only animal study conducted on the drug by the Romanian Health Ministry had found that the outcomes were "not adequate to justify the con-tinued use" of the drug.[15] After protests from Western researchers and some chil-dren's charities, the Romanian Health Ministry invited us to send a team to Romania to investigate. Our team found evidence of inadequate research and unethical proce-dures, and recommended that the Health Ministry ban the drug and halt the study.[16] Thankfully, the Ministry immediately followed our recommendations.[17]

This brings us back to claims made about Kemron, which presented a far more complicated situation than the one we encountered in Romania. Claims about its effectiveness had spread beyond Kenya and it was unclear whether or not Kemron was effective. Indeed, the initial published data on Kemron suggested that it held moderate promise. Moreover, Kemron raised a host of diplomatic issues as the word of the drug's alleged curative effect had reached Washington, DC, and led United States Senator Edward (Ted) Kennedy to request us to investigate the drug. We decided to invite David Koech, the Director of KEMRI and the individual making claims about the drug, to Geneva to discuss his findings. However, Koech refused to

[14] Ibid.

[15] "Romanians ban drug tested on AIDS babies," *The Toronto Star* October 29, 1990, A2.

[16] Global Programme on AIDS, "Press Release WHO/56: Clinical Trials of FLV23/A To Be Stopped," Geneva: World Health Organization, 29 October 1990.

[17] Rosie Waterhouse, "Drug tests on Aids babies halted," *The Independent*, October 28, 1990, 1.

make the trip unless we provided him a first class ticket (which was against WHO regulations). As a result, we never met with Koech. In addition, GPA commissioned a robust review of evidence of the drug's effectiveness, the results of which revealed conflicting data and non-replicability of the results in a number of small studies.[18] Consequently, in the end, we decided to support a randomized, placebo controlled, multicenter study to assess Kemron's efficacy comprehensively.[19] To reduce potential sources of bias (particularly confirmation bias), we located the study in Uganda, rather than in Kenya, because the latter had too much vested interest in the drug's success. Joep Lange, an AIDS researcher from Amsterdam who would soon be joining the program, served as outside consultant on all aspects of the study. The results showed definitively that Kemron had no impact on "disease progression, symptomatology, or any of the other efficacy parameters"; did not increase survival; and did not result in loss of HIV antibody seropositivity.[20] In other words, all the claims about Kemron had proven false.

The result of this trial was both disappointing and beneficial. It was disappointing because it would have been wonderful to have found a drug—any drug—that could do what the makers of Kemron claimed it could do; we were trying hard to find locally derived treatments for AIDS in Africa and elsewhere. It was beneficial in that it debunked a so-called AIDS cure and in a broader sense helped to establish GPA's credibility in designing and supporting clinical trials.[21] GPA could also now promote itself in something of a new role, that of an international arbiter which could maintain ethical and scientifically rigorous standards in international human subjects' research. This was important, since charlatans during this period of the pandemic often took advantage of desperate people living with AIDS, making a great deal of money promoting false drugs. Exposing these scams and helping countries navigate the ethical and technical pitfalls of research became a new priority for GPA and WHO.[22]

Beyond addressing false leads, we were also commited to conducting research on promising new therapies for HIV-infected persons living in low- and middle-income countries, and to making any drugs shown to be efficacious available at

---

[18] G. Kaiser, H. Jaeger, J. Birkmann, et al. "Low-dose oral natural human interferon-á in 29 patients with HIV-1 infection: a double-blind, randomised, placebo-controlled trial." *AIDS* 1992;6:563–9; M. R. Hulton, D.L. Levin, L.S. Freedman. "Randomised, placebo-controlled, double-blind study of low-dose oral interferon-á in HIV-1 antibody positive patients." *J Acquir Immune Def Syndr* 1992;5:1084–90; S.J. Sperber, D.J. Gocke, C.A. Haberzettl, et al. "Low-dose oral recombinant interferon-A in patients with HIV-1 infection: a blinded pilot study." *AIDS* 1993;7:693–7.

[19] World Health Organisation. Low-dose oral interferon alfa in the management of AIDS: still an experimental drug. Press release WHO/47. Geneva: WHO, 14 September 1990.

[20] E. T. Katabira, N. K. Sewankambo, R. D. Mugerwa, E. M. Belsey, F. X. Mubiru, C. Othieno, P. Kataaha, M. Karam, M. Youle, J. H. Perriens, and J. M. Lange, "Lack of efficacy of low dose oral interferon alfa in symptomatic HIV-1 infection: a randomised, double blind, placebo controlled trial," *Sex Transm Infect.* 1998; 74(4): 265–270.

[21] Michael Merson, "Report of the Director: Sixth meeting of the Management Committee, Geneva, 23–24 April 1991; Provisional agenda item 3," Geneva: Global Programme on AIDS, GPA/GMC(1)/91.3; 22 April 1991, 10–12.

[22] "Media Reaction: W.H.O. AIDS Expert Interviewed," October 31, 1990, 4.

affordable costs to such individuals. In other words, we were maintaining Jonathan Mann's committment in this area. In the early 1990s, there was only one drug on the market shown to delay HIV progression: azidothymidine (AZT).[23] Burroughs Wellcome produced the drug, and it was prohibitively costly for many living in industrialized countries, much less for those in low- and middle-income nations. This had been an issue I had faced during my first visit to Brazil (see Chapter 10).

In 1990, GPA began discussions with Burroughs Wellcome about making AZT more accessible to people in developing nations. We held our first formal meeting on October 19, 1990, when four Burroughs Wellcome representatives met in my office with David Heymann, Lars Kallings, Roy Widdus, and myself. The Burroughs Wellcome team was led by Keith Merrifield, Director of the Wellcome Foundation, who came across as a very sincere and well-meaning individual. Burroughs Wellcome had found its research efforts in several African countries to have been logistically difficult and of limited scientific value, but the company expressed interest in exploring with us the possibility that AZT might reduce perinatal HIV transmission. This, of course, was an important question in its own right (in fact, the company had just launched a study to that effect in the United States), but it also served as a potential entry point for them to have the drug used in Africa.

At the meeting, I explained that GPA was committed to making effective drugs available to all people with HIV, but that the high cost of AZT concerned us, as did a number of other issues. For example, there was much pressure on GPA to provide therapy to persons living in low- and middle-income countries, so research to determine whether the drug showed efficacy among adults in these countries was a top priority. However, we recognized that research on perinatal transmission was also needed. Accordingly, we offered our expertise in setting up research studies to examine both questions, with the understanding that the company would make the drug available and affordable in the countries where the research was conducted once the studies were completed.

Burroughs Wellcome, for its part, felt it had already lowered the cost of AZT considerably, and maintained that it could not reduce it further, owing to the fixed cost of production. Accordingly, it argued that the drug's short-term use for prevention of perinatal transmission—rather than for continuous treatment—was the best route to pursue in low- and middle-income countries. We pushed back on two fronts. First, we asked if it would keep supplying the drug to HIV-infected pregnant women after they delivered their babies. To us, the company had a moral and ethical obligation to do so. Second, we noted that other drug companies had found creative ways to work with WHO in making drugs affordable to everyone. For example Merck had made Ivermectin, a drug used to combat river blindness, freely available to African countries. Also, we argued, at lower costs Burroughs Wellcome would likely create much larger markets for the drug, and this would more than cover its production and supply costs. Without lowering the price, we argued, it would be very difficult for

---

[23] Stephen Inrig, *In a place so ordinary: North Carolina and the problem of AIDS, 1981—1997* by Duke University, 2007, 474 pages; 3321835.

GPA to endorse the use of AZT for perinatal prevention. We agreed to meet again in late 1990 for further discussion.

Our second meeting in December, 1990, was only with Merrifield and was held in London. He told us that Burroughs Wellcome would consider dropping its price, but it needed some guarantees on intellectual property rights, distribution mechanisms, laboratory-based surveillance, and counterfeit protections. However, there were clear limits to how low Burroughs Wellcome was willing to go, limits it argued were imposed by the costs of patient dose thresholds (500 mg/day) and market conditions in high-income countries. We also discussed the possibility of creating a special company to deliver AZT in low- and middle-income countries. We ended the meeting by agreeing to draw up some possible solutions to these issues by February 1991.

These negotiations prompted substantial debate within GPA. Over the next few months, we considered several questions: Should AZT even be GPA's priority? What role, if any, should GPA play in making it available? What should an AZT distribution program look like? Given the difficultly in providing everyone with drugs, how would GPA distribute AZT equitably? Widdus led us through this thinking process, with the assistance of consultants who provided baseline analyses on the need for AZT within countries, Burroughs Wellcome's market share, and the financial capacity of people to pay for the drug in the hardest hit countries. In the end, most of us felt AZT should not be GPA's priority, echoing Heymann's feeling that increasing access to medicines for other AIDS-related diseases (like esophageal thrush, tuberculosis, etc.) would be more cost-effective. However, a few members of our team, such as Marc Karam, (who was at the time head of our clinical research unit), felt that if such antiretroviral drugs were available, GPA had a moral and ethical obligation to find a way to provide them.

If we did help to make AZT available, we concluded, we needed to construct a clear mechanism for doing so. GPA staff developed two options, the first was for WHO to provide AZT at the lowest prices to certain hospitals in targeted countries. The second was to develop a WHO-supported company to carry out this function. With either option, we ran into the same financing reality: fewer than 13% of people with AIDS could afford AZT at its current market price in the hardest hit nations, and that number climbed only to 22% if we were able to encourage Burroughs Wellcome to significantly further reduce the price.

As it turned out, Burroughs Wellcome was unable or unwilling to move further on its price position. We did not know this, however, when we met with Burroughs Wellcome and 17 other companies developing AIDS drugs and vaccines in a 1 day conference on May 21, 1991 in Geneva. We stressed at this meeting the need for developing and producing "vaccines and drugs against AIDS … at a cost all can afford,"[24] and we prepared a six-page document to guide the discussion, which noted that the current pricing strategies that included profits and new research and development seed costs put the price of drugs like AZT out of reach for low- and

---

[24] Barton Gellman, "An Unequal Calculus of Life and Death," *Washington Post*, December 27, 2000.

middle-income countries. We recommended more flexible differential pricing strategies for the hardest hit countries, an idea that Widdus had long been promoting.

There was little in the way of a positive response from the pharmaceutical companies. They put forth three counter arguments: that they were only responsible for contributing their research competence and research products to the global fight against AIDS, and that "the broader responsibility for ensuring that such products are delivered to those they could benefit should be borne by society, particularly governments"[25]; that antiretrovirals could not be used safely in the developing world and were even doubtful that resources should be used to make such drugs available in these countries in view of competing health problems; and that Africa's social, political, and medical systems were greater barriers to access to these drugs than affordability. We convened the same group again a year later but made no further progress.

With regard specifically to Burroughs Wellcome, we continued exploring various options with the company regarding access to AZT over the next few years. In late 1992 and early 1993, the company offered to donate about $20 million worth of AZT, an amount that constituted about 5% of their expected 1993 sales. While this seemed very generous, our calculations (based on the donation amount [$20 million over 5 years] and unit price [$1 for a 100 mg capsule, 6 caps/day]) estimated that we could treat 9000 patients per year with the drugs. Considering a survival time of 24 months after AIDS diagnosis, the donation would cover only 22% of reported cases, and 5% of estimated cases in Africa (that is, it would have barely met the needs for the single country of Rwanda).[26] Given that Burroughs Wellcome only promised to provide the drug for 5 years, that countries receiving the drug would feel compelled to purchase additional quantities to treat those not receiving it, and that the proposal ignored larger issues of AZT distribution across Africa, we chose not to accept this offer. We believed that such a limited donation would risk causing considerable disruption in the public health infrastructure of participating countries by diverting scarce resources and creating pressure for increased access. While we continued working on perinatal prevention, our negotiations with Burroughs Wellcome come to an end in early 1993. At that time the company was confronting a host of issues, including patent challenges, potential competition from similar drugs made by other manufacturers, study results suggesting the limited effect of AZT monotherapy in delaying AIDS mortality, and questions about the cost-effectiveness of monotherapy.[27]

We had tried with these efforts to break through the access barriers with Burroughs Wellcome and with other pharmaceutical companies, but were unsuc-

---

[25] Ibid.

[26] Confidential memo; WHO Drug Negotions.; Jean Pierre Aboulker and Ann Marie Swart, "Letter to Lancet: Preliminary Analysis of the Concorde Trial," *The Lancet* 341: 889–890, April 2 1993.

[27] The FDA approved three other Nucleoside analog reverse transcriptase inhibitors (NARTI) in the early 1990s, including Didanosine (also called Videx, or DDI) approved in 1991; Zalcitabine (Hivid, dideoxycytidine, or ddC) approved in 1992; and Stavudine (also known as Zerit, or d4T) approved in 1994; Jean Pierre Aboulker and Ann Marie Swart, "Letter to Lancet: Preliminary Analysis of the Concorde Trial," *The Lancet* 341: 889–890, April 2 1993.

cessful. It would turn out that these early negotiating failures would help in subsequent discussions about drug pricing with Bristol-Myers Squibb and Glaxo-Wellcome in 1995, when research indicated that two-drug combination antiretroviral therapy (ART) was moderately effective in slowing the progression of HIV disease. However, it would not be until the turn of the century, when AIDS was ravaging much of sub-Saharan Africa, that the pharmaceutical companies realized the serious error they had made earlier in not devising schemes for differential pricing of their drugs for poorer nations. Thus, while GPA did not create any earthshattering alliances that directly resulted in low cost AZT, our discussions did lay the foundation for the eventual substantial drop in the costs of these drugs through the efforts of the Joint United Nations Programme on HIV/AIDS (UNAIDS) (see Chapter 17).

Notable at this stage as well was the lack of participation by Western AIDS activists in fighting for cheaper drug costs in Africa. On one hand, it seemed reasonable to expect them to mobilize on such an issue: the AIDS Coalition to Unleash Power (ACT UP) was an advocacy organization formed in 1987 in response to many of the frustrations in the gay community in the United States about the prohibitive pricing of AZT when Burroughs Wellcome first marketed the drug. On the other hand, Western AIDS activists had their hands full trying to obtain drugs and services for themselves, much less think about the needs of those in Africa. "I can't get AIDS medicine in the Bronx! Don't tell me about people in Africa," David Barr, of Gay Men's Health Crisis, told Eric Sawyer, an ACT UP pioneer and founder of Housing Works, the largest provider of housing for people with AIDS in the United States, in 1993. "It was self-interest," Sawyer recalled.[28] This was unfortunate, I often felt, since the kind of activism that had led to a number of successes for gay men in the United States—including the creation of a "parallel track" system for more rapidly enabling access to new antiretroviral drugs—would likely have greatly benefited those infected with HIV in Africa and other low-and middle-income regions.

Eric Sawyer was an exception. Early on he attended international AIDS conferences and spoke about AIDS activism, living with HIV, and housing issues faced by AIDS patients, and would meet persons living with AIDS (PLWAs) from low- and middle-income countries who told him about their difficulty accessing basic medicines. He eventually went on the board of The Global Network of People Living with HIV/AIDS (GNP+), founded the Global AIDS Action Committee of ACT UP, and in 1999 worked with Alan Berkman, a veteran civil rights activist in New York City and others to help form Health GAP (Health Global Access Program), which advocates for access to essential medicine. He subsequently joined UNAIDS as its Civil Society Partnership Adviser in 2008.[29]

We eventually made headway securing AZT for preventing mother to child transmission of HIV. The discovery, in 1994, that AZT successfully interrupted

---

[28] Barton Gellman, "An Unequal Calculus of Life and Death," *Washington Post*, December 27, 2000.

[29] Eric Sawyer, Interview with Carlos Motta, *We Who Feel Differently,* March 1, 2011. http://wewhofeeldifferently.info/interview.php?interview=100

perinatal transmission brought great excitement to the AIDS research community.[30] However, the AZT treatment regimen employed in that study had a number of fea- tures (high cost and treatment through the duration of pregnancy) which limited its general applicability. Under the leadership of Joep Lange (who by now had become Chief of our Clinical Research and Drug Development unit), GPA convened sev- eral meetings to discuss the possibility of evaluating AZT given near or at delivery (i.e., short-course therapy) rather then througout pregnancy. A large meeting of experts in the field held at WHO in June 1994 recommended that GPA support research to develop "simpler and less costly drug regimes in the full spectrum of HIV-infected pregnant women," and that such studies should be "randomized con- trol trials."[31] With AZT being so cost-prohibitive for regular use by HIV-positive adults in low-and middle-income countries, our aim was to determine if short- course therapy conferred any benefit over nontreatment.

The results were promising. A number of studies, which were conducted under Lange's leadership and guidance of the Steering Committee on Clinical Research and Product Development, showed that short-course administration of AZT signifi- cantly reduced mother to child transmission.[32] This approach led to widespread uptake of short-course AZT (as well as other antiretroviral drugs) for this purpose and resulted in the significant reduction of perinatal transmission worldwide. Also, one very important GPA-supported study (known as the PETRA study) undertaken in South Africa, Uganda, and Tanzania demonstrated that HIV-positive pregnant women who receive short-course ART to prevent mother to child transmission of HIV-1 must continue to receive treatment after delivery to minimize the risk of transmission from mother to child via breastfeeding.[33] The same study provided the best database available on the timing of HIV transmission through breastfeeding. This research would exacerbate our conflicts with the United Nations Children's Emergency Fund (UNICEF) over breastfeeding advice to HIV-infected mothers (see Chapter 13), but its impact on the larger pandemic was tremendously important.

These studies were not without controversy, however. Some of them would later come under scrutiny and criticism for their use of placebo (rather than a comparison with full-course AZT administration) in resource poor countries. In my view, these criticisms were unfair and unfounded and I published a letter to that effect in the *New England Journal of Medicine*.[34]

---

[30] E.M. Conner, R.S. Sperling, R. Gelber, et al "Reduction of maternal-infant transmission of human immunodeficiency virus type 1 with zidovudine treatment," *New England Journal of Medicine* 1994 331:1173–1180.

[31] Report of the WHO Meeting on Prevention of Mother to Infant Transmission of HIV By Use of Antiretrovirals, Geneva, 23–25 June 1994.

[32] N. Shaffer. et al. Short-course zidovudine for perinatal HIV-1 transmission in Bangkok, Thailand: a randomised controlled trial." *The Lancet* 353(9155):773–780.

[33] Petra Study Team. "Efficacy of three short-course regimens of zidovudine and lamivudine in preventing early and late transmission of HIV-1 from mother to child in Tanzania, South Africa, and Uganda (Petra study): a randomised, double-blind, placebo-controlled trial." *The Lancet.* 2002 Apr 6;359(9313):1178–86.

[34] Michael Merson., "Ethics of placebo-controlled trials of zidovudine to prevent the perinatal transmission of HIV in the Third World." *New England Journal of Medicine* 1998 Mar 19;338(12):836.

We played a similarly supporting role in testing potential HIV vaccine candidates. In 1990, when I joined GPA, several vaccine candidates (and more than 50 drugs) were in some stage of testing or development. GPA had yet to devise a comprehensive strategy by which to prioritize the numerous potential vaccine candidates in low- and middle-income countries. That said, Jose Esparza had started to lay the foundation for some important work we would do in development and testing of HIV vaccines.[35] Under his leadership, GPA targeted four countries as possible sites for the first HIV vaccine trials—Thailand, Uganda, Brazil, and Rwanda (Rwanda eventually had to drop out owing to the 1994 Civil War), and in 1991 GPA proposed that Thailand become the first site for testing HIV vaccines. This proposal sparked some controversy, with a few individuals even claiming that we were turning the Thais into "guinea pigs."[36] I tried to assuage these fears ("Those who think we are going to turn [the Thais] into guinea pigs have got it all wrong," I explained at a press conference in late 1991. "We gave countries the best assurances in the world [that our research would meet ethical standards]"[37]), but the controversy would drag on for a few years. Esparza worked tirelessly to assure everyone that GPA would only support trials conducted with the utmost safety and ethical rigor.[38] He worked closely with the local leaders of our vaccine sites to develop national AIDS vaccine plans, which included ethical guidance on conduct of vaccine studies.

These efforts culminated in October 1994, when we convened in Geneva a historic consultation on the Scientific and Public Health Rational for HIV Vaccine Efficacy Trials. Thirty-four individuals from ten countries attended, including participants from public health institutions, universities, the pharmaceutical industry, and community representatives. The purpose of the meeting was to: (a) review data on the safety and immunogenicity of selected HIV vaccines presently being evaluated in Phase I and Phase II clinical trials; (b) discuss the scientific, public health and feasibility considerations related to conduct of Phase III efficacy trials and HIV candidate vaccines; (c) make recommendations on initiation of Phase III trials using recombinant subunit envelope proteins (gp120 products) as immunogens; and (d) further develop broad guidelines for the conduct of international efficacy trials of HIV candidate vaccines. The key recommendation emanating from this consultation was that Phase III trials of vaccines that had not necessarily shown to be safe and efficacious in the vaccine manufacture country of origin should be allowed to proceed on a case by case basis in low- and middle- income countries, taking into account such factors as scientific criteria, public health considerations, feasibility of conducting the trial, strict adherence to ethical requirements, and the potential benefit to the population.[39]

[35] GPA Progress Report, No 6, May 1990 WHO.

[36] Anchalee Worrachate, "Thailand likely to become testing ground for new AIDS vaccines," *Agence France Presse*, October 15, 1991.

[37] Ibid.

[38] Jose Esparza, Interview by Michael, Merson Seattle, WA, October, 2001; "Jose Esparza," HIV Vaccine electronic (e) resource (HIVe), http://www.vaccineenterprise.org/hive/feature/935; David Heymann, Interview by Michael Merson, Geneva, October, 2001.

[39] World Health Organization, "Scientific and public health rationale for HIV Vaccine efficacy trials," *AIDS* 1995 9:WHO1-WHO4.

While this recommendation was unanimous, participants at the meeting debated vigorously about the suitability of the available HIV-1 gp120 vaccines (gp120 is a fragment on the envelope of the human immunodeficiency virus that binds to CD4 cells) for efficacy trials. Some attendees had particular concerns about the efficacy of these vaccines. They feared that if their efficacy was low, this could lead to higher rates of HIV infection in study participants receiving the vaccine because they might feel a false sense of security and increase their high risk behavior. Others at the meeting argued that even a vaccine with a relatively low level of efficacy might save thousands of lives.[40] In the end, it was decided to leave this to governments to decide. As John Moore, one of the meeting participants, wrote, "A consensus has been reached by WHO in a good faith effort to leave a decision for a Phase III trial of HIV subunit vaccines to national governments, and to support those who chose to do so. These governments are quite capable of deciding in their own best interests, so perhaps it is time for us to leave them to do so."[41]

This decision opened the way for an efficacy trial in Thailand 4 years later of a gp120 vaccine made by VaxGen in North America. Unfortunately, the trial ended with disappointing results, but the robust debate GPA had facilitated taught us a great deal and paved the way for future HIV vaccine trials. Moreover, it helped stimulate the Rockefeller Foundation to convene a meeting in 1994 at its venue in Bellagio, Italy, of several groups and researchers, including Esparza, to begin planning the establishment of what would turn out to be the highly successful, International AIDS Vaccine Initiative (IAVI). IAVI would be launched formally in 1996 as a product development partnership with the goals of creating financial incentives for pharmaceutical companies to invest in HIV vaccine development and develop vaccines of high efficacy. IAVI issued a "Call to Action" in 1997 and it's first Scientific Blueprint for AIDS Vaccine Development a year later, and has remained a key actor in HIV vaccine development. Esparza went on to work for UNAIDS and then joined the Bill & Melinda Gates Foundation in 2004 where he led its HIV vaccine development efforts for a decade.[42]

As for GPA, by 1994 and 1995 the program had laid the groundwork and built the infrastructure for conducting vaccine efficacy studies in Brazil, Thailand, and Uganda, and had launched field studies among high risk populations in these locations. While researchers in high-income countries conducted most of the preclinical and early-phase trials of vaccine candidates, by the mid-1990s GPA's work cultivating and preparing the above sites allowed Thailand and Brazil to join in the organization and implementation of Phase III trials of three vaccine candidates.[43] The development of the research infrastructure in these countries would play an important role in future vaccine studies.

[40] "HIV vaccines get the green light for Third World Trials," *Nature* October 20 1994, 371: 844.

[41] John Moore and Roy Anderson, "The WHO and why of HIV vaccine trials," *Nature* November 24, 1994, 372: 313–314.

[42] Jose Esparza, "A brief history of the global effort to develop a preventive HIV vaccine," *Vaccine* 2013 Aug 2;31(35):3502–18.

[43] The candidate vaccines included two different candidates based on gp 120 and one candidate based on the oligomeric V3-MAPS synthetic peptide.

During this time, Esparza's GPA Network for HIV Isolation and Characterization was also making significant strides. In 1992, Saladin Osmanov, a Russian virologist who was part of Esparza's team, had established a virus isolation network that for many years provided vital information on the characteristics of HIV strains circulating around the world, including their genetic variability, which was a key obstacle to the development of a broadly effective vaccine.[44] The network would go on to make important discoveries about HIV-1 genetic subtypes that led to a host of vaccine candidates based on those genotypes.

But for all our efforts to develop drugs to treat AIDS and vaccines to prevent HIV infection, GPA found itself increasingly dogged by people who did not believe HIV existed or, at best, that it did not cause AIDS. During my time at GPA, a movement of individuals and activists—some with impressive medical credentials—began publicly contesting the causal role between HIV and AIDS. While essentially all researchers did not doubt this causality, this did not deter the dissenters. This issue came to prominence at the 1992 International AIDS Conference in Amsterdam when there were reports that another virus (other than HIV) caused severe immunosuppression in adults which resembled AIDS clinically. This caused so much interest and excitement among the many journalists attending the conference that I was asked to debate the matter on the ABC TV program Nightline with Peter Duesberg, the University of California, Berkeley professor and leader of the AIDS denialist movement. I saw little value in participating in such a debate, and our communication director, Chris Powell, declined this request, arguing that it would only give credence to the denialist theory.

However, I did participate in a large and tumultuous press conference the next day, where I made a commitment for GPA to convene a scientific meeting as soon as possible to review these reports. Accordingly, we convened a meeting of experts in virology, immunology, and epidemiology in Geneva 3 months later. By that time a total of 80 such cases of severe immunosuppression in adults which clinically resembled AIDS had been identified through extensive surveillance efforts by CDC and GPA, only four of which had been from developing countries. The meeting concluded that cases of unexplained severe immunosuppression without HIV infection were rare, unlinked epidemiologically, not likely caused by a transmissible agent, and not a single disease entity.[45] The denialists did not win in this case, but they still proved difficult to defeat: by the end of the decade their movement would make substantive and devastating headway in South Africa when President Thabo Mbeki openly questioned the idea that HIV caused AIDS. The unfortunate result of all these claims was the considerable loss of lives.[46]

---

[44] Saladin Osmanov, William L. Heyward, José Esparza, "HIV-1 Genetic Variability: mplications for the Development of HIV Vaccines," *Antibiotics and Chemotherapy*, 1996, 48:30–38.

[45] Report of a Scientific meeting on unexplained Severe immunosuppression without evidence of HIV infection, Geneva, Sept 28–29, 1992.

[46] Nicoli Nattrass and Seth Kalichman, "The Politics and Psychology of AIDS Denialism," in Poul Rohleder, Leslie Swartz, Seth C. Kalichman, Leickness Chisamu Simbayi, Eds., *HIV/AIDS in South Africa 25 Years On.* ISBN: 978-1-4419-0305-1 (Print) 978-1-4419-0306-8.

Another challenge I had to face was coordination and collaboration between GPA and WHO's STD program. This was a more nuanced undertaking than it might seem. Despite GPA and WHO's STD program having considerable overlapping sets of interests, at the time WHO was grappling with "AIDS exceptionalism," that is "a set of policies treating HIV infection as fundamentally different from all other pub-lic health threats."[47] Generally speaking, this meant, among other things, adopting different testing, screening, and practice procedures than public health workers would normally apply to communicable diseases (such as, in the case of STDs, named reporting policies and partner notification).[48] (It also included the concept of specifically targeted funding to combat the disease, though that is not what we are referring to here.) The rationale behind this policy, which many developed nations had embraced, was that the coercive aspects of traditional communicable disease control were harmful in the context of a disease like HIV that had so much stigma and discrimination, and were therefore to be avoided. Traditional STD physicians were considered paternalistic, lacking roots in affected communities, and employ-ing coercive tactics including quarantine and contact tracing to identify partners of cases. AIDS practitioners and an alliance of "gay leaders, civil libertarians, physi-cians, and public health officials" instead championed voluntary, noncoercive, pub-lic health control measures that were anti-discriminatory and upheld the human rights of those affected with the virus.[49]

GPA's reluctance to work more closely with the STD Program stemmed from Jonathan Mann's embrace of AIDS exceptionalism and his ambivalence towards coordinating efforts in these two fields. Mann's feelings were not unique, however: A few weeks after being appointed GPA Director, I visited the AIDS Division at CDC in Atlanta to learn about their approaches to HIV prevention in the United States, and was surprised when Jim Curran and other CDC staff advised me to be very cautious about integrating STD and AIDS programs. The challenge, as Curran explained, was that AIDS exceptionalism had been largely embraced by public health practitioners and policymakers in the United States and Europe.

Despite his reservations about integrating AIDS programs with STD programs, Mann did eventually decide to at least explore the possibility. In July 1989, GPA brought 32 people from 21 countries together to develop consensus recommenda-tions on the coordination of the two fields. The group concluded that "STD and HIV prevention and control programs should work together to develop strategies and effective means for program interaction and mutual support."[50] Mann followed up on the recommendations from this meeting by inviting renowned STD specialist King Holmes from the University of Washington in Seattle, to consult with GPA

---

[47] Ronald Bayer, "Public health policy and the AIDS epidemic: an end to HIV exceptionalism?" *New England Journal of Medicine,* May 23, 1991, 324:1500–1504.

[48] Ibid.

[49] Ibid.

[50] WHO consensus statement, "Sexually transmitted diseases as a risk factor for HIV transmis-sion," *The Journal of Sex Research,* 1989, 26(2), http://www.tandfonline.com/doi/abs/10.1080/00 224498909551512#preview

about improving coordination between the two fields. From the time that Fakhry Assaad had launched WHO's AIDS program, Holmes had been critical of the way WHO and other agencies were ignoring linkages between STDs and HIV. Indeed, at the 5th International Conference on AIDS in Montreal in June 1989 (just a month before GPA's consensus meeting mentioned above), Holmes delivered a talk wherein he reviewed the epidemiological evidence connecting STDs and HIV, and warned about the consequences of international organizations neglect of these associations. In the wake of this talk, Mann met with Holmes and asked him "If you are concerned about this, why don't you come to GPA and help us develop a program?" Holmes, who was due a sabbatical leave from his university and wanted to spend time at WHO to learn more about its operations, agreed to visit and, in October 1989, began a consultation with GPA. His consultation overlapped with my first month as GPA Director.[51]

As a newcomer, I was unaware of the debate over AIDS exceptionalism. While I understood the concerns Curran and others had about the incompatible approaches between STD and HIV programs to control the two diseases, I felt that it made good public health sense—since sexual transmission was the primary mode of HIV infection—to integrate the implementation of these programs. Additionally, by early 1990, there was a growing body of evidence suggesting that persons with STDs were more susceptible to HIV. Also, some were even suggesting that male circumcision could prevent both STD and HIV transmission. Consequently, I supported the position Holmes was taking.

In bringing Holmes on board, Mann had asked him to define GPA's future approach to STDs. Holmes spoke with several GPA staff and sought advice from a number of consultants such as Jeff Harris (who was at that time the AIDS focal point at the United States Agency for International Development (USAID) and someone I had worked with in the CDD program), and Peter Piot (who at the time was a Professor of Microbiology and Public Health at the Institute of Tropical Medicine in Antwerp), to help him prepare a plan of action for GPA. Andre Meheus, a Belgian physician who directed WHO's Venereally Transmitted Diseases (VDT) program and had cautiously sought a collaborative relationship with GPA, found a receptive ear with Holmes. Holmes' work and the rapprochement he fostered between GPA and Meheus' STD program led to a second consultation in Geneva in July 1990 attended by 36 participants from 30 countries.[52] At this meeting, participants adopted a consensus statement based on a paper Holmes had prepared that called for "the close coordination, or where appropriate, the combining of AIDS and STD control programs...assisted by WHO."[53]

---

[51] King Holmes, Interview by Michael Merson, New Haven, CT, September, 2002.

[52] Global Programme on AIDS and Programme of STC, "Consensus Statement From the Consultation on Global Strategies for Coordination of AIDS and STD Control Programmes, Geneva, 11–13 July 1990," Geneva: World Health Organization, WHO/GPA/INF/90.2, 1990; http://whqlibdoc.who.int/hq/1990/WHO_GPA_INF_90.2.pdf

[53] Ibid.

GPA's Management Committee (GMC) approved the consensus statement at its meeting in November 1990. We then developed a plan that restructured the STD program as "a strengthened and distinct VDT unit" reporting to the Director of GPA. In August 1992 we recruited Piot to serve as GPA's Associate Director, with one of his responsibilities being the development and coordination of GPA's policies for STDs.[54] From then on, GPA began advocating for improved STD services in national short- and medium-term AIDS plans.[55] Also, that year GPA began cosponsoring a series of 2-week training courses on the management of STD programs developed by the Institute of Tropical Medicine in Antwerp and the London School of Hygiene and Tropical Medicine.[56]

Within 2 years, Piot made great strides integrating our AIDS and STD efforts. For example, GPA developed its own STD case management course that helped integrate STD/AIDS information into the knowledge and practice of health personnel that were treating outpatients and making first-level diagnosis of STDs.[57] We also included STD control in our course for national AIDS program managers and as part of national AIDS program reviews.[58] Subsequently, GPA developed a new public health strategy for STD control. In contrast to the traditional clinical approach which relied on treatment of STDs in specialized clinics, this new strategy emphasized: the promotion of safer sexual behavior, condom promotion, and appropriate health care seeking behavior; provision of effective STD case management throughout the general health system (not just in specialized STD clinics), and intensified STD services for populations at higher risk of infection. An additional key point of the strategy was the integration where possible of national HIV/STD and maternal and child health/family planning services, which allowed national AIDS programs to better reach women at what was for many their first point of entry in the health care system. The GMC commended GPA for its new STD strategy and urged that sufficient attention and resources continue to be given to HIV-related and non-HIV-related STDs in GPA and the rest of the UN system.[59]

Concurrently, the VDT unit in January 1994 changed its name to the Office of Sexually Transmitted Diseases and formally moved into GPA under Piot's direction, and we developed a detailed and comprehensive plan of work for implementation of this strategy.[60] This plan included preparation and validation of flowcharts for STD syndromic case management (where considerable effort was

---

[54] Global Programme on AIDS, 1987–1995 Final report with emphasis on 1994–1995 biennium, Geneva: World health organization, 1995, P. 50.

[55] Ibid.

[56] Ibid., 52.

[57] STD Case Management Course (WHO/GPA/TCO/PMT /95.18, A-G).

[58] Global Programme on AIDS, 1987–1995 Final report with emphasis on 1994–1995 biennium, Geneva: World Health Organization, 1995, 54.

[59] Ibid.

[60] Global Programme on AIDS, "Review of the Programme's activities in sexually transmitted diseases," Geneva: World Health Program, GPA/GMC/(10)/94.6, 1995.

made); improved and simplified laboratory diagnosis of STDs; development of a framework for assisting countries in ensuring the availability of STD drugs; and prevention and control of congenital syphilis. One of the most important pieces of the new STD strategy was GPA's adoption of the syndromic case management approach. The traditional approach for treatment of STDs required a patient to have a laboratory test when first seen by a health care worker and then to return to the clinic to obtain results and receive treatment based on the results. The syndromic case management approach used only a patient's specific clinical signs and symptoms to determine treatment without laboratory testing. This allowed health care workers to provide treatment when first seeing a patient with an STD, which was important as many patients did not return for their laboratory test results and thus never received treatment.

This stronger coordination and collaboration with the STD program made GPA's research in the area of HIV prevention even more important. Male condoms became an important deliverable to national AIDS programs, because of their important role in HIV prevention. One of our staff, Patrick Friel, an expert in male and female condom technology, worked closely with USAID and the United Nations Population Fund (UNFPA) to ensure quality control of condoms we were distributing to countries. GPA also led operational and behavioral research into the use and effectiveness of female condoms in settings where the product was acceptable to the population. This technology had great potential to give women more control over protecting themselves from HIV infection. One of the first female condom prototypes had been developed in the late 1980s by WHO's Special Programme of Research, Development and Research Training in Human Reproduction (HRP) in collaboration with the United Kingdom based company Chartex International, and licensed in Switzerland in 1992. Unfortunately, the response from national family planning programs to the product was limited, so ironically the same year the product was licensed HRP stopped supporting research on it. Thankfully, the situation changed early that year when GPA received a request from the government of Thailand to support a user effectiveness study of female condoms.

In fact, we went on to support several studies to determine the efficacy and effectiveness of female condoms.[61] Gratifyingly, the Thailand user effectiveness project we began supporting in 1994 found that two-thirds of the female sex workers studied reported satisfaction when using female condoms.[62] However, while those in the study using condoms were protected from STDs, they reported several obstacles

---

[61] Global Programme on AIDS, 1987–1995 Final report with emphasis on 1994–1995 biennium, Geneva: World Health Organization, 1995, 28.

[62] Supanee Jivasak-Apimas, Joseph Saba, Verapol Chandeying, Chuanchom Sakondhavat, Orawan Kiriwat, Sungwal Rugpao, Wiwat Rojanapithayakorn, Arnaud L. Fontanet, "Acceptability of the Female Condom Among Sex Workers in Thailand: Results From a Prospective Study," *Sexually Transmitted Diseases,* November 2001 – 28(11):648–654; http://journals.lww.com/stdjournal/Fulltext/2001/11000/Acceptability_of_the_Female_Condom_Among_Sex.7.aspx

with consistent utilization.[63] A second GPA-supported study was a multisite, multinational investigation of an intervention consisting of sexual negotiation, the empowerment of women, and female condom utilization. Undertaken at sites in Mexico, Senegal, Indonesia, and Costa Rica, the study showed that the economic dependence of women on men, along with problems in sexual communication, constrained women's safe-sex behavior, and suggested that female condoms could overcome these obstacles and enhance female empowerment.[64] While we and our collaborators felt that we had built a strong research basis for use of female condoms, their high price, difficulty in use, and requirement for mutual consent by the male partner has unfortunately limited their utility to help women gain full autonomy over their sexual lives.

The limitations associated with the use of male and female condoms (the former was under the control of the insertive partner and the latter required consent) compelled us to explore other technologies. In many settings, partners—and particularly women in more traditional societies or in abusive relationships—lacked the power to negotiate condom use. Married women in high-prevalence communities, for example, might lack the power or might open themselves to physical trauma if they requested their husbands wear condoms during sex. Consequently, GPA was among the first to support the development and evaluation of vaginal microbicides.[65] In 1993, following a GPA-sponsored consultation with industry and major national research agencies, we helped launch an interagency group on female microbicides (later dubbed the "International Working Group on Vaginal Microbicides"), which went on to play a critical role in the development of microbicide products.[66] Our own initial efforts to develop an effective vaginal microbicide were disappointing, primarily because the product we tested (Menfegol), like many of the earliest microbicide products, was found to irritate the vaginal epithelium and actually put women at higher risk of HIV infection. One positive aspect of the study was its successful

---

[63] Ibid.; Arnaud L. Fontanet, Joseph Saba, Verapol Chandelying, Chuanchom Sakondhavat, Praphas Bhiraleus, Sungwal Rugpao, Chompilas Chongsomchai, Orawan Kiriwat, Sodsai Tovanabutra, Leonard Dally, Joep M. Lange, Wiwat Rojanapithayakorn, "Protection against sexually transmitted diseases by granting sex workers in Thailand the choice of using the male or female condom: results from a randomized controlled trial," *AIDS* October 1998 – 12(14):1851–1859; http://journals.lww.com/aidsonline/Fulltext/1998/14000/Protection_against_sexually_transmitted_diseases.17.aspx

[64] "Sex and Youth: contextual factors affecting risk for HIV/AIDS; A comparative analysis of multi-site studies in developing countries," Geneva: UNAIDS, 1999; http://cedoc.cies.edu.ni/general/2nd_Generation%20(D)/Surveillance%20Guidelines/Behavioural%20Surveillance/Behavioural%20Study%20Results/Sex%20and%20youth%20factors.pdf

[65] Global Programme on AIDS, "Report of a Meeting on the Development of Vaginal Microbicides for the Prevention of Heterosexual Transmission of HIV, Geneva, 11–13 November, 1993," Geneva: World Health Organization, 1993, WHO/GPA/RIC/CRD/94.1.

[66] Global Programme on AIDS, 1987–1995 Final report with emphasis on 1994–1995 biennium, Geneva: World health organization, 1995.

use for the first time of colposcopy, a more accurate procedure for evaluating these products than just history taking.[67]

In 1994 and 1995, GPA collaborated with the aforementioned HRP program to devise research methods to evaluate and report on the efficacy and side effects of vaginal microbicides using a standard set of preclinical and clinical criteria.[68] Subsequently, GPA-supported studies of nonoxynol-9 based on these criteria.[69] These included two studies that assessed the safety of COL-1492, a nonoxynol-9 containing gel, which was readily available on the commercial market, low in price, and possessed in vitro activity against HIV. These showed the product to be safe using colposcopy,[70] but when tested in a large, randomized controlled trial in Benin, Cote d'Ivoire, South Africa, and Thailand, the product was not found to be efficacious and it was even shown to increase risk of HIV infection.[71] While these research efforts did not succeed in identifying an effective microbicide product, GPA had pioneered an important avenue for research that could give women more control over protecting themselves from HIV infection. It also positioned GPA as an advocate for these technologies and their link to female sexual empowerment on a global scale.

Hand in hand with these efforts on preventive technology, GPA devoted attention to research on population-level behavior and behavior change. The goal was to find behavioral interventions that would slow or prevent HIV transmission. As mentioned earlier, I believed GPA's best strategy would be to concentrate its resources on a few evidence-based approaches shown to have maximum impact on slowing the pandemic. However, my intention to have GPA "do a few things well, rather than be spread thin," presented a challenge, because GPA had several areas where it "needed to do a few things well," including diagnostics, prevention research, clinical research, drug development, and vaccine development and testing.

Building off of the KABP and PR surveys that Carballo had earlier supported, GPA's Steering Committee on Social and Behavioral Research in 1991 set out to help translate the survey information into pilot interventions that we hoped would impede

---

[67] J. Goeman, I. Ndoye, L.M. Sakho, S. Mboup, P. Piot, M. Karam, E. Belsey, J.M. Lange, M. Laga, J.H. Perriëns. "Frequent use of menfegol spermicidal vaginal foaming tablets associated with a high incidence of genital lesions." *J Infect Dis*. 1995 Jun;171(6):1611–4.

[68] *Colposcopy Manual* (RID/CRD/95.10); *Report of a Meeting on the Development of Vaginal Microbicides for the Prevention of Heterosexual Transmission of HIV* (WHO/GPA/RID/CRD/94.1.

[69] Global Programme on AIDS, 1987–1995 Final report with emphasis on 1994–1995 biennium, Geneva: World health organization, 1995, 27–28.

[70] L. Van Damme, V. Chandeying, G. Ramjee, H. Rees, P. Sirivongrangson, M. Laga, J. Perriëns. "Safety of multiple daily applications of COL-1492, a nonoxynol-9 vaginal gel, among female sex workers. COL-1492 Phase II Study Group." *AIDS*. 2000 Jan 7;14(1):85–8.

[71] Lut Van Damme, Gita Ramjee, Michel Alary, Bea Vuylsteke, Verapol Chandeying, Helen Rees, Pachara Sirivongrangson, Léonard Mukenge-Tshibaka, Virginie Ettiègne-Traoré, Charn Uaheowitchai, Salim S Abdool Karim, Benoît Mâsse, Jos Perriëns, Marie Laga, on behalf of the COL-1492 study group, "Effectiveness of COL-1492, a nonoxynol-9 vaginal gel, on HIV-1 transmission in female sex workers: a randomised controlled trial," *Lancet*, 360: 971–977, 2002.

sexual transmission of HIV.[72] We knew, for example, that condoms prevented sexual HIV transmission, but how could we improve their use among high-risk populations? As one test of this, we supported a city-wide intervention in Ciudad Juarez, Mexico, aimed at increasing condom use in men and spermicide uptake in women. Condom use jumped from 68 to 90%.[73] Also, it was known that the presence of some STDs, particularly those causing genital ulcers, were risk factors for HIV transmission, and that we needed to reach HIV/STD co-infected people and find the most cost-effective ways to treat both STDs and HIV infections.[74] Accordingly, we supported a pilot study in Zimbabwe that evaluated the risk of HIV transmission due to genital ulcer disease and other STDs.[75] These were very intensive projects and produced promising results; however, it was often challenging to translate outcomes from small research studies to the more general population. Indeed, scaling up any program can be challenging, but those related to human sexual behavior were particularly so, given the complexity of sexual behaviors and how especially difficult they are to change. For example, we were aware of several programs that had increased condom use among small groups of sex workers, but found it difficult to see similar success when we tried to expand the program from a local to a national setting. We were not always stymied, however. For example, in Ethiopia, we identified an effective pilot intervention that targeted sex workers and their clients that was successfully able to expand to 24 sites nationwide.[76] To facilitate national efforts, we published a series of documents in GPA's AIDS Series (i.e., AIDS Series Nos. 5 and 6) that helped guide program planners and managers (and their staff) in the development and evaluation of context-specific HIV interventions.[77]

Our unique research portfolio required a special type of leadership, and so in 1992, I asked Peter Piot to take on the role of directing our Office of Research. I had initially recruited Piot primarily to lead our efforts integrating the STD Program into GPA (as described earlier), but it soon became clear that he had the ideal qualifications to head up our research efforts as well. I felt this change made the best use of Piot's strengths, and would allow David Heymann, who had held that position, to concentrate on epidemiological research, a field where he clearly had the greatest knowledge and experience (when I left WHO in 1995, I urged Nakajima to appoint him as Director of WHO's Programme on Emerging and other Communicable Diseases).

---

[72] Global Programme on AIDS, 1987–1995 Final report with emphasis on 1994–1995 biennium, Geneva: World health organization, 1995, 14–15.

[73] Michael Merson, "Director, Programme on AIDS: Global AIDS Prevention and Control." Geneva. 5 August 1990, MHM1015, 10–12.

[74] Michael Merson, "Report of the Director, Fifth meeting of the Management Comnittee, Provisional agenda item 3: Geneva. 26–28 November 1990," Geneva: World Health Organization, 26 November 1990 GPA/GMC(2)90.3, 8–9.

[75] 1991 Progress Report, Global Programme on AIDS, World Health Organization, pg 91.

[76] Michael Merson, "Report of the Director: Sixth meeting of the Management Committee, Geneva, 23–24 April 1991; Provisional agenda item 3," Geneva: Global Programme on AIDS, GPA/GMC(1)/91.3; 22 April 1991, 8–10.

[77] Ibid, 14–15.

As we have noted, one of the key set of questions Piot and his team were under the greatest pressure to answer was in the field of behavioral research: How to achieve meaningful behavior change in order to reduce HIV transmission? How to get those at risk to practice safer sex? How best to encourage youth to practice abstinence or delay sexual initiation? How to increase condom utilization in high risk populations? How to measure whether condom distribution campaigns have reduced HIV infection rates, and how many infections were prevented?

These were important questions, and so to compliment the research that GPA was supporting in this area (described earlier), we thought it would be helpful to identify "success stories" in HIV prevention. Gary Slutkin, as Chief of Intervention Development and Support, led this effort to determine "what worked". We hoped that identifying these success stories would strengthen our guidance to countries, non-governmental organizations (NGOs), and other agencies (UN and otherwise) about how to design and implement effective interventions. "The next couple of years, [GPA] will be pressing on two or three or four specific approaches," Slutkin told reporters from the journal *Science* in late 1991, explaining his role in the process.[78]

Our goal was to create a menu of evidence-based, prevention interventions from which low- and middle-income nations could choose to fit the shape of their epidemic and the capacity of their health infrastructure, and which promised to be cost effective. As we explained in Chapter 9, GPA's intent was to include this menu in the materials and tools we were developing for national AIDS program managers, such as the program managers training course. We realized this was likely no easy task, as success stories, particularly in low- and middle-income countries, could be hard to find. Also, we were undertaking this effort before we had evidence of the successful national efforts in Uganda, Senegal, and Thailand described in Chapter 10.

There was another challenge. One of GPA's shortcomings, during its early years, was that it had not clearly demarcated which outcome variables it wished to measure to gauge effectiveness or success. While this was understandable in the face of a new disease, its inability to define what "worked" and the measures to document successful interventions had led to what some referred to as a "current of pessimism." With HIV numbers climbing ever higher, we needed to identify established metrics in HIV prevention that showed whether local and national efforts were having any effect, and also gave countries the ability to set targets for their programs. This type of information would be essential to include in the program manager's course.

Slutkin soon faced a number of challenges as he set out to identify effective programs. He found that these "successful" programs had not always had a rigorous evaluation design, so they were unable to clearly show that they resulted in any positive outcomes (the question of efficacy). Moreover, many of the interventions he looked at did not record HIV or STD rates as an outcome. A further challenge was that many of these "successful" programs were carried out in such

---

[78] Joseph Palca, "WHO AIDS Program: Moving on a New Track," *Science,* October 25, 1991, 254: 512.

highly select populations, or under such highly controlled conditions, that one could not know whether they would show similarly impressive outcomes when operationalized in the general population (the question of effectiveness).

Aware of these obstacles, but wanting to make this exercise as useful as possible, Slutkin set the bar for "success" as high as he could. First, he targeted only randomized studies of the interventions being evaluated. He recognized that this greatly limited the pool of studies from which he could draw, as randomized studies are difficult to perform and expensive to run. However, these were the interventions that had the rigor necessary to be promoted as efficacious. In studies lacking HIV and STD rates as outcome variables, Slutkin used proxy indicators, like increased condom use or other measures of behavioral change, although he recognized these often suffered from various types of bias. Slutkin chose not to use studies reporting only process outcomes (like number of condoms distributed or number of persons reached). Within those constraints Slutkin was able to create a working definition of program efficacy and effectiveness, identify the "hardest" evidence of success in the projects, establish the most reliable process indicators, and isolate the key elements of success so they could be operationalized for other programs. In the end, Slutkin was able to identify 15 randomized controlled interventions from "different communities in a range of countries," that met our methodological and ethical standards.

Slutkin's analysis drew seven conclusions from these success stories: (1) small-scale, targeted, interpersonal interventions (for example peer education with condom distribution) were effective; (2) contextualized/tailored messages were effective at reaching "hard-to-reach" communities; (3) implementing joint STD care and prevention programs promoted a mutually reinforcing effect of those programs; (4) social marketing was a robust mechanism for condom distribution; (5) mass media programs were most effective when inter-linked with community and interpersonal initiatives within an overall strategic framework; (6) HIV testing and counseling of couples in high-prevalence areas showed efficacy; and (7) legal and political barriers to sexual freedom, healthcare access, and condom utilization facilitated the success of AIDS programs.[79] Drawing on these conclusions, the report recommended that GPA produce "skeleton models" based upon "a minimum package of successful approaches and process indicators" that could be promulgated widely to reduce wastage and redundancy and build towards further improvement. Whatever the shortcomings of this analysis, this was the first time an effort had been made, at least globally, to articulate what "worked" in HIV prevention.

In the summer of 1992, GPA published Slutkin's report with the intent of showcasing some successes in HIV prevention and providing guidance to our partners and national programs. "We don't have to throw up our hands in despair or wait for a vaccine or treatment," I told participants at the 1992 International Conference on AIDS in Amsterdam. "We now have mounting evidence of what

---

[79] Michael Merson, Speech to World Health Assembly, A20/87/128, May 26–29, 1992.

works in prevention."[80] But I then concluded with one caveat: while we knew more about what worked, we still had "to put the political commitment behind it."[81] Slutkin's efforts were also part of our larger strategy to place GPA on a more robust public health footing, a push that also involved our support of research and our revised Global AIDS Strategy which emphasized Slutkin's evidence-based elements for HIV prevention.

We were aware that not all these prevention elements were easy or even welcomed. Some, like condom social marketing, challenged social and religious norms in a number of countries, often putting national leaders who might otherwise champion AIDS awareness into uncomfortable political positions. "Promoting the use of condoms can be a sensitive matter in many societies," I acknowledged in an interview with the *Associated Press* in the summer of 1992. "It must be done according to local customs and beliefs—but it must be done."[82] Of course, our goal was not just to give condoms away, because—as Slutkin's work indicated—"giving away condoms" en masse had little effect on outcomes. We needed national programs to adopt the targeted, evidence-based approaches that our analysis had identified. We also supported creative, pilot projects that ranged from social marketing condom campaigns to clever awareness-raising "gimmicks" (beginning in November 1991 we even began distributing "condom-containing key chains" ourselves, as GPA program staff, to increase awareness about AIDS and also to help make condoms, and hopefully their use, a ubiquitous phenomenon[83]). In addition, one of GPA's projects orchestrated by our High Risk Behavior Group under the leadership of Kevin O'Reilly (a behavioral scientist on secondment from CDC) showed that target inventions could change social norms in populations engaging in high risk behaviors, leading to decreased HIV transmission.[84] O'Reilly's work was emblematic of our effort at GPA to specifically link interventions to tangible outcomes.

I was proud of the work GPA staff undertook on evidence-based HIV prevention, so it was ironic that GPA developed a reputation during my leadership for not investing enough in social and behavioral research. This perception began early in my tenure, after one or more individuals orchestrated a letter-writing campaign directed at the WHO leadership and others expressing concerns that I "had no respect for the cultural or behavioral [aspects]" of AIDS and that I intended to "come in and deci-

---

[80] Ibid.

[81] Daniel Q. Haney, "AIDS Meeting Opens With Conflicting Visions on Stopping Epidemic," *The Associated Press*, July 19, 1992.

[82] Clare Nullis, "Health Agency Urges More Promotion of Condoms," *The Associated Press*, June 22, 1992.

[83] "WHO Gives Out Condom-Containing Key Rings," *The Associated Press*, November 28, 1991.

[84] Kevin R O' Reilly and Peter Piot, "International Perspectives on Individual and Community Approaches to the Prevention of Sexually Transmitted Diseases and Human Immunodeficiency Virus Infection," *JID*, 1996, 174 (Supplement 2), S214–S222.

mate the behavioral side of things."[85] Nakajima must have received some 50 letters expressing such concerns. I never learned who started the campaign, although it seemed most likely to be one or more individuals within or closely associated with GPA. This attack left me perplexed as to why such individuals had such a misconception of my intentions. I suspect that whomever was responsible likely assumed that I was "Nakajima's man" and sought to undo much of what Jonathan Mann had built. They must have also been unaware of our efforts in the CDD program to support a considerable amount of behavioral research.[86]

Unfortunately, this letter writing campaign created tension between me and Manuel Carballo, the leader of our behavioral research efforts. To help ease some of this tension, and, more importantly, because of his great knowledge of AIDS and of GPA, I invited him to serve as my Chief of Staff. Carballo, however, declined my offer. Eventually, over time the friction between us grew to the point where he sought another position in WHO (as WHO's Public Health Advisor, based in Sarajevo, responsible for the whole of Bosnia and Herzegovina). There was, in later years, a rapprochement between us. At the time we were in GPA together, Carballo told me, he did not think I understood what he was trying to do in the social and behavioral area, "My feeling was," Carballo explained, "that the clinical epidemiologist that you are, [you] didn't really want to understand."[87] "[I was] wrong—in hindsight wrong," Carballo would later admit, "but at that time that was my feeling."[88] Carballo's decision not to become my Chief of Staff was unfortunate, I think, because we likely would have mutually benefited from working more closely together.[89]

The rumblings over our real or perceived inattention to the cultural or behavioral aspects of AIDS[90] continued, and they caught the attention of enough outside observers that increasingly some in the donor community became dubious about GPA's ability to be "something good" ... and to handle a global pandemic for which few medical interventions existed.[91] The very reason Halfdan Mahler told me he had initially resisted committing WHO resources to AIDS—namely, that WHO had historically struggled to address diseases requiring behavioral solutions—was in a sense prophetic. Mann's decision to approach AIDS from an "expanded response" or human rights perspective had calmed some of these fears, but they surfaced again soon after Nakajima chose me to replace Mann. While most of our donors felt that I was a capable manager, some were worried that my skills and knowledge combined with Nakajima's interests might lead to us choosing a course that was too

[85] Thomas Coates, Interviewed by Michael Merson, New Haven, CT, February, 2002.

[86] Pertti J. Pelto and Gretel H. Pelto, *Anthropological Research: The Structure of Inquiry*. New York: Cambridge University Press, October 1978.

[87] Manuel Carballo, Interview by Michael Merson, New Haven, CT, November, 2002.

[88] Ibid.

[89] Ibid.

[90] Thomas Coates, Interview by Michael Merson, New Haven, CT, February, 2002.

[91] Progress report April 1991; Gill Walt, Interview by Stephen Inrig, Dallas, TX, September 23, 2010.

narrow. "[AIDS] was often still seen [by WHO] in fairly medical terms," remembers Gill Walt, who began serving as Vice-Chair of GPA's External Review Committee about 6 months after I joined GPA. "There were concerns among the donors who couldn't see any medical intervention available for HIV/AIDS … [that] the kind of social and cultural aspects of it were not being addressed sufficiently."[92] And so it is to GPA's efforts to attend to this "expanded response" that we now turn.

---

[92] Gill Walt, Interview by Stephen Inrig, Dallas, TX, September 23, 2010.

Chapter 12
Addressing Stigma, Discrimination, and Human Rights

Prison had not been part of Hans Paul Verhoef's travel plans.[1] It must, therefore, have shocked him profoundly when, on April 2, 1989, after a brief interrogation, Verhoef found himself in the custody of United States Customs officials. Behind bars at an immigrant holding tank in the Scott County jail in suburban Minneapolis, Minnesota, the Rotterdam native learned that he had been detained because of the drugs found in his luggage.

Unlike countless other drug smugglers detained at United States borders, however, Verhoef's story caused an immediate media sensation. After all, the man was not a criminal; the drugs found in his luggage were not illegal, and—for many, at least—his detention in the Scott County jail was outrageous. Verhoef was living with AIDS[2]; the drugs were for his treatment, and he was traveling to the National Lesbian and Gay Health Conference in San Francisco. But the presence of Verhoef's AIDS drugs revealed to officials his HIV status, signaling that he had fallen afoul of the relatively new United States immigration law that prohibited tourism and immigration by people living with AIDS.[3] His was the first public case of an immigrant being refused access to the United States on account of AIDS.

The Verhoef incident occurred before I joined the Global Programme on AIDS (GPA), but we mention it here because it was one of the first times discriminatory

---

Within this chapter the singular pronouns *I* and *my* refer to Michael Merson alone, whereas the plural pronouns *we* and *us* generally refer to Michael Merson and Stephen Inrig jointly. Where *we* or *us* refers to Michael Merson and his colleagues at WHO, the object of the pronoun is clarified by context.

[1] These paragraphs adapted from Stephen Inrig, "In a Place So Ordinary: North Carolina and the Problem of AIDS, 1981–1997," Duke University, PhD Dissertation, 2007.

[2] For the purposes of this text, we will use the term AIDS to encompass both AIDS and HIV unless otherwise specified.

[3] "Arrest of Dutch Visitor with AIDS Protested," *The Charlotte Observer*, April 5, 1989, 2A.

© Springer International Publishing AG 2018
M. Merson, S. Inrig, *The AIDS Pandemic*, DOI 10.1007/978-3-319-47133-4_12

AIDS policies gained international press attention in high-income countries. In many respects, Verhoef's experience was relatively minor compared to the stigma and discrimination endured by many on account of their HIV status. As we discussed in Chapter 6, people living with AIDS very commonly experienced stigma and discrimination that isolated them, and sometimes their families, from their communities.[4]

In Chapter 6, we also described how Jonathan Mann had focused many of his efforts around health and human rights issues in the years before he resigned as GPA Director. Upon my arrival in GPA, I quickly realized I needed to continue these efforts. Despite my reputation as Director-General Hiroshi Nakajima's contrarian to Mann's human rights perspective, and lack of experience working in the area of human rights, I wanted to maintain a focus on AIDS-related human rights concerns. I have already admitted that I was largely unaware of the politics of AIDS, and this was especially the case when it came to issues associated with AIDS-related stigma and human rights. That said, it did not take long for me to appreciate the central problem AIDS-related discrimination played in the pandemic and to understand why Mann had shifted his focus the way he did.[5] Unfortunately, AIDS's association with sexual taboos, sexual minorities, illicit drug users, and sex workers—along with the presumed lethality of the disease—led many communities and authorities to respond in very inhumane ways towards those afflicted with the disease, instituting laws and control measures counterproductive to the control of AIDS.[6]

I thus quickly understood—as Mann had come to realize—that individual behavior change as a prevention strategy alone was inadequate to slow the spread of AIDS and address the scope and potential impact of the pandemic. It was also necessary to

---

[4] M. Greeff, R. Phetlhu, L. N. Makoae, et al., "Disclosure of HIV status: experiences and perceptions of persons living with HIV/AIDS and nurses involved in their care in Africa," *Qualitative Health Research*, 2008, 18(3):311–324; A. N. Miller and D. L. Rubin, "Factors leading to self-disclosure of a positive HIV diagnosis in Nairobi, Kenya: people living with HIV/AIDS in the Sub-Sahara," *Qualitative Health Research*, 2007, 17(5):586–598; B. P. Ncama, P. A. McInerney, B. R. Bhengu, et al., "Social support and medication adherence in HIV disease in KwaZulu-Natal, South Africa," *International Journal of Nursing Studies*, 2008, 45(12):1757–1763; J. Iwelunmor, C. O. Airhihenbuwa, T. A. Okoror, D. C. Brown, and R. Belue, "Family systems and HIV/AIDS in South Africa," *International Quarterly of Community Health Education*, 2006, 27(4):321–335; T. A. Okoror, C. O. Airhihenbuwa, M. Zungu, D. Makofani, D. C. Brown, and J. Iwelunmor, "My mother told me i must not cook anymore—food, culture, and the context of HIV- and aids-related stigma in three communities in South Africa," *International Quarterly of Community Health Education*, 2007, 28(3):201–213; L. C. Simbayi, S. Kalichman, A. Strebel, A. Cloete, N. Henda, and A. Mqeketo, "Internalized stigma, discrimination, and depression among men and women living with HIV/AIDS in Cape Town, South Africa," *Social Science and Medicine*, 2007, 64(9):1823–1831; The Commission on Human Rights, "The Protection of Human Rights in the Context of Human Immunodeficiency Virus (HIV) and Acquired Immunodeficiency Syndrome (AIDS)" A/HRC/RES/16/28, 2011; K. Wood and H. Lambert, "Coded talk, scripted omissions: the micropolitics of AIDS talk in South Africa," *Medical Anthropology Quarterly*, 2008, 22(3): 213–233; C. I. Ulasi, P. O. Preko, J. A. Baidoo, et al., "HIV/AIDS-related stigma in Kumasi, Ghana," *Health and Place*, 2009, 15(1):255–262, 2009.

[5] Michael Merson, "Report of the Director, Fifth meeting of the Management Committee, Provisional agenda item 3: Geneva. 26–28 November 1990," Geneva: World Health Organization, 26 November 1990 GPA/GMC(2)90.3, 11.

[6] Ibid.

address the stigma and discrimination. What became a challenge for me was how to operationalize Mann's health and human rights approach beyond the individual perspective. By operationalize, I mean defining specific actions that could be taken by national AIDS programs to achieve specific human rights outcomes and to document the impact of these outcomes on HIV prevention and care. This meant GPA being able to give national AIDS program managers the ability to set human rights targets, determine if they were achieved, and calculate what impact this had on the epidemic in their country ideally in terms of HIV infections prevented or lives saved. Moreover, I felt, that if GPA failed to document how human rights violations increased vulnerability to HIV infection, and provide examples of how policies and actions that combatted discrimination reduced this vulnerability, then it would be difficult to convince leaders of national AIDS programs to give these approaches the financial support they needed. No doubt this was the manager in me, but I found myself frustrated because much of the health and human rights framework and language seemed inchoate when GPA tried to measure outcomes, ascertain causal influence, and determine impact.

To that end, in early June of 1990, a month after I became GPA Director, I decided to ask Mann about his intended plans to operationalize human rights within GPA and national AIDS programs. We met at my request at the Intercontinental Hotel coffee shop, a 5 min drive from the World Health Organization (WHO) headquarters in Geneva. It was the first time I had seen him since he had resigned. To my dismay, Mann gave me only vague answers to whatever questions I asked him. I attribute his reluctance in part to the suspicion and bitterness he was feeling towards me and WHO: this was less than 3 months after he had resigned from GPA and mere days after Abdelmoumene had notified Daniel Tarantola of his reassignment. But I also suspect that, in fact, operationalizing the health and human rights framework had proven rather difficult to do in practical terms, even for Mann.

To be fair, despite WHO having articulated a right to health concept in 1948 at the time of its founding,[7] there had been insufficient attention given to the practical implications and implementation of this concept. As Larry Gostin, a renowned human rights lawyer, would later write, "scholars … have failed systematically to examine the meaning and enforcement of social and economic rights."[8] While the United Nations Committee on Economic, Social, and Cultural Rights (CESCR) would eventually draft a more authoritative statement on the meaning of "the right to health," this did not come until 2000, a full decade after Mann had left GPA.[9] Moreover, in that 2000 statement, even CESCR acknowledged "considerable disagreement exists … as to whether 'health' is a meaningful, identifiable, operational, and enforceable right, or whether it is merely aspirational or rhetorical."[10] Indeed, even two decades after Mann's initial articulation of the health and human rights

[7] *Constitution of the World Health Organization.* Geneva: World Health Organization. 1948.

[8] Lawrence O. Gostin, "At Law: The Human Right to Health: A Right to the "Highest Attainable Standard of Health" *The Hastings Center Report*, Mar.–Apr., 2001, 31(2):29.

[9] General Comment 14, E/C.12/2000/4, 4 July 2000, available at <www.unhchr.ch/tbs/doc.nsf/>.

[10] Lawrence O. Gostin, "At Law: The Human Right to Health: A Right to the "Highest Attainable Standard of Health" *The Hastings Center Report*, Mar.–Apr., 2001, 31(2):29.

approach to AIDS, some of its most ardent proponents would publicly acknowledge that "it is difficult to find concrete examples of the benefits that have been derived from linking human rights norms and standards to public health imperatives."[11] This does not mean it is impossible or unimportant (the field has been more concretely defined today),[12] but it does help explain why, in 1990, it was not easy for me to see how or why Mann's health and human rights approach would be better at controlling AIDS than more traditional public health strategies.

Despite not having practical guidance or experience to draw upon, I tried my best to maintain a focus within GPA on health and human rights. For example, towards the end of 1990, GPA began hosting a series of regional workshops on ethical and legal issues related to AIDS. Then, in an attempt to operationalize a health and human rights framework, I invited the aforementioned Larry Gostin to Geneva (as Mann had done) in the summer of 1991 to teach our staff the basics of international human rights law and ways they could integrate human rights protections into national AIDS programs (the work Gostin did for GPA formed the foundation for his book, *Human Rights and Public Health in the AIDS Pandemic*, which he and Zita Lazzarini published in April 1997).[13] In conjunction with Gostin's efforts, in 1991 we hired a consultant, Fernando Chang-Muy, an expert on refugee law and policy, to develop a working relationship and set of objectives for GPA's collaboration with the United Nations Centre for Human Rights. Also, that November, GPA's European office held a pan-European consultation on AIDS in the context of public health and human rights in conjunction with the International Association of Rights and Humanity. This resulted in the Prague Statement that provided a consensus on strategies to ensure respect for human rights and ethical principles in response to the AIDS pandemic throughout Europe.[14]

While GPA took on the difficult challenge of operationalizing health and human rights, it was much easier to grasp Mann's earlier vision of a public health rationale that included antidiscrimination as a key component of the Global AIDS Strategy. As we explained in Chapter 6, Mann had been able to have the World Health Assembly (WHA), in May 1988, embrace this rationale by passing a resolution calling on all countries to prevent discrimination against people with AIDS.[15] Despite voting unanimously for this resolution, many nations still put restrictive regulations

---

[11] Sofia Gruskin and Laura Ferguson, "Using indicators to determine the contribution of human rights to public health efforts," *Bull World Health Organ* 2009;87:714–719.

[12] Benjamin Mason Meier, Adriane Gelpi, Matthew M. Kavanagh, Lisa Forman, and Joseph J. Amon. "Employing human rights frameworks to realize access to an HIV cure." *Journal of the International AIDS Society* 2015, 18(1).

[13] Lawrence O. Gostin and Zita Lazzarini, *Human Rights and Public Health in the AIDS Pandemic*, Oxford University Press, 1997, p. 1.

[14] "HIV/AIDS and Human Rights, International Guidelines from the Second International Consultation on HIV/AIDS and Human Rights," New York and Geneva: United Nations, 1998, HR/PUB/98/1, 57.

[15] Michael Merson, "Dr. Merson's Response to the WHA, May 15, 1990." Unpublished speech transcript.

and practices into place. This had frustrated Mann, particularly in light of the fact that Nakajima had been reluctant to satisfy Mann's requests to formally remind Member States of their commitments and responsibilities (indeed this refusal came to symbolize the divide between Nakajima and Mann on their approach to AIDS). Later, soon after I became Director, Nakajima made an about face and sent a *note verbale*[16] to all Member States recommending that each state reviews its national AIDS policies with a view to repealing discriminatory rules.[17] Whether this was a genuine effort on Nakajima's part to support the health and human rights concept, more of a cynical gesture to the concept, or a final comment on the division between Mann and himself, I do not know, but it was one of the early signals for me of the significant role that stigma and discrimination were playing in the spread of AIDS.[18] It also provided GPA with important leverage to continue our focus in this field.

The most concrete example of GPA's efforts in the area of human rights was our action against AIDS travel bans. Since the launch of GPA, several countries, including the United States, had ignored GPA's recommendations and instead passed laws restricting travel and migration of people with AIDS. The most notorious of these actions came in 1987 when the United States Congress unanimously passed a bill adding HIV/AIDS to the United States Public Health Service's list of dangerous and contagious diseases.[19] This effectively excluded HIV-positive foreigners like Hans Paul Verhoef from short-term entry into the United States, and it came at a time when efforts by AIDS activists and researchers against discrimination was starting to take off in the United States and other developed countries. GPA under Mann's leadership was, of course, a part of this movement.

The United States travel ban therefore became a focal point of controversy. Beginning in October 1989, the Red Cross Federation (RCF) in Europe started publicly voicing its concerns about the ban.[20] RCF had by this time adopted a position opposing such travel restrictions, and several members felt that United States travel restrictions were in conflict with its position, particularly if the United States failed

---

[16] A Note Verbale is a diplomatic communication prepared in the third person and unsigned: less formal than a note but more formal than aide-memoire. An aid-memoire is among other things a nonbinding document circulated among parties to remind them of the consequences of their prior commitments.

[17] Ibid.

[18] Hiroshi Nakajima, "Global Strategy For the Prevention and Control of AIDS: Report of the Director-General; Forty-Fourth World health Assembly, Provisional agenda item 19," Geneva: World Health Organization, A44/14;Dr. M.H. Merson, Lisbon, "WHO European Regional Meeting on Psychosocial Aspects of HIV/AIDS and Evaluation of Prevention Strategies," Lisbon, Portugal, MHMl, 1 June 1990, 4; Michael Merson, "Dr. Merson's Response to the WHA, May 15, 1990." Unpublished speech transcript.

[19] Philip J. Hilts, "U.S. to Ease Passport Curbs on Visitors Infected with AIDS Virus," *New York Times*, January 16, 1990; and Philip J. Hilts, "Bush May Support Easing AIDS Policy," *New York Times*, April 4, 1990.

[20] "The San Francisco Boycott: Leadership and Network Mobilization," in Leon Gordenker, Christer Jönsson, Roger A. Coate, and Peter Söderholm, *International cooperation in response to AIDS*. New York: Pinter, 1995, 119–127.

to make waivers available to HIV-positive individuals wanting to attend the 6th International AIDS Conference scheduled to be held in San Francisco in June 1990. As we described earlier in Chapter 8, this was one of the most difficult issues that I had faced during my 6-week period as Interim GPA Director. RCF members raised several questions with the United States government representatives: Would the United States truly make waivers available? What process would they make conference attendees go through to obtain the waivers? What consequences might there be for those unable to obtain waivers? What level of confidentiality would be assured to conference attendees with waivers both in the United States and when they returned to their home country?

Official answers from the United States government failed to assuage these concerns. After RCF representatives received no guarantees that the United States would safeguard "the confidentiality of HIV-positive people," RCF announced they would boycott the San Francisco conference—to the dismay of Mann and GPA.[21] Over the next several months, the intergovernmental Council of Europe, the *Comité France SIDA*, the European Parliament, over 80 AIDS organizations, and the governmental health agencies of France, Norway, Canada, Switzerland, and the United Kingdom joined in this boycott.[22]

As mentioned previously, Mann had not negotiated a solution to the controversy before he resigned, so brokering a resolution fell to me and my team.[23] For someone new to AIDS, I bore the difficult responsibility of negotiating an acceptable solution with the United States government that would allow the conference to continue as planned with participation of HIV-infected persons. Working with the Centers for Disease Control and Prevention (CDC), the International AIDS Society (IAS), and members of the United States Congress, we were able to convince the United States Immigration and Naturalization Services to adjust the travel ban in a way that allowed the Department of Health and Human Services to designate certain scientific conferences to be in the public interest and therefore eligible for a 10-day entry permit that did not ask about a traveler's HIV status. While this in no way addressed the fundamental discriminatory nature of the travel ban, it did modify the restrictions sufficiently enough, that GPA, IAS, and other institutions could maintain support for the conference. I must mention that the conference sponsors could not have secured the waiver without the assistance of James Mason, who at the time was the Director of CDC. Ultimately, 10,000 health workers and researchers from 74 nations were in attendance and listened to almost 2500 reports during the 5-day conference.[24]

---

[21] League of Red Cross and Red Crescent societies, Memorandum from Barbara Wallace to Andre Kisselev, 15 November 1989, Geneva; cited in "The San Francisco Boycott: Leadership and Network Mobilization," in Leon Gordenker, Christer Jönsson, Roger A. Coate, and Peter Söderholm, *International cooperation in response to AIDS*. New York: Pinter, 1995, 121.

[22] "The San Francisco Boycott: Leadership and Network Mobilization," in Leon Gordenker, Christer Jönsson, Roger A. Coate, and Peter Söderholm, *International cooperation in response to AIDS*. New York: Pinter, 1995, 119–127.

[23] Philip J. Hilts, "Bush May Support Easing AIDS Policy," *New York Times,* April 4, 1990.

[24] "International AIDS meeting to open in San Francisco," *Xinhua General News Service*, June 20, 1990, Item No: 0620025.

Much has been written on the 1990 conference elsewhere,[25] and we refer the reader there for greater detail. For me personally, the conference was the first time I had experienced the complex and contested world of AIDS activism. I was especially struck by the willingness of external advocacy groups to employ spectacular and theatrical strategies to gain attention.[26] The debates surrounding the conference and the travel ban made me immediately and irrevocably aware of the unique stigma associated with AIDS. On one hand, 100 advocacy groups, 3000 people, and 85 countries threatened to boycott an important International AIDS Conference over the United States government's discriminatory immigration policies.[27] On the other hand, the United States Immigration Service threatened to ban gay men from entering the country for the conference by enforcing an archaic, 1950s-era antigay law that blocked entrance to the country of "sexual deviants."[28] Never had I dealt with a public health issue so mired in controversy.

The conference itself was larger, and more diverse than I was accustomed to for international conferences focused on specific disease problems. And there were some surprises. For example, many months prior to the conference, GPA had agreed to organize a preconference session. When I arrived at the session, which I was to open as GPA Director, I was surprised to find the auditorium completely full. I had no idea how many were actually in attendance, but it felt like thousands. Moreover, it quickly became clear that I was viewed by many in the audience as an intruder, as the man who had replaced the beloved and highly respected Jonathan Mann. When I stepped up to the podium to open the conference, I don't think I have ever felt more unwelcome. Many in the audience were shouting insults at me, including a few whom I recognized as GPA staff. It was a tense, stressful, and difficult way to learn what it was like to be perceived as being on the wrong side of the fence at an AIDS conference.

The media added to this feverish atmosphere. I was scheduled to meet United States Secretary of Health and Human Services Louis Sullivan one morning for breakfast to discuss the final session of the conference. Sullivan wanted President George H. W. Bush to deliver the closing remarks, but he was not sure Bush would be willing to do so (Bush had been booed at a previous conference and consequently opted to skip the San Francisco conference and instead attend a fundraiser for Jesse Helms, the Senator who had ironically authored the HIV travel ban bill in the Senate).[29] As Sullivan was staying at a different hotel from me, he sent two United

---

[25] See, for example, Katherine E. Bliss. *The International AIDS Conference Returns to the United States: Lessons from the Past and Opportunities for the Future, July 2012*. Washington, DC: Center for Strategic and International Studies, 2012; Stephen Inrig, "In a Place So Ordinary: North Carolina and the Problem of AIDS, 1981—1997," Duke University, PhD Dissertation, 2007.

[26] Katherine E. Bliss. *The International AIDS Conference Returns to the United States: Lessons from the Past and Opportunities for the Future, July 2012*. Washington, DC: Center for Strategic and International Studies, 2012.

[27] Warren E. Leavy, "Visa Rules Eased for Foreigners with AIDS," *New York Times*, April 13, 1990.

[28] Philip J. Hilts, "Agency to Use Dormant Law to Ban Homosexuals from U.S.," *New York Times*, June 2, 1990, cited in Bliss. *The International AIDS Conference Returns to the United States*.

[29] Derrick Z. Jackson, "Bush adds insult to injury on AIDS," *The Boston Globe*, June 24, 1990, A2; Stephen Inrig, "In a Place So Ordinary: North Carolina and the Problem of AIDS, 1981—1997," Duke University, PhD Dissertation, 2007. 239.

States Secret Service agents to pick me up. The press must have become aware of this because they swarmed me as soon as I came out of the elevator. The Secret Service sped away as soon as I stepped into the car, and flew up and down the hills of San Francisco at breakneck speeds trying to lose the media, who were in hot pursuit. It was one of the most frightening car rides I have ever taken, all so I could meet with Secretary Sullivan privately. We had an amicable meeting and explored various scenarios for the closing session. After our meeting, Sullivan decided he would give the closing speech himself despite the anticipated protests.

The week was embroiled in controversy. Activists descended on the city, disrupting conference session after conference session, and spilling out into the streets in protest of both United States immigration policies and the perceived "lack of government response" to AIDS.[30] Fearing the protests might turn violent, police exerted a strong presence in and around the conference, and were accused of brutalizing activists during a protest in Golden Gate Park.[31] During the final session—and despite all the efforts Sullivan, others, and I had made to ensure the conference closed on a forward looking note—many in the audience turned their backs on Sullivan and drowned out his closing speech with boos, whistles, and horns.[32] It was a scene I would always remember. There would be many similar protests at future international AIDS conferences, but none like this one in its size, passion, and noise. I remember standing at the side, leaning on the wall and watching it, just amazed. I had no idea this went on at AIDS conferences. I would come to understand much of the activists' perspective as time went on, but this was a new experience for me, my initiation to the world of AIDS conferences and organized AIDS activism.

The San Francisco Conference educated me about the power GPA had—both the power of the purse and the power of public shaming—to enforce our antidiscrimination values. I believe that beyond all the rhetoric, in the long run, it was the practical enforcement of these values that resulted in the eventual adoption of less discriminatory health regulations and laws around the world. This meant that we would sometimes be forced to withdraw our cosponsorship and financial support of various meetings and international conferences. The next such incident occurred in Thailand 6 months after the San Francisco AIDS Conference. In February 1990, Mann had received an invitation from Princess Chulabhorn of Thailand for WHO to cosponsor, and for Mann to participate in an International Congress on AIDS at the Chulabhorn Research Institute in Bangkok in December 1990.[33] Nakajima himself had also received and accepted the invitation, agreeing that WHO would cosponsor the meeting and send five staff to participate.

---

[30] "International AIDS meeting to open in San Francisco," *Xinhua General News Service*, June 20, 1990, Item No: 0620025.

[31] Jane Gross, "Warily, San Francisco Braces for AIDS Forum," *New York Times*, June 17, 1990, A14.

[32] Ibid, See also Jane Gross, "Reporter's Notebook: City Hears Harmony, with A Few Jarring Notes," *New York Times*, June 24, 1990; Philip J. Hilts, "Jeers at AIDS Gathering Drown Out Health Chief," *New York Times*, June 25, 1990, cited in Bliss. *The International AIDS Conference Returns to the United States.*

[33] Michael Merson, "Letter to P. Vagliani, Re: International Congress on AIDS—Bangkok, 17–21 December 1990," World Health Organization, BPA/OOD/MHM/FP, Nov. 21, 1990.

However, as the conference neared, Thailand's HIV travel restrictions proved problematic. Back in August 1986, Thailand's Ministry of Interior had issued Ministerial Regulation No. 11, which prevented foreigners with AIDS from entering the country.[34] The rule remained in effect as the date for the conference approached, even though by this time the rising prevalence of AIDS in the country as a result of the commercial sex industry and injecting drug use had been well documented. Similar to the situation in the United States, the travel ban had and would continue to have little effect on Thailand's actual epidemic. After we pressed the Thai government on this point, we were informed on November 20 that it would remove the entry restriction on HIV-positive persons, though not for persons with clinical AIDS. We promptly informed the government that this policy was not acceptable and that it was necessary to allow visas to be issued to all HIV-positive persons, including those with AIDS, at least for the purpose of attending the conference. We cited resolution WHA 41.24 that called for avoidance of discrimination against HIV-infected people and persons with AIDS.[35] Not receiving a reply to our request from the Thai government, Nakajima informed Her Royal Highness on December 7—10 days before the conference—that unless the issue was satisfactorily resolved by the next day, WHO would not sponsor or participate in the conference.[36] Nakajima also informed WHO's Country Representative to Thailand that, if the situation was not resolved, he was to leave the country and "come to Geneva" during the period of the conference. On November 13, Nakajima was informed by the Permanent Secretary of Public Health that the Minister of Health had not been able to obtain the waiver. As a result, WHO issued a press release informing the world of its decision not to cosponsor or participate in the conference.[37]

This series of events and their eventual outcome was important for two reasons. First, it was the first time that WHO or any other United Nations (UN) agency had boycotted an international AIDS conference because of travel restrictions. The hard work done by Mann and Kathleen Kay to pass WHA Resolution 41.24 had made its mark. Second, despite his perceived lack of concern about discrimination against HIV-infected persons or support for the principles of human rights, and his fear of deeply insulting Her Royal Highness of Thailand, it was Nakajima who had made the final decision to boycott the conference. No doubt this decision was heavily influenced by GPA and by Sev Fluss, a Polish national and a senior administrator in the Director-General's office who had a strong interest in human rights, but the decision was Nakajima's to make and he made it. We also decided, soon thereafter and

---

[34] Uthai Sudsukh, "Letter to Dr. Nakajima, December 13, 2533 B.E. (1990), Ref. No. 0201/01/6479," 1–2; Michael Merson, "Letter to P. Vagliani, Re: International Congress on AIDS—Bangkok, 17–21 December 1990," World Health Organization, BPA/OOD/MHM/FP, Nov. 21, 1990.

[35] Michael Merson, "Memo: International Congress on AIDS, Bangkok, 17–21 December 1990" to SEARO Regional Director, Nov 22, 1990.

[36] Letter December 7 1990 from Nakajima to her Royal Highness Princess Chulabhorn.

[37] Uthai Sudsukh, "Letter to Dr. Nakajima, December 13, 2533 B.E. (1990), Ref. No. 0201/01/6479," 1–2; World Health Organization, "Press Release WH0/67: Statement on WHO's Decision Not to Participate in the International Congress on AIDS In Bangkok, 17–21 December 1990," Geneva, 13 December 1990; WHO Press Release WHO/67 13 December 1990.

for the same reasons, that we needed to change the venue of the 3rd International Conference on Health Promotion which we had originally scheduled to be held in the Philippines the following February.[38]

GPA and the international AIDS community continued to face the travel ban issue. In September 1991, at the 5th International conference of the Global Network of People Living with HIV/AIDS (GNP+) held in London, Jonathan Mann (who was now at Harvard University) announced that the 8th International Conference on AIDS, which was scheduled to be held in Boston the following summer and hosted by Harvard University with Mann serving as the conference Chair, would move to Amsterdam because of the United States government's HIV travel ban. "This decision is clearly, unequivocally, a result of US policy on HIV and immigration," Mann told conference attendees, "It is an extremely serious matter when America's oldest University has to leave the country to host a conference about a pandemic."[39] This action—jointly undertaken by WHO, IAS, and Harvard University—did little to change United States policy, however.

Indeed, a year later I experienced one of the most harrowing experiences of my life centered on the ongoing reality of the United States travel ban for people with HIV. In September 1993, I was invited by GNP+ to speak at the opening ceremony and in a panel discussion at the 6th International Conference of People living with HIV/AIDS being held in Acapulco.[40] The theme of the conference was "Communication and Solidarity for a Better Quality of Life," and a total of 270 delegates from 48 countries attended. I was scheduled to head to the airport shortly after my panel session. During the conference the attendees told me they would not allow me to leave unless I could guarantee that I would change the United States immigration law restricting entry of HIV-positive persons—as if I alone could somehow solve this problem. Many of them were angry that they had experienced great difficulty while transferring through the Miami airport to catch their flight to Acapulco. I could well understand their frustration, and had accepted their invitation to speak at the conference to show my solidarity and empathy with their plight. Moreover, during my talks, I had affirmed my opposition to mandatory HIV testing and had articulated my desire for more HIV-infected persons to serve on WHO advisory boards and in the leadership of more AIDS organizations. Despite these affirmations, and though having served as GPA Director for 3 years, I had underestimated their perception of me, "how do you wade through so much bullshit without getting a drop on you?" Aldyn McKean of the AIDS Coalition to Unleash Power (ACT UP) New York asked. "I don't buy it that you can't do what you say you want to do."[41]

[38] Michael Merson, "Report of the Director: Sixth meeting of the Management Committee, Geneva, 23–24 April 1991; Provisional agenda item 3," Geneva: Global Programme on AIDS, GPA/GMC(1)/91.3; 22 April 1991, 12–14.

[39] "International Conferences of People living with HIV: a Historical Overview" International Conference for People Living with HIV, 2008. http://2008.living2012.org/index.php?option=com_content&task=view&id=21&Itemid=37

[40] Ibid.

[41] "Communication and Solidarity for a Better Quality of Life," Report from the Sixth International Conference for People with HIV/AIDS, Acapulco, Mexico, September 23–28, 1993.

When it was time for me to depart for the airport, the participants formed a ring around me, physically preventing me from exiting the hall. Seeing that I was unable to negotiate my departure, Meurig Horton, a GPA staff member who accompanied me on the trip, broke through the ring giving me an open path to reach the waiting car of Cindy Robbins, the GNP+ President. She drove as fast as she dared to the Acapulco airport with some of the participants chasing us in their own cars. We were able to make it to the airport only 10 min prior to my scheduled departure, and I literally sprinted through passport control and onto the plane just as the doors were closing. On the flight home, I pondered what had brought on this confrontation and what I might have done to avoid it. I realize, reflecting on this experience now, that this was the desperate action of people who were living with a presumably fatal disease and enduring daily forms of brutal discrimination. While I was fully cognizant of the limits of my own power, they imagined I had some measure of leverage to influence policies that lay far outside of my control. This turned out to be not an uncommon experience for a number of health officials, particularly those perceived to have greater influence over United States research, health, or social policy.[42] While many of us agreed with the views of AIDS activists and advocates, we had to accept that expecting them to trust us, to trust me, was too much to ask.

The controversies that enveloped the San Francisco, Thailand, and Philippines conferences, and the associated protests, prompted GPA to initiate a systematic review and implementation of the WHA's antidiscrimination resolution (WHA41.24) in national AIDS programs. First, shortly after deciding to change the venue of the Philippines' health promotion conference, we undertook a systematic review of all legislation and regulations related to short-term travel of HIV-positive people in all countries.[43] GPA staff also began reviewing all medium-term plans and national AIDS program documents to ensure that GPA-supported national activities did not foster AIDS-related discrimination.[44] Furthermore, GPA continued implementing the plan, initiated by Mann prior to his resignation, of hosting regional consultations on the ethical, legal, and human rights aspects of AIDS.[45] At these consultations we discussed and agreed on priorities and follow-up activities for each region, explored innovative and effective solutions that various countries had devised to address particular concerns, and educated them on the international policies,

---

[42] Stephen Inrig, *North Carolina and the Problem of AIDS*. Chapel Hill, NC: University of North Carolina Press, 2011; Bob Roehr, "Anthony Fauci: A View from the Maelstrom of HIV/AIDS Research and Policy," American Association for the Advancement of Science (aaas.org), 16 May 2011, http://www.aaas.org/news/anthony-fauci-view-maelstrom-hivaids-research-and-policy

[43] Michael Merson, "Report of the Director: Sixth meeting of the Management Committee, Geneva, 23–24 April 1991; Provisional agenda item 3," Geneva: Global Programme on AIDS, GPA/GMC(1)/91.3; 22 April 1991, 12–14.

[44] Ibid, 16.

[45] Report of the Director-General "Forty-Fourth World health Assembly, Provisional agenda item 19: Global Strategy for the Prevention and Control of AIDS," Geneva: World Health Organization, 14 March 1991, A44/14.

principles, and information relevant to the ethical, legal, and human rights aspects of AIDS.[46]

We also maintained our collaboration with the United Nations Centre for Human Rights on its efforts to address AIDS-related discrimination at the UN and among Member States. This meant, for example, providing assistance and support to the United Nations Special Rapporteur on Discrimination against HIV-infected People and People with AIDS. It also included working with the Inter-Agency Advisory Group on AIDS (IAAG) to make recommendations on nondiscriminatory recruitment, insurance, and medical care for HIV-positive persons in the UN system, recommendations ultimately accepted by the heads of all UN agencies.[47] In addition, we established a concerted collaboration with the UN's Committee on Economic, Social, and Cultural Rights as it examined state reports on the right to health, giving particular attention to problems experienced integrating antidiscrimination policies into AIDS prevention and control efforts.[48]

Many of our activities in the area of health and human rights were headed up by GPA Deputy Director Dorothy Blake. She also worked with the World Bank and the International Monetary Fund (IMF) to gather evidence (and raise awareness) about the socioeconomic consequences of AIDS on developing economies.[49] Blake was particularly interested in and devoted special attention to the social and economic factors that put women, children, and sexual and ethnic minorities at greater risk of HIV infection. This meant designing interventions aimed at socially and economically empowering women, interventions that used frank messaging about the modes of HIV transmission, removed discriminatory policies, and educated adolescents and preadolescents about safer sex and harm reduction.[50] "Poverty makes whole

---

[46] The first regional consultation took place in Brazzaville in March 1990; the second in the Republic of Korea in July 1990; the third took place in Chile and the fourth to place in New Delhi, both in October 1990. A44/14; Report of the Director-General "Forty-Fourth World health Assembly, Provisional agenda item 19: Global Strategy for the Prevention and Control of AIDS," Geneva: World Health Organization, 14 March 1991, A44/14.

[47] Michael Merson, "Report of the Director, Fifth Meeting of the Management Committee, November 26, 1990" Geneva: World Health Organization GPA/GMC(2) 90.3, 1990; Report of the Director-General "Forty-Fourth World health Assembly, Provisional agenda item 19: Global Strategy for the Prevention and Control of AIDS," Geneva: World Health Organization, 14 March 1991, A44/14; Michael Merson, "Report of the Director: Sixth meeting of the Management Committee, Geneva, 23–24 April 1991; Provisional agenda item 3," Geneva: Global Programme on AIDS, GPA/GMC(1)/91.3; 22 April 1991, 12–14.

[48] Report of the Director-General "Forty-Fourth World health Assembly, Provisional agenda item 19: Global Strategy for the Prevention and Control of AIDS," Geneva: World Health Organization, 14 March 1991, A44/14.

[49] "WHO to co-sponsor international AIDS conference," *Agence France Presse*, September 12, 1991; "Malaysia Considering Internment of AIDS Victims," *The Associated Press*, September 19, 1991; Peter Starr, "Economic cost of AIDS to soar in developing countries: WHO," *Agence France Presse*, October 12, 1991; Sean Kelly, "AIDS Will Deplete African Work Force, WHO Doctor Says," *The Associated Press*, November 27, 1991.

[50] Alexander G. Higgins, "World Health Organization Revises Strategy to Meet AIDS Crisis Among Women," *The Associated Press*, January 28, 1992; "WHO shifts AIDS policy to focus on women," *Hamilton Spectator*, January 29, 1992, A4.

communities vulnerable to AIDS," we argued, as one example, in the revised Global AIDS Strategy, "by forcing men to leave their families in search of work, by leaving people hopeless enough to turn to the solace of drugs, and by making prostitution a survival strategy for women and children. AIDS then completes the vicious circle by making the community even poorer."[51]

As GPA developed the concept of the continuum of care, we understood the role that stigma and discrimination played in erecting obstacles to accessing care. Chapter 9 discussed ways GPA expanded its strategy in these areas during 1991 and 1992, but additional aspects bear mentioning. In May 1992, GPA pushed the WHA to adopt resolution WHA45.35, which stated emphatically that there was no public health rationale for arbitrarily limiting someone's human rights with measures like mandatory screening.[52] GPA formally accepted and adopted the "rights analysis" tool that Larry Gostin and Mann had developed through the Global AIDS Policy Coalition (see Chapter 13),[53] though we were unsure how to operationalize it. We also advocated for the formation of independent bodies to monitor AIDS discrimination laws at country level, provided countries with legal advice on their AIDS policies and practice, and wrote and distributed human rights-affirming literature and educational materials. Additionally, GPA promulgated our November 1987 Statement from a Consultation on Prevention and Control of AIDS in Prisons, calling for actions to combat discrimination of HIV-infected persons in prisons, along with our 1993 *WHO Guidelines on HIV Infection and AIDS in Prisons* which elaborated on the need to provide and maintain the continuity of prevention and care for incarcerated persons who were HIV-infected.[54] GPA was well aware of the severe discrimination often faced by HIV-infected persons in prisons around the world and felt they deserved particular attention.

In 1994, I hired Susan Timberlake, an American human rights lawyer, to lead our health and human rights efforts. Timberlake graduated from the University of Georgia Law School and received a degree in international law from Cambridge University before working at the United Nations High Commission for Refugees (UNHCR) in Geneva, from whence we recruited her. She concentrated her work specifically on health and human rights concerns, implementing a rights analysis and further cultivating GPA's relationship with the United Nations Centre for Human Rights. These and other efforts culminated in early 1995 in the publication of an *Aide-Memoire* from Nakajima on AIDS and human rights.[55] I think Timberlake did more than anyone else during my time as Director to build a credible health and

[51] Ibid.

[52] "HIV/AIDS and Human Rights, International Guidelines from the Second International Consultation on HIV/AIDS and Human Rights," New York and Geneva: United Nations, 1998, HR/PUB/98/1, 57.

[53] Jonathan Mann, "Letter to Michael Merson, July 1, 1993," Cambridge, MA: Harvard School of Public Health, 1993.

[54] WHO/SPA/INF/87.14; *WHO Guidelines on HIV Infection and AIDS in Prisons* (WHO/GPA/DIR/93.3).

[55] Global Programme on AIDS, "AIDE-Memoire: HIV/AIDS and Human Rights," Geneva: World Health Organization, 1995.

human rights program, though there were critics who still felt GPA was not doing enough in this area.

Looking back, I understand this criticism. As I have explained, we at GPA were not clear how to operationalize human rights actions into national AIDS programs, and so building a sufficient human rights programmatic response into GPA's operations was difficult.[56] Moreover, it would have likely required a significant modification of the mission of the program, and for human rights to become a major focus of many staff in GPA, not only the human rights officer. As Timberlake summarized her experience in GPA, "I think your heart and the hearts of people in GPA were very much in the right place, there was good support from you for anything I was trying to do. But I think that WHO had not taken on human rights in a programmatic way......It is hard to do (this) and it didn't happen in UNAIDS [Joint United Nations Programme on HIV/AIDS] either."[57] No doubt, there is much truth in what Timberlake said. Human rights deals intimately with a government's obligations and its citizens' entitlements, and requires holding nations responsible for their various agreed upon human rights obligations and commitments. The reality was, and is, that WHO has limited powers at its disposal to take such actions, being as it is a specialized UN agency interacting primarily with health ministries which often have limited ability to address larger societal and particularly human rights issues.

Would GPA have evolved differently in this area if Mann had not resigned as GPA Director? When I had an opportunity to ask him how GPA could have done more in the area of human rights at the 11th International Conference on AIDS in Vancouver in July 1996, just after he had given a plenary presentation on AIDS and Human Rights, Mann held up the Universal Declaration of Human Rights that was in his hand (he had referred to it in his presentation), implying that this charter would have served as the path to do so. But would this charter in itself been enough? It does not specify, for example, the practical steps governments in sub-Saharan Africa could take to realize the social, cultural, and economic changes that would lead to less discrimination against AIDS. We know that such changes—for example, the building of an "enabling environment" for AIDS prevention—usually occur slowly, and when they do translate into improved health, they often do so partially and over time. This does not mean public health practitioners should ignore issues like the empowerment of women or equal access to condoms, but because these reforms take time public health practitioners cannot depend solely on these changes for the success of their programs.[58]

---

[56] This paragraph taken from notes adapted from Merson's interview with Susan Timberlake. Susan Timberlake, Interview by Michael Merson, New Haven, CT, August, 2002.

[57] Susan Timberlake, Interview by Michael Merson, New Haven, CT, August, 2002.

[58] Revolutionizing the AIDS response: building AIDS resilient communities (aids2031 Social Drivers Working Group report). Worcester, MA: Clark University and International Center for Research on Women; 2010. Available from: http://www.aids2031.org/working-groups/socialdrive rs?view=resources#137 [accessed March 6, 2013].

I would give GPA's track record on health and human rights under my tenure a mixed grade. I feel we addressed human rights issues more than some give us credit for, though I admit we could have made greater efforts in their promotion and implementation. Also, while the efforts made for us by Larry Gostin, Fernando Chang-Muy, Ed Vela, and Lane Porter, among others, were helpful, I am certain that hiring a full-time person like Susan Timberlake to direct our efforts from the outset would have made GPA more effective in operationalizing human rights activities in national AIDS programs. Having not done so, I left GPA open to various criticisms about the sufficiency of our response in the area of human rights. However, this was not the only area where GPA was facing criticisms from the international community, as we will elaborate upon next.

Chapter 13
Challenges and Criticisms

On June 19, 1991, I mounted a podium in Florence, Italy to address a room full of AIDS[1] activists, researchers, and public health professionals attending the 7th International Conference on AIDS. It was mid-way through the week-long conference, and this group had gathered for a special session on the ongoing and future challenges facing national AIDS programs. My role was to open the session, and a palpable pall hung over the room: the Global Programme on AIDS (GPA) had just reported the most recent estimates of the global AIDS burden; more than 1 million people worldwide had now developed AIDS, and between 8 and 10 million people were infected with HIV. The speakers at that session, Jean Kalilani from Malawi, Ana Filgueiras from Portugal, and Steve Lwanga from Uganda, were to discuss key elements of national programs—prevention, care, research, and multisectoral action—with the aim of highlighting the role of multisectoral partnerships in mobilizing resources for the expanding pandemic.

As I looked out across the auditorium, I felt a deep desire to connect with those in the audience. A panoply of expressions filled their faces. Many new faces were spread throughout the room: the earnest, sometimes shell-shocked, faces of people who had, for the first time, come to this conference; sent because they or their government had recently been awakened to the disease threatening their land. I saw countless more familiar faces, as well: some allies, some critics, some curious, some neutral. These were often more burdened faces, expressing exhaustion both from the conference and the larger battle against this dreaded disease. They were the veteran scientists, activists, and public health professionals with whom I had become acquainted over this past year. Some looked at me through cynical eyes, some with outright derision, and not a few with camaraderie and a smile or nod of

---

Within this chapter the singular pronouns *I* and *my* refer to Michael Merson alone, whereas the plural pronouns *we* and *us* generally refer to Michael Merson and Stephen Inrig jointly. Where *we* or *us* refers to Michael Merson and his colleagues at WHO, the object of the pronoun is clarified by context.

[1] For the purposes of this text, we will use the term AIDS to encompass both AIDS and HIV unless otherwise specified.

© Springer International Publishing AG 2018
M. Merson, S. Inrig, *The AIDS Pandemic*, DOI 10.1007/978-3-319-47133-4_13

support. Any future success against AIDS (in GPA or elsewhere) depended on these people and the programs they ran, and it was with this in mind that I tried to fashion my words in a way that spoke to each of them: "A pandemic this extraordinary cries out for a truly extraordinary response," I said, trying to draw them into my vision of unified action.

> How can we account for the fact that the efforts made to date fall so far short of the mark? … How can we convey the measure of these 40 million lives that are at stake? Not even the Second World War—the biggest cataclysm of the twentieth century—produced this many casualties. Forty million—it is tantamount to a death threat hanging over the head of every last man, woman, and child in Uganda, Singapore, Australia, and Ireland. Surely this would cause an outcry. Surely this would prompt governments and donor agencies to allocate the resources needed to ward off disaster." I paused for a moment, as members of the audience responded with grunts or nods of agreement at the unfathomable indifference AIDS had elicited in many countries.

Then I worked to drive home my point:

> I am convinced that if we, all of us, take up and share the challenge, we have a chance to foil these dismal projections… Sharing the challenge means that individuals assume responsible behaviors that reduce their risk for HIV infection…Sharing the challenge means that individuals come together in communities to care for and support those affected and infected by AIDS…Sharing the challenge means that governments mobilize all their resources, both human and financial, to support communities and individuals in their fight against AIDS. Above all else, sharing the challenge means that the entire world must make a commitment to unite in a truly global alliance to mobilize the necessary technology, human resources, and political will. Future generations will expect no less from us.

With that, I ended my presentation, and our session on national programs began.

The speech marked something of "the end of the beginning" for me. I had been GPA Director for a little over a year. I had addressed the internal and external challenges faced by GPA and made a series of difficult but what I felt were essential changes to the program. Some of these changes meant the departure of a few key people who had built the program. Some meant acquiescing to internal World Health Organization (WHO) leadership about better aligning GPA with WHO's larger infrastructure. And some meant restructuring GPA's approach to focus more on objective outcomes and measurable management goals. In the end, I believed, this had and would put GPA on a stronger public health footing, better positioning it to provide health outcome deliverables to donor nations while upholding the core values espoused by Jonathan Mann and his team 4 years earlier.

The ensuing years had challenged these assumptions, however. I had not expected the complacency GPA would encounter from national leaders in the face of such a pressing pandemic. It took me time to realize that, for every tale we had of a President Museveni in Uganda or a Prime Minister Panyarachun in Thailand acting boldly on AIDS (see Chapter 10), there were countless other leaders remaining silent, living in denial, or taking a politically expedient route instead of facing the hard challenges that would have saved countless lives. As we mentioned in previous chapters, GPA also began facing mounting criticism about our efforts. In many cases, I had not expected these. Having labored for many years on public health issues largely hidden from the media spotlight, I had not anticipated the amount of criticism the press and other external actors would level upon us.

When I first joined GPA, Mann's concern about complacency seemed exaggerated to me and I don't think I realized the extent of the problem. Mann, of course, had done such a singularly effective job raising attention on AIDS that most people at WHO could only have dreamt of that kind of interest and support for their programs. Most were toiling away on diseases that never made the newspaper, much less the front page. Whatever those at WHO saw of AIDS on the global level, we would not have called it complacency. Yet Mann obviously sensed this growing complacency and warned against it in many of his speeches and press conferences.

But it was not long after I joined GPA that I realized how right Mann was. Indeed I found that, in high-income nations, the anticipation of new AIDS drugs and the lack of high infection rates among heterosexuals contributed to a waning fear of AIDS, while other health concerns, the end of the Cold War, and domestic issues related to economic growth began crowding AIDS out as a policy priority. At the same time, several low- and middle-income countries had yet to admit AIDS was even a problem.

Unfortunately, 1990 was precisely the wrong time for the world to become mired in complacency about AIDS. HIV infections continued rising: we estimated those with HIV to be about 6.5 million, but our models indicated we could expect as many as 40 million adults and children to be infected by 2000.[2] As we discussed in Chapter 10, the pandemic was broadening and diversifying, affecting high-income countries differently than low- and middle-income countries, and wreaking particular havoc in sub-Saharan Africa.[3] And the clusters of infection mushrooming in Thailand and Brazil suggested that AIDS was poised to explode across Southeast Asia and Latin America as well.[4] At GPA we were also worried about rising infection rates among African Americans in the United States, and drug users in both former Eastern Bloc

---

[2] Michael H. Merson, "The Global AIDS Epidemic: Current and Future Dimensions," WHO Global Programme on AIDS, mhm4/8 June 1990, 1–3.;Global Programme on AIDS, "The Problem, WHO Activities, and Financial Needs, June 1990," Geneva: World Health Organization, 1990, 2.14.1, 3, 6; "AIDS Carriers to Swell to 40 M. By 2000," *Jiji Press Ticker Service*, March 18, 1991; Celia Hall and Liz Hunt, "AIDS 'will be main cause of death in young women'" *The Independent* (London) November 28, 1990, 7; "1.5 million African women infected with AIDS," *Xinhua General News Service*, May 29, 1990, Item No: 0529034.

[3] Michael H. Merson, "The Global AIDS Epidemic: Current and Future Dimensions," WHO Global Programme on AIDS, mhm4/8 June 1990, 1–3; "Geneva," *The Times*, May 15, 1990; "1.5 million African women infected with AIDS," *Xinhua General News Service*, May 29, 1990, Item No: 0529034; WHO, "WHO Revises Global Estimates of HIV Infection: Ups Global Total to 8 to 10 Million," Geneva: World Health Organization, July 31, 1990, Press Release WHO/38, 1; Global Programme on AIDS, "The Problem, WHO Activities, and Financial Needs, June 1990," Geneva: World Health Organization, 1990, 2.14.1, 3.

[4] Michael H. Merson, "The Global AIDS Epidemic: Current and Future Dimensions," WHO Global Programme on AIDS, mhm4/8 June 1990, 1–3.; Global Programme on AIDS, "The Problem, WHO Activities, and Financial Needs, June 1990," Geneva: World Health Organization, 1990, 2.14.1, 3, 6; "AIDS Carriers to Swell to 40 M. by 2000," *Jiji Press Ticker Service*, March 18, 1991.

nations and in Western European metropolises.[5] Rising HIV incidence and prevalence rates among women across the globe likewise alarmed us: our forecasts predicted that women would constitute at least 40% of newly reported AIDS cases and
38% of estimated total HIV infections in the early 1990s.[6] Indeed, Jim Chin, GPA's
senior epidemiologist, warned that cause-of-death graph lines for women would go
"up at 45°," and he did not expect that trend to abate until the mid-1990s.[7] We estimated that over 3 million women of childbearing age had acquired HIV by the late
1980s, and that as a consequence at least 3 million women and children would die
from AIDS in the 1990s.[8] "The social, economic, and demographic impacts on
women" had largely been neglected, Chin and I noted.[9] The question was, how
could GPA effectively draw attention to the burgeoning problem?

We do not claim that AIDS was the only global disease beset by complacency. As
we mentioned, many of my colleagues and I at WHO had looked wistfully at GPA
for the funds and attention it had garnered during the time Mann led the program.
Indeed, there was a range of infectious diseases that affected more than a billion
persons living in low- and middle-income countries that would come to be called
"neglected tropical diseases." However, GPA's concern was about AIDS, and the
threat that one country's denial of its AIDS problem could pose to neighboring
nations, potentially thwarting global efforts to stop the spread of the disease.[10] To a
great extent, the long delay between HIV infection and the early signs and symptoms
of AIDS was our greatest enemy, because in both individuals and political leaders, it
is harder to incentivize prevention than a treatment or a cure.[11] Some of the denial
of and complacency towards AIDS stemmed from the fact that, from early on in the
pandemic, observers had conflated AIDS with homosexuality, taboo sexual behavior,
or drug use. Blanket associations between AIDS and these hidden, high-risk, and
often forbidden behaviors allowed countries to believe, falsely, that they were not at
risk for AIDS. They chose instead to believe (or say they believed) that people in

[5] Michael H. Merson, "The Global AIDS Epidemic: Current and Future Dimensions," WHO
Global Programme on AIDS, mhm4/8 June 1990, 1–3, 6; Charles Osgood, "CBS News Transcripts:
CBS This Morning, Friday, November 30, 1990," Celia Hall and Liz Hunt, "AIDS 'will be main
cause of death in young women,'" *The Independent (London)* November 28, 1990, 7.

[6] "1.5 million african women infected with AIDS," *Xinhua General News Service*, May 29, 1990, Item
No: 0529034; Michael H. Merson, "The Global AIDS Epidemic: Current and Future Dimensions,"
WHO Global Programme on AIDS, mhm4/8 June 1990, 1–3; Lawrence K. Altman, "U.N. Sees AIDS
Toll Surging Among Women and Infants," *The New York Times*, July 28, 1990, 1:24.

[7] Celia Hall and Liz Hunt, "AIDS 'will be main cause of death in young women,'" *The Independent
(London)* November 28, 1990, 7.

[8] WHO Issues New Estimates on Global AIDS Situation; Paediatric AIDS cases send estimates
soaring," Press Release WH0/49 25 September 1990, 1–2.

[9] Lawrence K. Altman, "U.N. Sees AIDS Toll Surging Among Women and Infants," *The New York
Times*, July 28, 1990, 1:24.

[10] Michael Merson, "Report of the Director, Fifth Meeting of the Management Committee,
November 26, 1990, Provisional Agenda Item 3" Geneva: World Health Organization GPA/GMC(2)
90.3, 1990.

[11] Michael Merson, "Report of the Director, Fifth Meeting of the Management Committee,
November 26, 1990" Geneva: World Health Organization GPA/GMC(2) 90.3, 1990, 12.

their culture did not practice these behaviors. In the meantime, AIDS continued spreading among those groups with often profound and devastating effects.[12]

One approach GPA took to deal with complacency was to cooperate with regional organizations to increase political will among Heads of State to confront the pandemic. As an example, in early 1992, I was asked by the United States Mission in Geneva to engage with the Organization of African Unity (OAU) for this purpose. OAU, located in Addis Ababa, Ethiopia, was formed in 1963 to coordinate and intensify cooperation among African states, many of which had recently received independence (in 2002 it was replaced by the African Union). I assigned this task to one of GPA's outstanding Technical Officers, Cyrilla Bwakira, who was from Burundi and at that time was our liaison with a number of countries in the Africa Region. Bwakira promptly organized a meeting in Abuja, Nigeria with Ministers of Health from nine African countries to discuss how the OAU could help raise awareness about AIDS. She followed this by organizing a regional meeting for all African Ministers of Health in Mbabane, Swaziland, that she and I both attended. At this meeting the Ministers unanimously drafted a resolution which, if adopted, would commit the Heads of State in Africa for the first time in the pandemic to "giving our fullest political commitment to mobilizing society as a whole for the fight against AIDS."[13] This resolution was then put forth by the government of Nigeria to the OAU Assembly of Heads of State in Dakar, Senegal, in July. The Heads of State agreed to discuss the resolution, though only in a closed session for fear of their comments being made public (Bwakira herself was barred from entering but listened to the debate in the interpreter's booth), and in the end the resolution was adopted.[14] It would take more than a resolution debated behind closed doors to obtain a real commitment from many African Heads of State to confront the pandemic, but it was at least a start. In June 2004, the OAU would adopt a second, far more comprehensive resolution on AIDS and the debate around this resolution was held in an open public session.[15]

Still, the complacency remained, and the lack of political commitment extended beyond national leadership. Other sectors of society failed to respond as well. I distinctly remember, in 1992, visiting the Vatican in Rome to explore the role the Catholic Church could play in the global response to the pandemic. I met with Cardinal Fiorenzo Angelini, the first President of the then newly created Pontifical Council for the Pastoral Care of Health Care Workers, which made him essentially the first proxy Minister of Health in the Vatican. We met in his small, barren office. I showed the Cardinal two graphic figures depicting the extent and projected gravity of the pan-

---

[12] Michael Merson, "Dr. Merson's Response to the WHA, May 15, 1990." Unpublished speech transcript.

[13] Organization of African Unity, Assembly of Heads of State, Twenty-eighth Ordinary Session, 29 June–1 July, 1992 AHD/Decl. 1 (XXVIII), AHD/Decl 1-2 (XXVIII), AHG/Res 206–217 (XXXVIII).

[14] Cyrilla Bwakira, Interview with Michael Merson, Johannesburg, October 12, 2013.

[15] Organization of African Unity, Assembly of Heads of State, Thirtieth Ordinary Session, 13–15 June 1994), AHG/Decl. 1-6, AHG/Res 228-233.

demic, particularly in Africa, where many in the Church were rumored to have been infected with HIV. He studied them for about 10 s, then tossed the papers in the air, looked at me, and said: "*Le problème n'est pas humain. Chacun doit trouver la voie.*" [The problem is not human. Each one must find his own way]. Was he telling me that the Church was not going to get involved in the pandemic? Was he saying that those with AIDS were sinners? I did not know. It would be 18 more years before the Vatican implied it would soften its stance and might condone the use of condoms in "some cases....with the intent of reducing the risk of HIV infection."[16] But even this small concession is very murky, and the Church has yet to provide clear guidelines on this issue. In any event, given the influence of the Catholic Church on the political leaders and lives of many living in sub-Saharan Africa, my encounter with Cardinal Angelini illustrated how difficult it would be for some political and religious leaders to speak openly about sex and condom use to prevent HIV infection, despite the intractable suffering caused by the pandemic.

This reticence among political and social leaders forced GPA to make sure that evidenced-based program management principles were included in national AIDS programs. To this end, GPA trained managers through our various planning, training, and program review efforts (see Chapter 9) so they could follow them even in the face of insufficient resources and meager political will.

On top of GPA's programmatic and managerial efforts, we also sought to garner support from global health leaders to fight complacency. At the end of 1990, I implored GPA's Management Committee to help combat AIDS-complacency: "Somehow we must combat this complacency and denial if we are really going to have an impact on the future course of this pandemic."[17] In those first years at GPA, I was particularly worried about Asia, so I visited a number of Asian countries with low HIV prevalence and where high-level officials often expressed little concern (with the exception of Thailand) about the threat of AIDS in their country. Almost a day did not go by during those first years where I was not wracked with fear that an African-scale pandemic would break out in parts of Asia before governments awoke to the problem.[18] But we at GPA often saw little change in response, and the denial and complacency persisted.[19] If African nations were only beginning to respond to

---

[16] Rachel Donadio and Laurie Goodstein, "After Condom Remarks, Vatican Confirms Shift," *The New York Times*, November 23, 2010. http://www.nytimes.com/2010/11/24/world/europe/24pope.html?pagewanted=all.

[17] Michael Merson, "Report of the Director, "Fifth meeting of the Management Comnittee, Provisional agenda item 3:Geneva. 26–28 November 1990," Geneva: World Health Organization, 26 November 1990 GPA/GMC(2)90.3, 12.

[18] Michael Merson, "Report of the Director, Sixth meeting of the Management Committee, Provisional agenda item 3:, Geneva, 23–24 April 1991," Geneva: World Health Organization, 1991, GPA/GMC(1)/91.3, 16; Michael Merson, "Report of the Director, Fifth Meeting of the Management Committee, November 26, 1990" Geneva: World Health Organization GPA/GMC(2) 90.3, 1990.

[19] Michael Merson, "Report of the Director, Fifth Meeting of the Management Committee, November 26, 1990" Geneva: World Health Organization GPA/GMC(2) 90.3, 1990; Michael Merson, "Report of the Director, Sixth meeting of the Management Committee, Provisional

the problem, we worried, how much greater would the devastation be if the much larger Asian nations failed to act?

I also sought the help of scientists to awaken national leaders to the threat of AIDS. In the May 28, 1993 edition of the journal *Science*, I invited scientists to join us in battling complacency on AIDS, imploring them to: educate others about the dangers of complacency; ensure that discussions about risk behaviors remained scientific rather than moralized; form collaborative research groups that crossed national, gender, class, and serostatus barriers; and concentrate on high-priority research issues (I proposed that these be: antiviral therapies; preventive technologies for women, minorities, and vulnerable people; improved therapies for comorbidities; and a more comprehensive understanding of the human immune system as a prerequisite for developing an HIV vaccine). "If the scientific community worldwide rises to these four challenges," I concluded, "we will have (an) historic opportunity—the opportunity to scale up application of what we already know works to slow the spread of HIV and to give even greater emphasis than in the past to new avenues for prevention."[20]

We tried other strategies as well in an effort to stress the potential profound severity of the AIDS pandemic. First, Chin began speaking about HIV prevalence rather than AIDS prevalence (i.e., infection rates rather than symptomatic disease rates) in many of his writings and presentations. He made this recalibration for both substantive and pragmatic reasons. Substantively, we at GPA knew by 1990 that HIV infection had a 10-year latency period, so reporting only national or global AIDS prevalence threatened seriously to under-report the pandemic's scope. Pragmatically, of course, we also knew that higher numbers generated more attention than lower ones, and the press seemed to love reporting on numbers. Making the case as strong as it could be, within the limits of science, was not a problem for me. As Chin has noted about this period, "HIV prevalence estimates made by staff of GPA/WHO from the late 1980s up to the mid-1990s were intentionally conservative."[21] This had to change, and we hoped that more alarming numbers would spur national and international leaders to grasp the need for desperate action.[22]

Second, with the help of celebrities, GPA promoted AIDS awareness. World AIDS Day played a particularly significant role in this effort. Mann had started World AIDS Day to raise awareness and confront ignorance and complacency

agenda item 3, Geneva, 23–24 April 1991," Geneva: World Health Organization, 1991, GPA/GMC(1)/91.3, 16.

[20] "AIDS researchers review progress," *United Press International*, May 27, 1993.

[21] James Chin, *The AIDS Pandemic: The Collision of Epidemiology with Political Correctness*. London: Radcliffe Publishing, 2007, 137.

[22] Michael Merson, "Report of the Director, Fifth Meeting of the Management Committee, November 26, 1990" Geneva: World Health Organization GPA/GMC(2) 90.3, 1990; Michael Merson, "Report of the Director, Fifth meeting of the Management Committee, Provisional agenda item 3, Geneva. 26–28 November 1990," Geneva: World Health Organization, 26 November 1990 GPA/GMC(2)90.3, 12; Michael Merson, "Dr. Merson's Response to the WHA, May 15, 1990." Unpublished speech transcript.

around AIDS (see Chapter 5) across the globe. As time went on, Chris Powell, our Director of Communications, Suzanne Cherney, and I all came to believe that World AIDS Day, if executed correctly, offered a unique platform to remind the global community that defeating AIDS required cooperation that crossed social and national boundaries.[23] Thus, GPA prioritized this event, selecting a timely theme each year, actively promoting events at country and global levels, and providing support materials for local activities. I recall doing countless interviews every World AIDS Day from early morning to late evening with television and radio stations around the world. There is no doubt that the early efforts by Powell and Cherney to make World AIDS Day a success helped it to become the important AIDS awareness vehicle it remains to this day.

Celebrities were often helpful in using their "star power" to garner attention around World AIDS Day events. My first such interaction with a celebrity was with Elizabeth Taylor. She and I shared the platform at a press conference immediately before the International AIDS Conference in San Francisco in June 1990. Since 1984 and the death of her close friend Rock Hudson from AIDS, Taylor had played a very important role spurring AIDS research, mobilizing AIDS funding, and raising awareness about the need for acceptance and compassion for persons living with AIDS in her position as the Founding National Chair and spokesperson for the American Foundation for AIDS Research or AMFAR (now called the Foundation for AIDS Research). I could never forget how much the press adored Taylor that day; it didn't matter what her talking points were or how well she delivered them: the press truly valued who she was and what she meant to the AIDS cause, and gave her maximum coverage. I realized from this experience that celebrities, if leveraged wisely, could give AIDS a public platform and raise awareness in ways that no public health professionals could achieve. I would see this again when I appeared with Liza Minnelli and the United States Olympic diver Greg Louganis at an AMFAR World AIDS Day event on December 1, 1993 at the United Nations (UN) in New York City (Picture 13.1).

There were other occasions as well. I vividly recall my meeting with Diana, Princess of Wales, who had made a name for herself in the AIDS world after she publicly shook the hand of a person with AIDS without wearing gloves in a London hospital ward in 1987, in order to reduce public fears about physical contact with people with AIDS. By the early 1990s Diana had started to travel to Africa, Asia, and South America to address world poverty, the global AIDS pandemic, and the plight of AIDS orphans. I met her at her Kensington Palace residence in London just before she was to make a trip to Africa in 1992. Also present was Michael Adler. Adler was a sexually transmitted disease (STD)[24] expert who helped guide Diana's work on AIDS from his position as Chairman of the National AIDS Trust in the United Kingdom (Adler, as we mentioned earlier, had also been nominated by his government

---

[23] "AIDS And The Status of Women: Challenges and perspectives for the 1990s," *WHO Feature*, October 1990, No 149, 2–3.

[24] For the purposes of this text, we use the term sexually transmitted disease(s) and the abbreviation STD rather than the other term sexually transmitted infection(s) or STIs.

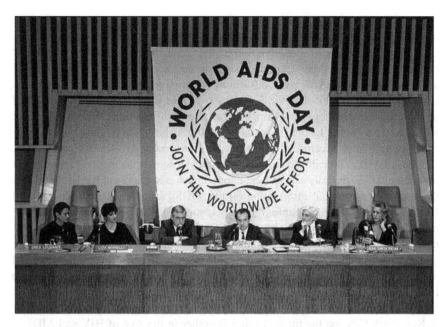

Picture 13.1 World AIDS Day commemorated at UN Headquarters, 12/1/93. In observance of World AIDS Day a panel discussion bringing together artists, entertainers, medical professionals, governmental and non-governmental organizations together to focus on advances made in combating the disease and specifically on the efforts of the arts and entertainment community to halt the spread of AIDS was held today at UN headquarters. *From left to right*: Greg Louganis, Olympic gold medalist, actor and AIDS activist; Liza Minnelli, actress, singer and AIDS activist; Michael Merson, Executive Director of the WHO Global Programme on AIDS; Bernard Gershon of ABC News Radio serving as Moderator; Mervin Silverman of the American Foundation for AIDS Research (AMFAR); and Ilka Tanya Payan, actress and member of the New York City Commission on Human Rights. 1/Dec/1993. Source: UN Photo/J Bu

for the GPA Director position). It was he who had asked me to brief the Princess on the status of the pandemic across the African continent. She was as elegant and graceful in person as she had looked on television, but seemed restless throughout our meeting—I had brought some data with me and tried to show it to her, but could tell she was having difficulty concentrating. I did not know of course that she would soon be separating from her husband, Prince Charles. We had tea, met for an hour or so, and I left her the information I had brought with me. I did not hear from her again, and was saddened when I learned of her fatal automobile accident in 1997. That tragic event reminded me of her restlessness during our meeting, and I often wondered what effect such a tumultuous public life must have had on her.

I also allied with sports figures to find new voices for the global fight against AIDS. Two of them, Arthur Ashe and Earvin "Magic" Johnson, both went public about their HIV-positive status in the early 1990s. Arthur Ashe was the first African American to make the United States Davis Cup Tennis team and the only African American male to win the singles title at Wimbledon, the US Open, and the

Australian Open. He had been infected with HIV through a contaminated blood transfusion he received during open heart surgery in a New York hospital in the early 1980s, shortly before hospitals routinely screened blood for HIV. He announced that he had AIDS in April 1992 and began to educate others about the disease. I appeared with him on ABC's Good Morning America on World AIDS Day that year, a few months before his death in February 1993. He was a remarkable, thoughtful figure. I was touched by his sincerity and desire to inform others about the risk of HIV infection. Before he died, he established the Arthur Ashe Foundation to Defeat AIDS, which later became the Arthur Ashe Endowment for the Defeat of AIDS, supporting AIDS education, training, and clinical research. Incidentally, throughout my time at GPA, the only one of the major television networks in the United States that reported substantial information on the AIDS pandemic was ABC; Marshall Hoffman, who directed a public relations company outside Washington, DC and helped us obtain interviews with United States television stations, could almost never get interviews on other major network morning shows.

In 1993, I met Earvin "Magic" Johnson, one of the most accomplished and popular professional basketball players of his era, when he joined me at "The International Symposium on AIDS '93" held in Tokyo. He was there to speak alongside David Ho, the well-known AIDS researcher from Rockefeller University in New York City, on the topic "Living Together in the Age of HIV and AIDS"[25] (Picture 13.2). Doctors first diagnosed Johnson with HIV in late October 1991, and his announcement 1 week later stunned the nation and reminded the world that heterosexuals and African Americans were vulnerable to contracting HIV. I first heard about Johnson's status while sitting in the Swissair lounge watching television at JFK Airport waiting to board my flight back to Geneva and was astounded. Would he be able to continue to play professional basketball (some prominent players were expressing fear about playing alongside him)? How easy would it be for him to become a global spokesperson for HIV awareness and protection? At the conference in Tokyo, Johnson seemed to show a slight reticence when talking about his status. We suspect this was due to a number of factors—his soft spoken personality, the difficult position in which he found himself personally, the positive image that the National Basketball Association (NBA) was trying to portray of itself, and the discomfort that American society has had historically talking openly about the sexuality and masculinity of African American men. In time, Johnson grew into his role as a global spokesman on AIDS, appearing with me again the following year at a conference in Geneva, and going on to establish the Magic Johnson Foundation, which invested considerable time and resources opening AIDS treatment clinics in underserved urban areas of the United States, and today is supporting educational and other types of activities that empower underserved urban communities.

---

[25] "Magic To Attend AIDS Meeting," *The Daily Yomiuri*, March 1, 1993, 2; Norma Reveler and Hiromi Sasamoto, "'Magic' Urges Japan To Fight AIDS; HIV Carriers Said To Battle Disease, Social Stigma," *The Daily Yomiuri*, March 26, 1993, 2.

Picture 13.2 The International Symposium on AIDS'93 Conference, Tokyo. February 1993. Michael Merson (*left*), Earvin "Magic" Johnson (*center*) and Ryoichi Sasakawa, Chairman of the Nippon Foundation (*right*), Photo courtesy of The Nippon Foundation

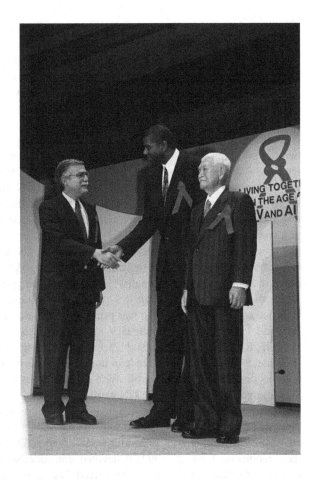

Because of his notoriety and the popularity of professional basketball, there was a great increase in HIV testing following Johnson's announcement of his HIV status (it rose by 60% in New York City alone). This gave me the idea of approaching the NBA to see if it would be interested in having HIV prevention messages posted in basketball arenas around the country.[26] More than anything else, I saw this as a teachable moment for youth. Unfortunately, the NBA remained unconvinced. "People don't come to a basketball game to hear about AIDS," the NBA's Commissioner's Office told me. "People pay a lot of money to come to these games and they don't want to hear about condoms." The league argued that they were trying to establish a positive family atmosphere at the games, and that pronounced messages about safer sex might work against that effort (I found a similar reluctance from American Express when it was selecting a theme for a global giving campaign—despite my efforts, it selected combating malnutrition rather than AIDS).

---

[26] Michael Specter, "How Magic Johnson Fought the AIDS Epidemic," *New Yorker*, May 14 2014.

The NBA did, however, mount an AIDS educational program for their players using experts from Johns Hopkins Medical Center after the league realized how much their players were at risk. While I was disappointed that our efforts to launch an information campaign within professional basketball arenas did not materialize, the NBA deserves much credit for the responsibility it showed in addressing AIDS risks among its players. Today, the situation is very different; the NBA now includes AIDS advocacy as a major part of its "NBA Cares" initiative.

Combating complacency certainly had its challenges… but I believed we were making some progress. These advances made our next challenge—dealing with the press—that much more frustrating. The international press corps often seemed more interested in covering squabbling and problems within the UN and WHO than in covering the expanding AIDS pandemic. Some of this surely stemmed from the resignation of Jonathan Mann, whom the press respected enormously. Some of this, however, was due to the fact that GPA had few success stories to share with them, and they built up a certain measure of disaster fatigue having covered story after story about extreme and seemingly endless suffering. AIDS also created some cognitive dissonance among journalists and readers: the global pandemic was largely a heterosexual phenomenon in low- and middle-income nations, while in North America and Western Europe it was primarily a disease of gay men and intravenous drug users. By the early 1990s, HIV rates seemed to have reached their peaks in many high-income countries, and since most of the international press corps came from these countries, the decrease in domestic concern about AIDS made it less of a global concern for them as well. With a global recession and the end of the Cold War, intrigue and reform in the UN garnered much greater attention. The challenge for GPA was continuing to find imaginative ways of presenting the pandemic to the press that would break through the hard shells of denial, apathy, and complacency.[27]

When the international press did write about AIDS, several issues consumed their reporting. First, in 1992, it devoted considerable attention to the external review of GPA and the response it received from donor governments and agencies (we discuss this in greater detail in Chapter 14).[28] Second, journalists focused on the emerging dysfunction within WHO. Several articles discussed criticisms of WHO's regional structure, and the way the personal ambitions or divergent approaches of the Regional Directors stymied effective use of WHO funds. The press was particularly critical of WHO's African Regional Director, Gottlieb Lobe Monekosso, alleging, as we noted previously, that he was abusing donor funds and was "up to no good."[29] Still other articles focused on stagnation in GPA funding and the delays or reductions this caused national programs: For example, Mboya Okeyo, medical officer of Kenya's AIDS Control Program, told reporters in 1992 that "he was hamstrung by 'this business of waiting around each year for money GPA does not

[27] Michael Merson, "Dr. Merson's Response to the WHA, May 15, 1990." Unpublished speech transcript.

[28] Mort Rosenblum, "U.N. AIDS-Fighting Agency Having Problems," *The Associated Press*, July 5, 1992.

[29] Ibid.

have.'"[30] It was undoubtedly true that GPA found itself in a real and growing resource crisis; however, it was also true that WHO's $87 million budget was less than the AIDS budgets of some American states.[31]

A number of reporters focused considerable attention on a third topic: WHO's perceived lack of urgency in responding to AIDS and the growing competition we faced from other bi- and multi-lateral organizations. Some articles criticized GPA, claiming we were treating AIDS "as yet another long-term problem" and had fallen short of our mandate to mobilize national authorities.[32] Others bemoaned that we had hopelessly picayune bureaucratic requirements that encumbered effective outreach and prevention.[33] Still others maintained that GPA strove to dominate the global response in ways that chafed other programs and prompted them to launch alternative programs outside our control. Not infrequently, these journalists would seek comments from Mann, now at Harvard University, or from Jim Sherry, the United Nations Children's Emergency Fund (UNICEF)'s Chief of Health Promotion and its key adviser on AIDS, and these individuals (particularly Mann) were only too ready with their critiques.[34]

It would be foolish to deny that there weren't problems. I had recognized many of these when I first came on board with GPA and the external review would call attention to several others. Controversy about various aspects of GPA's programs certainly dulled our impact and effectiveness. We were trying to reduce bureaucratic controls and ferret out any corruption, but there were challenges in doing so. Indeed, one of the main reasons, in 1992, that we recruited Peter Piot from his position in Antwerp to serve as Associate Director was to help improve GPA's effectiveness. "GPA went from nothing to something," Piot had explained to reporters after taking the job, "Now it must go from something to something good."[35] As a newcomer to AIDS, the magnitude and potential consequences of complacency impressed and dismayed me, particularly in light of the push Director-General Hiroshi Nakajima was making for regionalization.

One of our greatest challenges with the press was the real and perceived tensions emerging between GPA and Mann's newly formed organization, the "Global AIDS Policy Coalition" (GAPC) at Harvard University. As we mentioned, the press frequently sought out Mann's opinion on the global AIDS effort after he left GPA. His criticisms of the global response carried considerable weight in the court of public

---

[30] Ibid.

[31] "World Health's AIDS Chief To Appeal For More Funding," *The Associated Press*, July 16, 1992.

[32] Mort Rosenblum, "Combatants in Losing AIDS War Say Millions Will Die Needlessly," *The Associated Press*, July 5, 1992.

[33] Mort Rosenblum, "U.N. AIDS-Fighting Agency Having Problems," *The Associated Press*, July 5, 1992; Mort Rosenblum, "Combatants in Losing AIDS War Say Millions Will Die Needlessly," *The Associated Press*, July 5, 1992.

[34] Mort Rosenblum, "Combatants in Losing AIDS War Say Millions Will Die Needlessly," *The Associated Press*, July 5, 1992.

[35] Mort Rosenblum, "U.N. AIDS-Fighting Agency Having Problems," *The Associated Press*, July 5, 1992.

opinion and among some of GPA's donors. My relationship with Mann was certainly strained—as noted earlier, I first met with him soon after I had assumed the GPA Director position and, understandably at that time, he was very bitter towards WHO and very suspicious of me. I tried meeting with him again at the International Conference on AIDS in Amsterdam, in July 1992, but he was reticent to do so. Though 2 years had passed, I suspected his time after leaving WHO must have been difficult and he had not forgiven me for having taken his position.

GAPC consisted initially of nine individuals from nine countries who had met in the spring of 1991 to set goals for the coalition, discuss priorities, and elaborate an action plan.[36] This included Daniel Tarantola and Jeff O'Malley, who had worked with Mann in GPA. The group grew over the next few months, as did the goals of the organization, which came to be: provision of independent policy analysis on issues related to the pandemic; publication of an annual World AIDS Report; promotion of successful HIV policies and interventions; identifying and tracking trends in the pandemic; and stimulating international, multisectoral HIV policy research and analysis.[37]

As Mann developed GAPC, the press found a counter-narrative to our efforts at GPA. In fact, Mann had not been publicly critical of me or of GPA in the first several months after he had resigned. By the fall of 1991, the press began asking him about the global AIDS effort and his replies and criticisms began to sharpen and become more public. The target of Mann's earliest criticisms of GPA was our desire to focus our efforts in low- and middle-income countries. I explained this policy commitment in an interview with *Science* in the fall of 1991: "What I am trying to get [low- and middle-income nations] to understand is that if they wait for [AIDS] cases, it's too darn late."[38] When the press asked Mann about this, however, he argued that the approach was wrong-headed: "It's another level of denial that this is a global problem," Mann explained in the same *Science* article. "[It] put[s] the problem far away, and in a sense declares premature victory in some parts of the world, like the industrialized world."[39] This created a false sense of security about the pandemic, Mann believed. "Critics, including Mann," the *Science* reporter concluded, "argue[d] that Merson and WHO are trying to make AIDS into just another disease of the developing world, rather than the global problem they believe it to be."[40] Nothing could have been further from the truth. GPA was simply placing more emphasis on the parts of the world where the pandemic was already having devastating effects, or were likely to have them in the very near future.

What ensued, then, was a measure of competition in the press between GAPC and GPA. This continued to grow in late 1991, when Mann and his team met to plan

---

[36] Interim Report of the Global AIDS Policy Coalition to the Francois-Xavier Bagnoud Foundation," Global AIDS Policy Coalition, January 1, 1992, A20/372/54.

[37] Ibid.

[38] Joseph Palca, "WHO AIDS Program: Moving on a New Track," *Science,* October 25, 1991, 254: 512.

[39] Ibid.

[40] Ibid.

their first annual world AIDS situation report, dubbed *AIDS in the World*.[41] GPA published a report annually on the global AIDS pandemic and we were not opposed to other organizations doing likewise: The Panos Institute periodically published reports on AIDS, for example, as did the International Planned Parenthood Federation, the Institute of Development Studies, and the United States Agency for International Development (USAID).[42] Mann's group drew on many people previously associated with GPA in writing the GAPC report, which made it uniquely different in authorship from reports issued by other organizations. We responded to requests for information and documentation from Tarantola and the others working on the report.[43] Our chief concern, however, which we expressed to Mann and his group, was that the endeavor seemed duplicative, rather than complementary, with our work. On several occasions during the latter months of 1991 and early months of 1992, we suggested to Mann and Tarantola that they limit the scope of their report to the major topics that GAPC had decided to address. Instead GAPC published and promoted *AIDS in the World* as a comprehensive, "landmark publication" intent on tracking, "on an annual basis, the evolution of the pandemic, its effects, and the worldwide response."[44] This sounded very much like the purpose of our annual GPA report. Ultimately, to avoid confusion, we opted to reduce the scope of GPA's annual report and delay its publication to later in 1992, but we took the seemingly irreversible decision that Mann's group had made about its report and its stance towards GPA as an ominous sign.

In mid-1992, GPA came into public disagreement with GAPC in the press after GAPC openly challenged both GPA's projections for the pandemic and the larger nature of our strategy. In the spring of 1992, Jim Chin had predicted that, with the current incidence and prevalence rates for HIV and AIDS, we could expect about 10 million AIDS cases and 30–40 million HIV infections by the year 2000. At GPA, we felt those were careful and reasonable projections, based on the extent of our knowledge. That summer, GAPC came out with much higher estimates, projecting 25 million AIDS cases and between 100 to 120 million HIV-infected persons by the year 2000. It also projected that 42% of all infections would hail from Asia, substantially surpassing Africa, which GAPC projected would account for 31%.[45]

---

[41] Interim Report of the Global AIDS Policy Coalition to the Francois-Xavier Bagnoud Foundation," Global AIDS Policy Coalition, January 1, 1992, A20/372/54.

[42] *AIDS and the Third World*. London: Panos Institute, 1989; *AIDS & children: a family disease*. London: Panos Institute, 1989; *Triple jeopardy: women & AIDS*. London: Panos Institute, 1990; *The hidden cost of AIDS: the challenge of HIV to development*. London: Panos Institute, 1992; Sally Baden, "Women, HIV/AIDS and Development: Towards Gender Appropriate Prevention Strategies in South-East Asia And the South Pacific," Brighton, UK: Institute of Development Studies, University of Sussex, Report No. 5.

[43] Michael Merson, "Letter to Jonathan Mann, November 15, 1991," A20/372/54; Michael Merson, "Facsimile: Collaboration with Global AIDS Policy Coalition," Geneva: World Health Organization, January 8, 1992, GPA/PPC/OOD/SCH/jeb.

[44] Michael Merson, "Letter to Jonathan Mann, 9 January 1992," Unpublished Letter, GPA/PPC-A20/372/54.

[45] Daniel Q. Haney, "International AIDS explosion predicted by end of decade," *Chicago Sun-Times*, June 3, 1992, 3.

GAPC had arrived at these estimates using a Delphi method, which is a collective forecasting method that relies on a panel of experts to provide anonymous answers to a set of questions and then arrives at a collective "best guess" through iterative reassessment. In this case the questions were about the trajectory of HIV infections and AIDS cases. In light of his group's numbers, Mann "cited [our] projection of only 30–40 million cumulative infections by the year 2000 as an example of the underestimation that could impede progress."[46] To obtain his estimates, Chin had used a peer-reviewed model of HIV and AIDS estimations extrapolated from public health surveillance data, a WHO mathematical model, available HIV serological data, and national or regional HIV estimates.[47] Chin considered the Delphi method far inferior, and moreover from what we at GPA understood, GAPC had included less than 30 experts in making its estimates using the Delphi process. Nevertheless, the results appeared on the front page of the *New York Times* and other newspapers across the world, putting us on the defensive. After much thought, Chris Powell and I decided to make the case for GPA's more conservative and realistic estimates without confronting the accuracy of the GAPC estimates.[48] "Whether we're talking about 40 million or 100 million, what we need is support for national AIDS programs," I explained to reporters.[49] In my 5 years as GPA Director, there were few events that required so much time with the media.

More troubling, from our perspective, was that Mann used the differences in projected estimates to question the entire effort of GPA in the press. "This is a global epidemic that is heading out of control," Mann told reporters. "The current response cannot succeed, and must be changed, because it underestimates both the scope of the problem and what will be needed to deal with it." What was needed, Mann exclaimed, was new leadership and a new strategy. "The global strategy, the global leadership, is clearly not there," he told reporters.[50] "If we're not getting the global leadership from the World Health Organization, then we should demand it of them."[51] Claiming GPA's strategy was "too narrow, too limited, [and] too bureaucratic,"[52] Mann laid out his vision for a new Global AIDS Strategy; it had four parts: "make sure all countries apply effective prevention strategies; make sure all infected and ill people get the care and support they need; speed research

---

[46] Dolores Kong, "Grim Projections; Bold global AIDS strategy urged," *The Boston Globe*, June 8, 1992, 25.

[47] James Chin, M.A. Remenyi, F. Morrison, R. Bulatao. "The global epidemiology of the HIV/AIDS pandemic and its projected demographic impact in Africa," *World Health Stat Q*. 1992;45(2–3):220–7.; James Chin. "Global estimates of HIV infections and AIDS—early 1992." *Integration*. 1992 Jun;(32):22–3.

[48] Dolores Kong, "Grim Projections; Bold global AIDS strategy urged," *The Boston Globe*, June 8, 1992, 25.

[49] Kim Painter, "Estimate of AIDS virus cases triples," *USA Today*, June 4, 1992, 1A.

[50] Dolores Kong, "Grim Projections; Bold global AIDS strategy urged," *The Boston Globe*, June 8, 1992, 25.

[51] Ibid.

[52] Mort Rosenblum, "Combatants in Losing AIDS War Say Millions Will Die Needlessly," *The Associated Press*, July 5, 1992.

into treatments and a vaccine; [and] confront the social and health inequities that make societies vulnerable to a rapid spread of the virus."[53] At GPA, we felt this was exactly what we were doing.

Again, rather than attacking Mann, we tried to deflect his comments and explain GPA's efforts in a positive way. By 1992, GPA had updated the Global AIDS Strategy, and while I was willing to admit our limitations, I tried to turn the discussion to our strengths. "What is wonderful," I explained to reporters, "is we have a new global strategy that has been adopted by every country in the world and we are ready to move forward with it."[54] AIDS was a complex disease, I noted: "This is a hard disease, and we've only been at this for 5 years."[55] "To stop this disease on a dime is just not realistic. We don't have a magic bullet, we don't have a cure. We don't have a vaccine. We are dealing with sexual behaviors which will not change overnight."[56] Because of the methodological weaknesses in Mann's study, and the way it was being used to attack GPA, I decided to call Harvey Fineberg, at that time the Dean of Harvard's School of Public Health, to see if he could be of any help. Fineberg's response was that Mann, as a Harvard University professor, had the privilege of academic freedom and could say and publish what he wished. Whether Mann ever tried to do so, I do not know, but his Delphi study never appeared in the peer-reviewed literature.

I could not help but feel, at the time, that this open debate in the summer of 1992 represented a profound rift between Mann and the staff of GPA. That is, in attacking GPA, Mann was attacking so many of the people who had been so devoted to him. To me, that was the bitter irony of the whole conflict. But the discord with Mann that surfaced in the press also signaled a breach within the global response to AIDS. For all GPA's efforts identifying interventions that worked and designing management training to improve national programs, the clashes with Mann in the press publicly called into question our approach to the pandemic. And Mann was merely the most vocal among the voices of disquiet; there were others suggesting there might be better ways to fight the pandemic. Donors, already moving in a bilateral direction and growing increasingly dubious about GPA's ability to respond to the pandemic at country level, now began questioning if GPA was the best agency to coordinate the global effort against AIDS.[57]

The truth was that despite GPA's best efforts, regionalization, particularly in the African region (see Chapter 9), had taken some toll on our effectiveness. First, it

---

[53] Dolores Kong, "Grim Projections; Bold global AIDS strategy urged," *The Boston Globe*, June 8, 1992, 25.

[54] Daniel Q. Haney, "International AIDS explosion predicted by end of decade," *Chicago Sun-Times*, June 3, 1992, 3.

[55] Mort Rosenblum, "Combatants in Losing AIDS War Say Millions Will Die Needlessly," *The Associated Press*, July 5, 1992.

[56] Dolores Kong, "Grim Projections; Bold global AIDS strategy urged," *The Boston Globe*, June 8, 1992, 25.

[57] Global Programme on AIDS. *Progress report*. Geneva: World Health Organization, April 1991; Gill Walt, Interview by Stephen Inrig, Dallas, TX, September 23, 2010.

took essential staff out of countries needed to fight AIDS effectively. "Within 2 years [of the departure of Mann and his central management team], Gary Slutkin, noted in a 2000 article that "all 45 of the WHO African country staff had been removed. ... International funds became harder for the WHO to raise ... [and while] overall funding levels at country level may have been maintained ... they never achieved the level of funding or intensity that the Uganda program had realized".[58]

Second, even where regionalization in Africa did "succeed," it was primarily successful in bringing African programs into WHO's often inefficient regional orbit. "At GPA [there] is no sense of urgency," Uganda's AIDS director, Warren Naamara, complained to reporters in 1992, "If I need to organize a workshop, every detail must be approved."[59] I found myself pulled in different directions. On the one hand, Nakajima wanted GPA to work inside WHO's regional structure; on the other hand, working within that structure limited the effectiveness and timeliness of our support.

Given the ambiguous results of regionalization along with the tepid progress GPA was making against the mushrooming pandemic, it was not surprising that some donors were questioning their investment in GPA. A few of them had met with me in the early days after my appointment as Director to express considerable concern about the African region.[60] They would have preferred that GPA refrain from turning over responsibilities for country support to WHO's regional office for Africa (AFRO), owing to their concerns about that office's competence and misuse of funds as we described earlier in Chapter 9.[61] Now, little more than 2 years later, regionalization had sown a profound division between GPA and its donors. Indeed, as GPA expanded its program, it "was accompanied by a more critical attitude on the part of donors. ... Now, they started paying greater attention to the way the program was being managed, to the disbursement of and accounting for funds, and to the program's priorities and strategies."[62]

The donors had become more critical, also in part, because by this time many of them had developed their own bilateral AIDS programs, and their own experiences and budget constraints led them to demand more accountability for all their multilateral agency donations. There was also the growing sense among high-income nations that they no longer needed to fear a generalized epidemic in their own countries. This meant that WHO's global efforts became of less direct importance to them, which further increased their emphasis on bilateral rather than multilateral

---

[58] Elizabeth Fee and Manon Parry, "Jonathan Mann, HIV/AIDS, and Human Rights," *Journal of Public Health Policy,* 29(1).

[59] Mort Rosenblum, "U.N. AIDS-Fighting Agency Having Problems; With AIDS-Losing Battle." *The Associated Press,* July 5, 1992.

[60] Global Programme on AIDS. *Progress report.* Geneva: World Health Organization, April 1991; Gill Walt, Interview by Stephen Inrig, Dallas, TX, September 23, 2010.

[61] Global Programme on AIDS, "Sixth meeting of the Management Committee, Provisional agenda item 3: Report of the Director, Geneva, 23–24 April 1991," Geneva: World Health Organization, 1991, GPA/GMC(1)/91.3, 16.

[62] Bernadette Olowo-Freers, Gill Walt, et al., "Report of the External Review of the World Health Organization Global Programme on AIDS, January 1992," p. 6.

funding. We pursue this issue further in the next chapter. GPA's best strategy given this evolving scenario, I thought, was to continue positioning ourselves as the leader of the global AIDS effort, and to serve as a reliable authority of what strategies worked most effectively in AIDS prevention and care in low- and middle-income nations, where it was becoming increasingly clear the pandemic would be more severe. If donors were progressively skeptical about GPA's ability to deliver programs in the field successfully, I believed that at least they could count on us to be the gatekeeper of knowledge and expertise on proven strategies and to ensure a coordinated and unified response to the pandemic.

But, as we will see, donors were growing far less certain that GPA could ensure them a coordinated and unified response to AIDS.

Chapter 14
Growing Tensions Among United Nations Agencies

There was nothing to suggest that May 9, 1991 would be a significant day in the global fight against AIDS[1]. It was a day like any other, full of important global events: Saddam Hussein rejected the United Nations (UN) offer to send a UN police force to oversee Northern Iraq; the Indian government dispatched its army to the capital of Kashmir to prevent riots after security forces there had killed 14 people; and the Administrator for the United Nations Development Programme (UNDP) sent out the annual report and provisional agenda to the agency's Governing Council, ahead of its upcoming 38th session. Item #2 on the agenda was a discussion about UNDP's role in combating AIDS.

At first glance, it was not surprising that the UNDP Governing Council planned to discuss UNDP's current AIDS activities. As we elaborated earlier (see Chapter 5), UNDP had been involved in the global response since early 1988, when it had formed an alliance with the World Health Organization (WHO) to support national AIDS programs.[2] Since then, UNDP had slowly expanded its AIDS-related work. In 1990 it began concentrating its efforts on increasing "awareness of the development implications of the pandemic" by strengthening and expanding "the capacity of communities to respond to the pandemic," promoting and assisting "prevention, care, support, and treatment programs for women," and assisting "governments to develop effective

---

Within this chapter the singular pronouns *I* and *my* refer to Michael Merson alone, whereas the plural pronouns *we* and *us* generally refer to Michael Merson and Stephen Inrig jointly. Where *we* or *us* refers to Michael Merson and his colleagues at WHO, the object of the pronoun is clarified by context.

[1] For the purposes of this text, we will use the term AIDS to encompass both AIDS and HIV unless otherwise specified.

[2] UNDP Administrator, "Cooperation Against AIDS: Report of the Administrator," New York: Governing Council of the United Nations Development Programme, DP/1988/1/Add.1, 5 February 1988, Item 2 (a) of the provisional Agenda, http://web.undp.org/execbrd/archives/sessions/gc/OrgSp-1988/DP-1988-1-Add1.pdf.

© Springer International Publishing AG 2018   259
M. Merson, S. Inrig, *The AIDS Pandemic*, DOI 10.1007/978-3-319-47133-4_14

multisectoral HIV/AIDS strategies and to minimize the devastating consequences of widespread infection."[3]

But agenda item #2 was different, something new. Item #2 was not just about the further expansion of global AIDS efforts in support of the Global Programme on AIDS (GPA) and national AIDS programs. The background document for Item #2 announced that UNDP was launching its own global AIDS program: "The nature of the HIV/AIDS pandemic and its social and economic consequences demand a multisectoral and inter-disciplinary response," the document read, "UNDP has substantial responsibility within the United Nations system in the area of social and economic development and for the coordination of United Nations system programming. It carries these responsi-bilities also with respect to the HIV/AIDS pandemic."[4] The document included a policy framework with this announcement, one that outlined the short- and long-term goals of the program, its priorities, and the delivery mechanisms it would utilize going forward. UNDP did affirm that it would "seek technical and policy advice from WHO/GPA", and that this framework should be considered "consistent with the Global AIDS Strategy" established by GPA. However, and most importantly, the document also specified that UNDP would "facilitate donor coordination at the region and global levels" and "actively assist in the mobilization of human and financial resources required for assistance to communities and governments."[5]

What did this mean? Essentially, it meant that the global health community was about to have two UN agencies offering strategies and programs for fighting AIDS. At the 7th International Conference on AIDS in Florence 6 weeks later I called for the global health community to share the challenge of global AIDS. The question was: would GPA and UNDP be able to complement each other, or would they wind up competing against each other, especially for donor funding? WHO, and specifically GPA, had the responsibility for coordinating the AIDS response since the UN sys-tem had begun addressing the pandemic. With UNDP's announcement, GPA's lead-ership role in the response to the pandemic was about to be put to the test.

Coordination among any large agencies can be challenging, much less coordinat-ing a response against such a complex disease like AIDS. Since the late 1970s, WHO had sometimes found itself taking controversial positions on health issues where wide differences of opinion existed. This included, for example, disagreements with national governments (such as the United States) and international corporations (food and pharmaceutical companies) around policies related to breast milk substi-tutes and pharmaceuticals, as well as with UN agencies (such as the United Nations Children's Emergency Fund [UNICEF] and the World Bank) around the Bamako

---

[3] Annual Report of the Administrator for 1990 And Programme-Level Activities; Role of UNDP in combating HIV/AIDS: Policy framework for the response of UNDP to HIV/AIDS, Item 2 of the provisional agenda, Thirty-eighth session 3–21 June 1991 Geneva: Governing Council of the United Nations Development Programme, 9 May 1991, DP/1991/57.

[4] Ibid.

[5] UNDP Administrator, "Cooperation Against AIDS: Report of the Administrator," New York: Governing Council of the United Nations Development Programme, DP/1988/1/Add.1, 5 February 1988, Item 2 (a) of the provisional Agenda, http://web.undp.org/execbrd/archives/sessions/gc/OrgSp-1988/DP-1988-1-Add1.pdf.

Initiative (the Bamako Initiative was a program that sought to self-finance the development of each country's primary health infrastructure by selling drugs above cost and directing the profits to the infrastructure, privatizing and decentralizing drug purchasing in ways WHO felt detrimental to its Essential Drug Program).[6] Moreover, the recent collapse of the Soviet Union and its Central and Eastern Bloc satellites had thrown the Cold War "stability and predictability" into disarray, making it more difficult for WHO—whose structure depended primarily on partnerships with health ministries—to coordinate the actions of other UN agencies with regard to health and the social determinants of health in these volatile states.[7] The recognition of AIDS as a socially embedded disease meant that it required a "complex, multifaceted response" that adequately addressed "issues like discrimination, judicial reform, behavioral change, and prevention strategies that challenged cultural and religious norms."[8] This was not a natural fit for WHO. Thus, GPA faced considerable institutional dynamics working against effective coordination.

I was well aware of these coordination challenges when I started at GPA, but was optimistic I could address them. I had a long history working with the donors and other UN agencies and had established good relationships with them. In my years as Director of the Diarrheal Diseases Control Programme (CDD), for example, I had worked closely with UNICEF in promotion of oral rehydration therapy in dozens of countries, with UNDP in the establishment of a substantial research program to develop vaccines against cholera and other diarrheal diseases, and with the World Bank in providing support for construction of water and sanitation facilities in a number of countries. In fact, I had interacted with all of them in the creation of the Task Force for Child Survival (now the Task force for Global Health), which was established in 1984 to support a collaborative effort to improve child wellness and survival strategies.[9]

Thus, based on my past relationship with these agencies, I confidently started developing or expanding partnerships with them. One of the earliest GPA collaborations was with the World Bank. The World Bank, whose official name is the International Bank for Reconstruction and Development, has the dual role of development and reconstruction the world over. It raises funds through private financial markets and contributions from donor members, and makes interest-bearing and interest-free loans, credits, grants, and technical assistance to economically developing nations that otherwise would have been unable to obtain loans in the international marketplace.[10] From the 1960s through the 1980s, the World Bank's development mandate evolved beyond that of only economic growth to one that would "provide all human beings with the opportunity for a

[6] Fiona Godlee, "WHO in retreat: is it losing its influence?" *BMJ* 3 December 1994;309:1491–1495.

[7] Jon Liden, "The World Health Organization and Global Health Governance: Post-1990." *Public Health,* February 2014;128(2):141–147.

[8] Ibid.

[9] "About Us and Annual Report," Decatur, Georgia: The Task Force for Global Health, http://www.taskforce.org/about-us-and-annual-report.

[10] Jennifer Prah Ruger, "The Changing Role of the World Bank in Global Health," *American Journal of Public Health* January 2005, 95(1):60.

'full life' ... [by] meeting individuals' 'basic needs'." Consequently, starting in the 1980s, the World Bank took the historic step of investing in health, nutrition, education, and family planning.

The World Bank's first forays into AIDS began in 1986, building off a World Bank strategy paper on AIDS authored by Jean-Louis Lamboray, a public health specialist from Belgium who had long-standing experience and interest in Africa.[11] Around the same time, GPA, collaborated with Mead Over and Martha Ainsworth, two economists who led a small research office in the World Bank, on one of the first studies to assess the economic and demographic impact of AIDS in low- and middle-income countries.[12] I maintained close contact with Over during my Directorship. In fact, it was he who suggested I recruit Stef Bertozzi to GPA when, a few years into my Directorship, we began searching to add an economist to our policy team.

In the early years of GPA, Jonathan Mann himself had a somewhat ambivalent attitude towards the World Bank. The World Bank had initially wanted to work with GPA in undertaking cost-effectiveness evaluations of AIDS prevention interventions. Mann felt such research was important, and he was aware that some donors were calling for this type of evaluation, but he worried it might be too early to obtain meaningful data, as AIDS prevention programs were just starting in most countries. Instead, he tasked Roy Widdus with facilitating studies that evaluated the economic consequences of AIDS, while delaying the more critical cost-effectiveness analyses on GPA-supported interventions.[13]

Beginning in 1988, the World Bank began providing essential and substantial support to national AIDS programs in countries in Africa (Zaire, Uganda, Burundi, and Tanzania), South America (Brazil), and Asia (India, Indonesia).[14] As noted in Chapter 10, one of these, a $160 million loan made to aid Brazil's nationwide AIDS campaign, was one of the first to demonstrate an impact of a national AIDS program.[15]

---

[11] "HIV and AIDS: Projects & Programs—All Projects," New York: World Bank, 2016 http://www. worldbank.org/en/topic/hivandaids/projects/all?qterm=&lang_exact=English&os=220.

[12] Special Programme on AIDS, "Progress Report Number 2, November 1987," Geneva: World Health Organization, WHO/SPA/GEN/87.4, p. 12.

[13] Roy Widdus, Interview by Michael Merson, New Haven, CT, October, 2001.

[14] Mead Over, S. Bertozzi, J. Chin, B. N'Galy, and K. Nyamuryekung'e, "The Direct and Indirect Cost of HIV Infection in Developing Countries: The Cases of Zaire and Tanzania." In Alan Fleming, Manuel Carbalo, David W. Fitzsimmons, Michael R. Bailey, and Jonathan Mann, eds., *The Global Impact of AIDS*. New York: Alan R. Liss, Inc., 1988; A.A. Scitovsky and Mead Over. "AIDS: Costs of care in the developed and the developing world" *AIDS* 2 (Suppl 1): S71–81. 1988; A. Edward Elmendorf, Jean-Louis Lamboray, «Acquired Immunodeficiency Syndrome (AIDS): The Bank's Agenda for Action in Africa». Technical Paper, The World Bank, Africa Technical Department, October 24, 1988. (Unpublished); Thomas Land, "World Bank getting into fight against AIDS," *The Financial Post*, August 26, 1988, 1:13; Anaclet Rwegayura, "Health: African Countries Equipped to Carry Out AIDS Testing," *IPS-Inter Press Service*, September 16, 1988; National Council For International Health, "Press Briefing on Global AIDS Issues," *Federal News Service*, December 1, 1988; Global Programme on AIDS, "Progress Report Number 5, MAY 1989," Geneva: World Health Organization, WHO/GPA/DIR/89.4, p. 20.

[15] Thomas Land, "World Bank getting into fight against AIDS," *The Financial Post*, August 26, 1988, 1:13.

Unlike partnerships with most UN institutions, working with the World Bank required mostly individual level, one on one collaboration with the staff responsible for managing AIDS projects in specific countries or regions. GPA made it a point to provide, when requested, technical advice to these staff, whom it seemed were always under pressure to obtain the best return on investment.[16] I made an effort to cultivate relationships with these individuals, focusing mainly on those assigned to larger countries, like Jean-Louis Lamboray (Zaire), Anthony Measham (India), and Maureen Lewis (Brazil), as well as Ian Porter, Senior Public Health Specialist, from the Asia Technical Department. I remember Porter, in particular, because—having come from Australia—he had a keen appreciation of the impact the pandemic could have in Asia, and set up a regional project based in Thailand that focused on strengthening policy analysis and promoting policy dialogue in seven Asian countries. I also invested considerable time in 1993 working with Seth Berkeley (then at the Rockefeller Foundation) and Larry Summers (then Chief Economist at the World Bank), on a chapter devoted to AIDS that was included in the World Bank's first World Development Report dedicated to investing in health.[17] It was this World Development Report, incidentally, that would spur Bill Gates to become interested in global health and eventually to establish (with his wife, Melinda) the Bill & Melinda Gates Foundation.

As much as possible, in working with the World Bank, we sought to combine and leverage our respective funds to improve the health infrastructure of countries and develop sustainable AIDS interventions. Though we had some occasional disagreements on technical issues, for the most part, our relationship was constructive. To some extent, the World Bank played an important role in pushing us to address issues of effectiveness and cost-effectiveness in our support to countries. In fact, the World Bank's flexible country-based approach, and confidence in GPA's technical knowledge, made the agency initially resistant to the formation of the Joint United Nations Programme on HIV/AIDS (UNAIDS) (see Chapter 16).

GPA also developed a very cordial relationship with the United Nations Population Fund (UNFPA) and the United Nations Educational, Scientific and Cultural Organization (UNESCO). UNFPA's activities were led by Nick Dodd, who served as its liaison officer with GPA soon after the program was established, and a few years later became Chief of the agency's Maternal and Child Health Branch. UNFPA-supported programs focused on integrating AIDS activities into country-level AIDS programs, particularly those delivering maternal and child health/family planning services. By 1993, UNFPA had supported AIDS prevention in 93 countries, including general information and communication activities; in school and out-of-school AIDS education; supplying of condoms (done in close collaboration with GPA); and training within maternal and child health/family planning programs.[18] UNESCO had more limited resources to invest in AIDS-related activi-

[16] Terrance Lorne Mooney "Letter To: Director GPA; WHO/GPA Relations With The World Bank, 22 May 1989," Internal GPA Memorandum TM 1963/89, 6/192.

[17] The International Bank for Reconstruction and Development (The World Bank), *World Development Report 1993: Investing in Health.* New York: Oxford University Press, 1993.

[18] AIDS Update, 1993, A Report on UNPFA Support to the Area of HIV Prevention, United Nations

ties. Most of its efforts were in support of youth education programs delivered through schools, including a few joint projects with WHO in African countries. These were all examples of GPA's positive relationships and successful coordination efforts.

There were coordination challenges, however, with some of the larger UN entities, including the UN itself. As we discussed in Chapter 5, in the mid to late 1980s the UN had established two UN-wide committees to coordinate UN actions on AIDS. Initially, UN Secretary-General de Cuéllar had directed the UN's Department of International, Economic, and Social Affairs (DIESA) to establish a Steering Committee on AIDS to coordinate UN's AIDS-related activities. DIESA included "major UN departments", UNICEF, UNFPA, UNDP, and (eventually) WHO. It coordinated UN agencies in New York and communicated any UN-wide materials to the UN's Administrative Committee on Co-ordination.[19] Shortly thereafter, WHO Director-General Halfdan Mahler had established the Inter-Agency Advisory Group (IAAG) on AIDS with which both Mann and I were far more engaged.[20] Like most UN groups of this type, the IAAG lacked any authority and played only a marginal role operationally, though it provided a large forum for Mann to communicate and discuss AIDS policies, and I found it similarly useful.

One controversial issue that IAAG successfully took on during my tenure was the issue of mandatory HIV testing of UN peacekeeping troops. There was a great deal of pressure for this, as peacekeeping troops often came from countries with high HIV infection rates and were thus seen as a threat to countries where they were stationed (this was ironic, since host countries often already had high rates themselves). Instead of mandatory testing, IAAG developed a sound set of policies based on voluntary testing and prepared training courses and educational materials on HIV transmission and prevention for peacekeeping troops. This was one of the rare examples of successful UN-wide collaboration around AIDS, and it was in this context that I first met and worked with Kofi Annan, who at the time was UN Assistant Secretary-General for Peacekeeping Operations. Annan would later become UN Secretary-General and play an important role in the global AIDS effort, including the creation of the Global Fund to Fight AIDS, Tuberculosis, and Malaria (see Chapter 18). In the spring of 1994, Annan asked me to meet him at his New York office, where he requested that GPA provide AIDS medications to a few high ranking Indian military officers who had contracted HIV while serving in the UN Transitional Authority in Cambodia in 1992 and 1993. I explained that GPA did not provide direct care, including medications, to foreign nationals and thus could not be of assistance to the military officers. This interaction illustrated that, even when there were sincere efforts at cooperation, there were occasional misconceptions about GPA's role in the global AIDS response.

More complicated was our relationship with UNICEF. The relationship had many positive aspects: we never competed for funding, and UNICEF was for the

---

Population Fund.

[19] Christer Jonsson, "From 'Lead Agency' to 'Integrated Programming': The Global Response to AIDS in the Third World," *Green Globe Yearbook*, 1996, 65–72.

[20] Ibid.

most part comfortable with GPA as the lead agency in the global response. However, tensions emerged in two areas where we had overlapping, and sometimes conflicting, program differences: these were safer sex practices among youth (particularly condom use and condom promotion) and breastfeeding.

Since the 1960s, UNICEF had viewed national family planning programs focused on birth spacing and family size planning as essential components of maternal and child health, and had worked well alongside WHO and UNFPA in supporting these programs.[21] However, the Catholic Church had been an important supporter of UNICEF over the years, so in deference to Catholic doctrine on abortion and contraception, UNICEF in the 1980s and 1990s chose to remain somewhat neutral on particular methods of family planning and the supply of contraceptive technologies. Often, when such services were needed or requested, UNICEF worked through WHO or UNFPA to deliver them.[22] However, despite this caution, UNICEF still sometimes received criticism from the Church. In April 1990, for example, UNICEF had weathered some very vocal criticism from Archbishop Renato R. Martino, Permanent Observer of the Holy See to the United Nations, for the extent to which it might be participating directly in the provision of contraceptive and abortion services.[23]

Unlike UNICEF, GPA faced no religious constraints, and so we boldly and directly promoted condoms. As mentioned earlier, condom promotion was part of our broader vision of identifying a small number of simple, accessible, and inexpensive technologies to maximize AIDS prevention, and thus by the summer of 1992, we were strongly pushing condom uptake across the globe.[24] Drawing on the evidence amassed by Gary Slutkin and his team, GPA concentrated on supporting mass media campaigns and condom social marketing programs that had proved effective in different settings and produced results in a matter of months (see Chapter 11).[25] Under Patrick Friel's leadership, GPA also established an interagency working group on condom procurement and supply, and in 1989 published the first edition of the WHO Specifications and Guidelines for Condom Procurement.

UNICEF was reticent to join us in this effort, at least initially. Part of this reluctance stemmed from the aforementioned relationship with the Catholic Church, and, according to Neil Boyer (for many years the United States State Department representative on the WHO Executive Board), part was due to the fact that HIV-related condom use was associated with homosexuality, and some felt this might "tarnish UNICEF by going out and associating ourselves with this kind of thing."[26] To the

---

[21] *The Progress of Nations 1995* UNICEF, 8 June 1995; Stanley Johnson. *World Population and the United Nations*. Cambridge, UK: Cambridge University Press, 1987.

[22] Maggie Black, "The Children and the Nations, The Story of UNICEF," New York: UNICEF, 1986, 254.

[23] Archbishop Renato R. Martino, H.E., "Statement of H.E. Archbishop Renato R. Martino, Permanent Observer of the Holy See to the United Nations at the Meeting of the Executive Board of UNICEF," New York, Tuesday, 17 April, 1990.

[24] Clare Nullis, "Health Agency Urges More Promotion of Condoms," *The Associated Press*, June 22, 1992.

[25] Ibid.

[26] Ann Blackwood, Interview by Michael Merson, New Haven, CT, January, 2002; Neil Boyer,

extent that the Catholic Church played a role in this decision, I cannot say, but it was clear that early on UNICEF was reluctant to be seen as a promoter of condom use.

In early 1991, Jim Grant, UNICEF Executive Director, asked Jim Sherry, UNICEF's Senior Adviser for Program Strategy, if he "could wrestle with this AIDS thing." Sherry replied, "'I don't really want to get into AIDS. I don't see where it is going.' It seemed like a problem without a solution."[27] Eventually, in 1992, Sherry became more engaged and developed a five-element program for UNICEF on AIDS.[28] But I had hoped for a more aggressive stance from UNICEF on HIV prevention, largely because of all the agencies in the UN, it had the most operational strength at country level, particularly in mounting programs for youth, and I felt that this could have added significantly to our efforts.

A greater point of friction between UNICEF and GPA was the issue of breast-feeding and HIV. UNICEF had, for many years, committed itself to promoting breastfeeding as a means to lower infant mortality and morbidity, particularly from diarrheal diseases. In the 1960s and 1970s, however, there was mounting evidence that a number of developing countries were undergoing a "massive shift from breast milk to artificial means of infant feeding."[29] Since breastfeeding simultaneously lowered infant mortality and maternal fertility, observers worried that such shifts would have the dual effect of increasing infant mortality and population growth.[30] The issue garnered such concern in the 1970s that the World Health Assembly (WHA) took up the topic twice; the UN hosted a system-wide meeting in 1979; and WHO and UNICEF collaborated in 1980 to draw up an international code of marketing of breast milk substitutes, which the WHA adopted on May 21, 1981.[31]

In 1982, UNICEF launched its Child Survival Revolution, a program aimed at attacking the main sources of infant and child mortality through the universal adoption of a small number of simple, accessible, and inexpensive medical technologies.[32] These technologies included growth monitoring, oral rehydration therapy, breastfeeding, and immunization, which were arranged into the acronym GOBI (UNICEF would add three F's to the acronym the following year: food supplements, family

---

Interview by Michael Merson, New Haven, CT, January, 2002.

[27] Jim Sherry, Interview by Michael Merson, Geneva, October, 2001.

[28] Ibid.

[29] Resolution WHA27.43 (*Handbook of Resolutions and Decisions of the World Health Assembly and the Executive Board*), Volume II, 4th ed., Geneva, 1981, 58; *International Code of Marketing of Breast-milk Substitutes*. Geneva: World Health Organization, 1981, 5; James Grant, *The state of the world's children, 1982–1983*. New York: Oxford University Press, 1982, 14–16; Sara F. Matthews Grieco and Carlo A. Corsini, "Historical Perspectives on Breastfeeding; Two Essays," Florence, IT: UNICEF and Istituto degli Innocenti,1991.

[30] John Knodel, "Breast-feeding and population growth," *Science* 16 December 1977: *198(4322)*: 1111–1115.

[31] Resolution WHA33.32; Resolution EB67.R12; WHA34/1981/REC/1; WHA34/1981/REC/2, cited in *International Code of Marketing of Breast-milk Substitutes*. Geneva: World Health Organization, 1981, 5–7.

[32] James Grant, *The state of the world's children, 1982-1983*. Oxford, UK: Oxford University Press, 1982.

spacing, and female education).[33] Thus, the promotion of breastfeeding became one of UNICEF's key interventions throughout the 1980s.

WHO welcomed the GOBI-FFF effort: it put forth measurable outcomes, played to WHO's strengths as a technical organization, and complemented the push towards the Primary Health Care and Health for All by the Year 2000 goals adopted at the Alma Ata Conference. While serving as Director of the CDD Program, I welcomed the inclusion of oral rehydration therapy as a component of the Child Survival Revolution. However, in GPA, we were concerned about how to advise HIV positive women on breastfeeding practices since they could transmit HIV to their children through their breast milk. The first studies documenting HIV transmission through breast milk were in 1985, and through the late 1980s and early 1990s, our concerns about the rate of transmission through breast milk grew.[34] However, we still considered the probability of HIV transmission through breast milk to be relatively small, and for its part, UNICEF considered breastfeeding not to be "a significant means of transmitting AIDS" and that the "advantages of breastfeeding greatly outweigh[ed] the small risk that AIDS may be transmitted."[35]

However, our concerns heightened at a WHO/UNICEF Consultation on HIV Transmission and Breastfeeding held in April 1992. By this time, the evidence was mounting that the rate of HIV transmission through breastfeeding was much higher than we had thought, and in some countries the prevalence of HIV among women of childbearing potential had grown substantially.[36] Consequently, whereas GPA had in 1987 recommended breastfeeding in all but the most unique cases, the consensus statement adopted at our 1992 consultation was more equivocal and read as follows: "It is therefore important that the baby's risk of HIV infection through breastfeeding be weighed against its risk of dying of other causes if it is denied breastfeeding. In each country, specific guidelines should be developed to facilitate the assessment of the circumstances of the individual woman." In countries where "the primary causes of infant deaths are infectious diseases and malnutrition," breastfeeding should "remain the standard advice." In countries where this was not the case, "pregnant women known to be infected with HIV should be advised not to breastfeed."[37] In truth, we wanted to go further, to advise that all HIV-infected

---

[33] Ibid, 49–64.

[34] Ziegler et al, "Postnatal transmission of AIDS-associated retrovirus from mother to infant," *Lancet* 1(8434), 20 April 1985; CDC, "Current Trends Recommendations for Assisting in the Prevention of Perinatal Transmission of Human T-Lymphotropic Virus Type III/Lymphadenopathy-Associated Virus and Acquired Immunodeficiency Syndrome," *MMWR* 34(48), 6 December 1985; WHO, "Summary Statement on Breast-feeding/Breast Milk and Human Immunodeficiency Virus (HIV)," 1 July 1987.

[35] UNICEF, *The State of the World's Children, 1989.* Oxford, UK: Oxford University Press, 1989, 70.

[36] Philip J. Hilts, "Study Shows Passing AIDS in Breast Milk Is Easier Than Thought," *The New York Times*, August 29, 1991, B13; Dunn et al, "Risk of human immunodeficiency virus type 1 transmission through breastfeeding," *Lancet* 340(8819), 5 September 1992.

[37] Global Programme on AIDS, "Consensus Statement from the WHO/UNICEF Consultation on HIV Transmission and Breast-Feeding, Geneva, 30 April—1 May 1992," Geneva: World Health Organization, WHO/GPA/INF/92.1, 1–2.

women in every country opt for "nutritionally adequate breast milk substitutes" regardless of the main cause of infant mortality in their country, unless they could not obtain uninterrupted access to those substitutes, or the substitutes could not be prepared and fed to the children safely.[38]

But getting UNICEF even this far was a challenge for a couple of reasons. First, breastfeeding was a key component of the GOBI strategy and Grant's vision for child survival. GPA's new stance on breastfeeding threatened one of the lynchpins of his strategy. Moreover, UNICEF and WHO had recently launched a "baby friendly hospital initiative." This effort sought to ensure that all maternity units, whether freestanding or in hospitals, became centers of breastfeeding support. Consequently, there was a push to stop maternity units from accepting any free or low cost breast milk substitutes, feeding bottles, or teats. GPA's cautions on HIV and breastfeeding severely complicated, and even conflicted with these efforts.

In January 1991, about 15 months before our 1992 consultation, I had a heated discussion in my office with Grant and Sherry about breastfeeding and HIV transmission.[39] I showed them data which indicated that breastfeeding women infected with HIV before delivery might have transmission rates as high as 29%.[40] I recall going to the blackboard in my office and drawing figures to explain the physiological process by which breast milk could become infected, and showing them modelling data which suggested that breastfeeding could account for about 15% of all pediatric HIV infections in the world. Grant had a very difficult time accepting this reality. According to Sherry, he was just not convinced that there was a scalable strategy to address AIDS that trumped his larger nutritional concerns.[41]

The real tension, however, was not the data, Sherry later explained. UNICEF believed the data. "Our problem related to this whole issue of settings, we didn't want to give one set of recommendations in setting A and another set of recommendations in setting B ... If you are a middle class woman in Kampala, what setting are you in? How do you define the setting?"[42] Equally problematic was that GPA's advice about HIV testing made a coherent policy difficult for UNICEF. "We were running into [another] tension in UNICEF," Sherry explained. "We were saying, do people know their status? At the time the very strongly held view [in UNICEF] was that widespread [HIV] testing, even voluntary testing ...that the negative consequences of that were greater than the positive ones as there was no treatment available. [In contrast] GPA was arguing: 'if you are an HIV positive young woman, even without treatment, you have options, and knowing your status affects your options, and if you have young kids, you know in advance you could do something before you are sick.' That was really where we ran into the strong tension."[43]

[38] World Health Organization. HIV and infant feeding. *Guidelines for decision makers.* Geneva: WHO, 1998.

[39] Jim Sherry, Interview by Michael Merson, Geneva, October, 2001.

[40] Much of this came out the next year in Dunn et al, "Risk of human immunodeficiency virus type 1 transmission through breastfeeding," *The Lancet* 340(8819), 5 September 1992.

[41] Jim Sherry, Interview by Michael Merson, Geneva, October, 2001.

[42] Ibid.

[43] Ibid.

We at GPA were never able to get UNICEF to move further on the breastfeeding issue while I was Director. That said, on both the breastfeeding and condom promotion issues, our conflicts with UNICEF were technical ones; they were not over coordination. Still, these tension points indicated to us at GPA, and to our donors, that WHO's role in directing and coordinating the global AIDS response was not uncontested.

While our relationship with UNICEF was at times rocky, our relationship with UNDP was riddled with and thwarted by conflict. These tensions were in part due to the unique position UNDP held in the larger UN system, and in part to our overlapping interests. Established in 1969, UNDP was the largest intergovernmental technical assistance organization in the world, created to assist countries plan and achieve development priorities and to coordinate the various UN Specialized Agencies that had been set up independent of the larger UN system. The intent had been to have a single UN representative at country level...usually the UNDP Resident Representative...that would reduce the effort governments spent negotiating and coordinating UN development aid. Unfortunately, in practice, most UN agencies "continued to function autonomously."[44] By the "mid to late 1980s," according to Mina Mauerstein-Bail, an American program officer at UNDP who subsequently worked in the HIV and Development Program, the agency began "to go through a lot of reflection about its future directions, where it should go, what it should focus on … because its role as a central funding agency had already been eroding for some time."[45] When it came to health, UNDP—lacking technical expertise in the field—centered its limited health profile in its Division of Global and Interregional Programs (DGIP) in its New York headquarters, where it addressed cross-cutting issues like safe motherhood, tropical diseases research, and safe water. I had worked closely with DGIP during my years in the CDD program. In fact, DGIP had been one of the first major funders of the CDD program's research activities in the early 1980s.[46]

In the early years of GPA, UNDP provided important financial support to the program through its global and regional bureaus and country desks. As described in Chapter 5, in 1988 Halfdan Mahler and William Draper, the UNDP Administrator, signed a formal WHO/UNDP Alliance to Combat AIDS. This recognized WHO's role in directing and coordinating the global response to AIDS and UNDP's leadership in dealing with the social economic consequences of the pandemic and its role as coordinator of UN, in-country, operational activities. This Alliance was significant, as it allowed each agency to operate within its areas of strength and expertise, while creating a framework whereby WHO and UNDP could collaborate at country level. This facilitated working arrangements between ministries of health and

[44] Mike Bailey, "UNDP—healthy development? The case of HIV," *Health Policy and Planning*, 1994, 9(4):444–447.

[45] Mina Mauerstein-Bail, Interview by Michael Merson, New Haven, CT, September, 2002.

[46] Mike Bailey, "UNDP—healthy development? The case of HIV," *Health Policy and Planning*, 1994, 9(4):444–447.

finance and other relevant ministries with the WHO Representative and UNDP
Resident Representative. But UNDP soon viewed WHO's "biomedical"or public
health approach to be too limited and desired a broader response, which was exemplified by the subsequent launch of its HIV and Development Program in 1991.
Thus, by the early 1990s, as we illustrated at the beginning of this chapter, a breach
had developed between GPA and UNDP over AIDS strategy, a breach that would
begin a competition for resources and profoundly affect the shape of the global
response to AIDS in the years to come.

How did this happen? GPA had expanded so quickly in its first 18 months that
it outstripped WHO's institutional capacity to transfer funds as quickly as nations
demanded. The WHO/UNDP Alliance to Combat AIDS allowed GPA to draw on
UNDP funds in the short term without conforming to UNDP's usual accounting
procedures. But as time went on, tensions developed. The first, more subtle, strains
were between Jonathan Mann and Elizabeth Reid, who became the point person
for AIDS at the agency from her position as Director of UNDP's Division for
Women in Development between 1989 and 1991. While Reid and Mann shared
many affinities, especially as Mann evolved towards his health and human rights
framework, their positions were different enough and institutional loyalties strong
enough that, as Jeff O'Malley remembers it, "it was a very rocky relationship."[47]
Part of this must certainly have stemmed from the fact that, under Mann, WHO had
moved "away from its customary technical support role" and was now, with AIDS,
"executing as well as implementing."[48] But part of it also lay—despite Mann's
expansive view of the response—in the limitations that many saw inherent in
WHO's approach. As Mauerstein-Bail explained, "Some of the early responses
were obviously helpful to start mobilizing, but ... the response was in some ways
straight-jacketed and it was then very difficult to change it to a much broader-based
response, bringing in different partners."[49] In fact, according to Joe Cohen, Mahler's
Senior Policy Health Advisor, Reid "wanted to transfer the program to UNDP" as
early as 1987. Cohen, who considered AIDS fundamentally a medical problem,
would not hear of such a move. "I had a real dustup with a representative of
Australia [where Reid was from] ... because I refused to accept this. We had a
coordinating committee because of this link between medical epidemiology and
social epidemiology. However, this was predominantly a transmissible disease and
the other aspects resulted from that."[50]

This issue was exacerbated by the ascension of Hiroshi Nakajima to the WHO
Director-General position in 1988, and his desire to redirect GPA towards a more
biomedical approach and to exert more strongly WHO's primacy in coordinating
the global AIDS response. And changes were occurring at UNDP as well: Reid

---

[47] Jeff O'Malley, Interview by Michael Merson, New Haven, CT, September, 2002; Mike Bailey,
"UNDP—healthy development? The case of HIV," *Health Policy and Planning*, 1994,
9(4):444–447.

[48] Mike Bailey, "UNDP—healthy development? The case of HIV," *Health Policy and Planning*,
1994, 9(4):444–447.

[49] Mina Mauerstein-Bail, Interview by Michael Merson, New Haven, CT, September, 2002.

[50] Joshua Cohen, Interviewed by Michael Merson, New Haven, CT, August, 2002.

began pushing Draper and Tim Rothermel, the Director of the Division of Global and Regional Projects, for UNDP to have a greater role in the global response to the AIDS pandemic.[51] She found UNDP's secondary role increasingly unsatisfactory and frustrating, especially since it was developing "a complementary, but different, set of priorities in its [AIDS] policy framework." This was particularly true after 1989, when the UN General Assembly passed its "landmark resolution" (44/211) calling on national governments to take central responsibility for their own development. UNDP saw the resolution as a justification for its greater involvement on AIDS activities at country level, and consequently Draper appointed Reid as an HIV advisor in 1990. Over the next year the UNDP Governing Council passed several resolutions that embraced a more development-focused, multisectoral response to AIDS. This culminated in the establishment of the UNDP HIV and Development Program, which, as we mentioned above, was formally endorsed by UNDPs Governing Council in May 1991.

At the time I welcomed this move, hoping that it would allow UNDP to play a greater role in the global AIDS response and thus become a stronger partner able to provide more resources. I hoped that UNDP staff would take the lead in sectors other than health and that we could operate together, rather than as a subordinate or competitor. Funded through Dutch, Norwegian and, later, United States donations, the UNDP HIV and Development Program became operational on January 1, 1992.[52]

Despite my hopes, UNDP's establishment of an independent HIV program led to an unfortunate series of events. UNDP, for its part, saw Nakajima as an obstacle to an open and collaborative relationship because it felt he refused to allow GPA to collaborate on any HIV-related effort unless WHO served as the lead technical agency. WHO's primacy had been stipulated in the WHO/UNDP Alliance, and Nakajima was determined to maintain that relational hierarchy. UNDP staff had felt constrained by the Alliance and wished to pursue projects on its own which fell within its purview. With its new mandate, UNDP began developing and executing its own AIDS activities with GPA serving, at best (willingly or not), in a supportive role. This included UNDP country offices extending direct support to countries (rather than through WHO/GPA, as previously agreed in the Alliance), while UNDP's Regional Bureaus began initiating regional programs in Asia and Africa (sometimes duplicating the efforts of WHO's regional offices). The result was that staff from both agencies began viewing each other with increasing suspicion and acrimony, and the agencies began competing for AIDS funding and strategic primacy at country, regional, and global levels.

An early example of these competing visions that served as a precursor of what came later occurred in September 1990, even before UNDP had established its HIV and Development Program. At that time, UNDP earmarked over $600,000 for a project to support Ethiopia's AIDS Control Program.[53] While the program began as

---

[51] Timothy Rothermel, Interview by Michael Merson, New York, August, 2002.

[52] Mina Mauerstein-Bail, Interview by Michael Merson, New Haven, CT, September, 2002.

[53] Inyang Ebong-Harstrup, "Letter to T. Rothermel re: ETH/90/020-Assistance to AIDS Control Programme," Ethiopia: UNDP, 1991.

part of Ethiopia's GPA-structured Medium-Term Plan, UNDP sought to run this project and include WHO only in a supportive role.[54] Tensions quickly mounted over the role of the two agencies: could UNDP operate in the lead role? Did WHO need to be involved in the project at all? UNDP saw its project as emblematic of the fact that "HIV/AIDS [was] not just a disease problem but a development issue," and the agency argued that UNDP needed both to coordinate the program and mobilize resources for it.[55] WHO staff viewed the situation differently; they saw it as an attempt by UNDP to subvert WHO's coordinating and implementing role for AIDS efforts. It was around this time that Nakajima sent a fax to all WHO regional and country offices indicating that the organization was barred from participating in WHO/UNDP projects if WHO was not the executing agency. UNDP staff felt that Nakajima's instructions broke the collaborative spirit of the WHO/UNDP Alliance: "Nakajima broke the alliance," Mauerstein-Bail recalls. "I remember seeing this fax that went out to all country offices, saying 'if WHO is not the executing agency, you do not sign agreements with UNDP,' and I remember at the time we were developing this project … which was put on hold."[56] WHO's view was that the Ethiopian project was symptomatic of the larger problem of UN agencies in general, and UNDP in particular, actively competing for authority and resources to lead the response to the pandemic.

This conflict accelerated the agencies' deteriorating relationship; UNDP had put aside several hundred thousand dollars for the program and WHO delayed signing the agreement for several months. Eventually, UNDP redrafted the program plan to satisfy WHO's concerns. However, it began pushing to revisit the relationship between the agencies and, in 1992, WHO and UNDP revised their Alliance through a Memorandum of Understanding. This revision allowed UNDP funds to flow to national AIDS programs directly, and not only through the WHO Trust Fund for GPA.[57] I supported this change, feeling there was no reason to prevent UNDP funds from being given directly to national programs as long as UNDP sought WHO's advice in the design of these programs.

Then there was the issue of funding. While UNDP had a host of agency resources it could bring to the table, its funding proved more constrained. Its financial support to national AIDS programs relied on funds raised by its New York office, under Reid's leadership, as well as on "separately managed regional HIV programs" for Asia and Africa, which "were directed by the regional offices also located in New York."[58] What surprised me was that, despite UNDP's expressed interest in AIDS at the highest levels of the agency, Reid and her team obtained very little core budget support from UNDP and had only two small funding sources: Interregional

---

[54] "PAC Meeting: ETH/90/020—Assistance to the National AIDS Control Programme, August 27,1991".

[55] Basem Khader, "Note for Mr. Gomez: HIV/AIDS in Africa," New York: UNDP, October 10, 1991.

[56] Mina Mauerstein-Bail, Interview by Michael Merson, New Haven, CT, September, 2002.

[57] Mike Bailey, "UNDP—healthy development? The case of HIV," Health Policy and Planning, 1994, 9(4):444–447.

[58] Ibid, 446.

Program funds to be used for advocacy and training activities and Special Program funds allocated to support research.[59] With little organizational money for operations, Reid and her team felt compelled to seek funds aggressively from donor nations, which of course was precisely what GPA was doing. Thus, it was inevitable that the two agencies would find themselves in open competition for funds, resulting in further conflict. More on this below.

My personal relationship with Reid did not help matters. Reid was a specialist in development and women's rights. Before joining UNDP, she had had 25 years of professional development experience. She was the Australian representative to the United Nations Forum on the Role of Women in Population and Development in 1974, and the leader of the Australian delegation to the World Conference of the International Women's Year in Mexico City in 1975. Just before moving to New York, she had served as a senior consultant for Australia's national HIV/AIDS strategy. AIDS for Reid was not just a development issue; it was a very personal and ideological passion. It was a personal passion because she had lost her husband to AIDS as a result of a contaminated blood transfusion in Africa. [60] It was an ideological passion because AIDS in Africa so profoundly affected vulnerable women.[61] I had not had any interaction with Reid before joining GPA, but, as we mentioned earlier (see Chapter 9), within the first weeks of my becoming Director, I met her at a reception in New York. When Reid introduced herself, she immediately asked if I would consider hiring her as my Deputy Director. The request caught me completely by surprise, but I answered honestly and explained my intention to hire a woman from a low- or middle-income country (which I eventually did when I chose Dorothy Blake from Jamaica for the position). I often wondered what our relationship would have been like had I hired Reid as my Deputy Director. In any event, not long after that, she began to argue openly in various forums that money given to GPA could be better used at UNDP. She would even make this case at meetings of the GPA Management Committee, and also did so at a very important United States Congressional Forum on AIDS, established and hosted in 1991 by United States Representative Jim McDermott to rally Congressional support for global AIDS funding (where I also spoke, see Picture 14.1). Reid's attack on GPA—on our strategy, leadership role, and funding sources—was difficult for me to accept, and sometimes felt personal. Unfortunately, and often inadvertently, we could set each other off during meetings by drawing attention to what we saw as deficiencies in each other's viewpoints.

Thus there were several reasons for the breach with UNDP. UNDP had signed on to an Alliance with WHO which required that it serve in a supporting role to WHO, a role that it now wished to change. Since, as mentioned above, Reid had wanted to transfer the program to UNDP as early as 1987, it is not surprising that she would have objected to any perceived subservience by UNDP to WHO once she had

[59] Ibid.

[60] Timothy Rothermel, Interview by Michael Merson, New York, August, 2002.

[61] Ibid.

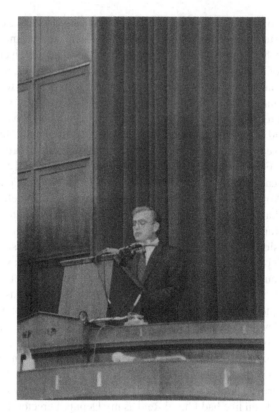

Picture 14.1 Michael Merson speaking at the United States Congressional Forum on AIDS, 1991. Photo courtesy of Melissa Ellison

authority over UNDP's activities.[62] She was not alone, of course. There were other UNDP staff like Gus Edgrin, Director of Program Policy and Evaluation, who wondered aloud, "Why aren't we getting more of the money that WHO is getting? Why aren't we more of a part of this, since we clearly have a role to play?" Moreover, in the period of UN reform following the end of the Cold War, UNDP was under pressure from donor countries to justify its role (and even existence) within the UN system. These pressures and differences made the feud with UNDP very real. While some observers have blamed this breach more on my relationship with Reid, which I admit had become strained, it seems very likely that the interagency squabbling would have occurred regardless of the nature of our personal relationship.

Beyond these agency-related or personal tensions, it was the case that UNDP and WHO had very different approaches to the pandemic. Reid championed what she called a "developmental" model—a bottom up, community-based response that addressed the social determinants of health. These, in her view, served as both a cause and consequence of the pandemic. As mentioned earlier, Reid often compared this approach with the "biomedical model" she (and others[63]) ascribed to WHO, "WHO's

[62] Joshua Cohen, Interviewed by Michael Merson, New Haven, CT, August, 2002.

[63] Fiona Godlee, "WHO in retreat: is it losing its influence?" *BMJ* 3 December 1994;309:1491–1495.

approach is a view of HIV transmission as the transmission of a pathogen from one individual to another," she told a reporter from the journal *Science* in 1994.[64] WHO's position was narrow, she claimed, neglecting the "socioeconomic factors such as poverty, access to health services, and the way male domination makes women vulnerable to infection, particularly in developing countries."[65] Reid was very articulate in her writings and speaking, and she believed GPA had an approach to AIDS with which she deeply disagreed. We at GPA, in turn, disagreed with her assessment, and we did not see these two perspectives as mutually exclusive—we felt both were important and had articulated as such in the Global AIDS Strategy. In fact, we looked to UNDP to operationalize the development approach within national AIDS programs, and were frustrated because it seemed that UNDP was only supporting small-scale community activities carried out by non-governmental organizations (NGOs) such as the Salvation Army. These activities largely focused on consciousness raising, community-based participatory interventions carried out by grassroots organization. A critical question for us was how we, or UNDP, could take such small programs to scale. We also wanted UNDP to help us figure out how countries could carry out development activities that produced measurable behavioral outcomes. If they could have provided any assistance in this regard, we would certainly have supported such efforts financially. Interestingly, this was similar to the dilemma GPA had faced in operationalizing Mann's human rights approach to AIDS (see Chapter 12).

To this day, I do not understand why Reid rejected so strongly the public health approach to AIDS prevention. After all, HIV was a transmissible virus that caused a classic sexually transmitted disease for which there were interventions that had been shown to be effective in research studies and later in countries like Uganda, Senegal, Thailand, and Brazil.[66] For Reid, the AIDS pandemic was primarily a symptom of a larger problem of vulnerability and social disruption, and until those underlying forces were addressed, she believed, the AIDS pandemic could not be stopped.

While these strategic differences were real, the issues related to funding and donor influence were far more consequential. As we mentioned earlier, Reid wound up relying on bilateral donor support for much of her program funding, as did GPA. "There were always financial uncertainties," Mauerstein-Bail remembered. "That was very difficult. I remember that quite a number of times … we'd have like 3 months left of funding."[67] Accordingly, UNDP began sending more and more AIDS project proposals to our donors. "UNDP was losing a lot of money at that time, in general," Marjory Dam explained, "[and Reid] was such a crusader, she could see the only way she was going to get money for what she was going to do was to get it the way [GPA was] getting it."[68] As a result, I found that when I would visit the United States Congress (see Picture 14.2) to meet with Congressional staff, or testify to the Senate or House of Representatives Foreign Operations sub-committee on Appropriations, the following day or week Reid would speak to the same

[64] Michael Balter "UN Readies New Global AIDS Plan," *Science*, 1994, 266:1312–1313.

[65] Ibid.

[66] Peter Lamptey, Interview by Michael Merson, Washington, DC, December, 2002.

[67] Mina Mauerstein-Bail, Interview by Michael Merson, New Haven, CT, September.

[68] Marjory Dam, Interview by Michael Merson, New Haven, CT, September 29, 2001.

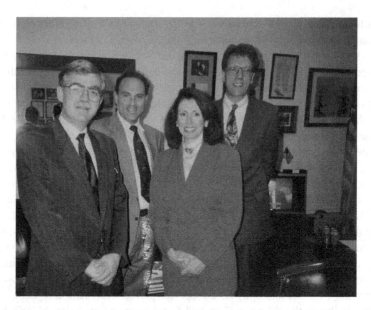

Picture 14.2 Michael Merson (far *left*), Gary Slutkin (second from *left*), Congresswoman Nancy Pelosi (second from *right*) and Chris Powell (far *right*). Office of Congresswoman Pelosi, 1991. Photo courtesy of Melissa Ellison

individuals or testify to the same committees.[69] While I tried never to criticize UNDP in my meetings or testimonies, Reid in contrast would frequently explain why UNDP was a better investment than WHO.[70] She would strategically use the differences between UNDP and WHO to illustrate what she saw as deficiencies in the WHO approach, and subsequently explain how these could be rectified with more designated funding to UNDP. With this approach, she succeeded in gaining support from Congressman McDermott to the point that McDermott recommended redirecting funds from GPA to UNDP. The result was that whatever opportunities there were for collaboration in our fundraising evaporated in front of the United States Congress.

A number of European donors also found themselves drawn to Reid's argument and the perspective she espoused. In May, 1992, for example, Portuguese Deputy Foreign Minister, Duarte Ivo Cruz, speaking on behalf of the European Community Presidency, indicated that the "E.C. [European Community][took] the view that AIDS, though a health matter, [was] closely linked to economic and social factors and therefore better managed by the UNDP."[71]

Unfortunately, over time, many donors became concerned that this tension between WHO and UNDP was hindering the overall global response. "We are concerned about divergences which have grown up in the process of getting the AIDS program started," Cruz had said at the May 1992 European Community meeting. "Matters like AIDS are evidently too important … to let differences of this kind

---

[69] Ibid.

[70] Ibid.

[71] "AIDS combat highlights rift over U.N. agencies' role," *Agence France Presse*, May 11, 1992.

arise between the UNDP and WHO in this field. This problem has to be settled rapidly"[72] "I recall," remembered Ann Blackwood (an official working with Neil Boyer in the United States State Department's Bureau of International Organization which had responsibility for WHO within the Department), "that there seemed to be a lot of duplication of effort among the agencies."[73] As the pandemic expanded, remembers Ken Bernard (at the time the Health Attaché in the United States Mission to WHO in Geneva), "You had UN agencies that had apparently, in the public eye, a divergent approach to dealing with the issue. Even at the time there were members of the Executive Board who were pounding their tables saying: 'This is a medical issue, doctors should be dealing with this! ... [but then] you had UNDP and other agencies saying: 'Wait a minute, wait a minute!'" [74] "I certainly got fed up at this point," Joe Decosas, who by then had taken over as Chair of the GPA Management Committee, remembered. "This just doesn't make any sense when the Director of the largest AIDS program has to spend 3 months in the US to defend his funding ... this was not an efficient way to support programs and do programs—it was too subjective to regional political influences."[75] Taken together, the growing tensions between UNDP and GPA, between Reid and myself, put a lot of pressure on GPA and called into question our ability to truly coordinate the global response, particularly among UN agencies.

The global health community thus found itself with two UN agencies offering different strategies for fighting AIDS, and competing for the same donor dollars. Moreover, this competition stoked existing concerns among donors about the funding they were providing to GPA. The early 1990s were difficult times for many economies: the first Gulf War and the global economic downturn of the early 1990s shrank international development budgets, compelling governments to reconsider their budget priorities. GPA certainly feared what this might mean for our budget, though in 1991 and 1992 GPA was able to maintain strong support from its donors.[76] In fact, the 17 governments funding GPA kept their funding levels stable, even as they expanded their own bilateral programs. In 1990, for example, we met our budget target of $90 million; in 1991, we again met our budget of $87 million. While some donors began reducing their funding, others made up the difference. Between 1991 and 1992, for example, the United States government increased its support to GPA from $21 million to $25 million. Still, by 1992, it was evident that we were likely reaching a ceiling with our budget.

As we explained in the previous chapter, GPA hit this ceiling, in part, because many donor nations had by then set up their own bilateral AIDS programs directed toward low- and middle-income countries. These had taken some time to establish. In the early years of the pandemic, many high-income nations had endured substantial pressure

---

[72] Ibid.

[73] Ann Blackwood, Interview by Michael Merson, New Haven, CT, January, 2002; Neil Boyer, Interview by Michael Merson, New Haven, CT, January, 2002.

[74] Ken Bernard, Interview by Michael Merson, New Haven, CT, February, 2002.

[75] Joe Decosas, Interview by Michael Merson, New Haven, CT, October, 2001.

[76] All numbers and citations in the following paragraph come from Marjory Dam, "Progress in the Global AIDS Effort," *The Washington Post*, August 11, 1992, Z4.

from activists in their countries to spend money on AIDS programs domestically and did not appreciate the potential global scope of the pandemic. Moreover, even if they had wanted to set up bilateral programs, they lacked the technical expertise and experience to address the challenges of AIDS abroad, which was not surprising given that it was a new disease. Instead, as we explained in Chapter 5, they had found it easiest to provide funding for GPA. GPA offered a quick, easy, and convenient mechanism by which to support global AIDS efforts, and Mann gave them every assurance that WHO could deliver whatever needed to be done.[77] By the early 1990s, however, donor nations had come to appreciate the potential global scale of the AIDS pandemic, in great part because of GPA's advocacy. Over this time, they were able to launch their own bilateral programs on AIDS, programs more aligned with their individual foreign policy commitments and priorities. Moreover, the emergence of several potential treatments for AIDS began making the disease seem, at least in high-income countries, less of an emergency. These factors—at home and abroad—meant that, by the early to mid-1990s, many donor nations regarded GPA, while still important, as less of a priority.

The problem for GPA was that AIDS was far from going away: countries were reporting an increasing number of HIV infections and AIDS cases, and a growing number of countries were seeking GPA's assistance and advice. Millions of persons infected with HIV during the 1980s were now becoming ill with AIDS. So, while GPA's budget from donors remained stable, a stable budget was insufficient to meet the increasing needs of many hard-hit countries. GPA thus encountered a unique situation: a balanced budget, which sounded positive but in fact was a huge problem. Back in 1987, contributions to GPA had totaled $33 million, but expenditures had only topped $17 million, allowing GPA to carry over a considerable amount of funds to the following year. By 1991, however, our contributions and expenditures both totaled $87 million. We had grown more efficient managing our resources, but the number of national programs had grown, and support demands had risen with them, not only for prevention but also for care. GPA had lost its financial cushion.

GPA's relationship with the United States Agency for International Development (USAID) provides a good example of how funding priorities were shifting among our donors. USAID was an essential partner with GPA in the global fight against AIDS. It provided on average between 25 and 30% of our budget in any given year. In fact, its hands had been tied: before I joined GPA, Mann had made the strategic move of obtaining an earmark from the United States Congress for WHO's AIDS program. This angered some at USAID, because it cemented GPA's role as a broker of the global AIDS response, and it diverted money that USAID staff would have preferred go to USAID (though there was no assurance it would have). As the *Washington Post*'s Bart Gellman related in a series of articles in 2000, "USAID focused much of its legislative energy on eliminating or reducing the earmark in order to recapture control of its budget."[78] "There were some battles between us and WHO as to who could spend the money better and hence who should get it, us or

[77] Joe Decosas, Interview by Michael Merson, New Haven, CT, October, 2001; Peter Piot, Interview with Michael Merson, New Haven, CT, October 26, 2002.

[78] Barton Gellman, "Death Watch: The Global Response to AIDS in Africa," *Washington Post,* July 5, 2000, A1.

WHO," remembered Brad Langmaid, who was Deputy Assistant Administrator in USAID's Bureau for Science and Technology in the late 1980s and oversaw the Agency's AIDS programs. "I think we [that is, USAID] held our own in those issues. We brought the WHO levels down considerably from the earlier earmark without totally damaging our relationship with WHO."[79]

One of the prime drivers in this effort was Duff Gillespie, who between 1986 and 1993 directed USAID's Office of Population. Gillespie, according to Gellman, felt that population control was by far a greater problem than AIDS in Africa, and worked assiduously to prevent population budget dollars from being used for AIDS (the population dollars were also a Congressional earmark). Investing in AIDS had significant downsides, Gillespie would later explain: the disease had no cure; program costs were exorbitant; interventions were not economical; clinicians lacked failsafe prophylaxis; and the afflicted were not inherently sympathetic.[80] His reluctance was a rare mistake in judgment for Gillespie, who was among the best USAID leaders at the time.

Still, despite USAID's resistance, I was very open to collaborating with Langmaid and USAID. I was particularly committed to working with them on lobbying the United States Congress for funding. While USAID's rules restricted it from doing so, WHO had considerable latitude in this area. This served both our interests, in that it allowed me both to preserve much of GPA's earmark and to advocate support for USAID's bilateral AIDS programs, which was mostly flowing to NGOs working in USAID priority countries. A number of GPA staff also collaborated with USAID to establish several new bilateral AIDS projects, such as the AIDS Public Health Communication project (AIDSCOM) and AIDS Technical Support project (AIDSTECH), even though these were financed with money from our earmark.[81] GPA also worked out a "soft earmark" strategy with USAID, by which we committed to using a portion of its contribution to GPA to support AIDS programs in some of the same countries where USAID-supported bilateral programs were present. Each year USAID would designate between 15 and 20 countries for this purpose, and I would meet quarterly with the USAID AIDS Coordinator (first with Jeff Harris, later with Helene Gayle) and other USAID staff to agree on these soft earmarks and how we could coordinate our efforts in these countries.

One of the key WHO staff, whom we have mentioned a number of times thus far, and with whom I worked closely on United States government matters, was Marjory Dam, WHO's External Relations Officer in Washington, DC. Dam was extraordinarily strategic, had Nakajima's full trust, and did an exceptional job representing WHO in Washington, DC. She often helped me navigate through the many minefields there, and we spent hours together strategizing the best ways to gain visibility, obtain support, and build relationships. That said, there was only

---

[79] Bradshaw Langmaid, Interview with W. Haven North, July 14, 1998, United States Foreign Assistance Oral History Program, 78.

[80] Barton Gellman, "Death Watch: The Global Response to AIDS in Africa," *Washington Post,* July 5, 2000, A1.

[81] Bradshaw Langmaid, Interview with W. Haven North, July 14, 1998, United States Foreign Assistance Oral History Program, 78.

so much Dam and I could do to increase our support from the United States government. And, unfortunately, GPA did not have a Marjory Dam in every donor country.

This last point is important because the social capital that GPA had built up was beginning to diminish. As we explained earlier, many donors had now had enough time to establish, like USAID, their own bilateral AIDS programs. As Ross Noble from the Canadian International Development Agency noted: "There is always more preference to channel money directly through channels where you can see the ground results and there is accountability … than trying to fund it through a multilateral organization."[82] This meant that donors were more likely to demand more accountability about use of their funds, and were now able to compare the effectiveness of GPA's programs with that of their own—particularly in countries where we were both working. "I think there was indeed the dissatisfaction of performance at country level [and] the executing capacity of WHO," Peter Piot remembered. This was more of a general WHO problem than one specific to GPA, Piot acknowledged, "The fact is that [WHO] is administratively not flexible enough, not flexible in terms of accountability. It is not set up to deliver any goods except publications and ideas and policies. That's what WHO does well."[83] Daniel Tarantola summed up the change in donor thinking like this:

> I think there was an erosion at the level of confidence that donors had placed in WHO… There was a better understanding also, thanks to WHO, about the alternatives, the fact that you could not only do condoms but attack HIV from a broader angle. The fact that you had groups like AIDSCAP, AIDSCOM, etc., which were putting USAID under pressure, saying why do you waste your money on those big UN things—why don't you give it to us? At least some of it will go back to the US tax payer, and so forth. So all these pressures combined, also the [British] ODA[Overseas Development Agency] … was already putting demands on WHO which were far stronger than they had ever been. … for WHO to now show evidence of declining HIV trends as a result of the money they had put, not realizing that they had put $15 million dollars in the whole basket and that three years later you could probably not show such results. So demands from them became unreasonable.[84]

And so, with high donor expectations, dwindling social capital, open competition between UN agencies, growing unhappiness with the WHO Director-General Hiroshi Nakajima, harsher external criticism, and an unabating pandemic, GPA found itself towards the end of 1992 with a brewing crisis with regard to its future. Donors and other agencies had begun questioning openly whether GPA's global effort was effective and, even more importantly, if it was the best entity to coordinate the global response. The donors had relied on GPA to coordinate the UN response, but increasingly other agencies began operating independently, raising fears of redundant programming and bureaucratic infighting. Whereas donors might forgive programmatic stumbles, they found interagency squabbling, bureaucratic infighting, and poor global coordination far less excusable, and of greater concern. These battles quickly became a key point of focus for international restructuring of the global response to the pandemic.

---

[82] Ross Noble, Interview by Michael Merson, Geneva, October, 2001.

[83] Peter Piot, Interview with Michael Merson, New Haven, CT, October, 26, 2002.

[84] Daniel Tarantola, Interview by Michael Merson, New Haven, CT, October, 2001.

Part III
Seeking Global Coordination
in a Pandemic

Chapter 15
Rethinking Global AIDS Governance

By early 1993, it was becoming clear that the global response to AIDS[1] had frayed considerably. Donors were expressing more dissatisfaction, United Nations (UN) agencies were bickering and competing openly for funds, and we at the Global Programme on AIDS (GPA) were struggling to engage and support an ever growing number of nations while our budget remained flat. All the while the pandemic rolled on, wrecking havoc in places least equipped to deal with the disease. The projections were only growing worse, for while we believed that as many as 40 million might be infected by the year 2000, we knew that without aggressive action the pandemic could cause even more damage. "Most of our estimates, unfortunately in the future if we have more data, will have to be revised probably upwards," our epidemiologist, Jim Chin, had warned reporters in 1991.[2]

With the hope of a unified global response now openly contested, GPA stakeholders began considering their next course of action. It was in this context that the donors began using the external review of GPA as a mechanism by which to review, and perhaps reform, the global AIDS response.

What was the external review of GPA? While the process began formally in the spring of 1990 (see Chapter 7), its origins in some ways stretched back to the very beginning of GPA. When interested parties first gathered with Fakhry Assaad and Jonathan Mann in 1986, the governments present were not all of one mind on how best to structure the global response to AIDS. For example, the Canadian mission advocated that the UN establish a multiagency, cosponsored program structurally equivalent to that of the Special Programme for Research and Training in

---

Within this chapter the singular pronouns *I* and *my* refer to Michael Merson alone, whereas the plural pronouns *we* and *us* generally refer to Michael Merson and Stephen Inrig jointly. Where *we* or *us* refers to Michael Merson and his colleagues at WHO, the object of the pronoun is clarified by context.

[1] For the purposes of this text, we will use the term AIDS to encompass both AIDS and HIV unless otherwise specified.

[2] CBS News Transcripts, "AIDS Conference Focuses On Spread Of AIDS In Asia," *CBS Evening News*, June 17, 1991.

© Springer International Publishing AG 2018
M. Merson, S. Inrig, *The AIDS Pandemic*, DOI 10.1007/978-3-319-47133-4_15

Tropical Diseases (TDR)[3] rather than a program housed solely in the World Health Organization (WHO). The UN had launched TDR in 1975 as a program based in and executed by WHO, but jointly sponsored by the United Nations Development Programme (UNDP), the World Bank, and WHO. Director-General Halfdan Mahler had been able to mollify the Canadians and those who supported its perspective by locating GPA in his office, giving it extrabudgetary standing, and permitting Mann to run it outside WHO's traditional system (as described earlier). As Joe Decosas explained, "GPA did not fit into what was expected of WHO. GPA had been pushed by the same donors into a program delivery mechanism which … looked somewhat doable because it had this independence within the WHO structure." [4]

While this independence did make a WHO-based global AIDS response appear "doable" during the first part of Mann's tenure, two problems eventually emerged. First, Mann and his team at GPA appear to have over-interpreted the donors' mandate for GPA and overestimated GPA's ability to direct and coordinate the global response. As we pointed out in Chapter 14, donors had needed GPA earlier in the pandemic, but as they developed their bilateral programs, their scrutiny increased substantially.[5]

Second, Hiroshi Nakajima's ascension to Director-General augmented donor concerns about the operations of GPA. Donors had consented to WHO's primacy, rather than a jointly sponsored program, on the basis of Mahler's willingness to permit its essentially autonomous existence outside WHO's bureaucratic structure. Nakajima, having been a WHO Regional Director, and unhappy with GPA's modus operandi under Mann, was unconvinced about the exceptional nature of AIDS and did not like the program functioning outside the regional office framework. "As soon as they started to get tied into the regional offices and the politics of WHO," Decosas recalled, "it became clear that GPA could not deliver institutionally."[6] There was particular concern, as we mentioned in Chapter 9, about the operational capability of the WHO regional office for Africa (AFRO) in Brazzaville.

This was the context in which the donors launched an external review of GPA, even before Mann resigned as Director. At GPA's Management Committee (GMC) meeting in November 1989, the GMC decided to undertake this review. In its April 1990 meeting, only 3 1/2 years after WHO established the AIDS program that was to become GPA, and just days after Mann's surprising resignation, the GMC prepared the detailed terms of reference for the External Review Committee (ERC).[7] [These appear in Chapter 8, and we include them here again for ease of reference (Fig. 15.1).] Chaired by Bernadette Olowo-Freers from Uganda, the ERC consisted of ten members with a wide range of public health, administrative, and academic backgrounds.[8] The group met for the first time in January 1991, and collected a large

[3] Joe Decosas, Interview by Michael Merson, New Haven, CT, October, 2001; Halfdan Mahler, Interview by Michael Merson, Geneva, October, 2001.

[4] Joe Decosas, Interview by Michael Merson, New Haven, CT, October, 2001.

[5] Ibid.

[6] Ibid.

[7] Michael Merson, "Report of the Director, Fifth Meeting of the Management Committee, November 26, 1990" Geneva: World Health Organization GPA/GMC(2) 90.3, 1990.

[8] Bernadette Olowo-Freers would later serve as UNAIDS Coordinator in Swaziland.

1. To review GPA's basic strategies and modes of operation, particularly mechanisms for operational support to national AIDS programmes, including their relevance to social and economic developments.
2. To assess GPA's accomplishments and contributions to global and national AIDS prevention and control efforts.
3. To assess the process used by GPA for priority setting, focusing on the relevance of the resulting priorities to all levels of programming
4. To review progress towards meeting targets
5. To assess the effectiveness, cost effectiveness, and efficiency of GPA's operation.
6. To assess the relevance of GPA activities to national health care systems, with particular attention to primary health care.
7. To assess the suitability of GPA's management structure, procedures, and priorities to enhance national and international efforts for AIDS prevention.
8. To assess GPA's activities and interactions with other parts of WHO at all levels, the UN system, and other institutions and organizations, including NGOs, concerned with AIDS prevention and control.
9. To consider the future role and priorities of GPA
10. To make recommendations relevant to the terms of reference.

Fig. 15.1 Terms of reference for external review. Source: Bernadette Olowo-Freers, Gill Walt, et al. *Report of the External Review of the World Health Organization, Global Programme on AIDS,* Geneva: World Health Organization, January 1992, pp. i–iii

amount of information between January and July 1991.[9] During those months, the ERC reviewed the program's activities, met with individuals from a large number of multilateral agencies, bilateral donors, private foundations, non-governmental organizations (NGOs), WHO Units in Geneva and the regional offices, GPA staff (past and present), and various GPA external advisory bodies (past and present). Between July and October 1991 the ERC prepared its findings and recommendations and, in November 1991, it presented an Executive Summary of its report to the GMC.[10]

---

[9] Bernadette Olowo-Freers, Gill Walt, et al. *Report of the External Review of the World Health Organization, Global Programme on AIDS,* Geneva: World Health Organization, January 1992, pp. i–iii.
[10] Ibid.

After clarifying certain issues raised by GMC members and considering a written response to the Executive Summary prepared by GPA, the ERC submitted its final report to the GMC in January 1992.

The report consisted of several chapters, including ones on the history of GPA, its structure and operations at country level, and its future. Most of the committee's findings did not come as a surprise to me. In fact, many of the report's findings mirrored those I had identified with Walt Dowdle (from the Centers for Disease Control and Prevention [CDC]) in our assessment of GPA back in 1990. However, it was Chapter 4 of the report—which covered GPA's relationships within WHO and with NGOs, donor organizations, and UN Agencies—that proved to be most important for the GMC and the donors in particular.[11] The ERC concluded that GPA suffered from weak management and imprecise and irregular donor expectations during its unprecedented growth in the first 5 years. While the ERC expected GPA's improved management and fiscal transparency to reduce the need for donor scrutiny, it felt our mandate as "UN leader in policy development and coordination" required clarification, reaffirmation, reform, and operationalization. Specifically, the ERC recommended that GPA restructure its collaborative relationships with UN agencies, donor nations, and other organizations to maximize their value and benefit.

The donors paid particular attention to the ERC's recommendations for reform. The ERC proposed that GPA increase collaboration with other UN agencies at the regional and national level to build "a broad and multisectoral response", and that we integrate NGOs more in the planning and implementation phases of programs. While the ERC still believed WHO/GPA should retain overall multisectoral leadership, it called on the GMC to form a working group that would collectively define WHO/GPA's leadership role, while articulating the complementary roles other agencies would play, and identify the best structure for maximal UN collaboration on AIDS in developing nations. This would result, the ERC concluded, in stronger interagency collaboration (especially between WHO and the United Nations Development Programme [UNDP]) and improve national program capacity.

The ERC suggested several options for strengthening UN collboration. These included creating: (1) an entirely new UN Agency for HIV/AIDS Care and Prevention; (2) a cosponsored WHO program accountable to the cosponsoring agencies rather than the Director-General of WHO; (3) a Steering Committee, like other UN committees, that coordinates agency-specific AIDS contributions; (4) a UN-sponsored Commission that worked to generate greater political commitment to fighting HIV/AIDS; (5) more bilateral agreements between UN agencies along the lines of the WHO/UNDP Alliance to Combat AIDS; and (6) a new multiagency alliance created between the major UN agencies. The ERC provided its thoughts on the strengths and weaknesses of each option, but ultimately it threw its weight behind the last option. It recommended that the UN create a new, multiagency alliance guided by a subcommittee of the UN system's Administrative Committee on Coordination (ACC). This was not an easy solution, the ERC recognized, but

---

[11] The following paragraphs summarize Chapter 4 of The Report of the External Review of the Global Program on AIDS, January 1992.

better collaboration between UN agencies was an urgent need and it felt this was the best route to that end.

I believed at the outset that the external review could play an important role in the structure of global AIDS governance going forward, and the GPA leadership team and I did not think the ERC recommendations would threaten the existence of GPA. Moreover, I felt such reviews are integral to good management, and I did not take this review personally or perceive it as unfair. I was pleased to see that the report acknowledged all the work we had done during the past 18 months to reorganize GPA to better address the global pandemic.

While it was clear from the review that GPA needed to address issues around interagency cooperation, we had a mounting pandemic on our hands, and we needed to move forward aggressively with our program activities. This meant, for example, enhancing our performance at country level, strengthening the management of national AIDS programs, addressing antiretroviral drug pricing, making advances in reducing maternal to child transmission of HIV, advancing blood transfusion safety, enhancing sexually transmitted disease (STD)[12] control, expanding our research, ensuring the continuity of care, and bolstering our antidiscrimination efforts. GPA staff continued to work diligently and tirelessly, despite considerable obstacles, to leverage the assets we had at our disposal to combat the pandemic, and I believed we were slowly making progress. To help with our planning, I invited Dowdle to return to Geneva again to help me think through ways to improve our program effectiveness.

If the external review prompted GPA to double down on its efforts, it sent the donors in a different direction, one that, in retrospect, proved to be a turning point in global AIDS governance. We do not believe the donors intended this outcome when they decided to undertake the review, but very soon after the report was submitted, a process was put in motion that would have substantive consequences for the global response and for the hundreds of persons working in GPA. As the situation evolved, it became more and more evident that by the end of the process, GPA might not remain in its current configuration, or exist at all.

Recall that the ERC had recommended that the GMC establish a working group to look into "the structuring of UN collaboration so that the level of quality of the response to AIDS match the scale of the problem."[13] At its November 1991 meeting, even without having the full report, the GMC chose to establish such a working group, tasking it to explore coordination of UN system activities in HIV/AIDS.[14] This ad hoc working group consisted of ten members, including six donor countries

---

[12] For the purposes of this text, we use the term sexually transmitted disease(s) and the abbreviation STD rather than the other term sexually transmitted infection(s) or STIs.

[13] Bernadette Olowo-Freers, Gill Walt, et al., *Report of the External Review of the World Health Organization, Global Programme on AIDS,* Geneva: World Health Organization, January 1992, page 42.

[14] Global Programme on AIDS, "Extraordinary Meeting of the Management Committee: Mechanisms for Global Level Coordination—Proposal for the establishment of an AIDS coordination forum, Geneva. 23–25 November 1992; Provisional agenda item 2." Geneva: World Health Organization, GPA/GMC(E)/92.3, 6 November 1992.

(France, Japan, Netherlands, Nordic countries, United Kingdom, United States), two developing countries (Congo, Mexico), the European Commission, and the Chair of the GMC (Joe Decosas from Canada). It was chaired by Ulf Rundin, Senior Adviser to the Health Division of the Swedish International Development Authority (SIDA), who represented the Nordic countries. Rundin, who had served as Executive Director of the UN Nordic Project, was greatly respected in international affairs as an authority on multilateral assistance and, perhaps more importantly, as an expert on reforming the UN at the end of the Cold War. Over a period of 4 months, Rundin's group met with the main UN agencies involved in AIDS (WHO, UNDP, the World Bank, the United Nations Children's Emergency Fund (UNICEF), the United Nations Population Fund (UNFPA), and the United Nations Educational, Scientific and Cultural Organization (UNESCO)). There was little consensus about what the UN General Assembly had actually intended when, in 1987, it had designated WHO as the UN agency responsible for directing and coordinating the global AIDS response. The agencies stressed the autonomous nature of their mandates and AIDS efforts. They talked about cooperation and coordination, but were resistant to any attempt to narrow the scope of their AIDS activities or accept the authority of any UN coordinating committees to negotiate a more efficient division of labor.[15] This included WHO.

The ad hoc working group interviewed both Nakajima and myself. It reported that, while I was very open to "discuss[ing] various operational models for improved cooperation," Nakajima resisted any perceived attempt "to undermine [WHO's] own narrow interpretation of the 'global leadership' role."[16] It also found that I thought WHO/GPA could best serve as lead agency going forward by providing the technical assistance and financial support functions it was already offering. I remember agreeing with the working group that GPA did not have the ability to implement all aspects of the global response on its own, and suggesting that either a cosponsorship or a global coordinating unit (to which I was more partial) might compensate for GPA's limitations.[17] In contrast to my interactions with them, the group indicated that Nakajima was less open to thinking beyond WHO.[18]

The working group heard comments from UNDP that indicated it was clearly at odds, philosophically, with WHO about how to structure the global response. UNDP asserted its own right to "'lead' the 'response to AIDS at country level'." Indeed, this had been UNDP's rational for establishing its own AIDS program in New York and openly competing with WHO for funding (see Chapter 14).[19] The working

---

[15] "AIDS Program Coordination, or: Should we be here if we want to get there?" Internal Memorandum from Josef Decosas to Cathy Mains, *Health and Population Directorate*, 13 January 1993, 2.

[16] Ibid.

[17] GPA Management Committee, "Management Committee Subcommittee Meeting—External Evaluation of the WHO/GPA: Merson Interviews." Geneva: World Health Organization, 1992, 2.

[18] Josef Decosas, "AIDS Program Coordination, or: Should we be here if we want to get there?" *Health and Population Directorate*, 13 January 1993, 2.

[19] "AIDS Program Coordination, or: Should we be here if we want to get there?" Internal

group reported that UNICEF and UNESCO were more collaborative, with UNESCO serving a marginal and largely scientific role in the educational sector and UNICEF generally aligned with WHO's approach but struggling to operationalize its program at country level.[20]

In April 1992, the ad hoc working group issued its report.[21] The report stated that "there is a general recognition that HIV/AIDS, a health problem for individuals, is also of wide-ranging developmental significance for society as a whole. Thus, the important social and economic factors associated with the transmission of HIV, as well as its prevention and care, require that all sectors must be seriously involved in responding to the challenge posed by the pandemic."[22] The group recommended (somewhat half-heartedly, according to Joe Decosas) that GPA establish "an AIDS Coordination Forum … to function as an inclusive consultative mechanism involving the UN agencies of the UN family, bilateral donors, developing countries, and international NGO networks."[23] Such a Forum would encourage information exchange, provide a facility to discuss interagency issues and concerns, develop consensus on major issues of policy and programmatic significance, and discuss mobilization of resources for AIDS-related activities. For the group, the best means to establish this Forum was to reformulate the Inter-Agency Advisory Group on AIDS (IAAG), which was one of the existing UN coordination committees on AIDS described in Chapter 14.[24]

The GMC, at its 8th meeting held in Geneva in June 1992, received the final report of the ERC, submitted it to the WHO Director-General, and requested GPA to report on actions taken in response to the recommendations within the report at its June 1993 meeting. The GMC also reviewed the recommendations of the ad hoc working group chaired by Rundin. It requested that GPA establish an AIDS Coordinating Forum (though not by expanding the IAAG, and not as a "permanent organization or decision-making entity"), with UNDP as the initial chair and WHO as the Forum's Secretariat. It also asked that GPA report back on the progress made

---

Memorandum from Josef Decosas to Cathy Mains, *Health and Population Directorate*, 13 January 1993, 3.

[20] Ibid.

[21] Ad Hoc Working Group of the GPA Management Committee, "Report of the Ad Hoc Working Group of the GPA Management Committee, Eight Meeting of the Management Committee, Provisional Agenda Item 6, 10–12 June 1992," Geneva: World Health Organization, April 24, 1992, GPA/GMC(8)/92.5.

[22] Ibid., 8.

[23] "AIDS Program Coordination, or: Should we be here if we want to get there?" Internal Memorandum from Josef Decosas to Cathy Mains, *Health and Population Directorate*, 13 January 1993, p. 3.

[24] Global Programme on AIDS, "Extraordinary Meeting of the Management Committee: Mechanisms for Global Level Coordination: Proposal for strengthening the Inter-Agency Advisory Group on AIDS (IAAG); Provisional agenda item 2, Geneva, 23–25 November 1992," Geneva: World Health Organization, GPA/GMC(E)/92.6, 6 November 1992; "AIDS Program Coordination, or: Should we be here if we want to get there?" Internal Memorandum from Josef Decosas to Cathy Mains, *Health and Population Directorate*, 13 January 1993.

in establishing this Forum at an extraordinary meeting of the GMC to be convened in November 1992 (the GMC called the meeting "extraordinary" because the committee normally only met once a year).[25] It further recommended that the current IAAG (which included UNICEF, UNDP, UNFPA, UNESCO, the World Bank, and WHO) continue as the primary United Nations systems committee for discussing issues of relevance to the concerned agencies. The GMC additionally requested GPA to "initiate and carry through a process to propose mechanisms (whether new mechanisms or development of existing mechanisms) for country-level coordination" that would: (a) strengthen national capacity; (b) increase the impact of donor funds; (c) leverage UN agency capacity to best meet national needs; and (d) expand public/private partnerships for HIV/AIDS work.[26] To achieve this, the committee asked GPA to rapidly assess existing instruments and mechanisms for coordinating assistance at country level and to undertake a few case studies of country-level coordination to confirm the findings of this rapid assessment. In July 1992, the Economic and Social Council of the United Nations echoed these conclusions about country-level coordination and strengthening the IAAG.[27]

As had been recommended, in November 1992, the GMC convened the "extraordinary meeting"[28] and made what turned out to be some crucial decisions. First, it recommended further strengthening the IAAG by requesting it to meet more often, have a rotating Chairmanship, and improve the accountability of its members. Second, searching for a better mechanism to improve coordination than the previously recommended AIDS Coordination Forum, it called alternatively for the establishment of a Task Force on HIV/AIDS Coordination to facilitate coordination of the response to the AIDS pandemic, consisting of 12 members (three developing countries, three donor governments, three UN agencies on the IAAG, and three NGOs) and with a 2-year operating budget of $1.3 million.[29] In fact, none of the proposals to improve coordination put forth at the meeting particularly impressed the donors and some of them advocated to postpone a decision. David Nabarro, the British representative and at that time the Chief Health and Population Adviser

---

[25] "AIDS Program Coordination, or: Should we be here if we want to get there?" Internal Memorandum from Josef Decosas to Cathy Mains, *Health and Population Directorate*, 13 January 1993, p. 4.

[26] Eighth Meeting of the Management Committee, Global Programme on AIDS, Geneva, 10–12 June 1992.

[27] Global Programme on AIDS, "Extraordinary Meeting of the Management Committee: Mechanisms for Global Level Coordination: Proposal for strengthening the Inter-Agency Advisory Group on AIDS (IAAG); Provisional agenda item 2, Geneva, 23–25 November 1992," Geneva: World Health Organization, GPA/GMC(E)/92.6, 6 November 1992; Global Programme on AIDS, "Extraordinary Meeting of the Management Committee: Mechanisms for Country-Level Coordination: Recommendations for improved coordination of HIV/AIDS related activities at country level; Provisional agenda item 2, Geneva, 23–25 November 1992," Geneva: World Health Organization, GPA/GMC(E)/92.5, 9 November 1992.

[28] "AIDS Program Coordination, or: Should we be here if we want to get there?" Internal Memorandum from Josef Decosas to Cathy Mains, *Health and Population Directorate*, 13 January 1993, p. 4.

[29] Ibid.

for the United Kingdom's [since-renamed] Overseas Development Administration [ODA], lamented that none of the options reflected what had been requested at the previous GMC meeting. Nevertheless, the GMC's decision to move forward with a coordination Task Force strongly suggested to some observers that a new global coordination mechanism would emerge and would likely exist outside WHO/GPA.[30] By the end of its meeting, the GMC worked out terms of reference for the new Task Force and proposed that it meet twice yearly thereafter, with its first meeting scheduled for February 1993.

At this meeting, the GMC also reviewed a report on country-level coordination that GPA had submitted at its request. The report included a rapid assessment of existing instruments and mechanisms for coordinating assistance and mobilizing resources for AIDS programs at country level, along with case studies of AIDS coordination in six countries—Chile, Congo, Senegal, Thailand, Tanzania, and Zambia. The report had some important findings: it documented that lack of coordination at country level was a major obstacle to national effective responses to the AIDS pandemic, and that coordination was not always felt to be of mutual interest to all concerned; it illustrated how bilateral donors, even more so than UN agencies, not infrequently wished their support to be used for activities outside the framework of national AIDS programs; it demonstrated the insufficient amount of national resources allocated to national AIDS programs; it noted the increasing independence of NGOs in the implementation of their activities; and it confirmed the more general social and economic constraints experienced by the health and social sectors of countries most affected by the pandemic. The report concluded by recommending that all countries should: form a national AIDS coordinating committee; adopt a national AIDS plan as a broad framework to be used for all those participating in and supporting the program; conduct common external reviews of programs that are accepted by all external support agencies; create coordinating groups of all external support agencies to facilitate their working more closely together; and form coordination groups of NGOs to enhance their involvement and interaction with national AIDS programs. It further proposed that GPA develop a framework for guiding principles for coordination at country level, based on these recommendations. It is worth noting that these identical coordination issues would persist and other observers would continue to recommend these same proposals for a decade or more, and they would eventually be incorporated by UNAIDS into its guiding principles of the "Three Ones (see Chapter 18)."[31]

At its first meeting, the now named Task Force on HIV/AIDS Coordination appointed "outsider" Nils Kastberg as its Chairperson for 1 year.[32] Kastberg was a Swedish national who had recently moved to Geneva to work in Sweden's UN mis-

---

[30] Christer Jönsson, "From 'Lead Agency' to 'Integrated Programming': The Global Response to AIDS in the Third World," Green Globe Yearbook 1996, 65–72.

[31] *"Three ONEs" Key Principles*. Geneva: UNAIDS, 2004, Conference Paper 1, Washington Consultation 25.04.04; http://data.unaids.org/UNA-docs/Three-Ones_KeyPrinciples_en.pdf.

[32] Christer Jönsson, "From 'Lead Agency' to 'Integrated Programming': The Global Response to AIDS in the Third World," *Green Globe Yearbook*, 1996, 65–72.

sion, where he was responsible for addressing Sweden's investment in various UN agencies. He had been asked by the Swedish government to lead its delegation to the extraordinary GMC meeting because another member of the Swedish delegation had been unable to attend. Kastberg had felt the proposal for a coordinating forum made little sense, and thought a task force of stakeholders would be better suited to obtain broader support for AIDS funding. Not only did his opinion prove influential, but ultimately the group looked to him to help guide its deliberations by making him its Chairperson.[33]

At this stage—that is, at the end of 1992 and the beginning of 1993—it was not clear where the future of AIDS global governance was headed. As we mentioned earlier, the dedicated staff of GPA were hard at work confronting the spreading pandemic. With the exception of GPA's senior management group, which continued to meet for 30 min every morning, few staff were aware of the work of the Task Force on HIV/AIDS Coordination or had any idea that within 2 years GPA would no longer exist.

It was at this time, however, that WHO Member States made an important decision which seemed at the time to be only indirectly related to global AIDS governance: they reelected Hiroshi Nakajima to a second term as WHO Director-General. While this might seem rather perfunctory, in fact the contest—Nakajima's opponent had been his previous Deputy Director-General, Mohammed Abdelmoumene— proved highly contested and controversial.

As discussed in Chapter 9, WHO had several structural flaws that many at the time ascribed to Nakajima. In reality, Nakajima's management style did not create these flaws, but it certainly exposed and exacerbated them. Since WHO does not direct health care or prevention services; it depends on collaborative alliances between itself and national governments and intergovernmental agencies.[34] This puts WHO at the whim of national health ministries and renders it often dependent on their interests, priorities, and institutional strengths, often limiting its ability to affect change.[35] Moreover, as we have explained elsewhere, WHO's budgetary constraints, regional structure, and bureaucratic requirements often hamper its ability to act quickly.[36] WHO's reliance—at the time—mainly on ministers of health, who were mostly male physicians, also made it slow to adopt to multisectoral concepts of health. This limited its flexibility to collaborate with other agencies and sometimes created a leadership vacuum that other agencies were all too willing to fill. Additionally, WHO's heavy reliance on extrabudgetary programs encouraged it to pursue vertical programs rather than ones that were more horizontal in nature and in line with the primary

[33] Nils Kastberg, Interview by Michael Merson, New York City, September, 2002.

[34] World Health Organisation. Basic documents. 39th edition. Geneva: WHO, 1992; Fiona Godlee, "The World Health Organisation: WHO in crisis," *BMJ* 26 November 1994;309:1424–1428.

[35] Fiona Godlee, "The World Health Organisation: WHO at country level—a little impact, no strategy," *BMJ* 17 December 1994;309:1636–1639.

[36] K. Lee and Gill Walt. *What role for WHO in the 1990s? Health Policy and Planning* 1992;7:387–90; External Review Committee, "Report of the External Review of the World Health Organization Global Programme on AIDS, January 1992. P. 56.

health care philosophy adapted at Alma Ata. This fragmented to a certain degree the response to health needs at the regional and national level. All of these structural problems existed in WHO regardless of who was Director-General.

While Nakajima's weaknesses highlighted many of these structural defects in WHO, his own shortcomings also caused great concern among donors. He had undeniable communication difficulties and a reserved demeanor which contrasted markedly with the compelling eloquence and magnetism of his predecessor, Halfdan Mahler.[37] While Nakajima's supporters believed his mollifying style suited the post-colonial, post-Cold War, pro-deregulation milieu of the early 1990s, his critics felt it reduced WHO's global influence.[38] Moreover, his critics considered Nakajima incapable of crafting coherent policies or providing strategic leadership. For example, Nakajima drafted a "new paradigm for health," which he tried to champion, but it appeared "either too complicated or too poorly articulated for most people to follow," according to a study of WHO under Nakajima by Fiona Godlee.[39] Nakajima was too wedded to the medical model, his critics contended. WHO could have recruited a more multidisciplinary set of leaders for an expanded response, but under Nakajima's leadership, WHO continued relying on physicians in positions of senior management.[40] "The main determinants of health—poverty, education, and environmental degradation— ... are too complex for us," Miroslaw Wysocki, WHO's Regional Advisor and Director of Poland's National Institute of Public Health, explained in a 1994 interview.[41] Nakajima's focus on a physician-led WHO caused a gap in addressing the social determinants of health.

These management flaws were no small matter: Mahler had been able to use his management style to offset WHO's structural weaknesses. For example, though Mahler convinced the World Health Assembly (WHA) in 1976 to decentralize WHO's budgeting structure by allocating 70% of WHO's regular budget to its regional and country offices (rather than the previous 30%), he was able to keep the regional offices from operating independently and maintained "one WHO" through his strong leadership and charisma. Nakajima, in contrast, had a more restrained style that allowed the autonomy of each region to foster balkanization and individualism.[42] Moreover, Nakajima's communication and management deficits, along with his past history as a Regional Director himself, made it essentially

[37] George Alleyne, Interview by Michael Merson, New Haven, CT, August, 2002; Manuel Carballo, Interview by Michael Merson, New Haven, CT, November, 2002.

[38] Fiona Godlee, "The World Health Organisation: WHO in crisis," *BMJ* 26 November 1994;309:1424–1428.

[39] Fiona Godlee, "WHO in retreat: is it losing its influence?" *BMJ* 3 December 1994;309:1491–1495.

[40] Denis Aitken, Interview (email) by Michael Merson, 2001; Lars Kallings, Interview by Michael Merson, New Haven, CT, September, 2002.

[41] Fiona Godlee, "WHO in retreat: is it losing its influence?" *BMJ* 3 December 1994;309:1491–1495.

[42] Fiona Godlee, "The World Health Organisation: The regions—too much power, too little effect." *BMJ* 1994, 10 December, 309:1566–1570; Fiona Godlee, "The World Health Organisation: WHO at country level—a little impact, no strategy," *BMJ* 17 December 1994;309:1636–1639.

impossible for him to reign in the Regional Directors,[43] which in reality created seven WHOs (headquarters and the six regional offices).

In his critics' minds, Nakajima's reserved personal style also allowed internal and external pressures to fragment WHO. His director appointments sometimes bypassed standard WHO procedures in ways that seemed arbitrary, capricious, and self-serving, these critics contended, eroding staff morale.[44] Meanwhile, his reserved managerial approach allowed interorganizational conflicts to ferment, as departmental disputes over territory and collaborative hierarchies fractured the organization.[45] Nakajima also appears to have had an aversion towards controversy with external agencies and donors, and this troubled many. In the decades before Nakajima's ascent, Mahler had spearheaded two efforts—WHO's Essential Drugs Program and its International Code of Marketing of Breast-milk Substitutes—that maintained WHO autonomy against considerable corporate and international (including United States government) pressure.[46] Observers suspected Nakajima might not prove so confrontational, and many critics felt these concerns were justified when Nakajima dropped Mahler's opposition to UNICEF's Bamako Initiative (see Chapter 13) and moved the Essential Drug Program out of the Director-General's office into its own division.[47] Some critics, concerned about WHO's standing relative to other UN agencies, felt Nakajima proved more willing than Mahler to acquiesce to other groups—particularly the World Bank—damaging both WHO's global standing and its influence over global health concerns.

However, we do not believe these criticisms tell the whole story. Nakajima was first and foremost a scientist, reflecting his study of pharmacology at the University of Paris, his medical degree and doctoral degree in medical sciences at Tokyo Medical University, and his position as a Research Director for Nippon Roche, the Japanese subsidiary of Hoffmann-LaRoche. He was thus highly knowledgeable in biomedical research and had great respect for the results of basic (laboratory) research. I found Nakajima quite personable. He and I occasionally traveled together and he would often ask about my family and I know he did the same to others. He was a very tra-

---

[43] Fiona Godlee, "The World Health Organisation: The regions—too much power, too little effect." *BMJ* 1994, 10 December, 309:1566–1570.

[44] Fiona Godlee, "The World Health Organisation: WHO in crisis," *BMJ* 1994, 26 November, 309:1424–1428; United Nations. Prevention of sexual harassment. Geneva: United Nations, 1994.

[45] Ibid.

[46] World Health Organisation. Resolution 23. In: 34th session of the World Health Assembly. Handbook of resolutions and decisions of the World Health Assembly and the Executive Board 1973–84. Geneva: WHO, 1985; Gill Walt and JW Harnmeijer. "Formulating an essential drugs policy: WHO's role". In: N. Kanji, A. Hardon, JW Harnmeijer, M. Mamdani, Gill Walt. *Drugs policy in developing countries*. London: Zed Books, 1992; Fiona Godlee, "WHO in retreat: is it losing its influence?" *BMJ* 3 December 1994;309:1491–1495.

[47] Nazneed Kanji, "Charging for drugs in Africa: UNICEF's Bamako initiative." *Health Policy and Planning* 1989;4:110–20; Gill Walt, JW Harnmeijer. "Formulating an essential drugs policy: WHO's role." In: N. Kanji, A. Hardon, JW Harnmeijer, M. Mamdani, Gill Walt. *Drugs policy in developing countries*. London: Zed Books, 1992; Unicef/HAI/Oxfam. Report on the international study conference on community financing in primary health care, Freetown, 23–30 September 1989. Amsterdam: HAI/Unicef, 1990.

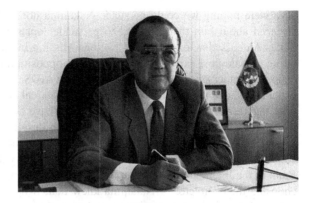

ditional Japanese man—thus perhaps not well understood by many in WHO at that time. He lost his first wife at an early age due to breast cancer and subsequently married a woman who worked in the United States Embassy in the Philippines. His limitations notwithstanding, we agree with George Alleyne, Regional Director of the Pan American Health Organization (PAHO) from 1995 to 2002, that Nakajima "was well intentioned and his view was, if you have all of these programs cooperating more fully with one another, under similar rules and regulations, … [one could have] more of a corporate approach to all of these things. Not just donors going off and giving money to TDR, to GPA—not appreciating that they were part of WHO."[48] Ralph Henderson, who had served as an Assistant Director-General under Nakajima, also felt Nakajima's strengths have been lost amidst the criticisms. "He was not micromanaging the program in any way," Henderson remembered. "He was letting the good programs run and thrive."[49] Alleyne felt that people, unfortunately, became suspicious of Nakajima because of his communication weaknesses and the fundamental structural flaws of WHO that were beyond his control. "History will treat Nakajima much more kindly than what occurred at the end of his reign, I am definite about that," Alleyne concluded.[50]

Whatever the case, these mixed (and often negative) feelings about Nakajima remained close to the surface as the 1993 election for Director-General approached. Many of Nakajima's critics worried that the Japanese government would manipulate the balloting at the Executive Board in the way they believed it had during the 1988 election (see Chapter 7). A number of high-income countries opposed his reelection. Many low- and middle-income countries supported him, however. Consequently, in late 1992, the United States government approached Japan about Nakajima withdrawing his candidacy for reelection.[51] United States State Department representative to the WHO Executive Board, Neil Boyer, explained:

[48] George Alleyne, Interview by Michael Merson, New Haven, CT, August, 2002.

[49] Ralph Henderson, Interview by Michael Merson, NH, February, 2003.

[50] George Alleyne, Interview by Michael Merson, New Haven, CT, August, 2002.

[51] World Health Organisation. Report of the Executive Board Working Group on the WHO response to global change. Executive Board, 92nd session. Geneva: WHO, 1993.

"We were hoping we could persuade Nakajima not to run because so much dirt surfaced about him that we tried to persuade Japan to withdraw him."[52] United States Ambassador to the United Nations Mission in Geneva Morris Abram even wrote to Nakajima expressing Washington's opposition to his reelection and criticizing his leadership in several areas, including AIDS.[53] Very aware of this criticism, Nakajima chose to interpret it in a broader historical context: "This [was] the first time that developing and developed countries have been divided very clearly," he told a reporter in 1994. But Nakajima felt that, despite the clear division of opinion, WHO's structure provided him leverage: "like the UN, WHO works on one country one vote, no matter how much money a country donates, not like the World Bank or the International Monetary Fund, which have weighted voting systems for choosing their Director."[54] Nakajima knew that, if he secured enough votes from low- and middle-income countries, he had nothing to fear from the high-income countries opposed to him. With these dynamics in mind, and despite determined opposition from many Western governments (later rumors would circulate that the United States ultimately voted for him), Nakajima retained his position as WHO Director-General, winning the election by a vote of 18–13 in the Executive Board.[55]

Immediately after the election, allegations of corruption surfaced again, with claims that the Japanese had bought the votes of representatives from low-and middle-income nations on the Executive Board. There were rumors that Japan had threatened to cut off fish imports from the Maldives and coffee imports from Jamaica if those countries did not support Nakajima.[56] For his part, Nakajima considered the claims merely political posturing, claiming that "the United States wants to impose its particular vision of the world's future upon the United Nations' humanitarian organizations."[57] His supporters also considered the allegations mere pretext, that Nakajima was simply "caught in the middle of a Washington power play for control of the organization."[58] But donor governments were unpersuaded by these statements and demanded an external audit of the organization. There were allegations, for example, that Japan had awarded contracts or favors to 21 of the 31 WHO Executive Board members. Fraud detection experts from the United Kingdom's National

---

[52] Ann Blackwood, Interview by Michael Merson, New Haven, CT, January, 2002; Neil Boyer, Interview by Michael Merson, New Haven, CT, January, 2002.

[53] Victor Ego Ducrot, "United Nations: Hiroshi Nakajima Remains WHO Director-General," *IPS-Inter Press Service*, January 20, 1993.

[54] Fiona Godlee, "The World Health Organisation: Interview with the Director-General," *BMJ* 1995, 3 March, 310:583–588.

[55] Victor Ego Ducrot, "United Nations: Hiroshi Nakajima Remains WHO Director-General," *IPS-Inter Press Service*, January 20, 1993.

[56] Douglas Martin, "Hiroshi Nakajima, Leader of WHO, Dies at 84," *New York Times*, January 28, 2013.

[57] Fiona Godlee, "The World Health Organisation: Interview with the Director-General," *BMJ* 1995, 3 March, 310:583–588; Victor Ego Ducrot, "United Nations: Hiroshi Nakajima Remains WHO Director-General," *IPS-Inter Press Service*, January 20, 1993.

[58] Victor Ego Ducrot, "United Nations: Hiroshi Nakajima Remains WHO Director-General," *IPS-Inter Press Service*, January 20, 1993.

Audit Office were called in to examine staff and payment records and found that the contracts—the largest of which was $150,000 to a member of the Executive Board from the Philippines—were technically legal but presented "a problem of ethics," in the words of the Board Chairman, Jean-François Girard of France.[59] While the audit "found financial mismanagement and misuse of the organization's funds," the auditors were unable to implicate Nakajima in any of these.[60] At the WHA in May, where all members of WHO have a vote, Nakajima's election to a second term was confirmed by a tally of 93-58. Never before in WHO's history had the WHA not voted unanimously in favor of a candidate for Director-General proposed by the Executive Board, illustrating the discontent that Nakajima fostered.

Very unhappy with the outcomes of both the Director-General election and the external audit, some high-income nations began calling for substantive reform of WHO's governance. There was precedent for this: during the late 1980s, the United States Government had made a serious effort at reforming the governing structure of WHO to give more authority to the Director-General. However, the Regional Directors were able to stymie these efforts by getting various Member States in their regions to object when the proposed reforms came before WHO's Executive Board. In the first half of the 1990s, a few donor nations held several international meetings to address the subject of global health governance and WHO's place in that constellation.[61] At these meetings, critics of WHO converged on some central themes: the need for coordinated international health initiatives; the necessity of a multisectoral, multidisciplinary approach to health; and the desire for a more flexible, less bureaucratically encumbered institution that could move more rapidly to address important issues like AIDS while retaining the foresight to help low- and middle-income nations develop their health infrastructure.[62]

With Nakajima's reelection in hand, it was clear that the future bode poorly for WHO in general and, I feared, for GPA in particular. The donor nations had lost patience with what they perceived as flaws in Nakajima's leadership. In a 2002 interview, Mahler's senior policy adviser Joe Cohen articulated exactly what I was thinking: "When [Nakajima] got reelected ... [GPA] was cooked. [The donors] wanted

[59] Douglas Martin, "Hiroshi Nakajima, Leader of WHO, Dies at 84," *New York Times*, January 28, 2013; Michael Sheridan, "World health chief faces fraud inquiry," *The Independent,* 28 February, 1993.

[60] World Health Organisation. Report of the external auditor to the World Health Assembly: allegations of possible financial irregularities during 1992. 46th World Health Assembly. Geneva: WHO, 1993.

[61] J. Frenk, J. Sepulveda, O. Gomez-Dantes, M.J. McGuinness, and F. Knaul. "The new world order and the future of international health." *BMJ* 1997;314:1404–7; Seventh Consultative Committee on Primary Health Care Systems for the 21st Century. "Health care systems for the 21st century." *BMJ* 1997;314:1407–9; R. Saracci. "WHO may need to reconsider its definition of health." *BMJ* 1997;314:1409–10 cited in Fiona Godlee, "WHO reform and global health: Radical restructuring is the only way ahead," *BMJ*, 1997; 10 May 314:1359.

[62] Fiona Godlee, "WHO reform and global health: Radical restructuring is the only way ahead," *BMJ*, 1997; 10 May, 314:1359.

vengeance and that was one way to do it—get GPA away".[63] My greatest fear was, as the health attaché in the United States Mission to Geneva Ken Bernard said, "no matter how good GPA was, with Nakajima at the helm, this was headed for disaster."[64]

It was against this backdrop that GMC's Task Force on HIV/AIDS Coordination began meeting in February 1993. At this point, several facts were clear: (a) the UN agencies now had a single UN Committee, the IAAG, and a commitment from the agencies to use it as a forum to work together to address their coordination problems; (b) cooperation between UNICEF and GPA had improved, but UNDP had continued "its initiative to build up a second global AIDS program"; (c) the GMC now had a functional Task Force with broad representation to address the coordination issue; and (d) the only way to avoid bureaucratic proliferation, program duplication, and agency competition was to create a "common dedicated accountability mechanism for UN-system AIDS programming."[65] The key question was whether the Task Force could agree upon a mechanism.

In early 1993, however, some Western donors and members of the Task Force came up with a creative idea for how donor countries could move towards such a mechanism. Joe Decosas proposed a way forward: "There is no reason why the World Health Assembly cannot formally delegate the governance of WHO's AIDS programming to the GMC, and why the UNICEF Executive Board and the UNDP Governing Council cannot delegate the governance of their AIDS related programming to a similar committee. There is also no reason why these committees could not be one and the same."[66] Several things had to be in place for this to happen, Decosas realized, but it was not inconceivable. The Task Force needed to get resolutions passed in the WHA and the governing bodies of other UN agencies mandating the creation of a common AIDS governance structure. "These struggles are … destroying the system," Decosas concluded. "Common governance is one way to stop this self-destruction."[67]

Not long after GPA's Task Force held its first meeting, donor nations took the situation into their own hands and held an informal meeting in London to agree on a strategy and formulate the next steps. The meeting was held on March 29, 1993, at the request of David Nabarro, and was chaired by the United States' Helene Gayle (who at the time was Director of the AIDS Division at USAID on secondment from CDC, Atlanta). The meeting included representatives from nine countries: the United States, Canada, Denmark, Norway, Sweden, Netherlands, Switzerland, the United Kingdom, and France.[68] WHO was not invited to the meeting and I did not

---

[63] Joshua Cohen, Interviewed by Michael Merson, New Haven, CT, August, 2002.

[64] Ken Bernard, Interview by Michael Merson, New Haven, CT, February, 2002.

[65] Josef Decosas, "AIDS Program Coordination, or: Should we be here if we want to get there? Internal Memorandum from Josef Decosas to Cathy Mains" *Health and Population Directorate*, January 13, 1993, p. 4.

[66] Ibid, p. 5.

[67] Ibid, p. 6.

[68] Victoria Ware, "Draft Minutes of the donor's meeting held on Monday 29 March 1993." Health and Population Division, Oversees Development Administration, London, April 2, 1993, unpublished document.

know it was even being held (I only learned about it weeks afterwards). All the participants agreed that the lack of cooperation on UN AIDS programming was symptomatic of larger UN dysfunction. According to the meeting's minutes, "general dissatisfaction was expressed with WHO/GPA—and the program being set up by other UN agencies—particularly UNDP—and their failure to work effectively together."[69] The conversation provided donor nations with a window of opportunity to institute common governance on this issue.[70] "The Canadians, the British, the Dutch, the French ... the Nordics, especially Swedish SIDA ... were all very determined to make a kind of breakthrough," Hans Moekerk, the Dutch representative to the GMC, remembered. "UNAIDS had not yet been named, but it was very clear that a number of people had unofficial instructions from the highest level in their governments."[71] The group agreed to a Canadian plan that proposed that the six major UN agencies cosponsor an AIDS program wherein "WHO/GPA should have a normative role" while the other agencies, including UNDP, would act "based on technical guidance drawn from WHO."[72] Although the group originally intended merely to propose the plan during the GMC meeting in May, by the end of the meeting they agreed that Canadian representatives would instead submit the proposal for discussion at the next WHA, in May, and then pursue its approval with the governing boards of the other UN agencies over the ensuing year.[73] As a "last resort," London participants agreed, donor nations would withdraw their funds from any agency refusing to coordinate and collaborate.[74]

Momentum now pushed the donors forward in this direction. By May, members of the London group had drawn up a version of Canada's cosponsored proposal and, in a move that surprised GPA and many Member States, the London group prepared a formal resolution for consideration by the WHA.[75] As Bernard told me "I was there, I sat with Nils [Kastberg] and I wrote the first resolution that went to the

---

[69] Ibid.

[70] Christer Jonsson, "From 'Lead Agency' to 'Integrated Programming': The Global Response to AIDS in the Third World," *Green Globe Yearbook*, 1996, 65–72.

[71] Hans Moerkerk, Interview by Michael Merson, New Haven, CT, August, 2002.

[72] Coordination of the UN system response to the AIDS pandemic: Position paper of the Canadian international development agency, March 10, 1993; Victoria Ware, "Draft Minutes of the donor's meeting held on Monday 29 March 1993." Health and Population Division, Oversees Development Administration, London, April 2, 1993, unpublished document.

[73] Josef Decosas, "AIDS Program Coordination, or: Should we be here if we want to get there? Internal Memorandum from Josef Decosas to Cathy Mains" *Health and Population Directorate*, January 13, 1993. Ware (Victoria Ware, "Draft Minutes of the donor's meeting held on Monday 29 March 1993." Health and Population Division, Oversees Development Administration, London, April 2, 1993, unpublished document.) *contra* Johnston. Joe Decosas. Interview by Michael Merson, New Haven, CT, October, 2001.

[74] Victoria Ware, "Draft Minutes of the donor's meeting held on Monday 29 March 1993." Health and Population Division, Oversees Development Administration, London, April 2, 1993, unpublished document.

[75] Clare Nullis, "WHO Assembly Likely to Approve Overhaul of AIDS Programs," *The Associated Press*, May 11, 1993.

Health Assembly in 1993."[76] As the proposal circulated among WHA members, about 38 nations expressed their support of the proposal.[77] When the resolution was shown to us at GPA, we expressed concern about some of its language, and the London group edited some of the more controversial sections.[78] As Bernard explained in our interview, "So David Nabarro came in the room and broke it loose. It was a difficult paragraph…He sat down, he pulled out his computer, he listened for 20 min, he typed up a quick paragraph …everybody looked at each other and said yes, I think that works."[79] During this process Kastberg and I discussed the steps that WHO and other UN bodies would need to take to move forward. When I gave my response on the floor of the WHA to the many comments from the delegates, I told them that I was "confident that the proposed study would strengthen the program's effort and clarify the responsibilities of WHO and the other UN bodies."[80] I felt I had no choice to do otherwise.

Passing this resolution would be a turning point. It was now clear that, no matter what we did to reform GPA, we were not going to satisfy the donors. They would always be critical of our African regional office, our capacity to operate efficiently within the traditional WHO structure, and our ability to coordinate effectively with other agencies. When I first accepted the GPA Directorship, I thought I could operate GPA well with it more closely incorporated into the WHO structure because of my previous experience at the Diarrheal Diseases Control (CDD) programme. It now appeared I had been too confident in this regard. Certainly, I had underestimated just how unsettling the changes in GPA would be to our donors, particularly with regard to Africa where the pandemic was most severe and our regional and country offices the weakest. Ultimately, I felt that if we had been given more time, perhaps we could have established credibility with our donors about our efforts in that region. Indeed, some within WHO felt that I should have fought harder against the creation of a new governance structure for AIDS by rallying developing countries in support of GPA and WHO. As Aleya Hammad (an Egyptian women with many years of experience working in WHO and senior adviser to Nakajima) later told me,

> If you had had said, look people are dying of AIDS, what morality do we have in giving up our responsibility for people dying of AIDS because we don't like Nakajima…to hell with Nakajima, Nakajima is not going to stay forever…but the program has to stay in WHO. Then they would have listened to you. They could have not said no…I would have called their bluff (about not giving you money) and I would have won the bluff."[81]

---

[76] Ken Bernard, Interview by Michael Merson, New Haven, CT, February, 2002.

[77] Clare Nullis, "WHO Assembly Likely to Approve Overhaul of AIDS Programs," *The Associated Press*, May 11, 1993.

[78] Christer Jonsson, "From 'Lead Agency' to 'Integrated Programming': The Global Response to AIDS in the Third World," *Green Globe Yearbook*, 1996, 65–72.

[79] Ken Bernard, Interview by Michael Merson, New Haven, CT, February, 2002.

[80] WHA Committee B records, pg 293.

[81] Aleya Hammad, Interview by Michael Merson, New Haven, CT, April, 2004.

But to have fought the donors as Hammad argued, to have pushed for more time, would have pitted me against almost all our donors, and I did not feel I would win such a battle. As Kastberg later put it to me, "You would have died a slow death."[82]

And I was not sure myself if I even wanted to fight this battle. After what was now 3 years in the GPA Director position, I was slowly coming to believe that a new mechanism for UN cooperation and AIDS governance might work better. "If the UN could not coordinate itself successfully around AIDS," I said to myself, "what could it coordinate?" I now wondered whether the donors had a new AIDS governance structure in mind when they set up the external review process, but when I later asked Kastberg if this was true, he said, "no, we didn't know where this was going."[83] Regardless, moving towards this new structure meant that GPA, as it was currently configured, would cease to exist.

On Friday, May 14, 1993, the WHA unanimously approved resolution WHA46.37 requesting the Director-General to study the "feasibility and practicability" of establishing "a joint United Nations programme on HIV and AIDS" in close consultation with the executive heads of UNDP, UNICEF, UNFPA, UNESCO, and the World Bank.[84] The resolution gave little time; it requested that the study results be submitted to the Executive Board of WHO in January, 1994. The resolution also requested that the GMC Task Force on HIV/AIDS Coordination participate actively in this study and that the Director-General produce several options for such a cosponsored program, taking into full account the views of the GPA Management Committee.[85] One key benefit of including such options was that it prevented "watered-down consensus formulations."[86] What was not clear to me was whether the many developing countries who signed on to sponsor the resolution realized that the donor community was now envisaging a completely new type of governing structure for AIDS. My hunch was that they thought it would result in more resources for them under the continued leadership and direction of GPA. In any event, the move towards the establishment of the Joint United Nations Programme on HIV/AIDS (UNAIDS) had formally begun.[87]

---

[82] Nils Kastberg, Interview by Michael Merson, New York City, September, 2002.

[83] Ibid.

[84] Christer Jonsson, "From 'Lead Agency' to 'Integrated Programming': The Global Response to AIDS in the Third World," *Green Globe Yearbook*, 1996, 65–72.

[85] World Health Assembly (1993), Resolution WHA46.37.

[86] Christer Jonsson, "From 'Lead Agency' to 'Integrated Programming': The Global Response to AIDS in the Third World," *Green Globe Yearbook*, 1996, 65–72.

[87] For a summary of events leading to the formation of The Joint United Nations Programme on HIV/AIDS (UNAIDS), which are discussed at length in the next chapter, see Appendix 4.

Chapter 16
End of the Global Programme on AIDS and the Launch of UNAIDS

The unanimous resolution adopted by the World Health Assembly (WHA), in May 1993, called on the World Health Organization (WHO) Director-General Hiroshi Nakajima to study the feasibility and practicability of establishing a joint and cosponsored United Nations Programme on HIV/AIDS.[1] This would be done in close consultation with his counterparts from five other UN agencies with whom the Global Programme on AIDS (GPA) had already been collaborating. It was clear that I would have to find someone sufficiently trusted by all six agencies to carry out this study and lead the consultation process. The best person to do this was, in my mind, Kathleen Cravero, GPA's External Relations Officer. Cravero was a very competent, straightforward individual who was ideally suited to this task. I mentioned earlier that I had tried unsuccessfully to recruit her to GPA as my senior policy advisor (see Chapter 9), but I eventually succeeded in doing so in 1992.

I had first met Cravero in the late 1980s when I was directing the WHO Diarrheal Diseases Control Programme (CDD). As the United Nations Children's Emergency Fund (UNICEF) Senior Health Adviser in UNICEF headquarters in New York, she worked as the focal point for diarrheal disease programming. Cravero had joined UNICEF in 1985 as the UNICEF Program Coordinator in Chad and served there for 3 years before moving to New York. She knew the UN system very well, had written the paper on UN coordination requested earlier by GPA's Management Committee (GMC), and was widely trusted as a fair-minded administrator and an honest broker. When I asked her to take on the responsibility of this study, she agreed. Cravero later told me, "I was kind of thrown into it, not really understanding AIDS very

---

Within this chapter the singular pronouns *I* and *my* refer to Michael Merson alone, whereas the plural pronouns *we* and *us* generally refer to Michael Merson and Stephen Inrig jointly. Where *we* or *us* refers to Michael Merson and his colleagues at WHO, the object of the pronoun is clarified by context.

[1] For a summary of events leading to the formation of The Joint United Nations Programme on HIV/AIDS (UNAIDS), which are discussed at length in this chapter, see Appendix 4.

© Springer International Publishing AG 2018
M. Merson, S. Inrig, *The AIDS Pandemic*, DOI 10.1007/978-3-319-47133-4_16

much…my job was more about coordination…that seemed to be where I could make the greatest contribution."[2] The process was a real challenge for her, "it seemed like it was a cross between responding and reacting…we were just being pulled in a whole lot of directions. It seemed that every agency had its own agenda and it was hard to separate individual agendas from institutional agendas."[3]

On May 17, 1993 Cravero convened in New York the first meeting of representatives from WHO, the United Nations Development Programme (UNDP), the United Nations Population Fund (UNFPA), UNICEF, and the World Bank (the potential cosponsors of the new program) to discuss a plan for moving forward. The meeting was attended by Mina Mauerstein-Bail from UNDP, Nick Dodd from UNFPA, Jim Sherry from UNICEF, and Anthony Measham from the World Bank. Only Measham, a Canadian physician who had spent 17 years at the World Bank and at the time was Chief of Policy and Research in its Health Population and Nutrition Division, was new to this process. All of them were guarded in their approach to the study and to the idea of a joint and cosponsored program.[4] No one from the United Nations Education, Scientific, and Cultural Organization (UNESCO) was able to attend the meeting, though UNESCO was the sixth potential cosponsor of the program.

Cravero also met individually over the next few days with individuals from UNDP, the American Foundation for AIDS Research (AMFAR), and the Bureau of International and Organization Affairs at the United States State Department (this included Deputy Assistant Secretary Melinda Kimble, who was responsible for policy development concerning UN agencies, and Ann Blackwood, who was responsible for WHO-related matters). Cravero convened a second meeting of the potential cosponsors in New York City on June 17, which this time was attended by representatives of all six agencies. The group decided to develop a proposal without the assistance of an outside consultant rather than conduct a formal study. Cravero agreed to prepare a four-to-five page draft summary of the options for such a program as part of the process.[5]

Contemporaneously with the preparation of this proposal the governing bodies of the potential cosponsors (except for the World Bank) needed to pass resolutions calling for a joint and cosponsored HIV/AIDS program, as had been done by the WHA. I contributed to this effort, beginning in June 1993, by making presentations on the global AIDS[6] burden and the need for better coordination to the various agency governing bodies at the time the resolutions were being considered.[7] But the brunt of the work fell to Cravero, who within a few months was able to secure

---

[2] Kathleen Cravero, Interview by Michael Merson, Geneva, October, 2001.

[3] Ibid.

[4] Cravero Trip report to NYC and Washington DC, May 16–19, 1993, May 26, 1993.

[5] Cravero trip report to NYC, June 10–18, 1993, prepared June 22, 1993.

[6] For the purposes of this text, we will use the term AIDS to encompass both AIDS and HIV unless otherwise specified.

[7] Michael Merson, "Fortieth Session of the UNDP Governing council, New York, 15 June, 1993: Statement," Geneva: World Health Organization, 1993Annex 1; Luis Maria Gomez, "Letter to Dr. Nakajima, June 9, 1993." UNDP, 1993, A20/372/7.

resolutions from the governing bodies of UNESCO, UNDP, UNICEF, and UNFPA.[8] Also, in August, the Economic and Social Council (ECOSOC) of the United Nations approved resolution 1993/51 requesting WHO's Director-General to report to ECOSOC in a year's time about "the possibility of establishing a joint United Nations Programme on HIV and AIDS."[9]

During the same time period, GMC's Task Force on HIV/AIDS Coordination (chaired by Nils Kastburg [see Chapter 15]) held its second meeting, where it focused on issues and problems related to AIDS coordination and discussed what form the new program might take.[10] The various agencies also worked individually on their own ideas about the shape and structure of the program. WHO in general and Nakajima in particular assumed WHO would be the implementing agency for the cosponsored program.[11] Concurrently, and to the concern of some observers, UNDP jockeyed to have itself positioned as the lead entity.[12] (As an aside, the vying between agencies made me aware that others outside WHO, particularly in UNDP and UNICEF, viewed my efforts skeptically. They suspected I was going to use the study to strengthen WHO's and my position in AIDS governance; this was not the case and was one reason I asked Cravero to do most of this work). Indeed, with each agency wanting the program to best suit its interests, the cosponsors could not reach consensus. Consequently, after six interagency meetings, on October 20 the potential cosponsors decided to put forward three options for the shape of a joint and cosponsored program (see Appendices 5 and 6).[13] Each option favored a different division of authority between the proposed program's headquarters Secretariat and the cosponsoring agencies. These can be summarized as follows:

- Option A: The Strong Secretariat option, which at the global level meant the "activities of the cosponsors are largely undertaken by a unified secretariat administered

[8] "Study of a Joint and Cosponsored UN Programme on HIV/AIDS, 20 October 1993," Geneva: World Health Organization, 1993.

[9] Commission on Human Rights Sub-Commission on Prevention of Discrimination and Protection of Minorities, "Forty-sixth session, Item 4 of the provisional agenda: Developments in the United Nations System Concerning HIV and AIDS; Report of the Secretary-General, 17 June 1994," New York: Economic and Social Council, E/CN.4/Sub.2/1994/8, 2.

[10] Global Programme on AIDS, "Second Meeting of GMC Task Force on HIV/AIDS Coordination; Provisional agenda item 3: Inventory and Summary Analysis of Coordination Issues and Problems Related to HIV/AIDS, 2 June, 1993." Geneva: World Health Organization, GPA/TFC(2)/93.2; Lindsay Knight. *UNAIDS: the first 10 years, 1996–2006*, New York: Joint United Nations Programme on HIV/AIDS (UNAIDS), 2008.

[11] Michael Merson, "Note For the Record: Meeting with the Secretary-General and Director-General, WHO, 22 June 1993." Geneva: World Health Organization, 1993, A20/372/30; Lindsay Knight. *UNAIDS: the first 10 years, 1996–2006*, New York: Joint United Nations Programme on HIV/AIDS (UNAIDS), 2008.

[12] Marjory Dam, "Letter to R.H. Henderson, RE: Report Accompanying House Foreign Operations Bill, 23 June, 1993," Washington, D.C.: Pan American Health Organization, 1993, A20/372/7; "Statement by the representative of Sweden on behalf of the Nordic Countries," UNDP Governing Council, 40th Session 1–18 June, Agenda Item 2(b) HIV, AIDS, and Development, 16 June 1993.

[13] Study of a joint and Cosponsored UN Programme on HIV/AIDS, WHO, October 20, 1913.

by WHO." Cosponsors have staff to convey guidance from the secretariat to individual agency staff at all levels and ensure integration of HIV/AIDS issues into their broader health and socioeconomic activities.

- Option B: The Medium Strength Secretariat option, which designated "selected areas of activities" to the secretariat administered by one of the agencies and vested with "the authority to provide policy and technical guidance and arbitrate areas of overlap." Cosponsors have staff to develop institutional policies and programs in response to their mandates, within a global policy and coordination framework.
- Option C: The Weak Secretariat option, which designated "a few key areas of responsibility ... [to] a small secretariat administered by WHO." Cosponsors have staff to develop institutional policies and programs in response to their mandates, within a global policy and coordination framework.

The various agencies differed—perhaps predictably—over which of these three options they favored. WHO supported option A; Elizabeth Reid and UNDP preferred option B (and argued that UNDP, instead of WHO, should serve as the administrating agency); and Jim Sherry and UNICEF advocated for option C.[14]

Why did WHO endorse option A? Option A seemed the most likely to maintain the soul and structure of GPA and preserve WHO's primacy in the UN response, since it established WHO as the administrator of the joint and cosponsored program.[15] Indeed, as notes from the first meeting of an internal WHO working group established by the Director-General to provide guidance on the establishment of the cosponsored program indicate, Nakajima believed that "the UN program [would] serve as WHO's technical program on HIV/AIDS." Indeed, WHO staff felt the working documents did not state this relationship between WHO and the joint and cosponsored program clearly enough and suggested that language in future documents should read that "WHO will implement most of its HIV/AIDS activities through this program."[16] It is important to stress how WHO interpreted Option A because it helps to explain why WHO did not—probably could not—have imagined what would happen over the next several years to WHO's role in the global response to the pandemic.

A critical event in this process was a meeting held at UN headquarters in New York on October 28, 1993, of the executive heads of each the six agencies with Boutros Boutros-Gali, the UN Secretary-General, to discuss the joint and cosponsored program. At this time, the six agency heads were: Jim Grant [UNICEF], Hiroshi Nakajima [WHO], Lewis Preston [World Bank], Nafis Sadik [UNFPA],

---

[14] Lindsay Knight. *UNAIDS: the first 10 years, 1996–2006*, New York: Joint United Nations Programme on HIV/AIDS (UNAIDS), 2008, 22, 28.

[15] Commission on Human Rights Sub-Commission on Prevention of Discrimination and Protection of Minorities, "Forty-sixth session, Item 4 of the provisional agenda: Developments in the United Nations System Concerning HIV and AIDS; Report of the Secretary-General, 17 June 1994, New York: Economic and Social Council, E/CN.4/Sub.2/1994/8, 2.

[16] "Recommendations of the Director-General's Working Group on the Establishment of a Joint and Cosponsored United Nations Programme on HIV/AIDS, 3 March 1994, Geneva: World Health Organization, 1994, 1.

James Gustave Speth [UNDP], and Federico Mayor Zaragoza [UNESCO]. I was the only additional person attending this meeting. Aleya Hammad, a WHO colleague and a fellow Egyptian, knew Boutros-Gali well through family connections and had briefed him on the likely plan to proceed with Option A. Boutros-Gali had initially wondered whether a new UN agency for AIDS was necessary, as Director-General Halfdan Mahler had told me had been the case when GPA had been established. However, as had been the case earlier, Boutros-Gali decided not to move in this direction because of the substantial costs involved. After about 20 min of discussion, Boutros-Gali went around the room and asked each of the six agency heads individually if they would pledge their full support to a strong collaborative relationship creating and implementing a joint and cosponsored program along the lines of Option A. Each of them pledged their fullest support. The discussion with Boutros-Gali thus "resulted in agreement on Option A."[17] Having listened to the group reach consensus and heard each agency head pledge full support for the program, I left the meeting feeling a great sense of optimism that we were headed for a truly united and collaborative global response to the AIDS pandemic.

Aware of the outcome of this meeting with the Secretary-General, the GMC Task Force on HIV/AIDS Coordination met on November 22–24 and gave its full support to Option A as "its vision is that of a UN Program providing a well-coordinated and focused global response to the HIV/AIDS pandemic with a joint secretariat servicing all cosponsors in this endeavor." Moreover, it concluded that "neither of the other two options meet basic requirements for a joint and cosponsored UN program on HIV/AIDS." It also called for greater clarity on: the governance of the program; the arrangements for a joint secretariat; UN program arrangements at country level; and the selection of the new program's Executive Director.[18]

The process now moved remarkably swiftly towards a final resolution. In early December, Cravero prepared a final, amended study report on the establishment of a joint and cosponsored program on HIV/AIDS for consideration by WHO's Executive Board at its January meeting.[19] Since Option A had "clearly emerged as the preferred option," the report to the Executive Board asked it to "consider the establishment of a joint and cosponsored United Nations Programme on HIV/AIDS in accordance with the preferred option and the measures proposed to launch it."[20] I introduced the report to the Executive Board on January 21 and provided considerable details about the proposed structure of the new program. I said "what was

---

[17] Hiroshi Nakajima, "Draft Study Report on the Establishment of a Joint and Cosponsored UN Programme on HIV/AIDS, 12 November 1993," Geneva: World Health Organization, 1993, GPA-A20/372/30; Lindsay Knight. *UNAIDS: the first 10 years, 1996–2006*, New York: Joint United Nations Programme on HIV/AIDS (UNAIDS), 2008.

[18] Letter from Nils-Arne Kastberg to Hiroshi Nakakima, 26 November 1993.

[19] World Health Organization, "Study of a Joint and Cosponsored United Nations Programme on HIV/AIDS, EB93/INF.DOC./5" (Geneva: WHO, 21, Dec. 1993.), 11.

[20] Ibid,; Commission on Human Rights Sub-Commission on Prevention of Discrimination and Protection of Minorities, "Forty-sixth session, Item 4 of the provisional agenda: Developments in the United Nations System Concerning HIV and AIDS; Report of the Secretary-General, 17 June 1994," New York: Economic and Social Council, E/CN.4/Sub.2/1994/8, 2.

before the Board was a proposal that would help countries accelerate their response, unite members of the United Nations system in support of that response, and ensure use of national and external resources." Twenty-one members then spoke in favor of the recommendations in the report, then the Director-General commented that he was in "full agreement with option A" and that "it was a historic moment, signaling a new approach to combating AIDS for years ahead."[21] The Board then adopted Resolution (EB93.R5) recommending "the development and eventual establishment of a joint and cosponsored United Nations Programme on HIV/AIDS, to be administered by WHO, in accordance with the preferred option."[22] It also requested that the governing bodies of the other agencies and ECOSOC endorse the establishment of this new program.[23]

In a donors meeting in Brussels, held a few days after the Executive Board meeting, the Task Force reported that "a consensus was reached among the secretariats of five of the organizations in favor of option A" (the World Bank had not formally agreed at this stage), and that they believed it "would provide the most effectively coordinated program and a unified approach by the cosponsors."[24] Over the next few months, the Task Force met twice to reach consensus on the structure and function of the cosponsored program. It was during this time that some of the implications of the joint and cosponsored program began to become clearer to senior leadership at WHO, which suggested that rather than bolstering GPA, GPA might, in fact, end up being closed down and WHO might no longer direct the global response to the AIDS pandemic.[25]

One issue that surfaced was the ECOSOC resolution passed in August 1993, requiring[26] WHO to submit a report to ECOSOC on the joint and cosponsored program.

---

[21] Proceedings of the Executive Board, Ninety Third session, Eighth Meeting, 21 January 1994, pages 85–95.

[22] Commission on Human Rights Sub-Commission on Prevention of Discrimination and Protection of Minorities, "Forty-sixth session, Item 4 of the provisional agenda: Developments in the United Nations System Concerning HIV and AIDS; Report of the Secretary-General, 17 June 1994," New York: Economic and Social Council, E/CN.4/Sub.2/1994/8, 2.

[23] ECOSOC serves as the central forum for discussing international economic and social issues, and for formulating policy recommendations addressed to Member States and the UN system. It is responsible for promoting higher standards of living, full employment and economic and social progress. ECOSOC was established under the UN Charter as the principal organ to coordinate economic, social and related work of the 14 UN specialized agencies, 10 functional commissions and five regional commissions. It also receives reports from 11 UN funds and programmes.

[24] "Annex 3: Views Expressed at an informal meeting of GPA donors, Brussels, 14 January 1994, on study of a Joint and Cosponsored UN Programme on HIV/AIDS," p. 13; Lindsay Knight. *UNAIDS: the first 10 years, 1996–2006*, New York: Joint United Nations Programme on HIV/AIDS (UNAIDS), 2008; "Structure for the Task Force Response on the Study of A Joint and Cosponsored UN Programme on HIV/AIDS."

[25] Paul Delay, Interview by Michael Merson, New Haven, CT, December, 2002.

[26] Commission on Human Rights Sub-Commission on Prevention of Discrimination and Protection of Minorities, "Forty-sixth session, Item 4 of the provisional agenda: Developments in the United Nations System Concerning HIV and AIDS; Report of the Secretary-General, 17 June 1994," New York: Economic and Social Council, E/CN.4/Sub.2/1994/8, 2.

On paper, this might seem uncontroversial: Article 62 of the UN Charter states that "The Economic and Social Council may make or initiate studies and reports with respect to international economic, social, cultural, educational, health, and related matters and may make recommendations with respect to any such matters to the General Assembly to the Members of the United Nations, and to the specialized agencies concerned," and WHO is a specialized agency. However, in reality, since the UN Charter had been written in 1946, a division had grown over time between the UN agencies in New York and the UN specialized agencies located throughout the world. On one hand, the UN agencies in New York—in this case UNDP, UNICEF, and UNFPA—have their own Executive Boards which report to the UN General Assembly, with ECOSOC serving as a coordinating authority for the economic, social, and related work of these agencies. On the other hand, the UN Specialized Agencies—in this case WHO (in Geneva), UNESCO (in Paris), and the World Bank (in Washington, DC)—are autonomous organizations that carry out functions on behalf of the UN and have their own governing bodies, which vary greatly in their structure. The specialized agencies participate in ECOSOC, but ECOSOC traditionally had had limited authority over them. WHO takes seriously its guidance and direction from its supreme governing body, the World Health Assembly, while the UN agencies take seriously the guidance they receive from the UN General Assembly and ECOSOC. It is within this context that a debate sprang up within WHO leadership as to how much attention WHO should give to the demands imposed upon it by ECOSOC.

An additional complicating factor was that, in its January 1994 resolution, WHO's Executive Board mandated that WHO obtain ECOSOC's approval as part of the cosponsoring process. Why did the Board require this? It was because the donor governments needed ECOSOC's approval in order to bring the other UN agencies into the jointly cosponsored program. Thus, this request by WHO's Executive Board was entirely reasonable. In reality, however, this decision would have profound effects on WHO, GPA, and the global response.

At the time, the Australian Ambassador to the UN, Richard Butler, was serving as President of ECOSOC. Butler had been part of an effort at the end of the Cold War to reform ECOSOC and make it more relevant. It was thus understandable that he wanted ECOSOC to have a leading role in the creation of the joint and cosponsored program on HIV/AIDS (now more and more being referred to as UNAIDS). Butler, who had a strong personality, cared about AIDS: he had seen its devastating impact while serving as Australian Ambassador to Thailand and Cambodia, and was a close colleague of fellow Australian Elizabeth Reid at UNDP. ECOSOC asked Butler, whose term as President lasted only for 1 year (i.e., throughout 1994), to continue leading ECOSOC's deliberation on UNAIDSs after his time as President ended. Thus, Butler played an important role in the transition from GPA to UNAIDS into 1995.[27]

As Butler explained in our interview, he saw the rationale for UNAIDS in relatively simple terms: "what we had on our hands was a fairly classic and deeply unsatisfactory case of competition between UN agencies … turf wars, duplication

---

[27] Richard Butler, Interview by Michael Merson, New Haven, CT, February, 2002.

of effort, refusal to communicate with each other."[28] Given that Butler considered AIDS an important issue, the internecine combat seemed absurd. "Of all subjects in the world where this should not be happening, HIV is surely the key one," Butler concluded. "[So] an attempt to bring about unity of action amongst the major actors in the UN system … struck me as being an utterly wholesome idea."[29] Butler was not alone in this perspective; he received particularly strong support from the Canadian delegation to the UN to make UNAIDS succeed; the United States, Sweden, the Dutch to some degree, and eventually the European Union all showed similar support. Butler was driven to demonstrate that UN reform and efficiency were possible, but I have no doubt he was also strongly committed to the fight against AIDS.[30] On a more personal note, Butler was not particularly impressed with Nakajima as a leader and, given the importance of AIDS, he felt the pandemic was perhaps better placed outside Nakajima's authority.[31] That said, in my various interactions with Butler, I did not think he considered me as one of Nakajima's "cronies," and believe he saw my dealings in the UNAIDS process as fair.

What was particularly important for our purposes, however, was the different views on governance that Nakajima and Butler brought to the table. As noted above, Nakajima was not pleased that WHO, as an organization, had to answer to ECOSOC. Nakajima felt aggravated by this subservience, and he frequently complained about the time I was expending to address and appease ECOSOC. In Nakajima's mind, the structuring of the joint and cosponsored program should proceed with WHO retaining primacy in the hierarchy of power.[32] Indeed, Nakajima wanted the phraseology about the program to specify "the establishment of a joint … programme on HIV/AIDS, to be administered by WHO."[33] This was the language that both the WHO Executive Board (in January) and WHA (later in May) had approved.

Butler saw things very differently. He understood that the raison d'être of the joint and cosponsored program was to circumvent turf wars and duplication of effort, and he considered Nakajima to be the classic embodiment of that problem. "I'd been exposed to [Nakajima] a couple of times," Butler explained in our interview, "… he was just a classic bureaucratic manipulator who couldn't give a tinker's fart about substance."[34] Butler felt that Nakajima was working "to make UNAIDS

---

[28] Ibid.

[29] Ibid.

[30] Ibid.

[31] Ibid.

[32] Michael Merson, "Note For the Record: Meeting with the Secretary-General and Director-General, WHO, 22 June 1993." Geneva: World Health Organization, 1993, A20/372/30; WHO "Press Release," Geneva: WHO, 21 January 1994.

[33] Commission on Human Rights Sub-Commission on Prevention of Discrimination and Protection of Minorities, "Forty-sixth session, Item 4 of the provisional agenda: Developments in the United Nations System Concerning HIV and AIDS; Report of the Secretary-General, 17 June 1994," New York: Economic and Social Council, E/CN.4/Sub.2/1994/8, 5.

[34] Richard Butler, Interview by Michael Merson, New Haven, CT, February, 2002.

subordinate to WHO... I had it very clear in my mind that the problem was Nakajima ... a man holding bureaucratic turf. My impression was that if we were going to get there, it was going to be over his dead body."[35]

It was in this context, then, in the summer of 1994 that ECOSOC took up the issue of the joint and cosponsored program. By this time, the UNESCO Governing Board, UNICEF Executive Board, and UNDP/UNFPA Governing Council had endorsed the establishment of the program, committing their agencies to its formation, and the World Bank had formally agreed to be a cosponsor. On May 9, 1994, the WHA discussed a report on the progress on the formation of the program submitted by the Director-General. An unusually large number of delegations (41 in total) made comments on or asked questions about the newly proposed joint and cosponsored program. These included questions about: the degree of commitment of the cosponsoring agencies; the mechanism for ensuring coordination at country level through the proposed "theme group" composed of the program's cosponsors and constituted by the UN Resident Coordinator (usually the UNDP Resident Representative); whether the current financial support being provided by GPA to national AIDS programs would continue; and the role of the WHO regional offices in the new program.[36] I did my best to address these questions, though all of them would soon surface as major areas of contention between the cosponsors once the new program started.

By this time, Kathleen Cravero had left WHO and taken up the position as the UNICEF Representative to Uganda. After her departure but before the ECOSOC meeting, the UN Interagency Group met twice to hammer out more details about the new program. Held in Annapolis, Maryland in April, and in Stockholm, Sweden in May, these meetings discussed the governance structure and then produced the Group's mission statement for the new program. The GMC, now under the Chairmanship of Hans Moerkerk from the Netherlands, had held its tenth meeting on May 24–26 in Geneva. It had expressed its strong commitment to the ongoing process of establishing the joint and cosponsored program on HIV/AIDS; recommended that the cosponsors proceed with the early establishment of the program's country level coordination mechanism; and extended the work of its Task Force on HIV/AIDS Coordination until the next meeting of the GMC in April, 1995.[37] The Task Force itself convened its fifth meeting immediately after the GMC meeting and discussed various aspects of the new program that required further consideration.[38]

On July 26, 1994, ECOSOC approved Resolution 1994/24, (see Appendix 7) calling for the establishment of a new Joint and Cosponsored Program that would:

(a) Provide global leadership in response to the epidemic;
(b) Achieve and promote global consensus on policy and programmatic approaches;

---

[35] Ibid.

[36] Summary Record of the 93rd WHA, Committee B, pp. 140–152.

[37] Global Programme on AIDS, "Report of the Tenth Meeting of the Management Committee, Geneva, 24–26 May, 1994." Geneva: World Health Organization, GPA/GMC(10)/94.14.

[38] Ibid.

(c) Strengthen the capacity of the UN system to monitor trends and ensure that appropriate and effective policies and strategies are implemented at the country level;

(d) Strengthen the capacity of national governments to develop comprehensive national strategies and implement effective HIV/AIDS activities at the country level;

(e) Promote broad-based political and social mobilization to prevent and respond to HIV/AIDS within countries, ensuring that national responses involve a wide range of sectors and institutions;

(f) Advocate greater political commitment in responding to the epidemic at the global and country levels, including the mobilization and allocation of adequate resources for HIV/AIDS-related activities.

Reading through the resolution's entire text, however, it is easy to see how ECOSOC's construction of the program might generate several tensions over governance. The program, according to Resolution 1994/24, would be co-owned, and both planned and executed in an equitable and collaborative fashion. "The co-sponsors will share responsibility for the development of the program," the resolution read, "contribute equally to its strategic direction, and receive from it policy and technical guidance relating to the implementation of their HIV/AIDS activities. In this way, the program will also serve to harmonize the HIV/AIDS activities of the cosponsors."[39] Also, whereas the original program proposal had said the program was "to be administered by WHO," the ECOSOC drafters had inserted the phrase, "The World Health Organization will be responsible for the administration in support of the program." Many observers felt this subtle shift in wording to be important, that ECOSOC was sending the clear message that WHO would not be directing or controlling the joint and cosponsored program. I had, perhaps naively, interpreted the revised wording to be no different from the original language, but for Nakajima it was a significant change. As he later told us, "When we woke up the next day, the text had been completely changed and it was going to vote in the afternoon. They took out the WHO leadership role and the head of UNAIDS had to be elected rather than WHO nominating the head, so that was the end of WHO's program."[40]

Importantly, the ECOSOC resolution made five other noteworthy requests. First, it stressed that the new program should prioritize country-level activities and initiate these as soon as possible. Second, it created a timetable of events that needed to occur before the program formally started and set the start date to be no later than January 1, 1996. Third, it called for the cosponsors to transform the Inter-Agency Working Group into a formally constituted Committee of Cosponsoring Organizations (CCO), functioning with a rotational chairmanship, that would oversee the transition process to full program implementation. Fourth, it called on the President of ECOSOC to organize "informal open-ended consultations" in conjunction with the CCO to determine the composition of the Programme Coordinating Board (PCB) which would oversee

---

[39] ECOSOC Resolution 1994/24.

[40] Hiroshi Nakajima, Interview by Michael Merson, Poitiers, October 13, 2002.

its governance, the program implementation plans, and other detailed program proposals. Finally, ECOSOC's resolution directed that the CCO begin recruiting a program Executive Director, whom the UN Secretary General would formally appoint.[41]

I had decided that I would not be a candidate for the position of UNAIDS Executive Director. The reasons were both personal and professional. From a personal standpoint, I was making two moves: looking to my future and moving on from my past. It had been a great privilege to lead the dedicated GPA staff as we took on what appeared to be one of the largest and gravest pandemics of our time. But it was difficult being such a controversial figure on so many fronts. I was controversial in some quarters for taking Jonathan Mann's place; in other quarters for my belief in following a public health approach to HIV prevention; and I grew only more controversial in still other quarters—and particularly within WHO—for the role I played in the closure of GPA and the birth of UNAIDS. This controversy would not have stopped had I stood to lead UNAIDS, and it was beginning to weigh heavily on me. Apparently, this was evident to some of those around me. Cravero, for example, remembers noticing my reactions during this period: "I felt that you became increasingly disheartened and frustrated at being kicked around on the outside for defending WHO and kicked around on the inside for not defending it."[42]

Standing for the UNAIDS job also did not make good organizational sense. There had been much interagency squabbling during my tenure, and the best chance to reduce this would be to bring in a new person who lacked my institutional baggage and close association with Nakajima, someone who would be acceptable to all the cosponsoring agencies. There were also donor countries that would have opposed my candidacy. While I felt I had a good working relationship with all of them, I knew they had divided opinions about me. Some liked my public health focus, others favored more of a human rights and development-based strategy and felt I focused too much on the former. I could also sense that, after Mann and myself, both Americans, the Europeans preferred a leader from one of the European countries. Moreover, it was clear to me that someone who had a solid history and reputation working in the AIDS field should lead the next phase of the global response to the pandemic. UNAIDS was to be a new program and would require a leader who would generate the same amount of admiration and respect from the staff that Mann had in GPA, as well as from AIDS experts and activists around the world.

I decided I would return home to the United States. I had lived abroad now for 18 years, almost 2 years in Bangladesh and the rest of the time in Geneva. Originally, I had planned to live abroad for only 2 years, but life and circumstances had taken me in a different direction. I had resigned from the Centers for Disease Control and

[41] Economic and Social Council 44th plenary meeting 26 July 1994 1994/24. Joint and co-sponsored United Nations programme on human immunodeficiency virus/acquired immunodeficiency syndrome (HIV/AIDS); Resolution 1994/24

[42] Kathleen Cravero, Interview by Michael Merson, Geneva, October, 2001.

Prevention (CDC) in 1992 after 20 years of service, was approaching my 50th birthday, and felt that I would like to spend my next decade at a university helping to inspire the next generation of global health scholars and leaders. D. A. Henderson, who had led the WHO Smallpox Eradication Programme and then became the Dean of the Johns Hopkins Bloomberg School of Public Health, counselled me that it might be difficult to find a position in academia if I waited much longer to return. By accepting the GPA position, I had already waited 4 years longer than I intended. Also by 1994, I had another incentive: my son, a senior in high school, wanted to attend university in the United States, and moving back would keep me closer to him. I also had aging parents who were in declining health. Thus, when Nils Kastberg called me a few months later to ask if I wanted to be a candidate for the UNAIDS position, I thanked him sincerely for his offer and told him firmly that I would be leaving Geneva as soon as I found a new position.

The ECOSOC decision in fact provided me with a deadline, an unavoidable transition date; it was now clear that on December 31, 1994, GPA would no longer exist. By chance or not, shortly after the ECOSOC resolution, Jerry Borrow, the Dean of the School of Medicine at Yale, contacted me to ask if I might have any interest in being the Dean of the School of Public Health at Yale, a role which also carried with it the position of Chair of the Department of Epidemiology and Public Health in the School of Medicine. Borrow and I met soon after for lunch in London, where he convinced me to apply for the position, and throughout the fall of 1994, I visited the school and met with faculty and the search commitee. By November, my desire to leave Geneva had become public[43] and in December I accepted Yale's offer and informed Nakajima of my decision. Somewhat to my surprise, Nakajima pressed me to remain at WHO and serve as one of his Assistant Directors-General with responsibility for emerging infectious diseases, flu pandemics, and the like. I believe his offer was sincere—we had maintained a good relationship and, despite the loss of GPA and the leadership of the global AIDS response, I think he trusted me. We had discussed a number of times during the previous year the process underway to create the joint and cosponsored program, and I had cleared with him all the major decisions being made about the new program and about GPA. But I really did not want to stay on, and so I told him that while I appreciated his offer, I intended to leave WHO. Soon after I agreed to terms with Yale, but before I had officially resigned from GPA, Larry Altman, the long-time health reporter at *The New York Times,* published comments made by Yale faculty that I would be moving there.[44]

Even without me in the picture, the selection of the first Director of UNAIDS turned out to be full of intrigues and a complex web of interactions between donor governments, the cosponsors (particularly WHO), and the UN in New York. ECOSOC's July resolution called on the CCO to "fill the position of Director … as soon as possible, through an open, wide-ranging search process, including consul-

---

[43] Michael Balter, "UN Readies New Global AIDS Plan," *Science,* November 25, 1994, 266:1312–1313.

[44] Lawrence K. Altman, "Yale Accepts Blame for Safety Lapses Linked to Lab Accident," *The New York Times,* December 13, 1994; See also Abram Katz, "Expert on AIDS coming to Yale," *New Haven Register,* January 13, 1995, A3, A5.

tation with governments and other concerned parties."[45] Within weeks of the ECOSOC resolution, Nakajima sent the heads of the other cosponsoring organizations a letter requesting the names of possible candidates.[46] Nakajima set a deadline for the nominations of mid-September, and proposed that the agency leaders discuss the list when they met on September 22nd. Donor nations and other stakeholders almost immediately grew concerned that this process had started moving forward within the UN system without the requisite "consultations with governments and other concerned parties."[47] Nakajima apparently did not wish to establish a formal search committee, however, but rather wanted to adopt a very informal "suggestion" process, and had not given any consideration to the form that any "consultations" should take.[48]

On September 5, Kastberg sent letters on behalf of the GMC Task Force to GMC members inviting them "to consult with your constituency on proposals for names of persons who could serve in the position as Director of the program."[49] He set October 10 as a date for submitting candidate names, and noted that "A possible role of the Task Force in the further consultations once a pool of names is available depends on whether the CCO wishes, or does not wish, such assistance. I will be informing the CCO of the Task Force's availability in this regard and await their decision following the September 22nd meeting of the CCO."[50] One day after CCO members were to have submitted their list of candidates to Nakajima, Kastberg wrote to Nakajima offering his assistance on the "consultation process for a Director, should the CCO so wish."[51] Kastberg included in the letter a consultation mechanism whereby the GMC Task Force could provide a list of candidates from which the CCO to choose. This process would retain the steps that the CCO had already taken to select the Executive Director while fulfilling ECOSOC's mandate for an open process. Kastberg explained his maneuvering to me, "At the time and I don't know if it is true or not, the thought was that Jim Grant and Nakajima had basically agreed to select Jesus Kumate (a highly respected pediatrician, and at the time the Secretary of Health in Mexico and Chair of the WHO Executive Board). Firstly I felt 'OK, it may be him or it may not be him, but this is not the way a selection should be done, if it is to be done in a transparent manner.' ... I certainly upset a lot of people when I really went way

[45] The Economic and Social Council, "44th plenary meeting, Resolution 1994/24: Joint and co-sponsored United Nations programme on human immunodeficiency virus/acquired immunodeficiency syndrome (HIV/AIDS) 26 July 1994.

[46] Hiroshi Nakajima, "Letter to Mr. Speth, August 1, 1994," Geneva: World Health Organization, 1994.

[47] Daniel Speigel, "Letter to Dr. Nakajima, September 1, 1994," Geneva: Permanent Representative of the United States of America to the United Nations, 1994.

[48] Based on hand-written notes written on Speigel letter. Daniel Speigel, "Letter to Dr. Nakajima, September 1, 1994," Geneva: Permanent Representative of the United States of America to the United Nations, 1994.

[49] Nils Kastberg letter to the GMC Task force, September 5, 1994.

[50] Ibid.

[51] Ibid.

beyond the Task Force mandate and sent a notification to all the Missions in Geneva saying, hey guys, submit CVs."[52] Kastberg's actions frustrated some, who felt he had taken action beyond the Task Force's mandate and that hundreds of applicants would deluge the Task Force with their CVs.

Perhaps owing to the pressure from disgruntled donor countries and recognizing the wisdom of Kastberg's approach, Nakajima and the CCO adjusted their plan and decided to incorporate more fully the recommendations of the GMC Task Force in their search for a new Executive Director. At its meeting on September 22, the CCO agreed that by October 15, Nakajima would receive from the Task Force a list of all possible candidates for the Directorship, which he would then forward to each of the other five cosponsors.[53] Each of the cosponsors, in turn, would then select two names from the list whom they would support, and, through an iterative process, the CCO would reach consensus on a candidate to put forward to the UN Secretary-General for appointment.[54] On October 14, Kastberg sent Nakajima the list of candidates the Task Force had received for the Executive Director's post. This list consisted of the following individuals:

1. Rita Arauz, Founder, Fundación Nimehuatzin, Nicaragua
2. Joe Decosas, Adviser, Canadian International Development Agency and previous Chair of the GPA Management Committee
3. Jonathan Mann, Previous Director of WHO's Global Programme on AIDS and Professor, Health and Human Rights, Harvard School of Public Health
4. Michael Merson, Director of the WHO's Global Programme on AIDS
5. Julio S. G. Montaner, National Health Research Scholar of Health Canada
6. Peter Piot, Director of Research and Intervention Development, WHO Global Programme on AIDS
7. Elizabeth Reid, Director of the HIV and Development Programme, United Nations Development Programme
8. Sergio Viera De Mello, Director of Political Affairs, UN Protection Force and Special Envoy of the UN High Commission for Refugees

Kastberg noted that this was only an initial list, that there was broad variability in the support for each of the listed candidates, and that "the process of identifying possible candidates has not yet been concluded in some key constituencies."[55] Having received this list of names, in mid-October Nakajima forwarded it to the

[52] Nils Kastberg, Interview by Michael Merson, New York City, September, 2002.

[53] GMC Task Force on HIV/AIDS Coordination, "Seventh Meeting, Provisional agenda item 2: Experiences from the Task Force Constituency Working Method, 17 February 1995," Geneva: World Health Organization, 1995, GMC/TFC(7)95.2.

[54] Committee of Cosponsoring Organizations, "Conclusions of the First Meeting, 22 September 1994, New York," CCO, September 29, 1994.

[55] Nils Kastberg, "Letter to Dr. Nakajima, 14 October 1994," Geneva: World Health Organization, 1994.

members of the CCO.[56] A total of ten more names were submitted by November 17, while three members of the original list asked to have their names removed from consideration.[57]

The process continued to be consumed in controversy, however, as some members of the CCO—as well as other stakeholders—felt the process was moving too quickly. On October 13, James Speth, the recently appointed Administrator of UNDP wrote a letter to the WHO UN Liaison Office in New York as well as to WHO and UNESCO. Speth noted that "while, as the minutes of this meeting indicate, we agreed that the names of candidates for this position would be submitted to us on 15 October by the Director-General of WHO ... the consultation process among our organizations and Member States seems to have been left rather unstructured." Speth asked that the process be delayed and called for a consultation to "ensure that the selection process is fully consultative, extensive, and transparent."[58] Nakajima took offense at such aspersions: "I am surprised at your comment on the need to ensure that the selection process is 'fully consultative, extensive, and transparent,'" Nakajima wrote Speth on October 17th. "We are adhering closely to the process agreed, and I trust that each agency will weigh the proposals carefully to ensure the best possible leadership for this important UN initiative." Still, Nakajima did note that the process would be ongoing. "Since the Task Force did not communicate to us the full list of candidates by 15 October 1994," Nakajima wrote, "it is clear that the selection process will be slightly delayed."[59]

Richard Butler, as we have noted, had little tolerance for what he considered the internal machinations of UN Geneva's political machine. Those based in Geneva were "running a process that would select this person, with an inevitable result," Butler believed. "The whole thing was a fix and I was not prepared to accept it. Therefore, I insisted that Permanent Representatives in New York be advised of the need to make this appointment and that States had the opportunity to advance candidates."[60] Butler, of course, had little confidence in the trustworthiness of Nakajima's actions, but he also suspected Kastberg of playing a similar game. Consequently, he himself hosted in New York City an open-ended consultation on October 25 to discuss the Directorship, and planned three more meetings on other topics (two in November on the PCB and UNAIDS structure, and another in

---

[56] Hiroshi Nakajima, "Confidential Letter to Executive Heads of UNDP, UNESCO, UNFPA, UNICEF, & World Bank, 17 October 1994" Geneva: World Health Organization, 1994, GPA-A20/372/30.

[57] GMC Task Force on HIV/AIDS Coordination, "Seventh Meeting, Provisional agenda item 2: Experiences from the Task Force Constituency Working Method, 17 February 1995," Geneva: World Health Organization, 1995, GMC/TFC(7)95.2.

[58] James Gustave Speth, "Letter to Mr. Andrew Joseph, Acting Director, UNO Office at the United Nations, October 13, 1994." New York, UNDP, 1994.

[59] Hiroshi Nakajima, "Letter to Mr. Speth, 17 October, 1994," Geneva: World Health Organization, 1994.

[60] Richard Butler, Interview by Michael Merson, New Haven, CT, February, 2002.

mid-December).[61] On November 7, Butler also invited "all the Permanent Representatives in New York" to send their recommendations for Executive Director to the GMC Task Force or the CCO.[62] "Butler sent out a communication [to all the stakeholders] saying, 'I will start the consultative process on this now,'" Kastberg remembers. "So I took a plane and came [to New York] and sent a letter to all the Missions here in New York, informing them that Butler had sent this letter as President of ECOSOC, and that we were very pleased that he was doing this consultation—but that I would just like to let them know that there had been considerable consultation already."[63]

For his part, Butler admits he was trying to make a political point by spearheading these consultations in New York: "I would argue that the text of the letter [was] impeccable in terms of procedures, but politically it said: 'You bastards are not going to run this from the bar at the Perle du Lac and the old boys' network, this is now going to be global and every Member State of the United Nations is going to be aware that there is a position there and if they've got a good candidate, they should put that person forward."[64] For Butler, it was the principle of the issue that mattered: "I'd sought to destroy [Kastberg's] process in Geneva for two reasons: one, because it was an insider process that was going to have an inevitable result and wasn't fair, and two, to make the point that this thing wasn't Geneva-based any more, it was now going global and it had the World Bank in it, the New York based agencies, and so on. This was to be a new kind of UN animal."[65]

Kastberg went along with Butler's move. "I extended the deadline that we had set in the Task Force by a couple of weeks and informed him that we would then proceed to send them results."[66] In fact, Kastberg did not find this extra time made much difference: "Only one additional name came," Kastberg maintained. "That showed how strong the consensus had been with what we had done."[67] By the end of November, Kastberg had received from stakeholders, members of the CCO, and representatives on the GMC Task Force a total of 14 candidates for the Executive Director position.[68] These included:

---

[61] Richard Butler, "Letter to Dr. Nakajima, 28 October 1994," New York: Economic and Social Council, 1994.

[62] GMC Task Force on HIV/AIDS Coordination, "Seventh Meeting, Provisional agenda item 2: Experiences from the Task Force Constituency Working Method, 17 February 1995," Geneva: World Health Organization, 1995, GMC/TFC(7)95.2.

[63] Nils Kastberg, Interview by Michael Merson, New York City, September, 2002.

[64] Richard Butler, Interview by Michael Merson, New Haven, CT, February, 2002.

[65] Ibid.

[66] Nils Kastberg, Interview by Michael Merson, New York City, September, 2002.

[67] Ibid; GMC Task Force on HIV/AIDS Coordination, "Seventh Meeting, Provisional agenda item 2: Experiences from the Task Force Constituency Working Method, 17 February 1995," Geneva: World Health Organization, 1995, GMC/TFC(7)95.2.

[68] In reality, the number was 16, but two individuals proposed by the CCO later maintained that "they had not been consulted and did not wish to be considered for the post." GMC Task Force on HIV/AIDS Coordination, "Seventh Meeting, Provisional agenda item 2: Experiences from the Task Force Constituency Working Method, 17 February 1995," Geneva: World Health Organization, 1995, GMC/TFC(7)95.2

 1. Dame Margaret J. Anstee, Former Undersecretary General of the United Nations
 2. Richard Butler, Australian Ambassador to the United Nations
 3. Margaret Catley-Carlson, President, Population Council, New York
 4. Helene Gayle, Associate Director, U.S. Centers for Disease Control and Prevention
 5. Lair Guerra de Macedo Rodrigues, Director, Brazil's National Program on Sexually Transmissible Diseases and AIDS
 6. Noerine Kaleeba, Founder of The AIDS Support Organization, Uganda
 7. Maureen Law, Director-General, Health Sciences-Division, International Development Research Center, Ottawa
 8. Michael Merson, Director, WHO's Global Programme on AIDS
 9. Peter Piot, Director, Research and Intervention Development, WHO Global Programme on AIDS
10. Elizabeth Reid, Director, HIV and Development Programme, United Nations Development Programme
11. Jesus Kumate Rodriguez, Secretary of Health of Mexico and chair of the Executive Board of WHO
12. Allan Rosenfield, Dean, Columbia University School of Public Health
13. Steven W. Sinding, Director, Population Sciences, Rockefeller Foundation
14. Jyoti Shankar Singh, Director, Technical and Evaluations Division, United Nations Population Fund[69]

Even at this stage, it was clear that some candidates had more support than others. Five CCO members, all the European Union countries, and three GMC members had supported Peter Piot, for example, and three CCO members and one GMC member had supported Kumate. Other nominees received only one or two votes. As Kastburg had suspected earlier, Nakajima supported the idea of Jesus Kumate as he felt "we didn't need somebody who knew how to run an HIV program—we needed more of a ministerial administrator, someone who [would] have more power over the donors and the agency heads."[70]

Kastberg began whittling down the list. I had already said I was not a candidate, so as soon as Kastberg called me to tell me that my name was on the list, I asked him to remove it.[71] For others, Kastberg required that they represent a constituency to remain in consideration. Thereafter, Richard Butler and Allan Rosenfield also removed themselves from consideration, followed in early December by an additional five of the 11

---

[69] Hiroshi Nakajima, "Letter to the Executive Heads of UNDP, UNESCO, UNFPA, UNICEF, and the World Bank: Summary of Status of Proposals For Candidates for Director of The Joint and Cosponsored UN Programme on HIV/AIDS." Geneva: World Health Organization, November 29, 1994, GPA-A20/372/30; Michael Balter, "UN Readies New Global AIDS Plan," *Science*, November 25, 1994, 266:1312–1313.

[70] Hiroshi Nakajima, Interview by Michael Merson, Poitiers, October 13, 2002.

[71] Michael Balter, "UN Readies New Global AIDS Plan," *Science*, November 25, 1994, 266: 1312–1313.

remaining candidates.[72] At this stage, by tabulation of the nominations, it was clear that there was "very broad support among Member States and non-governmental organizations for Dr. Peter Piot." As we mentioned, five out of the six members of the CCO had proposed Piot, and Piot also had the greatest level of support and acceptability.[73] Helene Gayle, had received the second greatest level of support. On December 12, 1994, Boutros Boutros-Ghali announced that he was appointing Peter Piot to direct the new joint and cosponsored program.[74]

Why had so many in the international community rallied behind Piot? Clearly, he was a highly respected AIDS researcher, had served as President of the International AIDS Society, had worked extensively in Africa, was fluent in French and English (and had working knowledge of other languages), and understood the medical, political, and developmental facets of the pandemic and the global response to it. Beyond that, donor nations on both sides of the Atlantic liked him as a person. Once, when Stef Bertozzi and I were taking Piot around to meet some of the important American health officials in the months after he had first joined GPA, he ran into an old family friend who happened to be Deputy Administrator for the United States Agency for International Development (USAID). "For me," remembered Bertozzi, "it was just emblematic of the fact that Peter had very good relationships and lots of [social] capital even though he hadn't been especially political until then."[75]

While Piot was amenable to the United States government, he was not its first choice. The nomination process had put the United States government in an interesting position; it had wanted to nominate one or more candidates, but the closed nomination process had made it difficult to do so. Even when Kastberg and Butler opened up the process in late October, it was undecided on who to nominate. As late as December 1, when there was lobbying for candidates taking place during the Paris AIDS Summit, which was being hosted by the French government to increase global commitment to AIDS…the United States was unclear about its choice. As it turned out, Gayle and Piot were both at the Paris Summit, and as Gayle explained,

[72] Hiroshi Nakajima, "Letter to the Executive Heads of UNDP, UNESCO, UNFPA< UNICEF, and the World Bank: Summary of Status of Proposals For Candidates for Director of The Joint and Cosponsored UN Programme on HIV/AIDS." Geneva: World Health Organization, November 29, 1994, GPA-A20/372/30; Hiroshi Nakajima, "Letter to the Executive Heads of UNDP, UNESCO, UNFPA< UNICEF, and the World Bank: Candidates for the Post of Director of The Joint and Cosponsored UN Programme on HIV/AIDS." Geneva: World Health Organization, December 8, 1994, GPA-A20/372/30. Those who removed themselves from the list included: Dame Margaret J. Anstee, Ms Margaret Catley-Carlson, Ms Noerine Kaleeba, Dr Maureen Law, Mr Steven W. Sinding.

[73] Hiroshi Nakajima, "Letter to the Executive Heads of UNDP, UNESCO, UNFPA< UNICEF, and the World Bank: Candidates for the Post of Director of The Joint and Cosponsored UN Programme on HIV/AIDS." Geneva: World Health Organization, December 8, 1994, GPA-A20/372/30.

[74] Office of the UN Secretary General, "Press Release: Dr. Peter Piot To Be Director of New United Nations Programme on HIV/AIDS," New York: United Nations, 1994, SG/A/596, BIO/2918, H/2864.

[75] Stefano Bertozzi, Interview by Stephen Inrig, October 22, 2010.

"when it became clear that Peter was going to be a candidate, I didn't take my candidacy further and our government backed Peter....I was not going to get into a competition with Peter, who I felt was poised to take this on. We agreed that having this not get into UN style politics was in the best interest of the program."[76]

Very soon after the Paris Summit the United States Ambassador to the United Nations in Geneva, Dan Spiegel, whom I had gotten to know quite well, called to ask my support of an American candidate, I had chosen not to support anyone openly, considered Piot eminently qualified, and had much respect for both Gayle and Rosenfield. I told Ambassador Spiegel that "I understand you want me to support your candidate, but Peter Piot is a great candidate, and you've got to come up with a candidate as great as Peter." At this stage in the process, the United States government would not have been able to muster the same level of support for its candidate as Piot was already garnering, and I did not feel there was anyone better than Piot to be the UNAIDS Executive Director.

My hunch is that the United States government likely knew this. Global AIDS efforts had been run by two Americans and, as I had surmised, there was understandably some resistance against there being a third. Its effort for an alternative candidate to Piot seemed consequently half-hearted, despite Gayle's considerable qualifications. Moreover, many in the American AIDS community had considerable confidence in Piot. Jim Curran, who was still leading the CDC Atlanta efforts on AIDS had known Piot for many years, having worked with him, as we described in Chapter 1 in the founding of *Projet SIDA* in the mid-1980. Piot also had an excellent relationship with the National Institutes for Health and the CDC and he "was the most accessible non-American you could have."[77] Moreover, Piot knew the UN system, had the necessary scientific stature, strong support from the Europeans and most of the UN agencies, and "as some colleagues added, he had fewer enemies than the other candidates."[78]

Very soon after Boutros-Ghali appointed him Executive Director of the new program, Piot found himself thrust into a cutthroat world of UN turfmanship. As Elisabeth Manipoud, a UNICEF representative to the UNAIDS transition team, would later comment, "One should never forget that this joint and cosponsored program was imposed on a number of very unwilling cosponsors who resented more coordination of their respective HIV/AIDS activities."[79] Very early on, Piot began seeing this first hand:

we were far ahead of our times in terms of working across the very diverse United Nations system, with its nearly 50 agencies and organizations covering about every aspect of society and governance. We were trailblazers for what is now a much more unified UN system than in the mid-nineties. But at times I truly felt I was meeting the worst aspects of human

[76] Helene Gayle, Interview by Michael Merson, August 10, 2014; Helene Gayle, Interview by Michael Merson, August 11, 2014.

[77] Stefano Bertozzi, Interview by Stephen Inrig, October 22, 2010.

[78] Lindsay Knight. *UNAIDS: the first 10 years, 1996–2006*, New York: Joint United Nations Programme on HIV/AIDS (UNAIDS), 2008.

[79] Ibid.

nature. For people working in the UN to be so wrapped up in issues of turf and ego and bureaucratic politics, in the face of a human problem so terrifying, well, it was deeply demoralizing and profoundly unethical.[80]

This truth bore itself out in the power struggle that subsequently ensued when the CCO began working on the governance structure of the cosponsored program. In late January and early February 1995, the CCO presented a plan for how the program would operate. One key issue was the constitution of the PCB, which the ECOSOC resolution had sought to bring under the authority of governments, but which the CCO (made up of the UN cosponsors) was trying to determine itself.[81] The GMC Task Force had recommended, with the support of Piot, that the PCB composition and other details be determined with external oversight ("If the CCO had been in control there would have been no accountability," Piot explained, "it would have been a matter of [their being] judge and jury").[82] At an informal ECOSOC consultation in late January, several governments expressed concern about the CCO's framing of program governance, particularly its construction of the relationship "between the program director, the CCO, and the PCB."[83] Throughout February, Butler, the GMC Task Force, Piot, and some governments all pushed for a more inclusive and externally representative PCB with NGO representation and equitable geographic distribution of government representation.[84] "The cosponsors tried to impose that I report to all of them together, collectively," Piot recalls. "[But] ECOSOC didn't buy [it] and that's where Richard Butler came in. He was the one who really killed that—so that I would formally report to the chair of the Board— the PCB."[85] Piot would report to the PCB, this coalition maintained, and the PCB— not the CCO—would "have ultimate responsibility for all policy and budgetary matters" and would represent the "interests and responsibilities" of all the stakeholders, not merely the cosponsors.[86] At the third CCO meeting in Vienna towards

[80] Peter Piot *No Time to Lose: A Life in Pursuit of Deadly Viruses.* New York: Norton, 2012, 228.

[81] "Report of the Committee of Cosponsoring Organizations to ECOSOC," Joint and Cosponsored United Nations Programme on HIV/AIDS, January 23, 1995, 28.

[82] Lindsay Knight. *UNAIDS: the first 10 years, 1996–2006*, New York: Joint United Nations Programme on HIV/AIDS (UNAIDS), 2008,; GMC Task Force on HIV/AIDS Coordination, "Seventh Meeting of the GMC Task Force on HIV/AIDS Coordination, Provisional agenda item 7: Information on Steps in the Decision Making Process on the Implementation of the Joint and Cosponsored UN Programme on HIV/AIDS." Geneva: World Health Organization, February 6, 1995, GMC/TFC/(7)95.7.

[83] Susan Holck, "Travel Report, 7 February 1995," Geneva: World Health Organization, A20/372/30.

[84] GMC Task Force on HIV/AIDS Coordination, "Seventh Meeting of the GMC Task Force on HIV/AIDS Coordination, Provisional agenda item 7: Status as regards ECOSOC Consultations of the Joint and Cosponsored UN Programme on HIV/AIDS." Geneva: World Health Organization, February 15, 1995, GMC/TFC(7)95.7 Add.1.

[85] Peter Piot, Interview by Michael Merson, New Haven, CT, October 26, 2002.

[86] GMC Task Force on HIV/AIDS Coordination, "Seventh Meeting of the GMC Task Force on HIV/AIDS Coordination, Provisional agenda item 7: Status as regards ECOSOC Consultations of the Joint and Cosponsored UN Programme on HIV/AIDS." Geneva: World Health Organization, February 15, 1995, GMC/TFC(7)95.7 Add.1.

the latter part of February, the CCO relented, claiming that it would "make every effort to work within the framework proposed by ECOSOC."[87]

Another key issue early on was the "joint" aspect of the program. UNFPA felt that the CCO plan had not indicated strongly enough that "all global-level activities on HIV/AIDS would be carried out through the joint program and that none of the cosponsoring agencies would undertake any HIV/AIDS activities outside the strategies, priorities, and workplan of the joint program."[88] The CCO had specified that "the joint program is not identical to the cosponsors' global response to the HIV/AIDS pandemic," but it was not clear from the document whether cosponsors could continue to run their own AIDS programs outside the joint program structure. UNFPA "was concerned that the other cosponsors would interpret the report as a 'green light' for continuing or initiating their own HIV/AIDS activities outside the joint program, a situation which UNFPA felt strongly would defeat the whole purpose of establishing the joint program."[89] If this happened, moreover, the new plan lacked any enforcement mechanism beyond PCB pressure, and neither the ECOSOC nor the GMC Task Force redrafted language to give it such a mechanism. For example, it was by no means clear whether Elizabeth Reid at UNDP intended to close down her HIV and Development Programme, as GPA was planning to do: "From your text [in response to US Government questions about Reid's program plans]," Piot wrote in March 1995, "it could be inferred that HIV and Development expects to continue its work, more or less unchanged ..."[90]

Upon reflection, there were critical moments (in late 1994 and early 1995) when those deciding—and I include myself—on the mechanisms and processes for UNAIDS could have done better. This was one such moment. Many individuals had worked on the UNAIDS formulation process for a year and had a number of ideas on how the program could be structured to ensure effective implementation and collaboration, but no one had found a solution on enforcement. The fact that UNAIDS lacked a mechanism to corral the cosponsors other than donor suasion would have immediate consequences both for shutting down GPA and establishing UNAIDS.

This brings to the fore a question that we and others have often asked: If Elizabeth Reid and I could have established a closer working relationship, would GPA have survived and UNAIDS never been created? Given Piot's similarly bumpy relationship with Reid, which we discuss in the next chapter, we believe that the potential for a more amicable working relationship between Reid and me would still have been limited. Yet even if we had established a better relationship, it is certainly possible that UNAIDS would still have been formed. As we have documented, there were other reasons—such as Nakajima's reelection and the lack of confidence in the

---

[87] James Gustave Speth, "Letter to Ambassador Butler, 5 March 1995," New York: UNDP, 1995, B/SS/F0008_HH.JJG.

[88] Peter Piot and Susan Holck, "Note For the Record: Meeting with Mr. Jyoti Singh and Dr. Nicholas Dodd, UNFPA, 30 January 1995."

[89] Ibid.

[90] Peter Piot, "Letter to Ms. Elizabeth Reid re: US State Department Request, 28 March 1995," Geneva: Joint United Nations Programme on AIDS, 1995, GPA-A20/372/30.

WHO regional structure—why the donor community had lost much of its confidence in WHO/GPA's leadership.

While I knew I was leaving WHO in late fall of 1994, and had formally announced as such towards the end of the year, it was not until March 30, 1995, that I planned to depart. The time between my announcement and my departure was relatively busy. The ECOSOC resolution required each of the six cosponsors to provide representatives "to work on the new program's structure, budgets and strategy."[91] I felt the best person to represent WHO in this process was Susan Holck, as she was very familiar with the workings of GPA and knew Piot well. She agreed do this and so I nominated her to the team. Then, I began working with Hu Ching Li, my Assistant Director-General, to decide who would take over for me as Interim GPA Director through the end of 1995 when GPA would close down. The most obvious option was Dorothy Blake, who was my loyal deputy and had been very committed to GPA. Unfortunately, she had a sometimes strained relationship with a number of our staff. Instead, I thought it best that she lead WHO's AIDS program which would start in January 1, 1996 after GPA closed down. For Interim GPA Director, I recommended Stef Bertozzi. Bertozzi was the youngest of our senior staff, but was highly respected and had good judgment and excellent personal relationships with just about everyone. I also thought he was very likely to join UNAIDS once it launched, which I reasoned should help in the transition process.

Bertozzi had joined GPA in the middle of his medical residency at the University of California, San Francisco. He attended medical school at the University of California, San Diego and earned a doctorate in health policy at the Massachusetts Institute of Technology (MIT), during which time (the late 1980s) he worked in Zaire and Tanzania in one of the World Bank's first AIDS projects. Not long after returning to the United States to complete his residency, Bertozzi was contacted by Doris Schopper in the Policy Unit at GPA and invited to come to Geneva. Soon after his visit Bertozzi agreed to join GPA's policy unit and serve as our in-house economist. In 1994, after Holck left GPA to join the UNAIDS transition team, I asked Bertozzi to serve as acting head of that unit. Then, once the Secretary-General formally chose Piot to lead UNAIDS, Bertozzi replaced him as head of our research division. "The decision that I think probably pissed people off the most was when this kid from Mike's Policy shop gets named to run the research group once Peter is selected," Bertozzi recalled. "It was an unpopular choice with the folks in the research group, without a question. And that included various senior people like Jose Esparza and David Heymann…There were people there that had many more years there and much more seniority—not just duration but who were at higher levels of position. That was a difficult situation and difficult to explain."[92] I thought it made good sense to appoint Bertozzi. He had performed well as head of the policy unit and the various unit leaders within our Research Division were mutually unacceptable to each other. Not only did I consider Bertozzi a highly competent manager; he was also a neutral

---

[91] Lindsay Knight. *UNAIDS: the first 10 years, 1996–2006*, New York: Joint United Nations Programme on HIV/AIDS (UNAIDS), 2008.

[92] Stefano Bertozzi, Interview by Stephen Inrig, October 22, 2010.

party who could mediate among camps of mutual disrespect. In the end, he performed outstandingly in his brief tenure as head of the research group.

Prior to my departure, Hu Ching Li appointed Bertozzi to take over GPA as Interim Director. Bertozzi, wisely in my opinion, asked to report to Hu Ching Li rather than directly to Nakajima. "I did not think highly of him," Bertozzi explained. "I wanted to have a boss that I could have a decent relationship with and who could handle Nakajima for me. I didn't feel that I would either have the appropriate influence or access to him that I needed to be able to run the program." Hu Ching Li agreed to these conditions as did Nakajima. Bertozzi was just 2 years out of his medical residency, had not yet received his Ph.D., and had been appointed as one of the youngest WHO Directors to lead one of the largest WHO programs about to close amid great controversy. "It was not popular," Bertozzi conceded.

Before I stepped down, however, I needed to address one final issue: the future of GPA staff. Importantly, back in 1993, as we at GPA were working on the joint and cosponsored program, we chose not to renew the contracts of any staff beyond December 1995.[93] By the late fall of 1994, staff morale was understandably becoming low as "UN administrators [were] not yet able to say who among GPA's 275 employees [would] be kept on and who [would] be let go."[94] Over the next several months, we verbally explained to GPA staff that their contracts were ending, but we were still unable to tell them what would happen next. It was, the *Geneva Post* noted, "the first time WHO has stopped a program but continued to work on the program's contents."[95] Of course, this was not my decision to make and so I tended to stay out of these discussions. However, on March 6, a few weeks before I left Geneva, I sent a letter to all staff explaining the termination of GPA and encouraged them "to apply for positions in the new program, as well as any vacancies in the [World Health] Organization" that might fit their skill set.[96]

Two days later, on March 8, Piot and the other members of the transition team met with GPA staff to answer questions about the transition. Tensions surfaced immediately. "The mood yesterday was somber," *Geneva Post* Sharmila Devi reported of the event. Some participants were upset with Piot's perceived aloofness "He seems to have become rather arrogant and doesn't want anything to do with us," one staff member reported, "He's betraying his old colleagues and he's betraying WHO." Others were quite disappointed with me: "One staff member asked why the WHO was prepared to hand over the remains of the GPA budget … 'But Merson

[93] Lindsay Knight. *UNAIDS: the first 10 years, 1996–2006*, New York: Joint United Nations Programme on HIV/AIDS (UNAIDS), 2008.

[94] Michael Balter, "UN Readies New Global AIDS Plan," *Science* November 25, 1994, 266:1312–1313.

[95] Michael O'Regan, "Two Hundred WHO Staff Served with notice to quit." *Geneva Post*, March 2, 1995.

[96] Micheal Merson, "Memorandum: WHO Global Programme on AIDS, March 6, 1995." Geneva: World Health Organization, 1995.

had no answer to that.'"[97] In fact, this was what the GMC had instructed us to do. To say the least, it was a very difficult time. GPA was an extrabudgetary program, its funds were drying up, and the program was closing down, so we had an obligation to inform the staff that they could not be guaranteed employment. Of course, they were welcome to apply for positions in another part of WHO or with UNAIDS, but we had not negotiated with Piot to take on any of the staff, and Piot was understandably wary of UNAIDS automatically inheriting staff from any of the cosponsors, particularly WHO. While staff were upset and demoralized, we felt that the only responsible action to take would be to give them time to prepare for a major transition in their lives, hence the reason for my sending the letter.

Obviously, this left Bertozzi with a challenging task. Many GPA staff never fully understood why the donors were abolishing GPA so soon after it had been established, especially at a time when the pandemic deserved full attention. More immediate for them was their concern about future employment. Would they join UNAIDS, would they transfer elsewhere within WHO, would they need to look for a position outside WHO? There was a problem, however, in that the March 6th letter came from me and not from WHO's Human Resources department. Bertozzi and I both thought this was the right thing to do, but as Bertozzi was to discover, it was "a combination of bad judgment and bad management." The bad management was something in which GPA and WHO leadership shared culpability: "It's fair to say that neither of us had done anything like it before," Bertozzi explained. In fact, WHO had never done this before. This is where the bad judgment came in, "mostly on the side of WHO," Bertozzi believed. Since this was such novel territory, "it was something that should have been negotiated at a higher level and planned for at a higher level, and anticipated better than it was." But, since the letter had come from me, from that point until the closing of GPA, Bertozzi did not find himself "in a collaborative role with WHO Human Resources. This was not a coordinated, termination of contract with planning for post contract issues. It was a very messy personnel situation."

The first week after I left, Bertozzi visited the European headquarters of Digital, the American computer company, which was located in Geneva and in the process of substantive downsizing.[98] Bertozzi sought out the head of Digital's Human Resources and asked him, "Help me to do this well. I have just taken over this program and my staff has all been fired." Digital's European Human Resources chief told Bertozzi, "Give them a generous relocation and an executive assistance package, and give them a few of hours to clean out their desks, 'cause the last thing you want is to have people that have been fired making the whole environment poisonous." Bertozzi left very discouraged because he felt WHO had done precisely the opposite: he had no package to offer GPA staff and "10 months of poison." What

---

[97] Sharmila Devi, "WHO Staff Left In Limbo Over Jobs," *The Geneva Post,* Thursday, March 9, 1995.

[98] Stefano Bertozzi, Interview by Stephen Inrig, October 22, 2010. Edgar H. Schein, Peter S. DeLisi, Paul J. Kampas, and Michael M. Sonduck, *DEC Is Dead, Long Live DEC—The Lasting Legacy of Digital Equipment Corporation.* San Francisco: Barrett-Koehler, 2003, 233–234.

neither Bertozzi nor I fully anticipated was what so many months of uncertainty could do to staff morale.

It was hard for GPA staff to be objective: They were "being fired in 10 months unless [they were] hired by the new program which is coming in to replace GPA," Bertozzi explained. "So psychologically, it is very normal that people have a high opinion of their own work and their ability and their likely desirability to a future program—so, rather than starting to actively look for work they passively assumed they will be desired by the new program." "It was a very difficult situation," Bertozzi concluded. "Human Resources was hopeless in providing them any sort of support ensuring them a healthy transition outside the program."[99] "A lot of [GPA staff] had difficulties because they didn't know whether they would have a job," explained Gunilla Ernberg.[100] The assistance provided by WHO's Human Resources would improve considerably over the next year.

For his part, Bertozzi collaborated very closely with the transition team setting up UNAIDS, and helped move a few GPA staff over to UNAIDS. One challenge was whether to have someone else in WHO take on their tasks or to have them continue their work with UNAIDS. One of the first to transfer was Purnima Mane, whom I had recruited from the Tata Institute of Social Sciences in Mumbai. Mane became Executive Director of UNAIDS' Policy, Evidence and Partnerships Department. Bertozzi would meet regularly with Piot and Mane and the UNAIDS' strategic team to plan the next steps in the transition. Since Bertozzi played such an intimate role in the transition process, there started to be "the perception among many GPA staff that [Bertozzi] had a fair amount to do with whether or not they transitioned." This created some conflicting emotions among those at GPA. "People felt they had to be incredibly positive about the new program, and incredibly positive about Peter, because they wanted him to hire them. But at the same time, [they felt] incredibly angry because he hadn't asked for them to be trickled over yet." The progress was slow throughout the year, but accelerated dramatically towards the end. But for those people who "hadn't made the transition, the more and more nervous they became about whether they would be making it."[101]

That last year, GPA took on no new projects. However, despite their circumstances, the GPA staff to their great credit continued working diligently on a bevy of ongoing projects: these included, for example, a multi-country, multi-site mother-to-child transmission prevention trial; a microbicide trial; an injection drug user project in Manipur; a sex worker project in Morocco and Madras. Most importantly, GPA also continued providing funds to multiple national AIDS programs. And, in the end, a number of highly competent people and important activities transitioned over to UNAIDS, rather than shifting to another part of WHO. This asymmetrical shifting struck Bertozzi for what it portended: "Lots of people were trickling over to UNAIDS; nobody was trickling into the rest of WHO. ... There was no attempt to give, for example, research projects to other parts of WHO. We could have peeled some of

[99] Stefano Bertozzi, Interview by Michael Merson, New Haven, NC, December, 2002.

[100] Gunilla Ernberg, Interview by Michael Merson, New Haven, CT, August, 2002.

[101] Stefano Bertozzi, Interview by Michael Merson, New Haven, NC, December, 2002.

those things off to other parts of WHO." But in fact the dissolution of GPA did not happen that way. Why? The truth is that, before this transition period, GPA had not been very successful in developing collaborative research with other parts of WHO, much less transferring its funds to them. Jonathan Mann and his team had, intentionally or not, discouraged this, and while we had tried to expand these collaborations over the past few years, they were not numerous.

Also, and unfortunately, problems developed between WHO and UNAIDS. In the weeks immediately after I left, UNAIDS "still had to work out the final negotiations about what role WHO would play administratively and other things, [so] there was still relative good will until that got settled," recalled Bertozzi. After that, however, the tension mounted. "Once those issues were settled, once there was no need to negotiate or play nice because WHO wanted to be the administrator of the program," Bertozzi remembered, "the resentment was given full opportunity to vent, and I recall very unpleasant meetings before the end of GPA with the Regional Directors and Nakajima in which the Regional Directors made it very clear that they were very angry and very resentful—very hostile to Nakajima for having let this happen ... Unfortunately that colored UNAIDS' beginning."[102] I heard later on from Aleya Hammad that they were also very hostile towards me. As she explained: "... when you are gone, the blame goes to you because you are not there...all of a sudden the Regional Directors went 180 degrees and told him (Nakajima) 'why did you let go of UNAIDS?' Then the axe came on your head....I said 'that is very easy because he is not here.' But at that time we were all accomplices. We all had a hand but nobody was guilty."[103]

A reasonable question to ask is why didn't Nakajima fight harder to keep GPA? Why didn't he fight harder to keep the leadership of the global response to the pandemic in WHO? There were at least two reasons, according to Claire Challat-Traquet, a close WHO colleague of Nakajima and an expert on tobacco control. First, he trusted the advice he received from me about the inevitability of UNAIDS. Second, Nakajima—perhaps because of his personality, perhaps because of his Japanese cultural values—never liked to show he was losing, or to show weakness. "To have fought and lost would have meant a complete loss of face, which [was] unacceptable."[104] Third, and this is my assumption, his government supported the formation of UNAIDS, possibly because the United States government was strongly advocating for its formation.

At the nascent UNAIDS, Piot was facing his own stresses. Hindsight here is clearer too. At the time, I felt the best thing I could do was to leave room for Piot to grow UNAIDS and to get out of the way, as is often best when leaders change. My focus was on the transition process and having the best people (Blake and Bertozzi) in leadership positions. Also, as I explained earlier, I had personal incentives to move on and needed to start my new position at Yale. With these factors drawing my

---

[102] Ibid.

[103] Aleya Hammad, Interview by Michael Merson, New Haven, CT, April, 2004.

[104] Claire Challot interview, Michael Merson.

attention away from WHO, I did not think as much as I should of about how to pro-vide a longer, more stabilized, and less internally contentious transition. I certainly had Nakajima's ear—he trusted me and listened to my advice. Perhaps I could have done more to smooth the transition from GPA to UNAIDS, to mollify the anger of the Regional Directors, to reduce the vicissitudes of WHO's support during the tran-sition period. I will always wonder if I should have stayed longer.

This raises another even more fundamental question. When it was decided to establish UNAIDS, the GMC decided concurrently to close down GPA and shift GPA's unspent resources to UNAIDS. Was this the right decision? As Helene Gayle later reflected,

> We all should have thought more about it. The part I think we got wrong was subsuming WHO's program within UNAIDS. I think that was the part because it essentially killed for 5 years WHO's AIDS program. This most affected the field, since that's where the countries go for their support. That was the piece---UNAIDS should have been a smaller secretariat and the WHO program remain. But the thinking was, since WHO was the lead organization or at least the largest organization, why have the two, since UNAIDS was going to be administered within WHO. That's the piece we didn't think through enough."[105]

Nils Kastberg had a little different take on this when we asked him why the GMC closed GPA, "That was probably because we had agreed that there needed to be some mainstreaming capacity, but what we also agreed was that UNAIDS should have a role in the selection of the mainstreaming staff, so that the agencies would not put useless staff in—quality control. What should have happened much earlier, perhaps, was that at the same time that UNAIDS was being created, the staff main-streaming for WHO should have been put in place."[106] We agree with Gayle and Kastberg. While there was surely the need for a more coordinated, effective, and powerful UN response to AIDS, the process used was too costly to WHO and, even more importantly, had a very deleterious effect on national AIDS programs. All of us involved in the process should have spent more time thinking about the best ways to preserve the best of WHO's input into the global response and build a strong col-laborative bridge between WHO and UNAIDS. It certainly would have made the situation easier for Piot. There will be some who may say this never would have been possible, but we should have tried harder, myself included.

Piot recognized that he needed sage advice during the transition on how best to establish UNAIDS. Thus, in early 1995, he began meeting with some outside advi-sors on a regular basis to get their perspectives on future steps. Moreover, with the shutting down of the formal UNAIDS transition team in February 1995, Piot pulled together his own, very competent, "preparatory team" to help guide the establish-ment and strategy of UNAIDS in the ensuing years. As part of this process, Piot and his team organized five regional consultations throughout the globe to obtain input and buy-in from the various donor nations, AIDS organizations, and other relevant

---

[105] Helene Gayle, Interview by Michael Merson, New Haven, CT, February, 2002.

[106] Nils Kastberg, Interview by Michael Merson, New York City, September, 2002.

stakeholders.[107] Some of the issues discussed were to define what UNAIDS was and what it would do, how it would be different from GPA, and what would happen once GPA closed down.

What made this somewhat difficult was that UNAIDS did not know its budget and the PCB (its governing board) had not yet met. The PCB had its first meeting in July 1995, after the elections to the Board had taken place. Each of the six cosponsoring organizations were represented, along with 22 countries (seven from Western European and other donor countries, three from Latin America and the Caribbean, two from Eastern Europe, five from Africa, and five from Asia) and five non-governmental organizations (NGOs) (three from developing countries; two from developed countries).[108] While NGO representation made up only 15% of the total PCB membership, it is notable—in the spirit of inclusion first fostered under Mann and carried through my tenure at GPA—that UNAIDS became the first UN entity with NGO representation as part of its governing structure.[109] In GPA, we invited NGOs to participate in the GMC, but they did not have voting privileges. What was also evident was the unprecedented power granted to the cosponsoring organizations. "We gave the UN agencies much more influence than was due," Kastberg later reflected. "Firstly, we recruited staff from among them. Secondly, they were members of the cosponsoring organizations, so they had some oversight even over the Executive Director of UNAIDS. Thirdly, we made them members of the PCB. It's unprecedented that UN agencies be given so much influence at all levels." The problem, from Kastberg's perspective, was that the cosponsors failed to uphold their portion of the implied social contract. "In spite of the fact that they were given all the elements for ownership and contribution ... in exchange for their full backing and support—they did not give it. They just used it to try to control and minimize ... instead of making this an element of full ownership and driving the whole AIDS agenda together towards the future."[110]

The key signal that the donors were now also far less supportive of UNAIDS came during the first PCB meeting, in a discussion about the program budget and donor support. Piot had "propose[d] a modest budget of 122 to 140 million dollars" for the 1996–1997 biennium, but the donor nations wanted far less. "Britain said 40 million," Piot recalled. "Some donors were really determined to keep this really small."[111] "They talked about a budget which was one third of what Peter Piot was [asking for]," Purnima Mane recalled, "and the Board was up in arms because there were so many different views that they had to ... call time-out for people to consult

[107] Purnima Mane, "Strategic Plan Development, 17 March 1995," Geneva: World Health Organization, 1995, UNAIDS/PM/er; Peter Piot, "Letter to Mr. Norberg: Strategic Plan Development," Geneva: World Health Organization, March 1, 1995.

[108] Christer Jonsson, "From 'Lead Agency' to 'Integrated Programming': The Global Response to AIDS in the Third World," Green Globe Yearbook, 1996, 65–72.

[109] Lindsay Knight. UNAIDS: the first 10 years, 1996–2006, New York: Joint United Nations Programme on HIV/AIDS (UNAIDS), 2008.

[110] Nils Kastberg, Interview by Michael Merson, New York City, September, 2002.

[111] Peter Piot, Interview by Stephen Inrig, Dallas, TX, February 2, 2011.

bilaterally because, otherwise, we would never have had consensus."[112] According to Mane, Piot confronted some of the donors with an ultimatum: "'Listen, you set this up.'" Mane remembers Piot saying. "'If you want it to succeed, you have to fund it right or I'm out'. He didn't have any staff and he was very, very firm. He said, '… this is non-negotiable because you're starting this up … to fail.'"[113] Piot was not alone in this. Kastberg reportedly told the Board: "Up to now, Sweden has always played a mediating role. I, as of today, cannot play a mediating role because for Sweden it's unacceptable to consider any budget that goes below US$140 million, [for] the first biennium of UNAIDS."[114] Jim Sherry, who would move from UNICEF to UNAIDS to serve in a senior policy position, likewise confronted the donors: "he gave a magnificent remark about: 'you set us up, you take your responsibility.'[115] Richard Butler remembers having "a major floor clash with Sally Shelton-Colby, the USA representative and Assistant Administrator from USAID at that meeting about the budget. … and then we withdrew to a private room and redid the budget according to serious goals."[116] The Board did in fact adjourn for about an hour according to Mane, and when it returned the members had been able to reach consensus on a budget within Piot's desired range.[117] During the break Piot had a heated discussion about the budget with David Nabarro, who headed the United Kingdom delegation and had played a key role in crafting the WHA resolution in 1993 that led to the establishment of UNAIDS.[118] "It was a big fight," Piot recalled, "but I won at the Board meeting."[119]

This debate must have sent a clear message to the cosponsors that the donors were not very committed to the agency they had just created. Sherry felt that donor nations liked the UNAIDS coordination concept but as soon as the various resolutions creating UNAIDS were passed, they dropped their political pressure. "They thought their job was done," Sherry explained. "[But] they never stayed with it in terms of serious governance, they never stayed with it in terms of what was required to move the governing boards and harmonize with the governing boards of the other agencies."[120] "I think that's probably right," Butler admitted, when asked if the donors and ECOSOC had decreased their pressure. "…The political impetus required to make it succeed has not been given to it."[121] For Piot, this experience was telling. It meant that "these

[112] Lindsay Knight. *UNAIDS: the first 10 years, 1996–2006*, New York: Joint United Nations Programme on HIV/AIDS (UNAIDS), 2008.

[113] Ibid; Peter Piot, *No Time to Lose: A Life in Pursuit of Deadly Viruses*. New York: Norton, 2012, 231.

[114] Lindsay Knight. *UNAIDS: the first 10 years, 1996–2006*, New York: Joint United Nations Programme on HIV/AIDS (UNAIDS), 2008.

[115] Gunilla Ernberg, Interview by Michael Merson, New Haven, CT, August, 2002.

[116] Richard Butler, Interview by Michael Merson, New Haven, CT, February, 2002.

[117] Lindsay Knight. *UNAIDS: the first 10 years, 1996–2006*, New York: Joint United Nations Programme on HIV/AIDS (UNAIDS), 2008.

[118] Peter Piot (Personal Communication, March 15, 2017).

[119] Peter Piot, Interview by Michael Merson, New Haven, CT, October, 26, 2002.

[120] Jim Sherry, Interview by Michael Merson, Geneva, October, 2001.

[121] Richard Butler, Interview by Michael Merson, New Haven, CT, February, 2002.

arrangements were being undermined by everybody—not everybody, but I certainly remember meetings with UNDP. WHO at that time was basically ignoring the creation of UNAIDS."[122] Having stood as a candidate for the job in good faith, Piot quickly realized he now faced both passive and active opposition. In October 1995, with 3 months left before UNAIDS' officially launched, five of the six agencies signed a Memorandum of Understanding agreeing to form the Joint and Cosponsored United Nations Programme on HIV/AIDS (the World Bank would sign later in 1996). Yet the doubts remained. "[After the] resolution in ECOSOC and so on—it was presented as if all this was agreed to," Piot recalled. "But it had not been agreed to."[123]

Piot experienced this most acutely in the transition with WHO at country level. While UNAIDS appointed a considerable number of GPA administrative staff working in Geneva, there were a number of country-level GPA staff that it could not hire, since UNAIDS would only be playing a coordinating role in countries rather than an implementing role as GPA had done. In the end, in total, according to Piot, about 30% of UNAIDS technical staff and almost all its administrative staff came from GPA. This had at least three consequences for UNAIDS. First, according to Piot, "the other cosponsoring agencies didn't like that." Second, keeping all these GPA staffers "made it harder [for Piot] to change cultures because they are the guardians of the culture."[124] And third, it meant that WHO was able to blame UNAIDS for what Piot considered was WHO's failure to ensure that country programs did not suffer during the launch of UNAIDS. "In the transition in countries," Piot explained, "the fact was that there were a lot of staff who couldn't be retained, because it was a totally different type of program—the communication about that came down to 'Blame it on UNAIDS. Sorry, we'd like to keep you, but we in WHO can't help you now.' ... Whatever went wrong was blamed on me."[125] Sherry offered an additional interpretation of WHO's actions: "If the people who should be doing the WHO work are now in UNAIDS, they haven't transformed themselves, they are competing [with WHO]. And WHO, who always had the good normative people— they had all gone to UNAIDS. So they basically withdrew from the battle for several years. It was like they had been whipped."[126]

Whether or not WHO had been whipped, GPA had been gutted. On December 31, 1995, the remaining GPA staff were terminated. GPA had come to an end. The program that 8 years earlier had been birthed in a spirit of passion and panic to respond to the global AIDS pandemic was no more.

Those who remained scrambled to draw on their political, social, and public health connections to find new positions. "There were a number of representatives from various countries with offices in Geneva coming in and insisting that WHO place their nationals," Bertozzi told us. "In several cases I think that was effective, [but] that worked against developing country people transitioning and in the favor

---

[122] Peter Piot, Interview by Michael Merson, New Haven, CT, October, 26, 2002.

[123] Ibid.

[124] Ibid.

[125] Ibid.

[126] Jim Sherry, Interview by Michael Merson, Geneva, October, 2001.

of some donor country nationals." Within 3 months, Bertozzi and Gunilla Ernberg confirmed, most people had found new jobs: "By the first quarter of 1996," Bertozzi recalls, "Many more people than in November 1995 ended up transitioning." UNAIDS had fewer posts than GPA, but it largely restricted its hiring pool to people from within the UN system, and most GPA staff who did not find a position in UNAIDS found other work in WHO. Ernberg felt more positive about the work WHO's Human Resources department did: "WHO was very supportive there—in helping to find jobs. The administration, the personnel department, they were extremely supportive. They spent a lot of time with us."[127]

Of course, not everyone was happy nor did everyone find work. "There were a number of people who did not have UN employment even though they found reasonable jobs elsewhere, who felt they were entitled to life-time UN employment and filed a lawsuit in order to get that back," Bertozzi explained. This proved to be about 40 people who sued for wrongful dismissal, seeking reinstatement at their previous pay grade and full back pay from the time of their dismissal. This legal fight dragged on for a considerable length of time. WHO ended up settling with the group for a little over $1 million. Bertozzi thinks this could have been avoided: "Just as I went to Digital, I should have sat down with [the Assistant Director-General responsible for finance and administration] Denis Aitken immediately—the three of us should have sat down before you left ... and said, 'We need an eleven-month plan for separation.'" This lawsuit was also unfortunate for UNAIDS as it further tainted its relationship with WHO. Moreover, WHO held back transferring $20 milion from GPA to UNAIDS in case it needed the money to cover potential damages that could have resulted from the lawsuit.

When I heard about the lawsuit, I certainly regretted what had happened. In retrospect, I wish that I had had the time and forsight to work with Bertozzi and our Human Resources on a transition plan for the staff. However, I was pleased to learn that in the end most of the staff found positions within or outside WHO and UNAIDS.

It would be unfair to GPA and those who worked so diligently for so long in the program to end the story of GPA on a sour note. So much of what GPA and its predecessors accomplish has gone unheralded in the wake of UNAIDS, the President's Emergency Plan for AIDS Relief (PEPFAR), and The Global Fund to Fight AIDS, Tuberculosis and Malaria. The reality is that GPA and its devoted staff achieved several major accomplishments at what was most likely the most challenging time during the pandemic. As highlighted in GPA's final report, veterans of GPA can proudly lay claim to GPA's central role in the early global fight against AIDS.[128] Far more than any other organization, GPA raised awareness of the threat posed by AIDS. Whether through the rousing speeches or media interviews of Jonathan Mann, the establishment of World AIDS Day (which is still celebrated), the comprehensive epidemiological reports of Jim Chin, or the strong support GPA offered

[127] Gunilla Ernberg, Interview by Michael Merson, New Haven, CT, August, 2002.
[128] Global Programme on AIDS, "Global Programme on AIDS, 1987–1995: Final Report with Emphasis on 1994—1995 Biennium." Geneva: World Health Organization, 1995.

non-governmental and human rights organizations, GPA performed a critical service sensitizing the global community to the looming crisis of AIDS. It also strongly motivated the UN, many intergovernmental organizations inside and outside the UN, and donor countries to become involved. Through its inauguration and continual refinement of its Global AIDS Strategy, GPA identified and pursued "a sound and coherent strategy for global action against HIV/AIDS."[129] Moreover, while casting a broad vision, GPA provided sound guidance on a myriad of technical issues that surfaced early in the pandemic. Of great importance and taken for granted today, GPA helped create a global open discourse around sex and illicit drug use and established sexual behavior as an important field of scientific research.

GPA also provided essential technical and financial support to almost all low- and middle-income countries in their establishment and implementation of their national AIDS Programs. From Fakhry Assaad through Daniel Tarantola to Gunilla Ernberg, thousands and perhaps millions of lives were saved as GPA guided countries through emergency, short-term, and medium-term plans to address the greatest needs of their affected populations. Some might disagree with this assessment, pointing to Africa where the WHO regional office was viewed at best as useless, and at worst, corrupt. What is beyond doubt, however, is that in providing its support to national programs, GPA always sought to improve its performance, realizing fully its accountability to its donors and to countries. There can be little doubt that the early success achieved by such countries as Thailand, Uganda, Brazil, and Senegal in controlling their epidemics was in great part a result of the assistance they received from GPA.

Because GPA's primary objective was to "Prevent Transmission of HIV," GPA devoted great attention to the development of prevention and surveillance approaches. Despite some criticism about GPA's "biomedical" focus and the views of some more conservative and religious organizations, the program never lost its emphasis on preventing HIV transmission through its promotion of "safer sex" practices (like condom use and partner reduction) and the uptake of harm-reducing, drug injection practices. GPA also played an important role in research and development and broad distribution of prevention technologies, such as male condoms, female condoms, and rapid diagnostic HIV tests. We also supported some of the earliest research in developing countries on behavioral approaches to HIV prevention, microbicides, and prevention of mother to child transmission using short course antiretroviral drug treatment, which lead to an understanding of the role of breastfeeding in HIV transmission. GPA also facilitated research at the national level more broadly by establishing priorities, identifying partner institutions, training behavioral researchers, ensuring laboratory quality, and providing research funding.[130] In the area of surveillance, GPA collaborated with the CDC to pioneer "Epinfo" and "EpiMap," software programs that facilitated research and analysis of surveillance data on HIV/AIDS.[131] And throughout, GPA strove to meet rigorous

---

[129] Ibid, 68.

[130] Ibid, 72.

[131] Ibid, 72.

ethical standards and employ the most cost-effective intervention strategies and technologies, respecting the full equity, dignity, and autonomy of its developing nation partners.[132]

GPA also deserves credit for the attention it gave to preventing HIV transmission by reducing the incidence of sexually transmitted diseases (STDs).[133] GPA brought together existing knowledge about the role STDs[134] played in HIV transmission, improved STD case management through development of diagnostic algorithms and syndromic approaches, and encouraged the coordination and integration of STD and HIV control efforts among primary health care providers.[135] There is a consensus today that strong STD prevention, testing, and treatment can play a vital role in comprehensive programs addressing sexual transmission of HIV.[136] As King Holmes has said, "how much progress has there been in vaccine development or in behavioral interventions or youth education…I think the move we made to mainstream or to integrate STDs into many programs had, at the national level, a substantial impact."[137]

Beginning with some of Fakhry Assaad's earliest efforts, creating successful strategies and programs to safeguard national blood supplies was one of GPA's crowning achievements. Blood-borne transmission is the most efficient mode of HIV infection, and its presence in the blood product network portends the greatest population-level risk. In light of this, GPA developed a framework and produced technical guidelines to ensure countries could safeguard their blood supply and blood transfusion services. These efforts increased public confidence in medically supervised blood services in numerous countries and greatly diminished the threat of HIV transmission via those means. GPA's actions had the additional benefit of safeguarding the overall safety of national blood systems from blood-borne infections transmitted similarly to HIV, as well as strengthening the adoption of universal precautions in health care settings.[138]

Importantly and, though not well appreciated, GPA was also the first to take up the challenge of developing a comprehensive paradigm for care and support for HIV-infected persons in developing countries at a time before antiretroviral treatment was available. This specified the various steps, transitions, and strategies for providing "care across a continuum" and home-based care. Some of this involved training health care workers on the safe care of people with AIDS. Beyond that, GPA developed and validated staging systems to ensure consistent clinical assessment for care of people with AIDS. We also articulated guidelines for treatment of

---

[132] Ibid, 69.

[133] Ibid, 69.

[134] For the purposes of this text, we use the term sexually transmitted disease(s) and the abbreviation STD rather than the other term sexually transmitted infection(s) or STIs.

[135] Ibid. 69.

[136] Ibid.

[137] King Holmes, Interview by Michael Merson, New Haven, CT, September, 2002.

[138] Global Programme on AIDS, "Global Programme on AIDS, 1987–1995: Final Report with Emphasis on 1994–1995 Biennium." Geneva: World Health Organization, 1995, 69, 72.

AIDS-related comorbidities, including tuberculosis, and opportunistic infections in resource-poor settings. In all this effort, GPA championed an emphasis on anti-discrimination as a means of ensuring ethical care management, effective linkage to care, and successful care adherence for and among people living with AIDS.[139]

The world also owes a great deal of appreciation to GPA in general, and Jonathan Mann in particular, for the emphasis GPA placed on anti-discrimination and human rights protections for people living with AIDS at a time when stigma against those infected and affected by AIDS was at its greatest. This is by no means a battle yet won, but few can deny that from the very beginning of the pandemic· Mann and GPA became essential catalysts in the movement to include vulnerability analysis and human rights protections in the implementation of public health interventions. As Daniel Tarantola said at the time of Mann's death: "Jonathan was a critical player … bringing together two worlds that had never spoken to each other: the world of doctors and scientists and medical officials, with the world of human rights activists and lawyers. They had two completely different jargons, and there was at first only cacophony. But now they speak."[140] Just as Amartya Sen has modeled the reciprocal relationship between development and freedom, Mann and GPA tried to operationalize the relationship between health and freedom.

This integration of health and human rights was perhaps best exemplified by the integration of activists and people living with AIDS into the formulation of global health governance. As we note above, UNAIDS is rightly lauded for being the first, and as of this writing only, UN agency to include civil society organizations in its governance structure. But it was GPA that laid that foundation by being the first WHO program to provide support directly to NGOs working at country level, and it is something for which GPA veterans can be truly proud.

In the late 1980's, at a time of great uncertainty as to the extent and impact of the pandemic, WHO provided much needed direction and leadership to the global response. While confronting what was primarily a health problem, it recognized from the onset that a multisectoral response was needed to ultimately control the pandemic and strove to achieve this through its own efforts, but more importantly, by promoting greater involvement of its UN partners. Perhaps in hindsight, GPA could have been more aggressive in promoting an expanded response and in welcoming and facilitating the involvement of other UN agencies, though as events developed, we suspect this would not have prevented GPA's dissolution and the establishment of UNAIDS.

However imperfect our efforts at GPA, the story of the global fight against AIDS should never be told without reference to the valiant efforts of GPA and its WHO predecessors, the Control Programme on AIDS (CPA) and the Special Programme on AIDS (SPA). As Suzanne Cherney (Picture 16.1), our Communications officer who had worked with so many GPA staff so aptly told me, "I will always remember being very impressed by the intelligence and level of achievement that I found

---

[139] Ibid, 69–70.

[140] Philip J. Hilts, "Jonathan Mann, AIDS Pioneer, Is Dead at 51", *New York Times*, September 4, 1998.

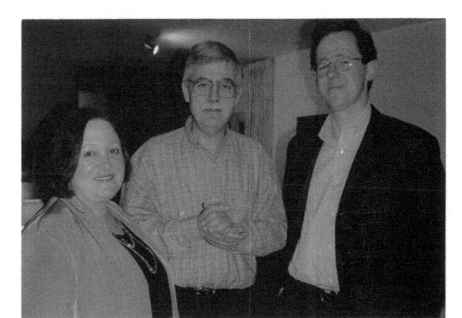

Picture 16.1 Suzanne Cherney, Michael Merson, and Stef Bertozzi in Geneva. Source: Michael Merson

among my colleagues—and their motivation: they were absolutely driven to do something about AIDS." [141]

As for me, my life had changed too. On December 12, 1995, the 1-year anniversary of Peter Piot's appointment as Executive Director of UNAIDS, I sat down and wrote him a letter. I was now happily situated at the Yale School of Public Health and working to develop an HIV research center. I promised to collaborate with UNAIDS if those plans went forward. More importantly, however, I sought just to reconnect after a particularly turbulent period in both our lives. The previous weekend, Cherney had visited New Haven, Connecticut, and had shared with me the tough time Piot was enduring with some of the cosponsors. For me, it was a time of hectic tranquility; it was nice to be out of the conflict I had undergone in my last years at WHO, as my days at Yale brimmed with activity. For Piot, it had clearly been a tumultuous year, and despite the excitement of the program launch, he would undoubtedly continue to battle in the years to come. I expressed hopes that he was "making progress recruiting good staff and winning [the] confidence of the donors," and that "even the cosponsors ha[d] accepted the reality of the program ... [and were] being supportive." I closed by giving him my support and, appreciating the sensitivities my involvement might entail, offering to help in any way I could. It would be some time though before I would have that opportunity.

---

[141] Email to Michael Merson from Suzanne Cherney, Aug 13, 2015.

Chapter 17
UNAIDS: Trying to Gain Traction

As Peter Piot looked out his hotel window across the harbor, he was in a pensive mood. It was the summer of 1996, and he was attending the 11th International Conference on AIDS in Vancouver, Canada. Piot had been Executive Director of the Joint United Nations Programme on HIV/AIDS (UNAIDS) for half a year, and this AIDS Conference served as something of his coming out party. To Larry Altman of *The New York Times*, a non-celebratory mood must have seemed out of place and out of character given the circumstances. The conference brimmed with a growing excitement about the promise of new combination therapy with antiretroviral drugs (ARVs). Indeed, as Altman met and mingled with other leading researchers at the conference, he had found their "hopes as high as the sun-drenched mountains surrounding [the] Canadian seaport."[1] New anti-HIV drugs—protease inhibitors—had just recently been approved by the United States Food and Drug Administration (FDA), and increasingly there were reports that they left people with AIDS[2] "bounc[ing] back from their deathbeds."[3] Some researchers struggled to contain their excitement. "We can't claim victory until the fat lady really sings," one prominent researcher told Altman. "She hasn't sung yet, but I think she is getting ready to sing."[4] "There's a period of excitement—and even optimism—that we haven't had before," AIDS researcher Paul Volberding told

---

Within this chapter the singular pronouns *I* and *my* refer to Michael Merson alone, whereas the plural pronouns *we* and *us* generally refer to Michael Merson and Stephen Inrig jointly. Where *we* or *us* refers to Michael Merson and his colleagues at WHO, the object of the pronoun is clarified by context.

[1] Lawrence K. Altman, " Exuberant Mood of AIDS Meeting Reflects Progress," *Contra Costa Times*, Sunday, July 7, 1996, D01.

[2] For the purposes of this text, we will use the term AIDS to encompass both AIDS and HIV unless otherwise specified.

[3] David Perlman, "A Bit Less Gloom in AIDS Battle—Optimistic backdrop to world conference," *The San Francisco Chronicle*—Friday, July 5, 1996, A1.

[4] Lawrence K. Altman, "Exuberant Mood of AIDS Meeting Reflects Progress," *Contra Costa Times*, Sunday July 7, 1996, D01.

© Springer International Publishing AG 2018

M. Merson, S. Inrig, *The AIDS Pandemic*, DOI 10.1007/978-3-319-47133-4_17

The San Francisco Chronicle. "It's possible today to dare think we might have the tools to eradicate the virus entirely from patients—that's still only a possibility, but it's now our goal."[5]

But Piot was more reserved. With the scenic port in view, Piot agreed that a more upbeat mood than usual pervaded the conference. "[The] advances in treatment and the emergence of evidence that AIDS prevention efforts—in Thailand and Uganda, for example—are beginning to pay off." Piot said in an interview.[6] But these facts did not bolster Piot's state of mind. These new therapies would likely have little impact on the AIDS pandemic: they were far too expensive. "The AIDS gap around the world remains," Piot told a San Francisco journalist. "Where the epidemic is at its worst people cannot hope to benefit from the new drugs."[7] 90% of people living with HIV resided in low- and middle-income countries, Piot explained. "At best, they can only dream of palliative treatment for some of the infections that AIDS causes."[8]

There was only one real hope, Piot told Altman: "Developed countries should act out of 'enlightened self-interest' to ensure adequate treatment of AIDS in the Third World." If they didn't, access to the new drugs would at best be partial, and partial access maximizes "the chances of resistant strains developing from improper use of drugs."[9] If developed nations wanted to avoid resistant strains of HIV eventually migrating back to them from the low- and middle-income countries, they needed to raise funds and lower drug prices. Piot felt that much of the responsibility for getting developed nations to take such action rested on his shoulders.

UNAIDS opened its doors on the first day of 1996, a year that would prove to be very important in AIDS treatment and prevention. It was in 1996 that researchers announced breakthroughs in AIDS treatment through a triple ARV regimen known as Highly Active Antiretroviral Therapy or HAART. The ensuing decrease in AIDS deaths and hospitalizations would suggest to many that a cure had been found for AIDS and that the end of the pandemic lay in sight.[10] While these claims proved sadly unfounded, HAART along with other advances in therapy gave Piot and others working in UNAIDS tremendous hope. In addition to these breakthroughs was the equally exciting news that HIV infections were starting or continuing to drop in several countries, including some developing nations like Thailand. The hard work of activists and health workers alike was starting to pay off, and UNAIDS stood poised to capitalize on these successes, a new organization for a new era in the battle against AIDS.

---

[5] David Perlman, "A Bit Less Gloom in AIDS Battle—Optimistic backdrop to world conference," *The San Francisco Chronicle*—Friday, July 5, 1996, A1.

[6] Ibid.

[7] Ibid.

[8] Ibid.

[9] Lawrence K. Altman, "Exuberant Mood of AIDS Meeting Reflects Progress," *Contra Costa Times*, Sunday, July 7, 1996, D01.

[10] Newsweek, around that time, had a cover entitled, "The End of AIDS."

Despite these very positive developments in AIDS care and prevention, UNAIDS faced considerable challenges. The pandemic continued to plague many countries, and it was uncertain whether UNAIDS would be able to slow its spread. Donors and cosponsors expected Piot and his team to advocate for increased political and financial support for AIDS, create an evaluation framework for national AIDS programs, organize country-level coordinating bodies (known as theme groups), and provide them with information on "best practices" for national AIDS strategies.[11] All this was expected at a time of shrinking budgets among donors, ongoing denial among affected countries, and a creeping apathy among Western nations. The frequently bickering UNAIDS cosponsors—the United Nations Children's Emergency Fund (UNICEF), United Nations Development Programme (UNDP), United Nations Population Fund (UNFPA), United Nations Educational, Scientific and Cultural Organization (UNESCO), World Health Organization (WHO), and the World Bank—had agreed to increase resources for AIDS, expand public/private partnerships, mobilize those resources and partnerships in affected countries, and coordinate with other cosponsors at the national level. However, having been forced into this agreement by donor nations, it still remained to be seen whether the vision of a joint and cosponsored program could actually become a reality.

UN theme groups were not unique to UNAIDS; they had been created by the UN in emergency situations. What was different with regard to UNAIDS was that the UN Theme Groups on HIV/AIDS were institutionalized mechanisms, permanent, rather than ad hoc and situational entities. The intent was that they would reduce duplication of effort and competition for funds in countries, allowing the UN to "speak with one voice" about AIDS in every country.[12] Their members consisted of a UNAIDS "Country Program Adviser", the heads of the various cosponsoring UN agencies in each country, donor representatives, and other interested parties (namely, national and international non-governmental organizations [NGOs]). Led by the Resident Coordinator—the highest-ranking UN official in each country and usually a UNDP employee—their task was to "plan, manage, and monitor" the actions of the different UN agencies in the country and coordinate the various AIDS "actors" at the national level. These theme groups were meant to bring the disparate assets of the various UN agencies together into a collective whole that would best support a country's specific AIDS-related needs. It was also thought that they might help make relationships between NGOs and governments more efficient as diverse NGOs all clamored for support.

---

[11] "HIV/AIDS: USAID and UN Response to the Epidemic in the Developing World; Report to Congressional Requesters, July 1998," Washington, DC: General Accounting Office, 1998, GAO/NSIAD-98-202.

[12] Lindsay Knight. *UNAIDS: the first 10 years, 1996–2006*, New York: Joint United Nations Programme on HIV/AIDS (UNAIDS), 2008.

An additional task of UNAIDS was to collect, model, and disseminate sound epidemiological data about the pandemic. One of the key concerns of the Global Programme on AIDS (GPA) Taskforce on HIV/AIDS Coordination during the latter years of GPA was that data on HIV and AIDS cases and deaths were coming from several different sources within the UN (WHO and UNDP) and external to it. For example, Jonathan Mann and his Global AIDS Policy Coalition (GAPC) had created its own surveillance system that differed widely from the one at GPA, and the United States Census Bureau had developed a unique HIV/AIDS Surveillance Data Base with funding from the United States Agency for International Development (USAID).[13] Within the UN, responsibility for collecting, modeling, and disseminating global HIV and AIDS prevalence and incidence rates transferred from WHO to UNAIDS in 1996. Robert Moodie, an Australian physician with years of field experience working for NGOs and the inaugural UNAIDS Director of Country Support, and Stef Bertozzi, now UNAIDS Deputy Director of Policy, Strategy, and Research, began working with staff at the Centers for Disease Control and Prevention (CDC), the United States Census Bureau, and GAPC to coordinate these different surveillance efforts. In November 1996, the UNAIDS/WHO Working Group on Global HIV/AIDS and Sexually Transmitted Infection Surveillance was created to generate the best available data on the pandemic. This group sponsored a 1997 meeting at the United States Census Bureau in Washington, DC, attended by the various stakeholders, to coordinate their country-level data and synchronize their data collection and analysis methodology. This group quickly congealed into the UNAIDS Reference Group on Estimates and Modeling, which in 1998 published its first set of authoritative HIV surveillance numbers for distribution at the 12th International Conference on AIDS in Geneva. Whereas before, WHO and UNAIDS had only been able to provide regional estimates of HIV prevalence, at the 1998 conference UNAIDS was also able to provide specific estimates for 180 different countries. This was clearly a very significant early achievement for UNAIDS.

Equally important, UNAIDS began to serve as the main reservoir for global AIDS policy and prevention strategies. For example, its Division of Policy, Strategy, and Research aimed to ameliorate the tensions that existed between GPA and UNDP by creating "multisectoral" approaches that spanned the biomedical and developmental perspectives. To help craft this expanded approach, UNAIDS brought together experts from cosponsoring agencies, service providers, policymakers, researchers, academics, and activists. It also made an effort to synthesize research on harm reduction techniques and on the "contextual, socioeconomic factors that determined the vulnerability of people," which included poverty, gender inequity, and the forces behind migration.[14] These documents were initially conceived as reference tools that fulfilled UNAIDS' original man-

---

[13] US Census Bureau, "HIV/AIDS Surveillance." Washington, DC: US Department of Commerce. Cited at http://www.census.gov/population/international/about/; accessed May 22, 2012.

[14] Lindsay Knight. *UNAIDS: the first 10 years, 1996–2006*, New York: Joint United Nations Programme on HIV/AIDS (UNAIDS), 2008, 63.

date to "achieve and promote global consensus on policy and programmatic approaches," through the specific identification, development, and advocacy of global best practices.[15] Sometimes, as UNAIDS Director of External Relations Sally Cowal noted, these devolved into little more than politically correct messages. "We never had billions of dollars to do our own research, so we fell back on the best practices and then we got to political correctness sensitivity," she recalls. Since UNAIDS had to rely on others for much of these best practices, they were of variable quality, a situation that Cowal lamented. "So I think we lost that sense of saying, 'We're the experts' ... I think we sort of lost our way there."[16] Nevertheless, despite these limitations, the series of "guidelines, updates and policy papers to case studies, handbooks, and examinations of particular challenges and responses" were heralded as UNAIDS' Best Practices Collection, which by the end of 2010 included around 150 publications across a broad range of topics.[17]

For national programs to be successful, Piot and his colleagues stressed the importance of courageous leadership. Perhaps the best example of this was President Yoweri Museveni of Uganda, his national program leaders, and innovative NGOs like The AIDS Support Organization (TASO), who had worked closely with GPA (see Chapter 9) and continued their strong relationship with UNAIDS. In December 1997, Piot lionized the Ugandans for their bold approach to AIDS.[18] Uganda's unflinching and comprehensive strategy, accessible and context-appropriate activities, considerable resource commitment, and strong national leadership proved to the global community just how successful a national anti-AIDS effort could be when political will aligned with evidence-based practices and robust support.[19] There were other examples: Mexico's President Ernesto Zedillo backing a UNAIDS-supported safer sex campaign in the face of vocal political and religious opposition; Thailand's sustained effort to control AIDS among its sex worker and injection drug user populations; Senegal's multisectoral response that brought religious communities and NGOs into the prevention effort (see Chapter 10).[20] Like GPA before it, UNAIDS encouraged research in behavioral and technological interventions, ranging from condom social marketing to sex worker empowerment to the development of vaccines

---

[15] Sue Funnell, "An Evaluation of the UNAIDS Best Practices Collection," Geneva: UNAIDS, November 1999, 1.

[16] Sally Cowal, Interview by Michael Merson, New Haven, CT, February, 2002.

[17] Lindsay Knight. *UNAIDS: the first 10 years, 1996–2006*, New York: Joint United Nations Programme on HIV/AIDS (UNAIDS), 2008, 64; "Learning from Experience," Geneva: Joint United Nations Programme on HIV/AIDS, January 19, 2007, http://www.unaids.org/en/resources/presscentre/featurestories/2007/january/20070119bestpracticehistory/. Accessed on May 22, 2012.

[18] Lindsay Knight. *UNAIDS: the first 10 years, 1996–2006*, New York: Joint United Nations Programme on HIV/AIDS (UNAIDS), 2008, 64.

[19] Werasit Sittitrai, "HIV Prevention Needs and Successes: A Tale of Three Countries," Geneva: UNAIDS, 2001, 9–14.

[20] Ibid, 5–19.

and vaginal microbicides. However, because of limitations in resources Piot decided that UNAIDS would not directly support research as GPA had done.[21]

UNAIDS also devoted considerable attention to mother to child transmission of HIV. Much had changed since GPA's conflicts with UNICEF in this area, and more specifically over breastfeeding in the early 1990s (see Chapter 13). The most significant development was that researchers in the United States had shown, in a multicenter randomized control trial, that initiating antiretroviral therapy (ART) to pregnant and lactating women substantially reduced the risk of mother to child transmission to rates below 10%.[22] Admittedly, the drugs were still expensive, and most women in developing nations were unable to afford them. Also, the CDC and Thailand's Public Health Ministry had jointly conducted a trial, supported first by GPA and then by UNAIDS, exploring whether a short course regimen of ART combined with breast milk substitutes reduced vertical HIV transmission among infected pregnant women.[23] Consequently in March 1998, USAID requested, and UNAIDS hosted, a consultation on the prevention of vertical HIV transmission, where the participants recommended that HIV-infected mothers receive a selection of "infant feeding options" if they chose not to breastfeed their infants, and receive support from their providers regardless of their choice.[24] While this was not the robust endorsement of breast milk substitutes for HIV-positive mothers that UNAIDS had hoped for, it was nonetheless progress. It would be some time before UNICEF moved more substantively on the issue, but at least two positive steps came out of this consultation: First, UNAIDS created a new task force with membership from UNICEF, UNFPA, and WHO—the Inter-Agency Task Team on Mother-to-Child Transmission—to "develop and publish

[21] Peter Piot, *No Time to Lose: A Life in Pursuit of Deadly Viruses*. New York: Norton, 2012.

[22] Centers for Disease Control and Prevention. "Zidovudine for the prevention of HIV transmission from mother to infant," *MMWR*, 1994 Apr 29;43(16):285–7; P.Cotton, "Trial halted after drug cuts maternal HIV transmission rate by two thirds." *JAMA*. 1994 Mar 16;271(11):807. J. Oleske, A. Bardequez, "Research shows AZT therapy reduces mother-child AIDS transmission." *New Jersey Medicine*, 1994 Apr;91(4):274; CDC. "Recommendations of the U.S. Public Health Service Task Force on the Use of Zidovudine to Reduce Perinatal Transmission of Human Immunodeficiency Virus." *MMWR*, August 05, 1994;43 (No. RR-11); 1–20; C. Peckham. "Mother to child transmission of the human immunodeficiency virus." *New England Journal of Medicine* 1995;333:298–302; "Zidovudine for the prevention of HIV transmission from mother to infant." *MMWR* 1994;43:285–7; Edward M. Connor, Rhoda S. Sperling, Richard Gelber et al. "Reduction of maternal-infant transmission of human immunodeficiency virus-type 1 with zidovudine treatment." *New England Journal of Medicine* 1994;331:1173–80; M. Rogers and Harold Jaffe. "Reducing the risk of maternal-infant transmission of HIV: a door is opened." *New England Journal of Medicine* 1994;331:1222–3.

[23] Jon Cohen. "Bringing AZT to poor countries." *Science* 269.5224 (1995): 624–6; "Ethics of Placebo-Controlled Trials of Zidovudine to Prevent the Perinatal Transmission of HIV in the Third World," *New England Journal of Medicine* 1998; 338:836–841.

[24] Arjan de Wagt, David Clark, "UNICEF's Support to Free Infant Formula for Infants of HIV Infected Mothers in Africa: A Review of UNICEF Experience," *Linkages*, April 14, 2004.

guidelines and recommendations" on mother to child transmission.[25] Second, in 1998 UNICEF began a pilot program in 11 countries that enabled governments to provide free formula to HIV-positive women.[26] Still, UNAIDS garnered considerable criticism for not pushing harder to develop a more evidence-based policy on breastfeeding.[27]

One reason that UNAIDS' supporters felt it stood a good chance of succeeding as an agency was that it would have more freedom than either UNDP or WHO had ever had to involve researchers, businesses, faith communities, people living with AIDS, and other parts of civil society in the battle against AIDS. Many of these relationships had started in the days of GPA and they grew further under UNAIDS. Key to many of them was the aforementioned UNAIDS Director of External Relations Sally Cowal, who excelled at the intensive process of building partnerships.[28] Cowal's experience in the United States State Department allowed her to think beyond the field of health, and she fully understood the value of involving broader communities. Piot hired Cowal after he met her in Geneva (she had recently served for 3 years as the United States Ambassador to the Republic of Trinidad and Tobago). Cowal understood the UN well, cared deeply about UN reform, and could help him navigate the American political system ("[Piot] wanted somebody who could tell him the difference between Jesse Jackson and Jesse Helms," Cowal told me). Thinking beyond health was essential, Cowal argued, because in the mid-1990s, AIDS had moved off many peoples' agenda. "I think there was this early flurry in the 1980s when we thought the girl next door was really at risk," Cowal explained.

> "But then [attention] really plummeted so that it was, by the time we got there, at least in terms of the United States, in 1995, it was off the charts. So to move it from off the charts, on the back burner, to 2000 when United Nations Ambassador Richard Holbrooke is saying, 'I think this is the most important crisis the world faces.' We were the ones who really made AIDS a security issue. I know that doesn't fit perfectly [with the public health model], but you've got to do something to wake people up. So how did we do that—well, I started on the Council on Foreign Relations and got Peter talking to breakfasts and really made some movement in saying, 'This is not a health crisis'."[29]

UNAIDS worked particularly hard to build relationships with nontraditional partners at the country level. To begin with, UNAIDS theme groups intentionally brought NGOs to the table. Beyond that, UNAIDS built off of the commitment of the Paris AIDS Summit (which had occurred in late 1994) to include people with HIV in

[25] Lindsay Knight. *UNAIDS: the first 10 years, 1996–2006*, New York: Joint United Nations Programme on HIV/AIDS (UNAIDS), 2008.

[26] Arjan de Wagt, David Clark, "UNICEF's Support to Free Infant Formula for Infants of HIV Infected Mothers in Africa: A Review of UNICEF Experience," *Linkages*, April 14, 2004.

[27] UNAIDS (2002). *Five Year Evaluation of UNAIDS*. Geneva, UNAIDS, cited in Lindsay Knight. *UNAIDS: the first 10 years, 1996–2006*, New York: Joint United Nations Programme on HIV/ AIDS (UNAIDS), 2008.

[28] Lindsay Knight. *UNAIDS: the first 10 years, 1996–2006*, New York: Joint United Nations Programme on HIV/AIDS (UNAIDS), 2008.

[29] Sally Cowal, Interview by Michael Merson, New Haven, CT, February, 2002.

national AIDS programs[30] and to make strong connections with networks of people living with HIV. UNAIDS' Community Mobilization Adviser, Noerine Kaleeba, helped establish relationships with these networks in Africa, Asia, and the Pacific Islands, ensuring that countries involved people with AIDS in the development and implementation of their national AIDS programs (Kaleeba had played a key role in creating one such network, TASO in Uganda,[31] and, as we described in Chapter 10, she hosted my first visit to that country in 1990). A prime example of this was a UNAIDS' program that helped strategically place people with HIV in government agencies, NGOs, and local businesses.

UNAIDS also forged relationships with communities of faith across the religious spectrum.[32] While GPA had involved a variety of religious groups as observers and participants in various consultations, UNAIDS made an intentional effort to "develop a broad-based coalition" of partners. Piot was initially critical of the church, but soon came to realize that "they are an essential part of that [coalition]."[33] UNAIDS Partnerships Development group worked with Protestant groups providing AIDS care and support in Southern Africa, partnered with Imams crafting AIDS prevention programs in Uganda, and collaborated with the Vatican and Catholic charities on development and social justice concerns across the globe (though they remained at an impasse on condoms).

UNAIDS also pressed hard to connect with the business community, both small local businesses and major multinational corporations. AIDS was relevant to these companies for a variety of reasons, but mainly because of AIDS-related health care costs, employee productivity, and domestic economic outlooks. With upwards of 37% of increased labor costs attributed to HIV-related absenteeism in some African businesses, national and multinational corporations could ill afford to ignore the problem. In 1996, UNAIDS hosted a meeting of business leaders to discuss the potential economic impact of AIDS and the importance of workplace AIDS prevention, and in 1997 the program hosted plenary sessions, panel discussions, and working group discussions on "business in the world of AIDS" at the World Economic Forum in Davos, Switzerland. The latter was far better attended than the session on the AIDS pandemic that I had participated in at Davos 5 years earlier. UNAIDS also supported innovative projects to create workplace AIDS prevention programs. Admittedly, before 2001 few major corporations organized such programs, but it was in these early years that UNAIDS developed the infrastructure for them.[34]

All these bridge-building efforts spoke to one of UNAIDS' primary missions: to overcome apathy and ignorance and raise awareness about the AIDS pandemic. The 11th International Conference on AIDS in Vancouver in July 1996 was the program's first big opportunity to combat the apathy that GPA had found so intractable,

---

[30]"Paris Declaration," Paris AIDS Summit - 1 December 1994, European Coalition of Positive People; http://www.ecpp.co.uk/parisdeclaration.htm

[31]Lindsay Knight. *UNAIDS: the first 10 years, 1996–2006*, New York: Joint United Nations Programme on HIV/AIDS (UNAIDS), 2008.

[32]Ibid.

[33]Ibid.

[34]Ibid.

while trying to explain the role the joint and cosponsored program would play in the global response to the pandemic. UNAIDS' task might have proved more difficult at earlier conferences, since most of them had carried the pall of pessimism and controversy (the 1994 conference in Yokohama, Japan perhaps stands out in this regard in the wake of the disappointing news about the short-term efficacy of azidothymidine (AZT) (see Chapter 11). As we mentioned earlier, the inauguration of UNAIDS coincided with an auspicious time in the world of AIDS treatment: the advent of protease inhibitors. Protease inhibitors targeted the viral protease enzyme and prevented the reproduction of virus.[35] The first protease inhibitor gained FDA approval in late 1995, and shortly thereafter a trial of two reverse transcriptase inhibitors produced by Glaxo Wellcome (the successor to Burroughs-Wellcome) with one of Merck's protease inhibitors showed dramatic decreases in viral load in the blood of subjects receiving these drugs.[36] Other companies found similarly dramatic results.[37] Thus, the halls of the 1996 Vancouver conference reverberated with the hope that this combination therapy might hold the promise of effective treatment.

While conference planners used "One World, One Hope" as the conference theme to cultivate this newfound spirit of promise, UNAIDS staff were also careful to highlight the costs associated with these new drugs (not to mention the earlier developed drugs). As mentioned above, UNAIDS was concerned that this optimism exuded by the AIDS community was potentially displaced because it was limited to people who could afford the new breakthroughs in therapy. "It remains unacceptable that people living with AIDS, especially but not only in the developing world, should have to live without the essential drugs they need for their HIV-related illnesses," Piot told conference participants, "Most of these drugs could be made accessible . . . if governments had the right drug policies."[38] With the new treatments almost certainly rendering HIV a manageable, chronic disease, Piot called on funders and researchers to "turn the global AIDS research agenda on its head. Nine out of 10 HIV infections occur in the developing countries, where people are desperate for a vaccine. Ignoring the research needs of 90% of the epidemic is not just unethical; it is irrational."[39] In taking this stance, Piot was following in the footsteps of GPA, as both Jonathan Mann and I had advocated at various levels to make AIDS

[35] Hung Fan, Ross Conner, Luis Villarreal, *AIDS: Science and Society*, 4th ed., Sudbury, MA: Jones and Bartlett Publishers, 2004. p. 62.

[36] Lawrence K. Altman, "3-Drug Therapy Shows Promise Against AIDS," *The New York Times*, January 30, 1996, C5.

[37] Lauran Neergaard, "FDA: New AIDS Drugs Are Promising," *The Charlotte Observer*, November 5, 1995, 2A; Lauran Neergaard, "FDA Panel Oks New AIDS Drug," *The Charlotte Observer*, November 8, 1995; John Schwartz, "FDA Panel Oks New AIDS Drug," *The Charlotte Observer*, November 8, 1995, 1A; Lauran Neergaard, "FDA Oks Drugs That Retard AIDS Virus," *The Charlotte Observer*, December 8, 1995, 10A; Lawrence K. Altman, "3-Drug Therapy Shows Promise Against AIDS," *The New York Times*, January 30, 1996, C5; Daniel Q. Haney, "AIDS Therapy With 3 Drugs Appears To Stall Disease," *The Charlotte Observer,* January 30, 1996, 4A.

[38] David Perlman, "Worry, Hope At AIDS Conference: Breakthroughs have too high a price for many," *San Francisco Chronicle*, July 8, 1996, A1.

[39] Ibid.

drugs more accessible to those in the worst-affected countries. He was also reflecting a growing movement to increase drug access. This was embodied best by Brazil's decision, at the end of 1996, to provide ART to people with HIV through its public health system (see Chapter 10).[40] Two years later, the movement spread to South Africa with the founding of The Treatment Action Campaign (on December 10, 1998), but in this case it was activists and not the government that mobilized "to ensure that people living with HIV got access to safe and effective treatment, anti-retroviral medicines in particular."[41]

UNAIDS advocated strongly for treament access following the 1996 conference. At the third meeting of UNAIDS' Program Coordinating Board (PCB) in 1996, Board members requested that UNAIDS increase its "activities in the areas of access to ART drugs."[42] Citing the "affordability gap" on AIDS-associated therapies, UNAIDS unveiled its HIV Drug Access Initiative the following November under the leadership of Joseph Perriens, a Belgian physician. GPA had recruited Perriens into the Clinical Research and Development Unit in 1992 and, over time and working closely with Joep Lange, he became one of the most knowledgeable persons globally on AIDS treatment and drug access. The Drug Access Initiative partnered with some of the leading pharmaceutical companies to increase access to ARVs in four countries (Chile, Uganda, Vietnam, and Côte d'Ivoire).[43] The project led to real, though marginal, cuts in the prices of some ARVs,[44] but more importantly, it showed that, "with moderate investment in the supply chain and in clinical service delivery, mainly training and some investment in laboratory infrastructure, it was possible to generate positive treatment outcomes with antiretrovirals in low-income countries."[45] Moreover, as Perriens later told me, he had "built a collaboration with the producers of ART that enabled them to test the ground as to whether differential pricing was a hugely risky strategy for them."[46] While UNAIDS was criticized for not including generic drugs in the original structuring of the Drug

[40] Francisco Inácio Bastos, Deanna Kerrigan, Monica Malta, Claudia Carneiro-da-Cunha, and Steffanie A. Strathdee, "Treatment for HIV/AIDS in Brazil: strengths, challenges, and opportunities for operations research," *AIDScience* Vol. 1, No. 15, November 2001, accessed at http://aid-science.org/Articles/aidscience012.asp

[41] Marcus Low, Catherine Tomlinson, Mara Kardas-Nelson, Kay Kim and Nathan Geffen, *Fighting for our lives: The history of the Treatment Action Campaign, 1998–2010.* Cape Town, SA: Treatment Action Campaign, 2010, 3.

[42] Lindsay Knight. *UNAIDS: the first 10 years, 1996–2006,* New York: Joint United Nations Programme on HIV/AIDS (UNAIDS), 2008, 68.

[43] *Access to drugs: UNAIDS Technical Update.* Geneva: UNIADS, October 1998, *WC 503.2,* 11.

[44] Gaston Djomand, Thierry Roels, Terence Chorba, "HIV/AIDS Drug Access Initiative: Preliminary Report," Projet RETRO-CI, May 2000. http://pdf.usaid.gov/pdf_docs/Pnacl667.pdf, accessed on May 24, 2012; B. Schwartländer, I. Grubb, J. Perriëns. "The 10-year struggle to provide antiretroviral treatment to people with HIV in developing countries." *The Lancet,* 2007, 368():541–546.

[45] B. Schwartländer, I. Grubb, J. Perriëns. "The 10-year struggle to provide antiretroviral treatment to people with HIV in developing countries." *The Lancet,* 2007, 368:541–546.

[46] Joseph Perriens, Interview by Michael Merson, Geneva, September, 2001.

Access Initiative, it eventually did incorporate them into the future plans for the initiative.[47] I also learned from Perriens that the initiative actually had its origins in 1995 near the end of GPA, which is when his discussions started with Glaxo Wellcome and Bristol Meyers Squibb. The subsequent and far more expansive Accelerating Access Initiative, launched in 2000, built upon the success of the Drug Access Initiative.[48]

In an effort to translate the optimism of the Vancouver Conference into a renewed global commitment to AIDS, UNAIDS in 1997 launched its "World AIDS Campaign." The idea behind this campaign was that, while World AIDS Day had focused attention on the global AIDS pandemic for 1 day per year, AIDS was truly a year-round problem that required a "year-round campaign." Building off World AIDS Day, UNAIDS planned to choose a different theme annually, which would incorporate advocacy and programmatic elements while allowing countries to tailor specific strategies to their national needs.[49] That first year, both to highlight an issue that all the cosponsors could support and to launch the campaign in the most socially acceptable fashion, UNAIDS chose the theme "Children living in a world with AIDS." Other themes in future years included: concentrating on men; discrimination; women and girls; and meeting global commitments in the fight against AIDS.[50] The reality was, however, that with the advent of protease inhibitors, UNAIDS found many Western activists still too preoccupied with drug access in their own countries to exert additional energy on the problem of access in the low- and middle-income countries.

This perception fueled the theme of the 12th International Conference on AIDS in Geneva in July, 1998, which focused on "the growing gap between the North and the South in access to treatment."[51] The mood at the Geneva conference resembled the pessimism that had hung over the earlier Yokohama Conference. This was largely the result of the realism that had set in about how much further progress was needed to make HAART available, and was a stark contrast to the optimism sparked at the Vancouver conference. Also, and as mentioned earlier, UNAIDS had just published country specific HIV and AIDS estimates for the first time drawing attention to the devastating effect the pandemic was having in low- and middle-income countries. This glum mood extended past the conference as UNAIDS found itself battling global inertia on several fronts, with Piot publicly decrying what he saw as "the gap between what we know we can do today and what we are actually doing."[52]

---

[47] B. Schwartländer, I. Grubb, J. Perriëns. "The 10-year struggle to provide antiretroviral treatment to people with HIV in developing countries." *The Lancet*, 2007, 368:541–546.

[48] Peter Piot *No Time to Lose: A Life in Pursuit of Deadly Viruses*. New York: Norton, 2012, 303–310.

[49] Lindsay Knight *UNAIDS: the first 10 years, 1996–2006*, New York: Joint United Nations Programme on HIV/AIDS (UNAIDS), 2008.

[50] Ibid.

[51] Ibid, 86.

[52] Ibid, 87.

One of the greatest challenges for UNAIDS from the outset was the inconsistent actions of the donor community. On one hand, donor countries had strong expectations about accountability. According to Piot, "the donors were constantly asking, 'Where are the results? What are you doing?'"[53] When it was established, its staff size was half that of GPA.[54] Stef Bertozzi explained UNAIDS' mentality: "We certainly had the sense we could be leaner and meaner. There was this sort of cowboy sense in the team that we were going to have a new way of doing things; that we were going to be able to be more effective per person and therefore more cost-effective and therefore in need of fewer resources."[55]

However, the donors would not provide substantive financial support for the program, curtailing UNAIDS' budget significantly: Piot's budget of $60 million per year was about 15% less than GPA's final budget had been.[56] Even then, however, it was difficult for Piot to raise this amount of funds. For example, Piot reported to the PCB in March 1997 that UNAIDS had only received 25% of the $18 million it had requested to fund cosponsor programs during the 1996–1997 biennium.[57] "Some donors were really determined to keep this small." Piot recalled.[58]

For Bertozzi, the donor actions were "completely unconscionable." "The rhetoric was not matched by the actions," he explained. "In theory they were doing this to strengthen the response. In practice they were cutting their funding. It was completely hypocritical."[59] Bertozzi acknowledged that establishing a program like GPA with a smaller budget was logical, but insufficient. The donors needed to "complement that with additional funds that went ... through UNAIDS back to the other agencies so as to create true mainstreaming with the necessary funds."[60] By mainstreaming, he meant that the cosponsors were to use existing funds within their organizations for activities undertaken on behalf of all the cosponsors. Others involved in the process put it more bluntly: Jeff O'Malley, who had become the Founder and Executive Director of the NGO International HIV/AIDS Alliance, told us that he thought "the donors, collectively, wanted a way out and the donors like nothing more than blaming a UN agency...the donors wanted to spend less."[61] "Everybody thought that UNAIDS should be the new GPA" Lars Kallings, who left GPA in 1993 to return home to Sweden, recalled, "but it didn't materialize and it was not thought to be so. In a way the donor

[53] Ibid.

[54] Michael Balter, "Global Program Struggles to Stem the Flood of New Cases," *Science*, June 19 1998, 280(5371):1863–1864.

[55] Lindsay Knight. *UNAIDS: the first 10 years, 1996–2006*, New York: Joint United Nations Programme on HIV/AIDS (UNAIDS), 2008.

[56] Michael Balter, "Global Program Struggles to Stem the Flood of New Cases," *Science*, June 19 1998, 280(5371):1863–1864.

[57] Lindsay Knight. *UNAIDS: the first 10 years, 1996–2006*, New York: Joint United Nations Programme on HIV/AIDS (UNAIDS), 2008.

[58] Peter Piot, Interview by Stephen Inrig, Dallas, TX, February 2, 2011; "Proposed Programme Budget, 1996–1997." Geneva: Joint United Nations Programme on HIV/AIDS, October 1995.

[59] Stefano Bertozzi, Interview by Michael Merson, New Haven, NC, December, 2002.

[60] Ibid.

[61] Jeff O'Malley, Interview by Michael Merson, New Haven, CT, September, 2002.

countries deceived the developing countries."[62] "In retrospect," Bertozzi would later conclude, "it was unrealistic and in some ways cruel for the donors to expect that UNAIDS would suddenly catalyse all this mainstreaming that would magically be squeezed out of the regular budgets of the cosponsors."[63]

In fairness to the donors, however, the cosponsors were not giving UNAIDS the support it needed. The different and often competing priorities of the six cosponsoring agencies made coordination at country level, much less at a global level, a difficult task. "[It] is like walking six cats on a leash," Mann explained to one journalist, when asked in 1998 about Piot's challenge.[64] Cosponsors across the spectrum resisted cooperation with UNAIDS and with each other. "It was incredibly difficult," Piot recalled when we interviewed him. "Nobody helped, really... I was in the system, so I went to activists, to NGOs, to help."[65] WHO's absence particularly troubled Piot and Bertozzi, "WHO did not even believe that we would start the program," Piot recalled. "I got one year to build up the organization, and they underestimated that I could do that, and didn't help also."[66] When serving as Interim GPA Director Bertozzi recalled "I even sat in a meeting with the assistant Directors-General and [Hiroshi] Nakajima where they were discussing how they could ensure the failure of UNAIDS so that it could come back to WHO."[67]

There was no doubt personal issues involved in the establishment of UNAIDS and the lack of support it received from WHO. UNAIDS was in part a response by Western donors against Nakajima. As Ken Bernard whom we mentioned earlier had played an important role in the establishment of UNAIDS, explained, "Since [AIDS] was clearly a health issue, we couldn't take it away and give it to UNDP, we couldn't move it to another agency, it was clear that WHO had primacy. However, what about an interesting idea of actually putting together a simple, small secretariat that can actually take over and be in charge, thereby making sure that Nakajima loses control. This was a Nakajima thing, but it was not punishment, it was based on incompetence."[68] As we explained in the previous chapter, losing GPA to UNAIDS did not sit well with Nakajima. "He was so mad about that," surmised Bernard. "He saw this as ripping the principle public health issue in the world today out of the principle public health agency."[69] Moreover, as we explained earlier, Nakajima was enduring profound criticism from within WHO—particularly the Regional Directors, who claimed that "Nakajima had sold WHO out."[70] Nakajima had already suffered a similar insult in 1992 with the founding of the Children's Vaccine

[62] Lars Kallings, Interview by Michael Merson, New Haven, CT, September, 2002.

[63] Lindsay Knight. *UNAIDS: the first 10 years, 1996–2006*, New York: Joint United Nations Programme on HIV/AIDS (UNAIDS), 2008.

[64] Michael Balter, "Global Program Struggles to Stem the Flood of New Cases," *Science, June 19 1998, 280(5371):*1863–1864.

[65] Peter Piot, Interview by Stephen Inrig, Dallas, TX, February 2, 2011.

[66] Ibid.

[67] Stafano Bertozzi, Interview by Stephen Inrig, October 22, 2010.

[68] Ken Bernard, Interview by Michael Merson, New Haven, CT, February, 2002.

[69] Ibid.

[70] Hu Ching Li, Interview by Michael Merson, New Jersey, August, 2002.

Initiative, seen by many in WHO as an attempt to take control of global vaccine development and delivery by the other partners involved (UNICEF, UNDP, the World Bank, the Rockefeller Foundation, and the Task Force for Child Survival).[71] Nakajima, therefore, felt little incentive to contribute to UNAIDS' success.

Others in WHO felt similarly spurned. There were rental problems, administrative problems, and the Regional Directors gave little cooperation in the regions.[72] George Alleyne, Regional Director for the Pan American Health Organization (PAHO) at the time, had conceptual difficulties with UNAIDS: "I thought that [AIDS] was a health problem and that it should have been managed by a health agency—and any coordination should have been done by a health agency."[73] Jo Asvall, WHO Regional Director for Europe during this period, remembered "we were absolutely furious because we said, 'Look, you think you are going to control this because you have the first chair [of the cosponsoring organizations], and so on. But you are very naïve if you think so.' ... So we were livid at that meeting—but he had already committed the WHO with the other UN leaders."[74] S. T. Han, then-Regional Director for WHO's Western Pacific region, told me "Judging from the situation prevailing at the time, when Dr. Nakajima's management of WHO was very much under scrutiny, one could surmise that the decision taken by the donor countries was based more on political rather than substantial considerations. I still strongly believe that it should have remained within WHO."[75]

After GPA closed down, WHO did, in fact, establish a very small AIDS program office in Geneva, with three staff members, while the Regional Directors largely established AIDS programs on their own, disconnected from WHO headquarters and only occasionally connected to UNAIDS.[76] Under the UNAIDS framework, WHO was to continue to support national sexually transmitted disease (STD)[77] and HIV prevention and control programs, and to integrate these efforts with other AIDS-related programs (Blood Safety, Tuberculosis, Maternal and Child Health, Reproductive Health, and Health Promotion) so the regional offices focused on these as well.[78] Dorothy Blake, who had been my Deputy

[71] William Muraskin, *The Politics of International Health: The Children's Vaccine Initiative and the Struggle to Develop Vaccines for the Third World* (Albany: State University of New York Press, 1998), cited in Theodore M. Brown, Marcos Cueto, and Elizabeth Fee, "The World Health Organization and the Transition From 'International' To 'Global' Public Health," *Am J Public Health.* 2006;96:62–72.; William Muraskin, "Origins of the Children's Vaccine Initiative: The intellectual foundations," *Social Science & Medicine* June 1996, 42(12): 1703–1719.

[72] See, for example, Dorothy Blake, "Signed Letter of Agreement between WHO and UNAIDS," Geneva: World Health Organization, May 13, 1996, JW/cch/A21/372/2.

[73] George Alleyne, Interview by Michael Merson, New Haven, CT, August, 2002.

[74] Joe Asvall, Interview by Michael Merson, January, 2002.

[75] S.T. Han, Interview by Michael Merson, New Haven, CT, August 30, 2012.

[76] Hu Ching Li, Interview by Michael Merson, New Jersey, August, 2002.

[77] For the purposes of this text, we use the term sexually transmitted disease(s) and the abbreviation STD rather than the other term sexually transmitted infection(s) or STIs.

[78] "First Planning Meeting on HIV/AIDS and STD, Geneva, 7–9 May, 1996: Regional Programme Statement for 1998–1999 programme budget," Geneva: World Health Organization, 1996, 4/6, 2; HIV/AIDS and Sexually Transmitted Diseases: WHO Policy and Strategic Orientations," Geneva: World Health Organization, May 1996, Rv. 12, 5.

Director, was appointed, upon my recommendation, as Senior Adviser on HIV/ AIDS and in this capacity served as WHO's primary contact person with UNAIDS. However, this turned out to be a rocky relationship. "My sense is that WHO gave it all up and stopped doing [its AIDS programs]," recalled Neil Boyer, the then United States State Department representative to the WHO Executive Board. "And when Peter [Piot] had relations with WHO it was [with] Dorothy Blake, who as it was explained to me, was very bitter and refused to let WHO staff talk to anyone from UNAIDS. Everything had to be channeled through her and she was being very restrictive and uncooperative."[79] Piot and Bertozzi did not see their interactions with Blake quite so personally: "My perception at the time [and] Peter's perception at the time," recalled Bertozzi, "was that she was doing Nakajima's bidding to make it as likely as possible that UNAIDS did not succeed."[80] Whether or not Blake was bitter herself, acting as Nakajima's proxy, or both, in trying to sabotage UNAIDS, she apparently felt that UNAIDS left WHO (and the other cosponsors) with an unclear identity and a vague work directive that lacked "concrete activities corresponding to objectives."[81] As Bernard put it: "We were just completely frustrated with WHO at the time—they weren't even doing blood safety, for heaven's sake. They had just abandoned anything to do with AIDS, it was like: "OK, I'm just out of here, have fun with UNAIDS, we're not doing this anymore."[82]

When Piot would meet with the Regional Directors, according to Nakajima's close colleague Claire Chollat-Traquet, they would complain that his presentations lacked clarity and precision and left them disappointed. Moreover, they wanted to keep and expand their own regional programs, and Piot was unable to provide them the financial support to do so. Also, according to Chollat-Traquet, they felt "UNAIDS was too focused on the social and development aspects of the pandemic and not paying enough attention to the public health aspects."[83] The hostility of the Regional Directors, the indifference of Nakajima, and the independence of the regional offices made it difficult for UNAIDS to establish a firm footing.

Thus, a corrosive spiral emerged: WHO headquarters resisted providing technical support to Piot and UNAIDS; Piot and UNAIDS in return chose to work with those groups who often operated outside WHO's traditional public health approach because they were the ones that wanted to collaborate. And when WHO's Regional Directors sought help from Piot and UNAIDS, they found it to be insufficient both technically and financially and thus did not deem UNAIDS worthy of further collaboration or support.[84]

---

[79] Neil Boyer, Interview by Michael Merson, New Haven, CT, January, 2002.

[80] Stefano Bertozzi, Interview by Michael Merson, New Haven, NC, December, 2002.

[81] Dorothy Blake, "WHO's Comments on UNAIDS Workplan; Memorandum to P. Piot," Geneva: World Health Organization, June 7 1996, As2-372-2.

[82] Ken Bernard, Interview by Michael Merson, New Haven, CT, February, 2002.

[83] Claire Chollat-Troquet, Interview by Michael Merson, New Haven, CT, August 12, 2002.

[84] Gunilla Ernberg, Interview by Michael Merson, New Haven, CT, August, 2002.

WHO cannot be held completely culpable in this estranged relationship, however. The reality was that Piot and his team felt, and we think rightly so, that for UNAIDS to succeed, it had to be perceived as different from GPA. This was made more difficult by UNAIDS' physical location—situated as it was on WHO's campus—and by the makeup of its staff. "There was for many of us this issue—we were defining ourselves as different," Bertozzi explained. "Needing to define oneself as the 'other' with respect to GPA … was an issue emotionally for people in the building to the extent that there was a split personality. Many of the UNAIDS staff were former GPAers—so it was a self-hatred kind of thing which was emotionally difficult. Peter himself had been GPA."[85] WHO staff who did not move over to UNAIDS complained about constantly hearing negative comments about WHO, and staff in UNAIDS felt considerable hostility towards WHO or GPA. On this count, Bertozzi demurs: "I think that if you create a new program in a very painful way, then there is a very understandable need to justify … causing the pain. Why did we need to shut GPA down? … Why couldn't it do what it was supposed to do? All kinds of things come into that, including that it wasn't being led the right way, that it didn't have the right people, it didn't have the right way of doing things (it was too bureaucratic and old school WHO)."[86] As Piot himself explains, "Retrospectively I made a mistake when I agreed that our program could be housed within the WHO campus. I should have broken more radically with their bureaucracy. The old WHO Global Programme on AIDS was still operational, and it was very uncomfortable to cohabitate between the past and the future."[87]

Whatever the explanation, the result could not have been more unfortunate: UNAIDS distanced itself from WHO, WHO virtually stopped its AIDS program, and tensions continued to flare between UNAIDS and WHO. The strain also occurred because UNAIDS needed other cosponsors to collaborate: UNICEF particularly feared that UNAIDS was or would be "GPA-lite."[88] However one wants to assign blame, the consequences were very unfortunate, the response to global AIDS was profoundly diminished at one of the most critical times in the pandemic's history, when it was likely that the annual number of HIV infections was reaching its peak.[89] "The right thing for WHO to have done," Bertozzi concludes, "was to say, 'We may have lost a battle here, it may have been damaging for the organization—but clearly the best way out of it is to show that UNAIDS will succeed because of WHO's support.'"[90] With UNAIDS being so closely aligned with WHO in mission

---

[85] Stefano Bertozzi, Interview by Michael Merson, New Haven, NC, December, 2002.

[86] Ibid.

[87] Peter Piot *No Time to Lose: A Life in Pursuit of Deadly Viruses*. New York: Norton, 2012, 226–227.

[88] Lindsay Knight. UNAIDS: the first 10 years, 1996–2006, New York: Joint United Nations Programme on HIV/AIDS (UNAIDS), 2008.

[89] Eleanor Gouw, "EPI Alert: Methods for estimating HIV incidence" *UNAIDS Quarterly Update on HIV Epidemiology* Geneva: UNAIDS, 1Q, 2010. http://www.unaids.org/sites/default/files/media_asset/epi_alert_1stqtr2010_en_0.pdf

[90] Stefano Bertozzi, Interview by Michael Merson, New Haven, NC, December, 2002.

and location, no other UN agency had as much opportunity to both ensure UNAIDS' success....and to take credit for UNAIDS' success. But that didn't happen, and it took some time for UNAIDS to make up the ground that had been lost during the transition from GPA.

Pausing here, I should say that I was unaware of these tensions. I heard very little from anyone in UNAIDS or in WHO during the first few years after my departure. I suspect this was because neither agency wanted to consider me a friend. On the one hand I was persona non grata within WHO for "giving up GPA,"and on the other hand UNAIDS wanted to demonstrate how it was different from WHO so was reluctant to seek advice from the former GPA Director. When I did hear about the tensions, as I reflected in the previous chapter, I wished that I could have done more before I left WHO to help UNAIDS and WHO avoid them.

The lack of cooperation from the other cosponsors also cannot be ignored here. As former United States Surgeon General Jocelyn Elders observed, "Collaboration is an unnatural act among non-consenting adults."[91] This was certainly true for UNAIDS.[92] At UNDP, for example, Elizabeth Reid seemed uninterested in collaborating with UNAIDS, maintaining a relatively rocky relationship with Piot and the rest of the organization.[93] Part of this stemmed from the fact that she disagreed with Piot's approach to the pandemic, just as she had previously disagreed with both Mann and myself. "You have a set number of things [to do] because you have to show that something is being done," Reid's Deputy, Mina Mauerstein-Bail, explained. "[And once they start, people tended not] to go back and say, 'well, was this the way to do it or not?' I remember Elizabeth saying that."[94] In Reid's opinion, Piot and UNAIDS were simply retracing GPA's steps, rather than rethinking the entire approach. Certainly Piot and UNAIDS were committed to addressing the issues around vulnerability that so concerned Reid and UNDP. "I make the distinction between getting a document out and having meetings," explained Mauerstein-Bail, "[and] actually working differently to facilitate things happening on the ground."[95] "And that was one of the reasons that her relationship with Peter was very difficult," Mauerstein-Bail concluded.[96]

In addition, Reid was dissatisfied with the final shape of UNAIDS. Her vision, recalled Jeff O'Malley, "was a very small UNAIDS secretariat that focused on global advocacy and a unified work plan, but with funding and technical staff posts spread amongst the cosponsors in their relevant technical areas."[97] Functionally, however, this meant that Reid and UNDP carefully guarded its mandate and were

---

[91] Christopher Wilson, "Finding the Middle Ground in a Spectrum of Collaboration," Presentation at the Knowledge Exchange Forum, 2010, Ottawa, ON, Canada, November 24, 2010. www.slideshare.net/cwilson_ottawa/phac-knowledge-exchange-forum-nov-2010. Accessed March 4, 2013.

[92] Ken Bernard, Interview by Michael Merson, New Haven, CT, February, 2002.

[93] Mina Mauerstein-Bail, Interview by Michael Merson, New Haven, CT, September, 2002.

[94] Mina Mauerstein-Bail, Interview by Michael Merson, New Haven, CT, October, 2001.

[95] Ibid.

[96] Ibid.

[97] Jeff O'Malley, Interview by Michael Merson, New Haven, CT, September, 2002.

reluctant to give it up for the sake of improved coordination and non-redundancy. Consequently, Reid continued to operate her UNDP HIV and Development Program essentially independent of UNAIDS.[98] Piot frequently tried to bring UNDP's program under the UNAIDS umbrella, but constantly met with resistance.[99] Bertozzi explained the practical implications of this stance:

> If you recall that, at the end of that year [1995] and at the beginning of the following year [1996], WHO had rolled over. GPA was being amputated from WHO and going into UNAIDS. UNDP in theory was doing the same thing, but in practice they weren't. They were fighting tooth and nail to keep their HIV unit as an HIV unit. So UNDP's HIV unit was not being amputated and folding into UNAIDS... The perception was, however true it is, that the fight and vision and operation between WHO and UNDP and their inability to present a unified and technical front to the world, were much of the reason why UNAIDS had to be created, so that meant that to be successful, UNAIDS needed to amputate them both. Then it could recreate them and mainstream them or whatever, but it needed to amputate them both. Now, since UNDP wasn't going along, we couldn't be in a position of pushing [technical programs back] into WHO while fighting UNDP to cut [its HIV program] off. Because then it appeared to be a personal issue with the leadership of the HIV unit. It would have been inconsistent... [This went on] for a very long time.[100]

Thus, according to Bertozzi, one of the reasons why UNAIDS had difficulty at the outset in leading the global response was that UNDP still had its own independent AIDS program. That while the donors had forced WHO to close down GPA, they had not forced UNDP to abandon its program. Essentially, for the first few years of UNAIDS, UNDP had leverage to undermine and circumvent UNAIDS. Ironically, the result remained the same: the divisive competition between UNDP and GPA that helped necessitate the creation of UNAIDS morphed into competition between UNDP and UNAIDS, severely impeding UNAIDS' initial efforts. It also illustrates all too well how the donor community failed to support the organization it had created supposedly to enhance the global response to the AIDS pandemic. It would not be until Reid (at UNDP) and Nakajima (at WHO) left their respective positions after 1998 that UNAIDS could begin to make real progress.

UNICEF also had mixed feeling about the establishment of UNAIDS. In part, as we mentioned, this stemmed from its suspicion that UNAIDS—having recruited many GPA staff, being located on the WHO campus, and thus having the potential to absorb so much of the GPA/WHO culture—would merely become GPA-lite. UNICEF, being one of the strongest and most well-known UN agencies, sought to safeguard its own role by promoting UNAIDS structures most aligned with its own self-interest.[101] As explained earlier (see Chapter 16), Jim Sherry, UNICEF's representative to the interagency group that helped to create UNAIDS, held strong views with regard to

---

[98] The UNDP HIV and Development Program continued its own independent way of operations. It would continue in this fashion until early 1998.

[99] See, for example, Peter Piot, "Letter to Elizabeth Reid: US State Department Request, March 28, 1995." Geneva: Joint United Nations Programme on AIDS, 1995, GPA-A20/372/30.

[100] Stefano Bertozzi, Interview by Michael Merson, New Haven, NC, December, 2002.

[101] Gillian Holmes, Interview by Michael Merson, Geneva, October, 2001; Nils Kastberg, Interview by Michael Merson, New York City, September, 2002.

the responsibilities of the secretariat in the joint and cosponsored program.[102] Similar to Reid at UNDP, Sherry had wanted a small, relatively weak UNAIDS secretariat—in his case, one largely confined to knowledge sharing—and so he was displeased with the decision to create a more robust organizational structure. This latter approach, Sherry felt, was too bureaucratic, though he realized that UNICEF's preferred option could be seen as insufficient to address the complex problems that the pandemic presented.[103] While UNICEF's opposition was not inconsequential, it had much less of an impact than UNDP's, because as Bertozzi explained, "UNICEF lacked an HIV unit (unlike UNDP), so its noncompliance, however real, remained largely conceptual."[104] Moreover, Sherry's opposition could not have been too severe, since he joined UNAIDS as Senior Advisor to the Executive Director soon after the program launched.

Several of these collaboration issues eventually worked themselves out at country level through the launch of the aforementioned UN theme groups on HIV/AIDS. There were a number of challenges to making this happen, though. The first was getting all the UN cosponsors around the same table, something a UN Resident Coordinator could not necessarily achieve. In some countries, the cosponsors were more concerned about guarding their "territory" than in providing one UN voice to advise and support governments in combating AIDS. Additionally, country-based staff of the various UN cosponsors felt little accountability for the theme group's success. For example, in Dominican Republic, the cosponsoring agencies worked well together, even initiating joint projects, while in others like Honduras and India, the agency representatives rarely met.[105] Clement Chan-Kam, who had joined the Country Program Support team at GPA in 1991 and became head of UNAIDS' Asia Pacific region, explained some of the tensions: "You might have a supportive theme group Chair but you might have a Resident Coordinator who's at odds with the theme group Chair. You might have a very strong civil society … perpetually in combat with authority and you are kind of caught between the two."[106] Piot and the UNAIDS staff eventually addressed these issues by having each of the cosponsor's headquarters send information on the roles and responsibilities of the theme groups to their field staff. However, the theme groups' success was still at the mercy of the individual whims, personalities, and interests of the staff in each country.

The second challenge was that each UN agency had already developed its own relationships with different government ministries in the years before UNAIDS was established. Bringing coherence to these different relationships and experiences was by no means easy to achieve. For many UNAIDS Country Program Advisors (CPAs),

[102] Marjorie Dam, Interview by Michael Merson, New Haven, CT, September 29, 2001.

[103] Helene Gayle, Interview by Michael Merson, New Haven, CT, February, 2002; Nils Kastberg, Interview by Michael Merson, New York City, September, 2002.

[104] Stefano Bertozzi, Interview by Michael Merson, New Haven, NC, December, 2002.

[105] "HIV/AIDS: USAID and UN Response to the Epidemic in the Developing World; Report to Congressional Requesters, July 1998," Washington, DC: General Accounting Office, 1998, GAO/NSIAD-98-202.

[106] Lindsay Knight. *UNAIDS: the first 10 years, 1996–2006.* New York: Joint United Nations Programme on HIV/AIDS (UNAIDS), 2008, 50.

this was the most difficult part of their work. For example, Tony Lisle, a former Save the Children Fund manager who served as one of UNAIDS's first CPAs in the Lao People's Democratic Republic, not only had to contend with the head of one cosponsoring agency who refused to meet with him, but also with Ministry of Health staff who had been advised by this same individual not to cooperate with him.

A third challenge was that these theme groups brought with them no extra resources, but did generate a host of expectations: some inflated, some more pessimistic. A number of theme groups did bring together representatives from donors, UN agencies, and NGOs who had previously not had (or not felt they had) any role to play in addressing the AIDS problem in a given country. While this helped national AIDS programs adopt an expanded approach to AIDS, it also meant that these parties (particularly NGOs) felt disappointed when these programs under-delivered. Also, there were some donors and recipient nations who considered theme groups "an untested and untried mechanism" that carried considerable startup costs and logistical expenses at the time of a widening and worsening pandemic.[107]

A final challenge was the dramatic drop in funding that national AIDS programs faced. In the 1994–1995 biennium, GPA had provided about $29 million in financial support to national programs, funds that were used by many program managers to maintain their staff and program activities. In 1996, with the launch of UNAIDS, such funds were no longer available, either from the theme groups or UNAIDS, leaving program managers understandably upset and greatly concerned. "There is a considerable decrease in financial support to the national program from UNAIDS compared to GPA in the past," wrote B. Sadrizadeh, Director of Integrated Control of Disease in the WHO Eastern Mediterranean regional office in Alexandria, Eygpt, in an October 1996 letter to Dorothy Blake. "UNAIDS support is less than one quarter of what GPA used to provide."[108] "The thing the countries looked at most critically was, here we were with GPA and we could count on a certain quantum of resources coming to us," George Alleyne recalled. "Now this new agency is formed and we cannot see the same quantum resources. That of course hurt them and several of the programs slowed—our (regional) program … was shrunk down to virtually very little."[109]

Had the developing countries known that the establishment of UNAIDS would have gutted GPA's financial support to national programs, it is unclear if they would have voted for the World Health Assembly resolution calling for the establishment of the joint and cosponsored program. We suspect they would have not done so. But that was not the whole story. Reflecting back on the process, Mauerstein-Bail from UNDP noted: "Just the meetings alone [to establish UNAIDS] … went on for 2 years…So time was lost then, and then just setting up a new institution took time.

[107] Ibid.

[108] B. Sadrizadeh, "Letter to Dorothy Blake, Re: Committee of Cosponsoring Organization (CCO), 24 October 1996, New York," Geneva: World Health Organization, 1996, A21/87/3.

[109] George Alleyne, Interview by Michael Merson, New Haven, CT, August, 2002.

They had a handful of people … added all together, 3 to 4 years were lost… in terms of working on the epidemic, time was lost."[110]

Tragically, this picture of lost momentum was cemented—at least symbolically, by the death of Jonathan Mann and his wife, Mary Lou Clements, a vaccine scientist, when their Swissair plane flying from New York to Geneva crashed off the coast of Nova Scotia on September 2, 1998. Mann was headed to WHO to meet with the new Director-General of WHO, Gro Bruntland, Peter Piot, and others, to discuss the possibility of his joining UNAIDS in some capacity.[111] Clements, whom I knew well from her earlier days conducting diarrheal diseases vaccine research, was attending an HIV vaccine meeting at UNAIDS. (Jose Esparza, who organized this meeting, has kept Clements' name badge). I learned about Mann's death through a phone call from Robin Ryder, an epidemiologist and infectious disease physician who had taken over Mann's position in *Projet SIDA* after he left for WHO, and who was on my faculty at the Yale School of Public Health. I was very shaken by the news. Later that evening I sobbed for hours while watching the television coverage of the accident and seeing Mann's picture repeatedly flashing across the screen.

Though we both remained active in AIDS work, Mann and I had seen each other just once in the 3 years since I left GPA... in 1996, at the International AIDS Conference in Vancouver. In the intervening years I had successfully set up an AIDS research center at Yale with funding from the National Institute of Mental Health, while Mann had become the Director of the Francois-Xavier Bagnoud Center for Health and Human Rights in the Harvard School of Public Health. Then, in January 1998, he was named the founding Dean of the Allegheny University School of Public Health (now Drexel School of Public Health), located in Philadelphia. Mann's trajectory since resigning from WHO in 1990 had been filled with highs and lows: he had launched a journal on health and human rights, organized the first world conference on health and human rights, and had done considerable work to address various aspects of the global AIDS pandemic through his Global AIDS Policy Coalition. However, despite the prominence and cache Harvard provided him, he had lost the platform, budget, and infrastructure that his position at GPA had afforded him. The move to Philadelphia offered a future of new possibilities, though the school's shaky financial state (unrelated to Mann) might have given him some trepidation about what he could achieve there. I suspect he was looking forward to new options and greater plans when he boarded the plane with his wife bound for Geneva.

The Harvard School of Public Health hosted a memorial service for Mann on September 27, 1998. I struggled over whether or not to attend and, in the end, decided not to do so. Why? I feared that it might upset those in attendance who may still have resented that I had succeeded Mann as GPA Director, and who possibly believed there was bad blood between us. Thus, they might have found my presence hypocritical, and I certainly did not desire to be a distraction. What none of them knew was that Mann and I had reached something of a rapprochement in October 1995

---

[110] Mina Mauerstein-Bail, Interview by Michael Merson, New Haven, CT, October, 2001.

[111] Peter Piot, *No Time to Lose: A Life in Pursuit of Deadly Viruses*. New York: Norton, 2012, 249.

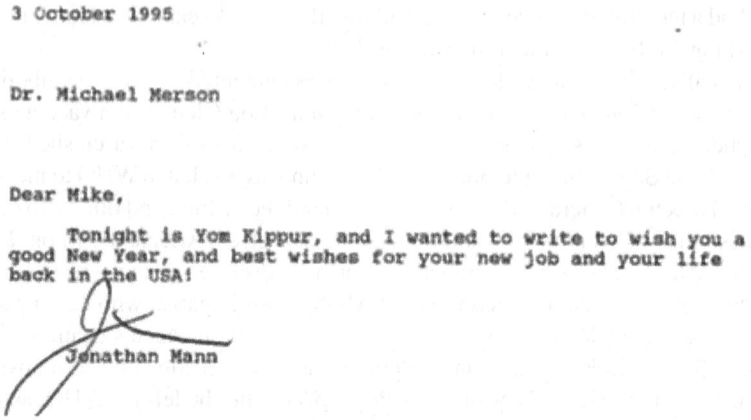

3 October 1995

Dr. Michael Merson

Dear Mike,

    Tonight is Yom Kippur, and I wanted to write to wish you a
good New Year, and best wishes for your new job and your life
back in the USA!

Jonathan Mann

Fig. 17.1 Letter from Jonathan Mann to Michael Merson. Source: Michael Merson

when, 6 months into my time at Yale, Mann sent me a letter on the Jewish High holiday of Yom Kippur (the Day of Atonement) wishing me the best for the future (Fig. 17.1). It was a nice gesture, I felt, and I thought that perhaps in time we could have found ways to work together. I had never fully understood why he chose to leave GPA and was hoping that, when I wrote this book, I would have an opportunity to ask him whether given the chance, he would have done things differently. Unfortunately, I never had that opportunity. I did attend the memorial service for Mary Lou Clements, which was held on September 16 at the Johns Hopkins School of Public Health. I briefly met Mann's family there and expressed my condolences, though I was not comfortable doing so. I had no idea how they felt about me and I felt a measure of guilt, that in the years after receiving his letter, I did not reach out and try to build better ties with him. His tragic death certainly symbolized the end of an era in the global fight against AIDS. It was a sad reminder that so much had been lost and many great challenges remained.

Chapter 18
UNAIDS: Finding its Place in Congested Waters

While the late 1990s were at times difficult for the Joint United Nations Programme on HIV/AIDS (UNAIDS), there were signs that the situation was improving. Two changes occurred that would help alter the global AIDS[1] landscape and strengthen UNAIDS. First, the World Health Organization (WHO) underwent a change in its leadership. In 1998, WHO's Executive Board nominated the Prime Minister of Norway, Gro Harlem Brundtland, to succeed Hiroshi Nakajima as WHO Director-General. Nakajima had decided not to seek a third term, a decision applauded by the United States and other countries. He had lost support from most African nations after attributing the relative scarcity of Africans in executive positions in WHO to their difficulty in conceptualizing and writing reports.[2] Initially, Brundtland was cautious about expanding WHO's AIDS activities, not necessarily keen on collaboration with other United Nations (UN) agencies, but not wanting to upset the donor governments who had established UNAIDS and helped greatly to advance her election.[3] However, the now-declining price of antiretroviral drugs (ARVs) implicitly demanded that countries improve their health systems to facilitate access to them. (Ironically, these developments required much greater WHO involvement in the global response, causing one to wonder whether the move to UNAIDS would have occurred if Highly Active Antiretroviral Therapy [HAART] had been discovered and made affordable a few years earlier.)

Within this chapter the singular pronouns *I* and *my* refer to Michael Merson alone, whereas the plural pronouns *we* and *us* generally refer to Michael Merson and Stephen Inrig jointly. Where *we* or *us* refers to Michael Merson and his colleagues at WHO, the object of the pronoun is clarified by context.

[1] For the purposes of this text, we will use the term AIDS to encompass both AIDS and HIV unless otherwise specified.

[2] Douglas Martin, "Hiroshi Nakajima, Leader of W.H.O., Dies at 84," *The New York Times,* January 28, 2013; Craig Turner, "U.N. Health Agency Director Says He'll Resign," *Los Angeles Times*, May 01, 1997.

[3] Ken Bernard. Interview by Michael Merson, New Haven CT, February, 2002; Henderson, Ralph. Interview by Michael Merson, NH February 2003.

© Springer International Publishing AG 2018

M. Merson, S. Inrig, *The AIDS Pandemic*, DOI 10.1007/978-3-319-47133-4_18

Consequently, over the next 2 years, Brundtland and UNAIDS' Executive Director Peter Piot, who by this time was keen to devolve many of UNAIDS' activities to the cosponsors, agreed that WHO should substantially enlarge its AIDS program staff and seek more resources from UNAIDS to provide more technical advice and support to countries.[4] By the end of 2001, WHO's AIDS program had expanded from its original three staff (in the immediate post-Global Programme on AIDS [GPA] era) to approximately 50 individuals situated in an HIV Department under the direction of Bernhard Schwartlander, a medical epidemiologist from Germany who had served as UNAIDS' Director of Evaluation and Strategic Information and led UNAIDS' efforts to integrate various HIV and AIDS surveillance data. In May 2003, Schwartlander released the first Global Health Sector Strategy on HIV/AIDS, written in response to a request from the World Health Assembly (WHA).[5]

The second change which occurred was that, by 1998, Elizabeth Reid was no longer at the helm of the United Nations Development Program (UNDP) HIV and Development Program; she had moved to Papua New Guinea to be the UN Resident Coordinator and Resident Representative for UNDP. While this did not remove all the existing tensions between UNDP and UNAIDS, it did open the way for better coordination among the cosponsors. This was facilitated by Piot's openness to having the cosponsors implement AIDS activities within their areas of expertise.[6] Thus, after 1998, UNAIDS began expanding its organizational breadth and depth as it evolved from "an underfunded substitute" for the UNDP and GPA AIDS programs to a viable entity coordinating UN AIDS activities and engaging the broader AIDS community.[7]

In the United States, the situation was changing for the better as well. Political conservatives like North Carolina Senator Jesse Helms had long stood as opponents to the UN, its programs, and the United States Agency for International Development (USAID)'s support of them and similar endeavors. He had engineered a freeze in the payment of the United States dues to the UN during most of the 1990s.[8] Helms was therefore no friend to UNAIDS or the larger fight against global AIDS. "Helms was a constant thorn in our side," recalled Paul DeLay, who, after working for 4 years for GPA in Malawi, joined USAID's Division of Global HIV/AIDS at USAID in 1991, becoming its Division Chief in 1997.[9] (He later served from 2003 to 2012 as the Deputy Executive Director of the Program Branch at UNAIDS). But in the late 1990s, with Christian activists like evangelist Franklin Graham and pop star Bono (Paul David Hewson) softening up Helms' resistance, and a new pool of

---

[4] Peter Piot.Interview by Michael Merson, New Haven, CT, October 26, 2002.

[5] Global Health-Sector Strategy for HIV/AIDS 2003-2007. Department of HIV/AIDS Family and Community Health, World Health Organization.

[6] Bertozzi SM, Martz TE, Piot P. "The evolving HIV/AIDS response and the urgent tasks ahead." *Health Affairs*. 2009 Nov–Dec;28(6):1578–90.

[7] Ibid.

[8] Greg Behrman, *The Invisible People: How the U.S. Has Slept Through the Global AIDS Pandemic, the Greatest Humanitarian Catastrophe of Our Time.* New York: Free Press, 2004, 160.

[9] Ibid, 73.

AIDS-conscious policy-makers—like the United States Ambassador to the UN, Richard Holbrooke, and Chair of the United States Senate's African Affairs Subcommittee, Tennesse Senator (and physician) William Frist—coming into leadership, the United States began taking a more proactive stance towards global AIDS.[10] As we have documented (see Chapter 14), the United States played an important role in funding global AIDS efforts through its support of GPA and UNAIDS and its bilateral programs, but this enhanced interest, particularly by political conservatives, would open the global response to a new set of opportunities. Still, these remained potential rather than kinetic changes, and in the meantime the pandemic worsened. As 1998 dawned, UNAIDS estimated that almost 12 million persons had died from AIDS since the start of the pandemic and that more than 30 million more were living with the disease. The earlier period of retrenchment at the international level had proven very costly for so many.[11]

The tide began to turn the following year. In July 1999, after a trip to Africa where he saw first-hand the breadth of devastation AIDS was wreaking on the continent, United States President Bill Clinton, along with Vice President Al Gore, launched the interagency "Leadership and Investment in Fighting an Epidemic" (LIFE) initiative.[12] Aimed at expanding United States funding for global AIDS activities in the hardest-hit countries, the effort led to a bi-partisan bill appropriating over $200 million for global AIDS in fiscal years 2000 and 2001.[13] Then, based on the work of Ambassador Holbrooke, Piot, and others, Gore chaired a UN Security Council Session on AIDS on January 10, 2000.[14] This was the first time the UN Security Council had broached a health topic, and it was, in Piot's words, "a defining moment;

---

[10] On the role of Ambassador Holbrooke and Senator Frist, see Greg Behrman, *The Invisible People: How the U.S. Has Slept Through the Global AIDS Pandemic, the Greatest Humanitarian Catastrophe of Our Time.* New York: Free Press, 2004, 158–165, 277–282; On the evolution of Jesse Helms, see Greg Barker, "Interview with Franklin Graham," in *Frontline: The Age of AIDS*, ed. Renata Simone (United States, 2006); Cathleen Falsani, "Bono's American Prayer," *Christianity Today*, February 21, 2003; Cathleen Falsani, "Mother Africa," *Christianity Today*, February 21, 2003; "Washington Wire," *Wall Street Journal*, September 22, 2000, A1; "Names & Faces," *The Washington Post*, June 14, 2001, C03; Jesse Helms, *Here's Where I Stand: A Memoir.* New York: Random House, 2005; Senator Jesse Helms, "S.2845: An original bill to authorize additional assistance to countries with large populations having HIV/AIDS, to authorize assistance for tuberculosis prevention, treatment, control, and elimination, and for other purposes. 106th US Senate, July 11, 2000; Senator Jesse Helms, "S.AMDT.4018 to H.R.3519: To authorize additional assistance to countries with large populations having HIV/AIDS, to provide for the establishment of the World Bank AIDS Trust Fund, to authorize assistance for tuberculosis prevention, treatment, control, and elimination, and for other purposes," 106th US Senate, July 26, 2000; Senator Jesse Helms, "S.2943: An Act to authorize additional assistance for international malaria control, and for other purposes," 106th US Senate, July 27, 2000.

[11] S.M. Bertozzi, T. E. Martz, P. Piot. "The evolving HIV/AIDS response and the urgent tasks ahead." *Health Affairs*. 2009 Nov–Dec;28(6):1578–90.

[12] Greg Behrman, *The Invisible People:* New York: Free Press, 2004, pp. 207, 209–211.

[13] William Clinton, "Statement on Signing the Global AIDS and Tuberculosis Relief Act of 2000, August 19, 2000," Washington, DC: Government Printing Office, 2000, 1651.

[14] Lindsay Knight. *UNAIDS: the first 10 years, 1996–2006*, New York: Joint United Nations Programme on HIV/AIDS (UNAIDS), 2008, 105.

finally AIDS was recognized as a threat to global security."[15] In the ensuing months, the Clinton Administration formally declared AIDS to be a threat to national security and on May 10, 2000, Clinton signed Executive Order 13155 aimed at helping countries in sub-Saharan Africa gain greater access to AIDS-related drugs and technologies.[16] At almost the same time, a group of Congressional Members, led by Iowa Republican Congressman Jim Leach and 30 cosponsors, submitted a bill titled the Global AIDS and Tuberculosis Relief Act of 2000, which among other things directed the Secretary of the United States Treasury to establish, within the World Bank, an AIDS Trust Fund to which it would allocate $300 million over 2 years to fight the AIDS pandemic in Africa.[17] After evangelist Franklin Graham secured the support of Helms, the measure passed the House and Senate and President Clinton signed it into law on July 26, 2000.

While the United States Congress ultimately failed to follow through on this particular measure, it did put into play the idea of providing substantial support for global AIDS efforts. With news coming out of Brazil that the government had substantially reduced its AIDS deaths and hospitalizations by providing HAART at no cost to HIV-infected individuals, and with offers by generic drug manufacturers in India to make HAART available at costs 95% below the market rate (see Chapter 10), the idea of launching some form of drug assistance fund for developing nations became not only attractive, but feasible as well.[18] During the 13th International AIDS Conference in Durban, South Africa in July 2000, which was the first international AIDS conference to be held in a low- or middle-income country and thus more than any other conference focused on the gravity of the pandemic in Africa, the attendees debated the relative priority that should be given to AIDS prevention versus treatment. This debate was now possible in light of the rapidly decreasing prices of ARVs, a trend that was accelerated as a consequence of drug access activism at the conference. I attended this conference and will never forget the keynote addresss given by Edwin Cameron, a judge on the Constituional Court of South Africa and an HIV-positive gay man, calling for universal access to ARVs. His words reverberated throughout the halls.[19]

It was at this conference as well that Jeffrey Sachs, then Director for the Center for International Development at Harvard, floated the idea of a global fund that could help countries carry out both strategies synergistically. That same month at the G8

---

[15] Peter Piot, "Commentary: 2001: a turning point in the epidemic," in *AIDS at 30: Nations at the Crossroads*. Geneva: Joint United Nations Programme on HIV/AIDS (UNAIDS), 2011, 23.

[16] B. Gellman. "AIDS is declared threat to US national security." *Washington Post*, 30 April, 2000 cited in Lindsay Knight,. *UNAIDS: the first 10 years, 1996–2006*, New York: Joint United Nations Programme on HIV/AIDS (UNAIDS), 2008, 108; http://www.gpo.gov/fdsys/pkg/FR-2000-05-12/pdf/00-12177.pdf.

[17] Rep James A. Leach. Global AIDS and Tuberculosis Relief Act of 2000 H.R.3519 [IA-1] (introduced 1/24/2000), http://thomas.loc.gov/cgi-bin/bdquery/z?d106:HR03519:@@@D&summ1& accessed on May 31, 2012.

[18] J. L. Antunes, E. A. Waldman, C. Borrell, "Is it possible to reduce AIDS deaths without reinforcing socioeconomic inequalities in health?" *Int J Epidemiol*. 2005 Jun;34(3):586–92.

[19] Edwin Cameron, "The Deafening Silence of AIDS," Plenary Presentation speech transcript for the 13th International AIDS Conference, July 2000.

summit in Okinawa, Japan, Ken Bernard, who was then the Senior Adviser for Security and Health on the United States National Security Council, and several other "senior government officials," agreed that a new global fund might be an effective vehicle to launch a multilateral assault on the pandemic.[20] Coming out of that Okinawa meeting, Bernard held a follow-up meeting in December 2000 that addressed funding AIDS, Malaria, and Tuberculosis—"three diseases that kill more than a million people a year each and for which there is no vaccine."[21]

By 2001, the idea had taken on its own momentum. Piot considered two events pivotal to this momentum.[22] The first came in February 2001, when the leaders of Caribbean nations signed the Caribbean Partnership Commitment, which helped launch the Pan-Caribbean Partnership against HIV/AIDS.[23] This called attention to the need for programming and infrastructure support among developing nations struggling against AIDS. The second came in April 2001, at the Special Summit of the Organization of African Unity (OAU) in Abuja, Nigeria, where African leaders agreed to the Abuja Declaration, which affirmed the emergency status of AIDS in Africa. It was, in Stef Bertozzi's words, a "collective breaking of the silence on AIDS by African leaders."[24] Equally important at the conference was the speech delivered by UN Secretary-General Kofi Annan, which issued a call to action around several AIDS care and prevention priorities, including: preventing further spread, minimizing mother to child transmission; increasing access to care and treatment; finding a cure/vaccine; and protecting the rights of those affected.[25]

Shortly after the Abuja Declaration, on May 11, 2001, Kofi Annan joined then United States President George W. Bush on the White House lawn to announce the goal of creating a global fund to fight HIV/AIDS, malaria and tuberculosis. Bush further announced that the United States would committ $200 million to support this new worldwide fund.[26] In addition, the momentum growing out of the earlier UN Security Council session on AIDS chaired by Gore and the September 2000 UN Millennium Summit (which adopted the Millennium Development Goals, one of which was to combat HIV/AIDS) compelled the UN General Assembly to announce it would hold a UN General Assembly Special Session (UNGASS) on HIV/AIDS in

---

[20] Greg Behrman, *The Invisible People:* New York: Free Press, 2004, 256; Ken Bernard. Interview by Michael Merson, New Haven CT, February, 2002.

[21] Ibid.

[22] Peter Piot, "Commentary: 2001: a turning point in the epidemic", in *AIDS at 30: Nations at the Crossroads*. Geneva: Joint United Nations Programme on HIV/AIDS (UNAIDS), 2011, 23.

[23] Ibid.

[24] S. M. Bertozzi, T.W. Martz, P. Piot. "The evolving HIV/AIDS response and the urgent tasks ahead." *Health Affairs*. 2009 Nov–Dec;28(6):1578–90.

[25] Peter Piot, "Commentary: 2001: a turning point in the epidemic", in *AIDS at 30: Nations at the Crossroads*. Geneva: Joint United Nations Programme on HIV/AIDS (UNAIDS), 2011, 23; S. M. Bertozzi, T.W. Martz, P. Piot. "The evolving HIV/AIDS response and the urgent tasks ahead." *Health Affairs*. 2009 Nov–Dec;28(6):1578–90.

[26] Kofi Annan calls for a 'war chest' to fight HIV/AIDS globally." May 11, 2001. C-SPAN. Available at https://www.c-span.org/video/?c4514657/kofi-annan-may-11-2001

June 2001, 2 months after the OAU summit.[27] On the day prior to UNGASS, the Kaiser Foundation sponsored a symposium on HIV prevention and care at which I was invited to speak, my last AIDS presentation at a UN-related event. The UNGASS meeting was, as the newly appointed UNAIDS Deputy Executive Director, Kathleen Cravero, would say, "a high point for everyone."[28] Not only did UNGASS formally recognize "AIDS as one of the big global issues of our time, not just a public health issue," but it resulted in a Declaration of Commitment on HIV/AIDS.[29] The Declaration formally committed countries to attaining the UN's specific Millennium Development Goal on AIDS by 2015, provided a specific guide for measurable action and outcomes, and reoriented the global community to understand that fighting AIDS required billions, rather than millions, in resources.[30]

The Declaration also added much impetus to the previous discussion at the G8 Summit in Okinawa the year before about the creation of a mechanism to increase global commitment to address the AIDS pandemic. This led to the decision by the G8 countries in their meeting in July in Genoa to establish a new Global Fund to Fight HIV/AIDS, Tuberculosis and Malaria (The Global Fund), along with a commitment to "make the Global Fund operational before the end of the year" and provide $1.3 billion towards its operations.[31] Over the next few months, with the support of the G8 countries, the Bill & Melinda Gates Foundation, and a few other donors, Kofi Annan created a Transitional Working Group for the Global Fund with an Interim Secretariat in Brussels. Thereafter, representatives from 43 countries and organizations met in three consultative meetings to decide upon the Global Fund's governance, country processes, and accountability. It was, Piot would later conclude, a "shift towards collective responsibility."[32]

In January 2002, the Global Fund to Fight AIDS, Tuberculosis, and Malaria[33] was formally launched as a public–private partnership intended to raise and distribute funds to combat these three diseases. Based in Geneva, the Global Fund was structured as a funding instrument, though its staff gave some technical support to

[27] United Nations General Assembly , "Fifty-fifth session, Agenda item 60(*b*); 55/2: United Nations Millennium Declaration," New York: United Nations, September 18, 2000, A/RES/55/2.

[28] Lindsay Knight. *UNAIDS: the first 10 years, 1996–2006*, New York: Joint United Nations Programme on HIV/AIDS (UNAIDS), 2008, 110.

[29] Declaration of Commitment on HIV/AIDS: United Nations General Assembly Special Session on HIV/AIDS, 25–27 June 2001. New York: United Nations, 2001.

[30] Peter Piot, "Commentary: 2001: a turning point in the epidemic", in *AIDS at 30: Nations at the Crossroads*. Geneva: Joint United Nations Programme on HIV/AIDS (UNAIDS), 2011, 23; S. M. Bertozzi, T.W. Martz, P. Piot. "The evolving HIV/AIDS response and the urgent tasks ahead." *Health Affairs*. 2009 Nov–Dec;28(6):1578–90.

[31] G-8 Communique, Genova, July 22, 2011, paragraph 15.

[32] Peter Piot, "Commentary: 2001: a turning point in the epidemic", in *AIDS at 30: Nations at the Crossroads*. Geneva: Joint United Nations Programme on HIV/AIDS (UNAIDS), 2011, 23.

[33] S. M. Bertozzi, T.W. Martz, P. Piot. "The evolving HIV/AIDS response and the urgent tasks ahead." *Health Affairs*. 2009 Nov–Dec;28(6):1578–90. J. L. Antunes, E. A. Waldman, C. Borrell. "Is it possible to reduce AIDS deaths without reinforcing socioeconomic inequalities in health?" *Int J Epidemiol*. 2005 Jun;34(3):586–92.

projects and programs it funded in countries. Some had hoped the Global Fund would have a very small secretariat, something similar to that of the much-heralded Global Alliance for Vaccines and Immunizations (GAVI). Instead, it developed a relatively large intergovernmental structure consisting of a Partnership Forum, Governing Board, Fund Secretariat, Technical Review Panels, and a Technical Policy and Program Support Group. Initially, some policy-makers intended to limit the Global Fund to AIDS, but Bernard convinced them that addressing tuberculosis and malaria as well would have substantial positive health and infrastructure benefits.[34] Had the Global Fund only focused on AIDS, its Secretariat might have been attached to UNAIDS and its financial operations run by the World Bank. But such a scenario would likely have never been acceptable to WHO. Moreover, from the experience of Bernard and others who had championed the structure, the concept had moved well beyond AIDS before it emerged as a proposal during the earlier G8 meeting in Okinawa.

Those who helped drive the creation of the Global Fund saw it as an important complement to UNAIDS. In any given country, UNAIDS and its cosponsors would help that country set up, develop, implement, and evaluate its national AIDS program. As Bernard explained, UNAIDS "makes sure that the national plan is vetted widely… [that] the best practices are set down, the local circumstances are taken into account, the national plan is written."[35] UNAIDS could co-ordinate how the various UN agencies contribute to execution of the plan. Then, according to Helene Gayle, (who eventually left government service to direct the AIDS program at the Bill & Melinda Gates Foundation) "there ought to be a strong WHO program that provides technical expertise and funding to the programs at the country level that deal with health issues…there ought to be a strong UNICEF that does country programming related to youth and mother-to-child."[36] Thus, the Global Fund's role, according to Bernard was, "intended not to deal so much with the planning, the advocacy, etc. but to deal with actually getting money on the ground to implement those parts of the national plan which need money."[37] "It's an evolution of strategies," Gayle concluded, "[strategies] that can work together to have greater strength ultimately at the country level, then I think they don't have to be seen as competitive."[38]

While this all sounded very logical, the Global Fund's relationship to UNAIDS would not be so simple. For example, it was unclear how the Global Fund would relate to the UNAIDS global appeal for funds, whether the Global Fund Secretariat or UNAIDS staff would help countries prepare funding proposals, what the relationship was at country level between the UNAIDS theme group and the Global Fund Country Coordinating Mechanism (CCM), and how the Global Fund's monitoring and evaluating framework would relate to that of UNAIDS. Some even wondered whether the establishment of the Global Fund called into question the rationale for

---

[34] Ken Bernard. Interview by Michael Merson, New Haven CT, February, 2002.

[35] Ibid.

[36] Helene Gayle. Interview by Michael Merson, New Haven, CT, February 2002.

[37] Ken Bernard. Interview by Michael Merson, New Haven CT, February, 2002.

[38] Helene Gayle. Interview by Michael Merson, New Haven, CT, February 2002.

UNAIDS existence. Had the donor community, which 7 years earlier had dissolved GPA and established UNAIDS in order to improve the UN response to the pandemic now decided that UNAIDS was no longer sufficient and that it needed to set up a new mechanism to support the global response?

Even though these various questions existed, most would agree that over time the Global Fund has had a very positive impact. Between its founding and 2011, it had approved over $23 billion in grants on AIDS, tuberculosis, and malaria and to health infrastructure projects in almost 150 countries. In total, the Global Fund had allocated over $12 billion and distributed at least $8 billion for AIDS programs, with almost all the funds being given to low- and middle-income countries and over half to countries in sub-Saharan Africa. The Global Fund balanced its AIDS disbursements in the following ways: 36% for HIV treatment, 29% for prevention, 22% for health system strengthening and program management, and 7% for enabling environments and other priorities. Based on its trends in funding, by 2015 it intended to provide about 30% of the international target for ARV treatment (i.e., covering 5.5–5.8 million people).

Despite the Global Fund's productivity, clouds began to gather over its operations towards the end of its first decade. In the fall of 2010, concerns started to surface about its senior management, funding to China and other large middle income countries, mission drift, and efficiency of spending.[39] Moreover, the global economic recession had put considerable pressure on the budgets of many low- and middle-income countries and caused a decline in the commitments from richer countries to the Global Fund. While pledges at the third replenishment conference were considerable (about $11.7 billion), they came at a reduced pace from previous years and were insufficient to meet the expected demands. Interestingly, the Global Fund found itself in a position somewhat similar to that of GPA (in terms of the amount of funds it had versus the needs of countries) in the early 1990s.

On top of these concerns about management and slow-down in contributions, 2011 also brought charges of corruption. Some of these charges had emerged earlier: the Global Fund relies on CCMs to create proposals and implement grants and contracts through local fund agents (LFAs) at country level. Countries with strong actors on their CCMs and weak (or even corrupt) LFAs were ripe for poor accounting practices at best or fraud at worst. The United States Government Accountability Office (GAO) had drawn attention to these vulnerabilities as early as 2003, but it was not until early 2011 when it identified misappropriation of its grants in several African countries ($34 million of alleged fraud). As news of these financial irregularities spread, several prominent donor governments began reviewing or suspending their previous pledges and financial commitments.

Concerns worsened throughout 2011, as "external reviews detailed the Global Fund's deficient managerial practices, weak oversight of investments, and ineffectual board governance. An alarming, $2-billion-plus financial shortfall, revealed

---

[39] Todd Summers, Lessons from the Global Fund, June 2015 Center for Strategic and International Studies (http://csis.org/files/publication/150624_Summers_LessonsGlobalFundReform_Web.pdf).

suddenly at year's end, reflected the worsening global economy, overly optimistic forecasting by the Global Fund secretariat, and flagging donor trust and confidence in the Global Fund itself."[40] The United States, which had been the major donor to the Global Fund, maintained its commitment but instigated substantial reforms. Towards the end of 2011, the Global Fund adopted a broad reform strategy, which involved tighter financial controls and accountability mechanisms, stronger vetting practices, and a shift in expectations for the Global Fund's grant managers from risk avoiders to impact investors. There were also many long overdue staffing changes.

This revised framework clarified the Global Fund's role vis a vis UNAIDS. The Global Fund revised its priorities such that grant management accounted for about 75% of its functions (as compared to only about 50% before the 2011 reforms). Its Board named a new and highly-regarded Executive Director, Mark Dybul, who had been the first Director of the President's Emergency Plan for AIDS Relief (PEPFAR). It put a new funding model in place and staff morale improved. Donor confidence in the Global Fund increased as reflected by the reasonable success of the fourth replenishment conference in December 2013 that secured funding from 2014 to 2016. By the end of 2015, in countries where the Global Fund invests, the AIDS death rate declined more than 45%, from 1.9 million in 2004 to 1.1 million in 2015, and access to ARVs rose from 3.3% coverage in 2005 to 45% in 2015. Also, from 2000 to 2015, the number of HIV infections declined by 37%.[41] The Global Fund's future seems bright, though this will depend upon how well it achieves its next 5-year strategy with an increased emphasis on strengthening health systems and reaching key populations, and whether it receives the full 3 year replenishment of $12.9 billion pledged by the donor community in 2016.[42]

Another important development following the establishment of UNAIDS was a decision by the World Bank to ramp up its AIDS efforts. The World Bank had been the last of the inital group of UN agencies to cosponsor UNAIDS, and while some of its representatives had strongly supported UNAIDS' work, others had a more tepid view. In fact, World Bank loans designated for AIDS-related activities fell from $67 million in 1994 to $41.7 million in 1997.[43] In 1999, after Debrework Zwedie and Hans Binswanger raised attention about the human and security costs associated with the pandemic, the World Bank began devoting more institution-level attention to the problem.[44] Zwedie had served as the Program Manager of Ethiopia's

---

[40] Stephen Morrison and Todd Summers, "Righting the Global Fund" Center for Strategic and International Studies, February 2012, p. 1. https://csis-prod.s3.amazonaws.com/s3fs-public/legacy_files/files/publication/120228_Morrison_RightingGlobalFund_Web.pdf.

[41] The Global Fund. Accessed on April 29, 2017 at https://www.theglobalfund.org/en/

[42] A. Usher. "Global Fund replenishment meeting nears target amount." *The Lancet*, 388, 10051, 1265.

[43] Lindsay Knight. *UNAIDS: the first 10 years, 1996–2006*, New York: Joint United Nations Programme on HIV/AIDS (UNAIDS), 2008, 117–118.

[44] Debrework Zewdie. Interview by Michael Merson, New Haven, CT September 2002; Lindsay Knight,. *UNAIDS: the first 10 years, 1996–2006*, New York: Joint United Nations Programme on HIV/AIDS (UNAIDS), 2008, 117–118.

AIDS program in the early 1990s (where I first met her) and then worked with USAID's AIDSCAP program in Kenya before she joined the World Bank in 1994 as a reproductive health adviser. The World Bank almost immediately asked Zwedie to serve as its representative on the CCO of UNAIDS, while she pushed to increase the World Bank's interest in and engagement with UNAIDS and the larger problem of AIDS.[45]

In May 1999, Zwedie opened a new department on AIDS in the World Bank's African region, and in September 2000 it launched its Multi-Country HIV/AIDS Program for Africa (MAP).[46] MAP's overarching goal was to increase access to AIDS care, treatment, and prevention among vulnerable populations according to each nation's needs.[47] Within this framework, MAP made available $500 million in grants and loans to non-governmental agencies (NGOs), private entities, and community organizations, as well as governments in September 2000 and again in February 2002. In 2001, the World Bank expanded its MAP program to the Caribbean region. A review conducted in 2007 concluded that the program "had supported the scaling up of HIV services in a catalytic manner."[48] Subsequently, the World Bank decided that for the poorest nations its support for AIDS projects could be up to 100% grant financed. In 2004, the World Bank entered into a partnership with the Global Fund, UNICEF, and the Clinton Foundation to make it possible for developing countries to purchase high-quality AIDS medicines at low prices, and established a Treatment Acceleration Project to pilot public sector/civil society partnerships to scale up treatment. By 2012, the MAP program alone had committed $2 billion to 33 countries and several multinational ventures. Through August 2013, the World Bank provided $4.6 billion for AIDS activities. In 2010, Zwedie went on to be the Deputy Director of the Global Fund until her departure in late 2014.[49]

Just over 2 years after the launch of MAP, and a mere 13 months after the creation of the Global Fund, on January 28, 2003, George W. Bush announced in his State of the Union address, between a paragraph on the war in Afghanistan and a paragraph on the war against terror, that the United States would immediately launch a 5 year, $15 billion President's Emergency Plan for AIDS Relief (PEPFAR). This initiative, which was a year in planning and a reflection of the growing interest in global AIDS among political conservatives described earlier, provided support for HIV prevention, treatment and care activities. PEPFAR would focus its efforts on 15 countries (12 in Africa), where 60% of people with AIDS in low- and middle-income countries live. Part of the logic behind the program was to unify

[45] Debrework Zewdie. Interview by Michael Merson, New Haven, CT September 2002.

[46] Ibid; Lindsay Knight. *UNAIDS: the first 10 years, 1996–2006*, New York: Joint United Nations Programme on HIV/AIDS (UNAIDS), 2008, 117–118.

[47] Devi Sridhar, Danielle Kuczynski, and Kristie Latulippe "Background Report for UNAIDS Transition Working Group." New York and Oxford UK: Center for Global Development, 21–22.

[48] The Africa Multi-Country AIDS Program 2000–2006: Results of the World Bank's Response to a Development Crisis, The World Bank—May 27, 2007.

[49] *Meeting the Challenge: The World Bank and HIV/AIDS,* World Bank, April 2012, 2.

into one operational structure all the disparate branches of the United States government that provided assistance to AIDS activities in developing countries. A key component of PEPFAR was a decision to disperse its funds under specific rules mandated by the United States Congress, some of which ran counter to advice put forth by the multilateral agencies. Most notable, Congress required PEPFAR to direct 20% of its budget to prevention and mandated that one-third of that 20% be directed to abstinence-only programs. With its prevention dollars, PEPFAR supported the ABC approach to prevention (Abstain, Be faithful, and Correct and Consistent use of Condoms) first implemented in Uganda's successful national AIDS program (see Chapter 10). Another important aspect of PEPFAR was that decisions on how its funds would be used were to be made in country by the United States Ambassador and not in Washington, DC.

In July 2008, Bush signed a bill reauthorizing PEPFAR and expanding its funding to $39 billion through fiscal year 2013. This reauthorization pushed PEPFAR into a new phase, where it focused more on building local capacity and developing country ownership—one of the steps that some critics said GPA had failed to do. The principle mechanism used by PEPFAR to accomplish this was Partnership Frameworks—"joint strategic roadmaps on AIDS" between the United States and partner nations. These frameworks allow partner nations to be more involved in identifying and prioritizing their needs, and then demarcating the division of roles between the two parties to meet the program's goals for each country. This meant that PEPFAR had something of a new footing, evolving from an "emergency" response to one concerned about sustainability and effectiveness, with a shift away from its initial focus on 15 countries to a broader model covering up to 65 countries each year. To the concern of some, PEPFAR funds "flat-lined," as the program attempted to integrate AIDS care and prevention into larger health systems. In 2011, United States Secretary of State Hillary Clinton announced the goal of creating an "AIDS-free generation" and in 2012 released a blueprint for achieving this goal.[50]

In fiscal years 2014, 2015, and 2016, $6.8 billion was appropriated for PEPFAR as the program continued to receive bipartisan support in the United States Congress. The fiscal year 2017 budget for PEPFAR is slightly less.[51] Its strategy has also shifted somewhat, placing an even greater emphasis on treatment and delivering on the promise of "an HIV-free generation" by reaching populations at greatest risk. This means that the program is now putting more resources into areas with the most HIV infections, while reducing resources in others, some of which still have considerable rates of infection, a somewhat risky approach.[52] There is also concern that countries receiving a substantial amount of PEPFAR support may become too dependent on this funding, severely compromising their national programs should they not be diversified enough to weather eventual cutbacks in United States

---

[50] PEPFAR. *Fiscal Year 2014–2016 PEPFAR Funding; October 2014.*

[51] www.pepfar.gov/funding/budget.

[52] Andrew Green, "Obama Dreams of an AIDS Free Generation," *Foreign Policy*, April 18. 2016.

investment.[53] Accordingly, PEPFAR (and the Global Fund) are assisting countries to mobilize more domestic resources to put toward their AIDS efforts.

There is no doubt that PEPFAR's investment has been significant. As of September 30, 2015, the program was supporting life-saving Antiretroviral Therapy (ART) for 11.5 million men, women, and children,[54] and has a target of putting 12.9 million persons on treatment by the end of 2017.[55] Also, in 2016, PEPFAR (along with the Bill & Melinda Gates Foundation and other organizations) launched a $385 million DREAMS project aimed at reducing HIV infections among adolescent girls and young women in ten sub-Saharan African countries, where new HIV infections continue to rise at an alarming rate, driven in part by the prevalent practice of older men, who were most likely infected through sex with HIV-infected women of their own age,[56] engaging in sex with younger women. DREAMS is delivering a core package that combines evidence-based approaches that go beyond the health sector, addressing the structural drivers that directly and indirectly increase girls' HIV risk, including poverty, gender inequality, sexual violence, and a lack of education.[57] Today, PEPFAR and the Global Fund together account for over 90% of donor funding for the AIDS response in the world's highest-burdened and lowest-resourced countries, and are committed to working together to invest resources in a coordinated, complementary, and synergistic manner eliminating duplication in their efforts to the extent possible. They, along with the World Bank are also committed to addressing the larger health system concerns that are essential for providing and maintaining treatment for all those with HIV infection.

What about WHO? In 2003, less than 6 months after Bush announced the creation of PEPFAR, Lee Jong-Wook began a 5-year term as the new Director-General of WHO succeeding Gro Bruntland who declined for personal reasons to seek a second term. Within a few months of taking office, he declared that his top priority would be the extension of AIDS care to 3 million persons in low- and middle-income countries by the end of 2005. Brundtland had first announced the project, termed the "3 by 5" Initiative at the 2002 International AIDS Conference in Barcelona.[58] "3 by 5"'s objective was to treat half of those lacking treatment at that time in developing nations. As this represented an almost tenfold increase in those

---

[53] S. Resch, Theresa Ryckman, R Hecht, "Funding AIDS programmes in the era of shared responsibility: an analysis of domestic spending in 12 low-income and middle-income countries." *Lancet Global Health* 3: 452–461, 2015.

[54] PEPFAR web site: http://www.pepfar.gov/funding/index.htm; WHO web site: http://www.who.int/hiv/en/.

[55] US President's Emergency Plan for AIDS Relief, Fact Sheet, 2015 United Nations General Assembly Sustainable Development Summit, September, 2015; http://www.pepfar.gov/documents/organization/247548.pdf.

[56] Tulio de Oliveira, et al. "Transmission networks and risk of HIV infection in KwaZulu-Natal, South Africa: a community-wide phylogenetic study." *The Lancet* HIV 4.1 (2017): e41-e50.

[57] *DREAMS: Working Together for and AIDS Free Future for Girls and Women*. Washington, DC: PEPFAR http://www.pepfar.gov/documents/organization/252380.pdf accessed on 8 August 2016.

[58] Lindsay Knight. *UNAIDS: the first 10 years, 1996–2006*, New York: Joint United Nations Programme on HIV/AIDS (UNAIDS), 2008, xx.

then receiving care, it seemed an almost herculean task, one which would call for profound infrastructure-building in WHO itself. WHO aimed to accomplish this audacious plan by training 1 million health workers in the most affected countries in the delivery of AIDS care and use of ARVs. Among other factors, the feasibility of the program hinged on provision of generic ARVs at greatly reduced cost. To help in this process, in April 2002 WHO had placed ARVs on its Model list of Essential Medicines. The program also demanded that WHO raise considerable new financial resources, and that it mobilize staff to assist in this effort. In a bold move Lee recruited Jim Kim (current President of the World Bank) from the Harvard School of Public Health to lead this program.

The "3 by 5" initiative was unable to attain its goal. Only approximately 1 million people were receiving ART by 2005. However, the goal was reached 2 years later.[59] The target had proved "excessively aspirational," Kevin De Cock, then Director of WHO's HIV/AIDS Department, told reporters. But, he noted, "reaching the target even two years late is quite a remarkable achievement."[60] Perhaps the biggest legacy of Lee's effort was that it drew attention to the need for strengthening health systems to ensure access[61]…and, most importantly, it brought WHO back as an actor in the global response to the pandemic.

Growing out of the aspirational "3 by 5" initiative, WHO put forth a 2006–2010 plan for universal access and, in 2010, it launched a new health system financing effort, the Path to Universal Coverage, under Lee's successor, Margaret Chan.[62] As part of this effort, in June 2010, WHO teamed up with UNAIDS to launch Treatment 2.0, a program that promoted universal access to ART as both a treatment and preventive intervention. This program expanded upon the lessons WHO learned from "3 by 5" and established five priority areas of work: drugs, costs, diagnostics, service delivery, and community mobilization.[63] Treatment 2.0 was also an attempt to align WHO's strategies with larger UNAIDS strategies. At the time of this writing, WHO's Department of HIV/AIDS consists of some 30 professional staff in Geneva and six in the regional offices working with a number of consultants and assistants.[64] It also incorporates WHO's efforts on sexually transmitted diseases (STDs)[65] and includes the Global Hepatitis Program. The Director of the Department, Gottfried Hirnschall, an Austrian public health physician, took up his position in May, 2010

---

[59] Thomas Maugh, "World AIDS plan meets '3 by 5' goal—two years late," *Los Angeles Times*, June 3, 2008.

[60] Ibid.

[61] Udani Samaresekera, "Margaret Chan's vision for WHO," *The Lancet,* 369(9577):1915–1916.

[62] David Holmes, "Margaret Chan: Committed to Universal Health Coverage," *The Lancet*, September 8, 2012, 380(9845:879; Udani Samaresekera, "Margaret Chan's vision for WHO," *The Lancet,* 369(9577):1915–1916.

[63] WHO Department of HIV/AIDS & UNAIDS, *The treatment 2.0 framework for action: catalysing the next phase of treatment, care and support.* Geneva: World Health Organization, 2011.

[64] WHO HIV/AIDS Organigram, September 2014, http://www.who.int/hiv/aboutdept/hiv_organigram_sep2014.pdf?ua=1.

[65] For the purposes of this text we use the term sexually transmitted disease(s) and the abbreviation STD rather than the other term sexually transmitted infection(s) or STIs.

after a decade working for WHO primarily in Geneva and Latin America in various AIDS program-related positions. Hirnschall became the 11th individual in just 30 years to head WHO's efforts on AIDS and is the person to have held this position the longest.[66]

WHO claims to be "leading the health sector response to HIV" and in many ways it is. The Department operated under a Global Health Sector Strategy on HIV/AIDS for the period 2011–2015 and its core activities included synthesizing evidence on the effectiveness, feasibility, and safety of HIV interventions and approaches; guiding the HIV research agenda; improving the availability and quality of HIV-related medicines and diagnostics tools; setting norms and standards for scaling up HIV prevention, diagnosis, treatment, care and support services; and monitoring and reporting on progress in the health-sector response towards achieving universal access to HIV services, including coverage and impact of these services. An updated strategy for the period 2016–2021 was adapted at the WHA in May, 2016 and similarly focuses on delivery, quality, and coverage of HIV services.[67] In 2016, the Department published important new guidelines for treating and preventing HIV infection, which provided updated guidance on the diagnosis of HIV infection, the care of people living with HIV, and the use of ARVs for treating and preventing HIV infection.[68]

Two important new actors have been added to the global response to the pandemic. One has been multinational pharmaceutical companies, who had functionally denied HIV-infected persons in poorer nations' access to ARVs in the latter half of the 1990s because of their high prices. In 1999, the Bristol-Myers Squibb Foundation launched *Secure the Future*, a $100 million project that used a variety of mechanisms to expand access to care for persons living with AIDS in resource-poor countries, build treatment capacity in those regions, and support programs focused on women and children.[69] The following year, the Merck Company Foundation and the Bill & Melinda Gates Foundation donated $50 million each to launch the African Comprehensive HIV/AIDS Partnership (ACHAP) in Botswana. Merck also donated a number of its ARVs and in 2010 donated an additional $50 million to the program. ACHAP's goal was to support the national AIDS program in Botswana, namely, by "rapidly advancing HIV/AIDS prevention programs

---

[66] Bernhard Schwartlander. Interview by Michael Merson, January 3, 2015.

[67] Global health sector strategies on HIV, viral hepatitis and sexually transmitted infections, for the period 2016–2021. Sixty-ninth world health assembly. Agenda Item 15.1, WHA69.22 May 28, 2016 http://apps.who.int/gb/ebwha/pdf_files/WHA69/A69_R22-en.pdf.

[68] Consolidated guidelines on the use of antiretroviral drugs for treating and preventing HIV infection. Recommendations for a public health approach-Second Edition. WHOhttp://www.who.int/hiv/pub/arv/arv-2016/en/.

[69] R. Sebastian Wanless, John Damonti, Phangisile Mtshali, and Patricia Doykos, "Public-Private Partnerships: From Theory to Practice," in: Marlink RG, Teitelman ST, eds. *From the Ground Up: Building Comprehensive HIV/AIDS Care Programs in Resource-Limited Settings*. Washington, DC: Elizabeth Glaser Pediatric AIDS Foundation; 2009. http://ftguonline.org/ftgu-232/index.php/ftgu/article/view/2057/4110, accessed on June 4, 2012.; "Globalization, Partnerships, and Health" in *Analysis of experience*, pp,10–14.

(including male circumcision), health care access, patient management, and treatment of HIV" in that country.[70] The partners selected Botswana because it had one of the highest adult HIV prevalence rates in the world, a viable existing health care infrastructure, and strong political support to address the epidemic. The program was highly successful in reducing HIV-related mortality.[71]

ACHAP signaled the emergence of the Bill & Melinda Gates Foundation as a prominent player in the global fight against AIDS. Founded in 1994, the Gates Foundation invested more than $15 billion in global health by 2013.[72] Today its Global Development, Global Health, and Global Policy and Advocacy Division supports a wide range of global health projects. While many of the Foundation's projects are research oriented, it has supported two important HIV/AIDS delivery programs that have illustrated that HIV treatment and prevention services can be successfully delivered with high impact. One was the aforementioned ACHAP in Botswana. The other was the AVAHAN project in India to which the Foundation committed $338 million. This initiative aimed to reduce HIV transmission and the prevalence of STDs in vulnerable high-risk populations, notably female sex workers, men who have sex with men (MSM), and transgender individuals living in six States of India, through prevention education and services such as condom promotion, STD management, behavior change communication, community mobilization, and advocacy. Indications are that it has also been a great success.[73] While the Gates Foundation has been at times criticized for a lack of transparency and for distorting the focus of health systems, it's focus on developing and testing new HIV prevention methods must be commended (its greatest commitment has been investing in the development of an HIV vaccine), as well as its support to a wide array of partners working to combat global AIDS, including the Global Fund.

All of this varied financial support and program commitment was a very welcome set of developments, as it meant that by 2004 the world had at least seven major "actors" significantly involved in the global AIDS response (namely, WHO, UNAIDS, PEPFAR, World Bank, the Global Fund, the Bill & Melinda Gates Foundation, and the United Nations (bolstered by its Millennium Development Goals). However, all had their own mandates, funding sources, and governance structure with no mechanism to ensure consistency in their policies and practices. In addition, some countries lacked the capabilities to provide the necessary coordination

---

[70] Globalization, Partnerships, and Health" in *Analysis of experience*, pp,10–14; Ilavenil Ramiah and Michael R. Reich, "Building effective public–private partnerships: Experiences and lessons from the African Comprehensive HIV/AIDS Partnerships (ACHAP)," *Social Science & Medicine,* July 2006, 63(2): 397–408.

[71] M Farahani et al, "Outcomes of the Botswana national HIV/AIDS treatment programme from 2002 to 2010: a longitudinal analysis," *The Lancet Global Health*, 2(1):e44–e50, January 2014.

[72] "What We Do," Bill & Melinda Gates Foundation, gatesfoundation.org http://www.gatesfoundation.org/What-We-Do.

[73] M. Pickles et al., "Assessment of the population-level effectiveness of the Avahan HIV-prevention programme in South India: a preplanned, causal-pathway-based modelling analysis," *The Lancet Global Health*, 1(5):e289–e299, November 2013; Gates Foundation 2000 Annual Report, pp. 28–31. I served on the Advisory Board for both this project and ACHAP.

and leadership and were often overwhelmed with meeting the reporting requirements of many donor institutions and international and bilateral agencies.

How to coordinate or at least bring more closely together these voices? Through a series of consultations at country, regional, and international levels in 2002 and 2003, UNAIDS sought to reach consensus on a number of issues. Coming out of one of these meetings, the International Conference on AIDS and Sexually Transmitted Infections in Africa, held in September 2003 in Nairobi, Peter Piot started distilling a set of principles that could guide future coordination. The result was UNAIDS' "Three Ones" framework, which called for (a) one consensus AIDS action framework for each country, (b) one national AIDS coordinating authority for each country, and (c) one consensus monitoring and evaluation system for each national program. Participating bodies all approved these tenets at the Consultation on Harmonization of International AIDS Funding in Washington, DC in April 2004. Piot intended the "Three Ones" not as a mere catchphrase, but rather as a fundamental framework for health governance at country level.[74] Absent a true accountability mechanism, this agreement seemed the most effective way of ensuring collaboration (or at least noncompetition) at country level. Of course, the limiting factor would be the extent to which donor agencies would incorporate the "Three Ones" into their own plans and performance indicators.

In March 2005, Piot and UNAIDS tried to increase buy-in from the largest donors to the "Three Ones" at a London meeting cosponsored by the United Kingdom, the United States, France, and UNAIDS and entitled "Making the money work: the 'Three Ones' in Action". The conference was quite contentious, but one of its few positive outcomes was the formation of the Global Task Team on Improving Coordination among Multilateral Institutions and International Donors co-chaired by UNAIDS Director of the Country and Regional Support Department, Michel Sidibé, and the Swedish AIDS Ambassador, Lennarth Hjelmaker. Despite its unwieldy name, the aim of the Global Task Team (GTT) was to improve "the institutional architecture" of the global AIDS response and to "streamline, simplify, and further harmonize procedures and practices" at country level.[75] In June 2005, the GTT documented the persisting problems in coordination among multilateral institutions and international donors and put forth a set of recommendations that sought to empower inclusive national leadership and ownership, bring about greater alignment and harmonization among the major actors, achieve a more effective multilateral response, and ensure more accountability and oversight in the global and national response. One of its recommendations was for the UNAIDS CCO to commission an independent review of the UNAIDS governance structure. With a growing number of important bilateral, multilateral, and intergovernmental players in the

---

[74] Lindsay Knight. *UNAIDS: the first 10 years, 1996–2006*, New York: Joint United Nations Programme on HIV/AIDS (UNAIDS), 2008.

[75] Global Task Team on improving AIDS coordination among multilateral donors and international donors." Geneva: UNAIDS, 2006. http://www.unaids.org/en/media/unaids/contentassets/documents/programmes/programmeeffectivenessandcountrysupportdepartment/GTT_en.pdf Accessed on June 2, 2012.

field of global AIDS, it was becoming increasingly difficult for UNAIDS to fulfill its coordinating mandate.

While the sea of new agencies and the clamor of their voices made coordination more difficult, UNAIDS found that many of these voices converged on at least one theme: the need for a global scale up of ART. The push for scale up sprang from two developments. First, it had become clear that, despite early doubters, low- and middle-income countries could deliver ARVs to their populations.[76] Second, the combined effort to reduce ARV prices—particularly through the work of former US President Bill Clinton and the Clinton Health Access Initiative (CHAI)—had lowered prices to a level where these countries could conceive of managing AIDS as a chronic disease. By the end of 2003, then, the global AIDS community shifted considerable attention to the issue of treatment scale up. The primary concerns were financing the drug acquisitions and ensuring a quality distribution and delivery mechanism. Health infrastructure belonged, as a practice boundary, to WHO, and it was for this reason that the "3 by 5" program and Treatment 2.0 efforts focused so specifically on treatment access.

Treatment access made considerable sense from a treatment and prevention standpoint. As Bertozzi noted, managing HIV with drugs "improve[ed] and prolong[ed] the quality of life of people with HIV" in countries where they previously would have died. Since reducing an individual's viral load not only improved their lives but reduced their infectivity, the role of treatment scale up could have the important additional benefit of prevention. Treatment scale up was not without its tradeoffs, however. The entire process—reducing the prices, securing the financing, bolstering the infrastructure—was expensive. The moral imperative behind scaling up treatment inevitably pushed prevention down the priority list, yet the costs inherent in treatment scale up "underscored the enormous costs of *not* preventing HIV."[77] Then, finally, despite the very commendable access goals promulgated by efforts like the "3 by 5" program, UNAIDS acknowledged in 2006 that new infections outstripped the most optimistic scale up goals by three to one. As Kevin de Cock, cautioned in his speech at the 16th International AIDS Conference in 2006 in Toronto, "we cannot treat our way out of the epidemic."[78] Without robust HIV prevention, treatment scale up alone was still a losing game.

The news on prevention had been mixed, however. Vaccine development had proved difficult owing to the mutability of HIV, the high variability between HIV isolates, and the difficulty in stimulating a reliable and appropriate antibody response in humans.[79] One vaccine candidate, Merck's V520, at first appeared promising and was evaluated in a 15-site trial of about 3000 recipients, but ultimately—and

[76] Bob Herbert, "In America: Refusing to Save Africans," *NY Times,* June 11 2001.

[77] S.M. Bertozzi, T.E. Martz, P. Piot. "The evolving HIV/AIDS response and the urgent tasks ahead." *Health Affairs.* 2009 Nov–Dec;28(6):1578–90.

[78] Ibid.

[79] David I. Watkins "Basic HIV Vaccine Development." *Top HIV Med* , Mar 2008,16 (1): 7–8.

disappointingly—failed to show efficacy.[80] A subsequent efficacy trial in Thailand (RV144) of two previously failed vaccines (Sanofi Pasteur's ALVAC-HIV [vCP1521], and Genentech's AIDSVAX B/E) reported approximately 30% protection against HIV acquisition, although a Bayesian reanalysis of the results suggested that the vaccine may not be as protective.[81] At the time of this writing, a large-scale efficacy trial is underway in South Africa to evaluate a modified version of the RV144 vaccine using components of HIV strains circulating in Southern Africa. Many additional candidates are also under development.[82]

The hunt for an effective microbicide has also been a challenge. As we explained earlier (see Chapter 11), GPA had supported several efforts to identify and develop an effective microbicide, but the trials stemming from these and other efforts produced disappointing results. At least two more recent trials have shown modest protection (around 30%) in women older than 21 years (but not in younger women), using a vaginal ring containing the antiretroviral dapivirine. One other candidate, 1% tenofovir gel, showed modest efficacy in a trial whose data were released in 2010, but subsequent trials did not confirm this finding.[83] This continues to be an area of great interest to researchers and AIDS activists. Research is underway on developing a vaginal ring that will both prevent HIV and act as a contraceptive.

In something of a surprise, during the past decade-and-a-half, male circumcision has emerged as an intervention that confers a highly protective effect on men who have sex with HIV-positive women. Beginning in the late 1980s, researchers led by Canadian medical microbiologist, Allan Ronald, working in Kenya found in cross-sectional and case-control studies that male circumcision dramatically decreased HIV infection rates.[84] Ronald and his colleague Stephen Moses had approached me when I was GPA Director about supporting more research on circumcision. We carefully considered their request, but decided that efficacy trials would be difficult and the evidence at the time was not compelling enough for us to take this on. In hindsight, we should have done so. In the mid-2000s, three randomized trials provided definitive evidence that male circumcision reduced the risk

---

[80] F.H. Priddy, D. Brown, J. Kublin, K. Monahan, D.P. Wright, J. Lalezari, S. Santiago, M. Marmor, M. Lally, R.M. Novak, S.J. Brown, P. Kulkarni, S.A. Dubey, L.S. Kierstead, D.P. Casimiro, R. Mogg, M.J. DiNubile, J.W. Shiver, R.Y. Leavitt, M.N. Robertson, D.V. Mehrotra, E. Quirk, for the Merck V520-016 Study Group, "Safety and immunogenicity of a replication-incompetent adenovirus type 5 HIV-1 clade B gag/pol/nef vaccine in healthy adults," *Clin Infect Dis.* 2008 Jun 1;46(11):1769–81.

[81] Peter B. Gilbert, James O. Berger, Donald Stablein, Stephen Becker, Max Essex, Scott M. Hammer, Jerome H. Kim and Victor G. DeGruttola, "Statistical Interpretation of the RV144 HIV Vaccine Efficacy Trial in Thailand: A Case Study for Statistical Issues in Efficacy Trials," *Journal of Infectious Diseases*, 203(7): 969–975.

[82] HIV Vaccine Research: An Update. May 2016. http://www.avac.org/sites/default/files/resource-files/HIVvax_research_update.pdf.

[83] Microbicides for HIV Prevention: An Introductory fact Sheet. April 2016. AVAC Global Advocacy for HIV Prevention. http://www.avac.org/microbicides/basics.

[84] Larry Krotz, *Piecing the Puzzle: The Genesis of AIDS Research in Africa,* Winnipeg, Manitoba: University of Manitoba Press, May 1, 2012.

of heterosexually acquired HIV infection in men by approximately 60%.[85] This led to a consensus that male circumcision should be a priority for HIV prevention in countries and regions with heterosexual epidemics and high HIV and low male circumcision prevalence. While progress in its uptake has been slower than desired, by the end of 2015, 11.7 million men had been circumcised in East and Southern Africa through voluntary male circumcision services, which will have averted 452,000 HIV infections by 2030.[86] Hence, while some progress has been made in developing a vaccine and vaginal microbicides, and in the uptake of adult male circumcision, we still do not have highly effective and feasible population level approaches to prevent HIV transmission.[87]

Compounding the difficulties of identifying effective prevention strategies, UNAIDS continued to face considerable challenges to behavior change interventions in numerous countries owing to social conventions and taboos around risk behaviors and stigmatization of persons living with AIDS. There were also differences in opinion of what worked in HIV prevention. For example, considerable attention was given to Uganda's ABC prevention strategy (Abstinence, Be faithful, and Correct and Consistent use of Condoms).[88] Rather than viewing these strategies holistically or contextually, considerable debate—often ideologically motivated—broke out over which of the three components was most responsible for Uganda's apparent success. This led to a hyper-focus on condom distribution in some

[85] H.A. Weiss, M.A. Quigley, R.J. Hayes. "Male circumcision and risk of HIV infection in sub-Saharan Africa: a systematic review and metaanalysis." *AIDS*. 2000 Oct 20;14(15):2361–70; N. Siegfried, M. Muller, J. Volmink, et al. "Male circumcision for prevention of heterosexual acquisition of HIV in men." *Cochrane Database Syst Rev*. 2003;(3):CD003362; B. Auvert, D. Taljaard, E. Lagarde, J. Sobngwi-Tambekou, R. Sitta, A. Puren. "Randomized, controlled intervention trial of male circumcision for reduction of HIV infection risk: the ANRS 1265 Trial." *PLoS Med*. 2005 Nov;2(11):e298. Erratum in: *PLoS Med*. 2006 May;3(5):e298; R.C. Bailey, S. Moses, C.B. Parker, et al. "Male circumcision for HIV prevention in young men in Kisumu, Kenya: a randomised controlled trial." *Lancet*. 2007 Feb 24;369(9562):643–56; R.H. Gray, G. Kigozi, D. Serwadda, et al. "Male circumcision for HIV prevention in men in Rakai, Uganda: a randomised trial." *Lancet*. 2007 Feb 24;369(9562):657–66; S.M. Bertozzi, T.E. Martz, P. Piot. "The evolving HIV/AIDS response and the urgent tasks ahead." *Health Affairs*. 2009 Nov–Dec;28(6):1578–90.

[86] "Voluntary Medical Male Circumcision for HIV Prevention - An Interview with Emmanuel Njeuhmeli. Posted October 26, 2016" by *PLOS Collections*. http://blogs.plos.org/collections/vmmc-2016-interview/. Accessed 27 February 2017.

[87] B. Auvert, D. Taljaard, E. Lagarde, J. Sobngwi-Tambekou, R. Sitta, A. Puren. "Randomized, controlled intervention trial of male circumcision for reduction of HIV infection risk: the ANRS 1265 Trial." *PLoS Med* 2005;2:e298–e298; R. C. Bailey, S. Moses, C. B. Parker, et al. "Male circumcision for HIV prevention in young men in Kisumu, Kenya: a randomised controlled trial." *Lancet* 2007;369:643–656; S. Rerks-Ngarm, P. Pitisuttithum, S. Nitayaphan, et al. "Vaccination with ALVAC and AIDSVAX to prevent HIV-1 infection in Thailand." *New England Journal of Medicine* 2009;361:2209–2220; Q. Abdool Karim, S.S. Abdool Karim, J.A. Frohlich, et al. "Effectiveness and safety of tenofovir gel, an antiretroviral microbicide, for the prevention of HIV infection in women." *Science* 2010;329:1168–1174.

[88] Bureau for Global Health, "The ABCs of HIV Prevention," Washington, D.C.; U.S. Agency for International Development, August 2003. Accessed at http://info.worldbank.org/etools/docs/library/166065/Uganda-ABC%20Model.pdf.

quarters, and an overemphasis on abstinence-based strategies in others, rather than on the use of approaches tailored to the risk behavior of the population.[89]

To push for more varied approaches, in 2004 UNAIDS moved forward on two new prevention fronts. First, UNAIDS partnered with other stakeholders to launch the Global Coalition on Women and AIDS (GCWA), which aimed at increasing the focus on HIV-related needs and vulnerabilities of women in national AIDS programs.[90] Beginning in 2005, GCWA began providing theme groups and national programs with funds to jumpstart or reinforce prevention programs aimed at or including women.[91] Second, the following year, in a response to a request from its Program Coordinating Board (PCB), UNAIDS presented a comprehensive policy on HIV prevention. While heated debate ensued, by the end of the meeting every Board member save for Russia and the United States had signed on to it (the United States broke specifically over needle exchange guidance). While the policy did not resolve conflicting values and opinions, it did represent a broad-based bill of fare about best practices in prevention upon which national programs could draw to improve their outcomes. The policy also furthered movement in these programs beyond nationwide, general awareness campaigns to the adoption of more targeted and focused prevention efforts.[92]

One of the most important and more recent developments has been research on the role that preexposure prophylaxis with ARVs (PrEP) could play in the prevention armamentarium.[93] Put simply, PrEP is the concept that high-risk seronegative individuals can be protected from HIV infection by taking oral ARVs on a daily basis.[94] Results from well-controlled studies (i.e., the iPrEX study; the Partners PrEP study) showed the efficacy of PrEP. In the IPrEX study, conducted at 11 sites in nine cities in six countries, PrEP reduced HIV infection by about 40% among MSM (and up to 73% among those with good adherence).[95] In the Partners PrEP study, undertaken in Kenya and Uganda, serodiscordant couples (couples in which

---

[89] Hearst N, Chen S. "Condom promotion for AIDS prevention in the developing world: is it working?" *Stud Fam Plann*. 2004 Mar;35(1):39–47; Malcolm Potts, Daniel T. Halperin, Douglas Kirby, Ann Swidler, Elliot Marseille, Jeffrey D. Klausner, Norman Hearst, Richard G. Wamai, James G. Kahn, and Julia Walsh, "Reassessing HIV Prevention," *Science* 9 May 2008: 749–750; Paul R. "Tailoring AIDS Prevention," *Science* 19 September 2008: 1631.

[90] Lindsay Knight. *UNAIDS: the first 10 years, 1996–2006*, New York: Joint United Nations Programme on HIV/AIDS (UNAIDS), 2008, 213.

[91] Ibid, 216.

[92] Bertozzi SM, Martz TE, Piot P. "The evolving HIV/AIDS response and the urgent tasks ahead." *Health Affairs*. 2009 Nov–Dec;28(6):1578–90.

[93] Robert M. Grant et al. "Preexposure Chemoprophylaxis for HIV Prevention in Men Who Have Sex with Men," *New England Journal of Medicine* 2010; 363:2587–599.

[94] Nelson L. Michael, "Oral Preexposure Prophylaxis for HIV—Another Arrow in the Quiver?" *New England Journal of Medicine* 2010; 363:2663–2665.

[95] WHO, "WHO issues first guidance on use of antiretrovirals by HIV-negative people at high risk to prevent infection," Geneva: WHO, July 20, 2012. Accessed http://www.who.int/mediacentre/news/notes/2012/hiv_medication_prep_20120720/en/.

one person is HIV positive) achieved 75% protection.[96] Several concerns mitigated this initial optimism, however, including concerns about: adherence; medication-use fatigue; long-term safety alongside comorbid conditions; compensatory declines in other preventive behaviors; and feasibility implications (cost and implementation) in large populations.[97] However, in 2012 WHO issued its first guidance on how high-risk HIV-negative persons could use ARVs to prevent infection,[98] and in 2014 the United States Public Health Service did likewise.[99] Provided there is good adherence, PrEP is now viewed as an effective prevention option for all populations at substantial risk of HIV infection.[100] One option being studied to increase adherence is the use of long-acting products given intramuscularly.[101]

An even greater achievement, however, and one that was heralded by *Science* as the breakthrough of the year,[102] was the release in May 2011 of the results of the HPTN O52 study which showed a 96% reduction of HIV transmission within sero-discordant couples assigned to taking ARVs.[103] In other words, HIV-positive individuals taking ARVs were more than 20 times less likely to infect their partners than untreated ones. The study was conducted in three sites across Africa, Asia, and the Americas, enrolled 1763 serodiscordant couples, and took 6 years to complete. These findings, according to Tony Fauci at the United States National Institute for Health (NIH) "convincingly demonstrates that treating the infected individual—and doing so sooner rather than later—can have a significant impact on reducing HIV transmission."[104] It was now, many felt, not unreasonable to ask whether the beginning of the end of AIDS was in sight a prediction made 5 years earlier by Julio Montaner.[105]

---

[96] Ibid.

[97] Nelson L. Michael, "Oral Preexposure Prophylaxis for HIV—Another Arrow in the Quiver?" *New England Journal of Medicine* 2010; 363:2663–2665; S. M. Bertozzi, T.E. Martz, P. Piot. "The evolving HIV/AIDS response and the urgent tasks ahead." *Health Affairs*. 2009 Nov–Dec; 28(6):1578–90.

[98] WHO Media Center." WHO issues first guidance on use of antiretrovirals by HIV-negative people at high risk to prevent infection." Geneva: World Health Organization, July 20, 2012.

[99] PreExposure Prophylaxis for the Prevention of HIV Infection in the United States, US Public Health Service 2014 http://www.cdc.gov/hiv/pdf/PrEPguidelines2014.pdf.

[100] "Oral Pre-Exposure Prophylaxis, Putting a new choice in context," Geneva: UNAIDS, 2015; WHO Expands Recommendation on oral pre-exposure prophylaxis of HIV infection (PrEP). Policy Brief. WHO, November 2015 http://www.who.int/hiv/pub/prep/policy-brief-prep-2015/en/.

[101] D Margolis et al., "Long-acting intramuscular cabotegravir and rilpivirine in adults with HIV-1 infection (LATTE-2): 96-week results of a randomised, open-label, phase 2b, non-inferiority trial," The Lancet (2017).

[102] J Cohen, "Breakthrough of the year HIV Treatment as Prevention," *Science* 23 December 2011;334(6063):1628.

[103] M Cohen et al., "Prevention of HIV Infection with Early Antiretroviral Therapy," *New England Journal of Medicine* 2011; 365:493–505.

[104] HIV Prevention Trial Network Press Release, May 12 2011.

[105] Montaner, Julio SG, et al. "The case for expanding access to highly active antiretroviral therapy to curb the growth of the HIV epidemic," *The Lancet* 368.9534 (2006): 531.

After more than two decades of existence, UNAIDS has become a large enterprise and a key advocate for global action on AIDS. Eleven UN agencies now cosponsor the organization, the original six (WHO, UNDP, UNESCO, UNFPA, UNICEF, World Bank) plus the International Labor Organization, World Food Programme, United Nations High Commission for Refugees, United Nations Office on Drugs and Crime, and UN Women (see Appendix 8). UNAIDS continues to have a broad mandate, captured in its five core functions: leadership, communication and advocacy; effective partnerships for impact and sustainability; strategic information for planning, monitoring, and evaluation; coordination, coherence, and convening; and mutual accountability.[106]

In 2011, UNAIDS launched an ambitious strategy for "Getting to Zero," a broad, multisectoral framework that outlined the roles of the cosponsors (and the UNAIDS Secretariat) to combat the pandemic by reaching the "Three Zeros," zero new deaths, zero new infections, and zero discrimination. Getting to Zero focused attention on the health sector of Member States and treatment of HIV infection, and linking health systems with other sectors "to tackle the social, economic, cultural and environmental issues that shape the epidemic and access to health services."[107] Some were critical of the framework and viewed it as "excessively aspirational" (much like WHO's "3 by 5") and a ploy to ensure funding during lean economic times. Despite this concern, there was agreement that careful planning and investment in health systems could not help but enable a sustainable response to the pandemic. In 2011, at a high-level meeting on AIDS the UN General Assembly adopted a Resolution whereby UN Member States committed to universal access to HIV prevention, treatment, care, and support by 2015 and the elimination of HIV and AIDS.[108] Following this Resolution, UNAIDS and PEPFAR jointly launched the Global Plan towards the elimination of new HIV infections among children by 2015 and keeping their mothers alive in 21 priority countries in sub-Saharan Africa. By 2015 this effort resulted in a 60% reduction in new HIV infections among children (since 2009, the baseline year for the Global Plan). Countries with the highest reductions were Uganda, South Africa, and Burundi who decreased new infections by 86%, 84%, and 84%, respectively. In all the countries, 80% of pregnant women living with HIV accessed ARVs to prevent HIV transmission, and among these women, 93% were accessing lifelong therapy.[109]

In 2016, UNAIDS adopted its 2016–2021 Strategy, "On the Fast Track to End AIDS," which outlines the essential features required in the global AIDS response to end the AIDS pandemic as a public health threat by 2030. The Strategy aims to advance progress towards reaching UNAIDS' vision of the "Three Zeros." As in the

---

[106] UNAIDS Programme Coordinating Board. Thirty-seventh meeting, Agenda Item 4. UNAIDS Unified Budget, Results and Accountability Framework 2016–2021. October 20, 2015 http://www.unaids.org/sites/default/files/media_asset/20151103_UNAIDS_UBRAF_PCB37_15-19_EN.pdf.

[107] UNAIDS 2011–2015 Strategy. Getting to Zero. Geneva: UNAIDS http://www.unaids.org/sites/default/files/sub_landing/files/JC2034_UNAIDS_Strategy_en.pdf.

[108] 65th Session of United Nations General Assembly, Resolution 65/277, July 8 2001.

[109] On the Fast-Track to An AIDS-Free Generation. UNAIDS and PEPFAR. 2016.

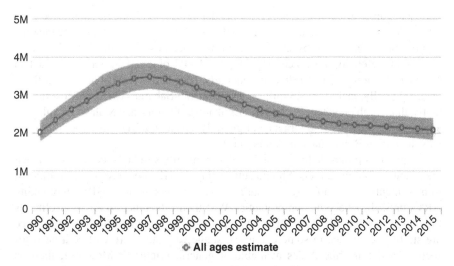

Fig. 18.1 New Global HIV Infections (all ages estimate). Source: UNAIDS

past, its focus remains on the strategic directions of prevention; treatment, care, and support; and human rights and gender equality.[110] At another high-level UN meeting in June, 2016, the UN General Assembly endorsed the same highly ambitious goal of ending the AIDS pandemic by 2030.[111] The Political Declaration included a set of specific, time-bound targets and actions by 2020. This includes a commitment that by 2020, 90% of all people living with HIV will know their HIV status, 90% of all people with diagnosed HIV infection will receive sustained ART, 90% of all people receiving ART will have viral suppression (90-90-90 targets).[112]

There is, at the time of this writing, considerable optimism that the global health community can reach these targets, which have now been widely adopted. Globally, new HIV infections have fallen 40% since their peak in 1997 (Fig. 18.1) (and in children by 70%), and the number of AIDS-related deaths has decreased by 45% since its peak in 2005.[113] In addition, 85 countries have come close to eliminating mother-to-child transmission of HIV,[114] and by 2016, 70% of people living with HIV were aware of their status.[115] Furthermore, ART distribution and uptake has

[110] *On the Fast Track to end AIDS*. UNAIDS 2016–2021 Strategy http://www.unaids.org/sites/default/files/media_asset/20151027_UNAIDS_PCB37_15_18_EN_rev1.pdf.

[111] Political Declaration on HIV and AIDS: On the Fast-Track to Accelerate the Fight against HIV and to End the AIDS Epidemic by 2030. A/RES/70/266. 8 June 2016.

[112] Prevention GAP report. UNAIDS 2016. http://www.unaids.org/sites/default/files/media_asset/2016-prevention-gap-report_en.pdf.

[113] Ibid.

[114] Michel Sidibe. "Charting a path to end the AIDS epidemic." *Bulletin of the World Health Organization* 2016;94:408. doi:http://dx.doi.org/10.2471/BLT.16.176875.

[115] Ending AIDS: Progress Towards the 90-90-90 Targets. UNAIDS 2017 http://www.unaids.org/sites/default/files/media_asset/Global_AIDS_update_2017_en.pdf.

slowly begun to affect the global AIDS pandemic. By 2015, the number of persons with access to ART was double that in 2010 and a staggering 22 times more than the number in 2000.[116] And, by 2016, 19.5 million persons (53% of all HIV-infected individuals) globally were accessing ARVs and 44% of all HIV-infected people had viral suppression.[117] Since 1995, consequently, ART had averted at least 7.6 million deaths globally, including 4.8 million deaths in sub-Saharan Africa.[118] Most importantly, three high prevalence countries (Zimbabwe, Zambia, and Malawi) are already approaching the 90-90-90 targets and globally seven countries have met these targets, including Botswana and Cambodia.[119, 120]

Despite this progress, the global health community still has much to do to reach these new ambitious targets. Should self-testing for HIV be more widely promoted to help identify HIV-infected persons? Will many persons with HIV delay taking ARVs until they become symptomatic? Will their adherence to ARVs decline as they no longer feel ill?[121] Additionally, reports of alarming rates of drug resistance are starting to surface in some countries, suggesting that there will be a need for second- and third-line ARVs available at generic pricing.[122] Moreover, there is growing unease that these highly optimistic targets are not realistic and this may lead to complacency in the global response.[123] Of particular concern is that, at the time of this writing, the annual rate of new adult HIV infections has levelled out at 1.8 million new infections for the past 5 years.[124] Clearly, prevention deserves greater attention. Clearly, global messaging on AIDS needs to refrain from declaring victory too soon, yet global leaders still need to provide hope that we can end the AIDS pandemic, and they must emphasize what the global community needs to do to achieve this goal.

Today, UNAIDS operates under a Unified Budget, Results and Accountability Framework (UBRAF), as a successor to its Unified Workplan and Budget, that maximizes coherence, coordination, and impact of the UN's response to AIDS by combin-

---

[116] Ibid.

[117] Ending AIDS: Progress Towards the 90-90-90 Targets. UNAIDS 2017 http://www.unaids.org/sites/default/files/media_asset/Global_AIDS_update_2017_en.pdf.

[118] Ibid., See also "The Gap Report" Geneva: Joint United Nations Programme on HIV/AIDS (UNAIDS), July 2014 UNAIDS / JC2656.

[119] Ending AIDS: Progress Towards the 90-90-90 Targets. UNAIDS 2017 http://www.unaids.org/sites/default/files/media_asset/Global_AIDS_update_2017_en.pdf.

[120] PEPFAR Latest Global Results. 2016. Accessed on May 4, 2017 at https://www.pepfar.gov/documents/organization/264882.pdf

[121] Kim, Sung-Hee et al. "Adherence to Antiretroviral Therapy in Adolescents Living with HIV: Systematic Review and Meta-Analysis." *AIDS (London, England)* 28.13 (2014): 1945–1956. *PMC*. Web. 8 Aug. 2016.

[122] The TenoRes Study Group, "Global epidemiology of drug resistance after failure of WHO recommended first-line regimens for adult HIV-1 infection: a multicentre retrospective cohort study." The Lancet Infectious Diseases, 2016, 16(5):565–575, http://www.thelancet.com/journals/laninf/article/PIIS1473-3099(15)00536-8/abstract.

[123] Sarah Boseley, "Hope for the "end of AIDS" is disappearing experts warn," *The Guardian*, 31 July 2016.

[124] Ending AIDS: Progress Towards the 90-90-90 Targets. UNAIDS 2017 http://www.unaids.org/sites/default/files/media_asset/Global_AIDS_update_2017_en.pdf.

ing the efforts of the cosponsors and the UNAIDS Secretariat. UBRAF is structured around a business plan, results and accountability framework with clear measures of achievement, and core budget for the cosponsors and UNAIDS Secretariat ($485 million for 2016–2017).[125] At country level, its role is to leverage, not replace funding to national programs from the cosponsors or governments. As Lisa Carty, Director of the UNAIDS office in Washington explained, UNAIDS should be seen as an "accelerator" (focusing on policy, future vision, aspirations) and a "gap filler" (assuming technical functions where UN cosponsors do not have responsibility such as human rights, civil society, monitoring, and evaluation). Most recently, it engineered the adoption of the Political Declaration by the UN General Assembly, set the vision for the Fast Track 90-90-90 global targets, and is assisting countries to establish, track and report on their achievements. UNAIDS' annual report provides the only complete set of global data on AIDS and is essential in helping to monitor and evaluate progress on the global response. Advocacy and a strong voice for civil society remain two of its strengths. UNAIDS views its main partners as host governments, the bilaterals (United States Government is a main partner through PEPFAR), and the Global Fund. UNAIDS' greatest challenge remains coordination within the UN system, particularly at headquarters level and with WHO. As Carty put it, it is "still not perfect, but there is significant learning along the way."[126] Additional challenges are the variability of its technical assistance and normative guidance and difficulty in confronting some governments, particularly in Eastern Europe.

What about the verdict on the success of UNAIDS? In our view, UNAIDS has an impressive list of accomplishments. Many observers credit UNAIDS, and Peter Piot in particular, with ensuring that AIDS remained in the global consciousness and on the international policy agenda, even in countries traditionally unconcerned for the populations most affected by the pandemic.[127] In many ways, Piot's greatest successes—advocacy and fundraising—were very similar to those of Jonathan Mann's. As Piot admitted, "Our achievements were not so much inside the UN system but in the world at large, which is what ultimately counted."[128]

Some have questioned the emphasis UNAIDS places on its advocacy role, but few have denied its effectiveness for the cause. More controversially, perhaps, UNAIDS has been successful in championing AIDS exceptionalism—that because AIDS existed at a unique intersection of disease severity, biomedical complexity, social devastation, and sociostructural vulnerability, it demanded an exceptional financial and public health response. As exemplified by its recent role in championing the Political Declaration, UNAIDS has successfully argued that investment in a disease with such widespread implications invariably improves the general condi-

---

[125] UNAIDS Programme Coordinating Board. Thirty-seventh meeting, Agenda Item 4. UNAIDS Unified Budget, Results and Accountability Framework 2016-2021. October 20, 2015 http://www.unaids.org/sites/default/files/media_asset/20151103_UNAIDS_UBRAF_PCB37_15-19_EN.pdf.

[126] Lisa Carty. Interview by Michael Merson, Durham, NC, October 8, 2012.

[127] Devi Sridhar, Danielle Kuczynski, and Kristie Latulippe "Background Report for UNAIDS Transition Working Group." New York and Oxford UK: Center for Global Development/Global Economic Governance Programme, 2008. Used with permission.

[128] Peter Piot, *No Time to Lose: A Life in Pursuit of Deadly Viruses*. New York: Norton, 2012, 374.

tion of health systems, human rights, vaccine development, drug pricing, and intergovernmental program coordination.[129] Some feel it is unfair for one disease to have attracted funds disproportionate to its impact, while others maintained that AIDS' rising tide lifted other boats and was even the genesis of the growing academic field of global health.[130] As a consequence, UNAIDS came to embody more than any other UN agency the promise of multisectoral responses to global problems and, in its ideal form, symbolized what an expanded and coordinated response might look like. This was particularly poignant when UNAIDS, and again Piot specifically, spoke out on behalf of society's most vulnerable—those whose individual and collective levels of health and vulnerability were dominated by social, political, and economic structures beyond their control. This last stance was courageous. Promoting access to condoms and clean needles, much less promoting the rights of women, MSM, and sex workers, flew in the face of countless laws, values, traditions, and convictions. UNAIDS endured as much criticism for deferring to national or donor sensitivities as for contravening them, but it deserves much credit for holding as high as possible the principles of human rights in all its efforts.

UNAIDS' track record in providing technical guidance and coordination is more equivocal.[131] Its surveillance efforts and collection and dissemination of best practices provided valuable insight into the pandemic's shape and strategies to fight it, though a few questioned the validity of its numbers or the effectiveness of its strategic and technical guidance.[132] Piot made a strategic decision early on in his tenure to allow the cosponsors to take the lead in providing guidance in their areas of expertise, and after a few years had only a small number of technical experts on the UNAIDS staff. While this was not what was initially envisioned in Option A during the establishment of UNAIDS (Option A envisioned a strong technical Secretariat similar to that at GPA [see Chapter 16]),[133] he felt it was the best way of ensuring maximum cooperation from the cosponsors, particularly of those working at headquarter level. As a coordinating body, UNAIDS has provided "a singular focus in the multilateral architecture," and maintained a "remarkably unified" response when compared to responses to other problems or disease entities, and has maintained a measure of

---

[129] Bayer, Ronald, "Public health policy and the AIDS epidemic: an end to HIV exceptionalism?" *New England Journal of Medicine,* May 23, 1991, 324:1500–1504.

[130] Allan M. Brandt, "How AIDS Invented Global Health," *New England Journal of Medicine* 2013; 368:2149–2152.

[131] Devi Sridhar, Danielle Kucyznski, and Kristie Latulippe "Background Report for UNAIDS Transition Working Group." New York and Oxford UK: Center for Global Development/Global Economic Governance Programme, 2008. Used with permission.

[132] Craig Timberg, "U.N. to Cut Estimate of AIDS Epidemic," *Washington Post,* November 20, 2007, Accessed at http://www.washingtonpost.com/wp-dyn/content/article/2007/11/19/AR2007111900978. html; Devi Sridhar, Danielle Kucyznski, and Kristie Latulippe "Background Report for UNAIDS Transition Working Group." New York and Oxford UK: Center for Global Development/Global Economic Governance Programme, 2008. Used with permission. Accessed at http://www.cgdev.org/doc/UNAIDS_Leadership_11_03_08.pdf; Five-Year Evaluation of UNAIDS: Final Report, Conclusions and summary of recommendations," Geneva: UNAIDS, 2009, http://data.unaids.org/pub/basedocument/2009/20090609_sie_fieconclusions_summary_of_recommendations_en.pdf.

[133] See Appendix 5 and 6

independence not enjoyed by many of its cosponsors.[134] The broad nature of the AIDS pandemic called for cooperation across many domains of expertise. This may have resulted in some delay in articulation of certain policies or positions, but to some extent this is inevitable for an organization coordinating the views of so many UN agencies. While UNAIDS enables its cosponsors, with their varying views on the biomedical, development, and human rights approaches to combating AIDS to live under one roof, it is unclear how well UNAIDS actually coordinates their efforts. In any event, UNAIDS lacks any substantive mechanism to hold bilateral and international institutions accountable when they choose not to coordinate, especially those wielding disproportionately large influence or with substantial resources, such as PEPFAR and the Global Fund (both of which were created more than 5 years after UNAIDS was established).[135] Since 2011, UNAIDS has taken steps to be a more efficient and effective organization and reduced its expenditures considerably. However, in 2016, it announced it had a shortfall of 30% in donor support, its first major funding crisis since the early days of its creation, which will likely cause it to rethink its priorities in the global response.[136]

In April, 2008, amid the promise and peril of fighting global AIDS, Piot announced that he intended to step down as UNAIDS Executive Director. Few noticed the statement or commented on it, but by the summer of 2008, after 13 years as head of UNAIDS, UN Secretary General Ban Ki-moon announced that Piot would be leaving his position. In 2008, at a High-Level Meeting on HIV/AIDS, Ban lauded Piot as a "tireless leader who has been at the vanguard of the response to AIDS since the earliest days of the epidemic."[137] The pandemic was not over, but Piot felt he had achieved a great deal. He was credited, concluded Larry Altman, "as the person most responsible for making Heads of State understand the political, economic and social ramifications of a pandemic that rivals the worst in history."[138] It was hard to deny this. When Piot started UNAIDS, the global health community was spending $250 million on HIV in developing countries; by 2008 that number topped $10 billion. In 1996, Piot had struggled to gain political traction on the issue; in 2008, critics claimed that global leaders paid too much attention to AIDS. In 1996, the cost of HAART drugs was outside the reality of 90% of the world; by 2008 some countries were giving the drugs away free or at vastly reduced cost.

---

[134] Devi Sridhhar, Danielle Kucyznski, and Kristie Latulippe "Background Report for UNAIDS Transition Working Group." New York and Oxford UK: Center for Global Development/Global Economic Governance Programme, 2008. Used with permission.

[135] Ibid.

[136] UNAIDS, "Press release: UNAIDS Board underlines the need for accelerated action and increased investment to end the AIDS epidemic by 2030," Geneva: UNAIDS, 1 July 2016 accessed at http://www.unaids.org/en/resources/presscentre/pressreleaseandstatementarchive/2016/July/20160701_PCB38.

[137] Daniel Bases, "Head of UN's AIDS program Piot to step down," *Reuters*, Tue, Jun 10, 2008. http://mobile.reuters.com/article/idUSN1039123320080610?irpc=932 accessed on June 5, 2012.

[138] Lawrence K. Altman, "Leaving Platform That Elevated AIDS Fight," *The New York Times*, December 30, 2008.

Did Piot have regrets? Certainly. He admitted UNAIDS' numbers were not perfect: they had overestimated Asia and underestimated Eastern Europe and some African nations. He wished he could have persuaded Russia to provide methadone replacement therapy for injection drug users; that he could have moved the Catholic Church further on condoms; and that he could have convinced South Africa's Thabo Mbeki that HIV caused AIDS. Particularly striking were his views on UN coordination.[139] In a telling remark, Piot showed his skepticism "as to whether the current UN coordination governance could ever be effective operationally, despite the goodwill of many, if not most, staff." As he explained:

> The two main obstacles for delivering as one UN were the institutional interests of individual agencies— careers, political influence, budgets— and the incoherence and volatility of its Member States, which not only had different, sometimes mutually exclusive, interests, but which also lacked internal coherence, as they promoted different agendas in different UN agencies depending upon which national department they represented. My conclusion on UN coordination was that **it was a collective failure** [emphasis ours], and that the international community either goes for some bold mergers and acquisitions as the current plethora of institutions is too expensive, or that it accepts that pluralism is a strength, as long as only effective and well-managed institutions are supported and others closed down. The creation of new institutions outside the UN system to fix problems of the UN is not a solution, as much as I worked to make the Global Fund to Fight AIDS, Tuberculosis and Malaria a success.[140]

More than regret, however, Piot had appreciation … appreciation for the sacrifice, teamwork, and cooperation that AIDS had brought out in the global community. At his last session as leader of UNAIDS, Piot chided the media for their penchant at seeing conflict in AIDS and in the AIDS community and for not appreciating the coming together of such a multifaceted coalition of actors. "Where else would you see all these different groups?" Piot asked those gathered. Then, to sum up what he had tried to embody during his time at UNAIDS and GPA and the International AIDS Society before that, Piot ended with a quote from Indian novelist Arundhati Roy:

> "To never simplify what is complicated or complicate what is simple. To respect strength, never power. Above all, to watch. To try and understand. To never look away. And never, never, to forget."[141]

---

[139] On Russia and Mbeki, see Ibid; on abstinence, see S.M. Bertozzi, T. E. Martz, P. Piot. "The evolving HIV/AIDS response and the urgent tasks ahead." *Health Affairs*. 2009 Nov-Dec;28(6):1578–90.

[140] Peter Piot, *No Time to Lose: A Life in Pursuit of Deadly Viruses*. New York: Norton, 2012, 373.

[141] "Dr Peter Piot delivers final report to UNAIDS' governing board as Executive Director," UNAIDS, 16 December 2008. http://www.unaids.org/en/Resources/PressCentre/Featurestories/2008/December/2008121623rdPCB/ accessed on June 5, 2012.

Part IV
Lessons Learned and the Future of the Global Response

Chapter 19
Conclusion

On July 17, 2014, Malaysian Air Flight MH17 was shot down over Ukraine during military actions related to Russia's annexing of Ukraine's Crimean peninsula. Tragic in its own regard (the attack killed all 298 people on board), the loss of innocent life on the flight was compounded for those in the AIDS[1] and global health communities when word emerged that its passengers included AIDS researchers and activists on their way to Melbourne, Australia, to attend the 20th International AIDS Conference.[2] Among the losses was Joep Lange, who had led the Global Programme on AIDS (GPA)'s clinical research and drug development activities (see Chapter 7).[3] Since leaving GPA in 1994, Lange had served as President of the International AIDS Society, promoted early and aggressive treatment of HIV infection, and become a strong advocate for access to low-cost treatment by calling for "a greater focus on health systems and on the integration of HIV services" and

---

Within this chapter the singular pronouns *I* and *my* refer to Michael Merson alone, whereas the plural pronouns *we* and *us* generally refer to Michael Merson and Stephen Inrig jointly. Where *we* or *us* refers to Michael Merson and his colleagues at WHO, the object of the pronoun is clarified by context.

[1] For the purposes of this text, we will use the term AIDS to encompass both AIDS and HIV unless otherwise specified.

[2] Ian Neubauer, "Top AIDS Researchers Killed in Malaysia Airlines Crash," *Time Magazine*, July 18, 2014, http://time.com/3003840/malaysia-airlines-ukraine-crash-top-aids-researchers-killed-aids2014-mh17/*AccessedJune18,2016.*http://www.cbc.ca/news/world/malaysia-airlines-mh17-what-we-k.

[3] Ibid.

© Springer International Publishing AG 2018
M. Merson, S. Inrig, *The AIDS Pandemic*, DOI 10.1007/978-3-319-47133-4_19

championing pre-exposure prophylaxis (PrEP).[4] "'You could usually get a cold Coke in a sub-Saharan village,' he observed. 'So there was no reason why you shouldn't be able to get anti-AIDS drugs to the same place.'"[5]

The loss of Lange and others on the MH17 flight was a powerful reminder of the remarkable people engaged in global health, many of whom I was fortunate to have worked with in GPA. Lange and others, in the words of United States President Barack Obama, were "focused on what can be built rather than what can be destroyed."[6] The purpose of this book has been to explore how different people, institutions, and nations have sought to respond to the AIDS pandemic, and the factors that have supported or hindered those efforts. Often what provided the best support has been the relentless commitment to humanity as exhibited by Lange and others on board that doomed flight. Often, what has most hampered these efforts seem petty in the big picture: personal disagreements between individuals; the supremacy of national over international interests; and the desire to retain complete autonomy over one's little piece of institutional pie.

But the reality is that, since the first reported AIDS cases in the early 1980s, almost 78 million people have acquired HIV and 35 million persons have died of AIDS-related causes.[7] Within 5 years of its discovery, the AIDS pandemic posed a substantial challenge to the global health community.[8] The initial discovery of the disease among marginalized persons who often engaged in socially taboo practices rendered it ripe for stigma and discrimination, and the extent to which it had spread only heightened these challenges. HIV often existed at the intersection of a host of factors that rendered many populations vulnerable to infection while at the same

---

[4] Julio S. G. Montaner, Peter Reiss, David Cooper, Stefano Vella, Marianne Harris, Brian Conway, Mark A. Wainberg, D. Smith, Patrick Robinson, David Hall, Maureen Myers, and Joep M. A. Lange, for the INCAS Study Group, "A Randomized, Double-blind Trial Comparing Combinations of Nevirapine, Didanosine, and Zidovudine for HIV-Infected Patients: The INCAS Trial," *JAMA*, March 25, 1998, 279(12): 930–937. doi:10.1001/jama.279.12.930; H. Schuitemaker, M. Koot, N.A. Kootstra, M.W. Dercksen, R.E. de Goede, R.P. van Steenwijk, et al. "Biological phenotype of human immunodeficiency virus type 1 clones at different stages of infection: progression of disease is associated with a shift from monocytotropic to T-cell-tropic virus population." *J Virol.* 1992;66:1354–60; Zach Dubinsky, "Malaysia Airlines Flight MH17: AIDS scientist Joep Lange did pioneering research with Canadians," *CBC News*, July 18, 2014 http://www.cbc.ca/news/world/malaysia-airlines-flight-mh17-aids-scientist-joep-lange-did-pioneering-research-with-canadians-1.2710793; Chris Beyrer, Stefano Vella, and David A. Cooper, "In memoriam: Joep Lange MD, PhD," *J Int AIDS Soc.* 2014; 17(1): 19401; Zach Dubinsky, "Malaysia Airlines Flight MH17: AIDS scientist Joep Lange did pioneering research with Canadians," *CBC News*, July 18, 2014 http://www.cbc.ca/news/world/malaysia-airlines-flight-mh17-aids-scientist-joep-lange-did-pioneering-research-with-canadians-1.2710793; Chris Beyrer, Stefano Vella, and David A. Cooper, "In memoriam: Joep Lange MD, PhD," *J Int AIDS Soc.* 2014; 17(1): 19401; "Obituary: Joep Lange," *The Economist*, July 26, 2014.

[5] "Obituary: Joep Lange," *The Economist*, July 26, 2014.

[6] Barack Obama, "The President Makes a Statement on Ukraine," Whitehouse.gov, July 18, 2014, https://www.whitehouse.gov/photos-and-video/video/2014/07/18/president-makes-statement-ukraine

[7] UNAIDS Fact Sheet 2016 http://www.unaids.org/sites/default/files/media_asset/UNAIDS_FactSheet_en.pdf.

[8] Ibid.

time blocking them from effective prevention and compassionate care. What type of organization or effort did the global community need to respond appropriately to the complex human crisis that was—and is—the global AIDS pandemic?

In this book, we have related the various paths that the global health community has taken over the years to answer this question. The first solution settled upon and arrived at through a process of abdication, opportunism, and consensus—was that the World Health Organization (WHO) should direct and coordinate the global response to the pandemic. This sprang from the tireless efforts of first Fakhry Assaad and then Jonathan Mann at WHO headquarters in Geneva. They initially had to overcome resistance from senior WHO officials, who were reluctant for WHO to take on a "social" disease thought primarily to be a "first world" problem. Ultimately, and unfortunately, 5 years passed before WHO Director-General, Halfdan Mahler agreed to view AIDS as a disease worthy of WHO's global attention. Discussions ensued as to whether a United Nations (UN) cosponsored program or new agency might be best to address such a complex and socially controversial problem. Eventually convinced of the importance and gravity of the disease, and viewing it first and foremost as a health problem, Mahler fought to keep the response housed within WHO. Recognizing the sizable challenge and inherent weaknesses of WHO's governance and structure, Mahler gave Mann considerable autonomy establishing GPA, allowing it to operate directly out of his office in ways similar to the successful Smallpox Eradication Program a decade earlier.

Mann, more than anyone else, informed the world about the catastrophic pandemic that lay ahead, and established GPA as the prime entity directing and coordinating the global response to the pandemic. He rapidly recruited a large and highly dedicated staff and raised a considerable amount of resources from donor governments, giving GPA the ability to rapidly help governments in nearly all low- and middle-income countries establish national AIDS programs. He also formulated a Global AIDS Strategy, providing HIV policy and prevention guidance to all countries. Working with the blessing of Mahler, Mann leveraged the resources of other UN and international organizations while maintaining WHO's authority.

A mere 3 years after GPA was established, many of the program's donors and observers, had become dissatisfied with the program's performance. The pandemic, meanwhile, continued to expand unabated. Mann's leadership was simultaneously inspiring and challenging to people both inside and outside WHO. Some saw his approach as insufficient to the challenges ahead, while others found fault in WHO's structure, its new leadership under Director-General Hiroshi Nakajima, and its penchant to see AIDS through a strictly biomedical lens. Blocked bureaucratically from implementing a program with a strong focus on human rights and frustrated by the constraints placed on him by Nakajima, Mann abruptly resigned as GPA Director in March 1990, strongly criticizing Nakajima in the process.

Many deeply lamented Mann's departure from the global stage, and his resignation opened up the question about the primacy and leadership of WHO in the fight against AIDS. It was during this transition that other UN agencies launched their own AIDS efforts, the most important of which was the United Nations Development Programme (UNDP)'s HIV and Development Program. It was also around this time that many donor nations began investing more energy and resources in their own bilateral AIDS programs. Moreover, there was growing dissatisfaction with Nakajima himself, who many considered incompetent and more concerned with preserving WHO's way of operating than ending the AIDS pandemic. His controversial reelection to a second term as Director-General caused great consternation among many of GPA's donors.

As Mann's successor, I found myself in a very challenging situation: I was associated with an increasingly unpopular Director-General, was inheriting staff with fierce loyalty to Mann, and did not have anywhere near the charisma that he possessed.[9] Nevertheless, GPA moved forward: we placed a strong emphasis on traditional public health approaches and program management to improve national programs, established solid initiatives in such areas as comprehensive care, sexually transmitted diseases (STDs)[10], and blood safety, carried out a robust research agenda, and did our best to provide accountability for the resources we received. However, after conducting an external review of the program, GPA's oversight body decided to close down GPA despite its brief tenure and create a new global AIDS governance structure in its place, one they felt would ensure better coordination and collaboration particularly among the UN agencies.

After months of discussions to find the most appropriate programmatic alternative, the donor community settled on the establishment of a new joint and cosponsored program on HIV/AIDS, which became known as UNAIDS. GPA closed down on December 31, 1995, and UNAIDS opened its doors the next day amidst much excitement. Problems soon arose, however, when Peter Piot—the Executive Director of the new program—realized that some of the UN cosponsors, despite their agreement to the formation of UNAIDS, had little interest in supporting the program. Also, donor nations were neither willing to compel them to work together nor provide the budgetary resources the program needed.

The situation dramatically changed around the turn of the last century when Highly Active Antiretroviral Therapy (HAART), which had been discovered in 1996, became available and affordable. In 2001, the UN General Assembly adopted a declaration at a special session that committed Heads of State to seriously fight the pandemic, following which a number of agencies and organizations committed substantial additional resources. Over only a few years, a number of institutions, some of them new, stood alongside UNAIDS, each with their own assets and vision about the appropriate global response. These included the World Bank, the Global Fund to Fight AIDS, Tuberculosis and Malaria, the United States government's President's Emergency Plan for AIDS Relief (PEPFAR) program, a newly committed WHO, and the Bill & Melinda Gates Foundation. WHO had far less resources at its disposal than all the other organizations. While the donors and UN

---

[9] Dennis Altman, the Australian human rights activist, referred to as a "poisoned chalice." Denis Altman, Interview by Michael Merson, November 2, 2001.

[10] For the purposes of this text, we use the term sexually transmitted disease(s) and the abbreviation STD rather than the other term sexually transmitted infection(s) or STIs.

cosponsors had originally designated UNAIDS to take the lead in coordinating the global response, it was clear by the mid 2000s that despite Piot's hard work and impassioned advocacy, UNAIDS would only play a limited though important role, serving as the global health community's main multi-lateral contributor and as a major global champion for the response. Beyond whatever limitations UNAIDS may have had, advances in AIDS treatment, the desire by donors to have greater control over their resources, and the significant increase in funds from various organizations generated an increasingly patchwork response globally and in countries. This again raised questions about the most effective way to move forward against the pandemic.

Within the last few years, the situation has changed. The discovery that early treatment with antiretroviral therapy (ART) could not only effectively prevent death from AIDS but also prevent transmission of the virus has raised tremendous hope and optimism that the "end of AIDS" is in sight. The existence of effective treatment reenergized the AIDS response and fostered a new political declaration of commitment to fight AIDS by Member States at a high-level UN General Assembly Special Session in 2011. At the 20th AIDS International Conference in Melbourne in August 2014, the UNAIDS Executive Director Michel Sidibé, who succeeded Piot, let the world know that "The AIDS epidemic can be ended in every region, in every country, in every location, in every population and every community."[11] This goal was endorsed at another high-level UN General Assembly Special Session in 2016. While this goal may not be fully attainable and is fraught with many challenges, not the least of which is complacency, there are reasons to think that it might be possible to end the AIDS pandemic as a major public health threat by 2030.[12]

A UNAIDS-Lancet Commission report on Defeating AIDS-Advancing Global Health published in June 2015 laid out a series of guiding principles and recommendations to achieve this goal.[13] It will require, not just significant increases in access to ART, but also scale up in prevention programs, such as male circumcision, PrEP (Pre-exposure prophylaxis), prevention to mother to child transmission, behavioral interventions and—ideally—an effective HIV vaccine. Additionally, despite the progress made destigmatizing AIDS and its associated behaviors, there remains a constant threat that nations will take measures that threaten the human rights of HIV-positive persons (like the punitive laws recently adopted in Uganda).[14] AIDS advocates must confront these policies. Furthermore, we must also give greater attention to up-stream, structural interventions, such as a reduction of gender-based violence and access to social protection programs. Finally, many of

---

[11] Kate Kelland, "Global AIDS epidemic can be controlled by 2030, U.N. says," *Reuters*, Wed Jul 16, 2014.

[12] WM El-Sadr et al., *Science* 11 July 2014: Vol. 345 no. 6193 p. 166; Michel Sidibe, "The sustainable development agenda and the end of AIDS," *Lancet*, 386: 108–110, July 11, 2015.

[13] "A UNAIDS-Lancet Commission on Defeating AIDS-Advancing Global Health," *Lancet*, 11 July, 2015, 386(9989):171–218.

[14] Somini Sengupta, "Antigay laws gain global attention; countering them remains challenge." *NYT*, March 1, 2014.

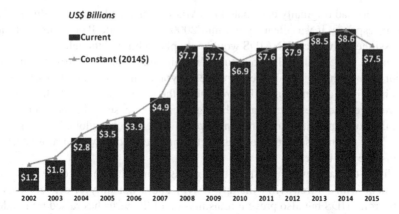

Fig. 19.1 International HIV assistance from donor governments: disbursements, 2002–2015. Source: Jennifer Kates, Adam Wexler, Eric Lief, "Financing the Response to HIV in Low- and Middle-Income Countries: International Assistance from Donor Governments in 2015," Kaiser Family Foundation and UNAIDS, 2016.

the weaknesses that inhibited the global response during the past three decades remain today, including: short-term funding cycles of donors; inadequate coordination between international institutions; insufficient harmonization with national agendas and structures; duplication in evaluation reporting; insufficient attention to prevention; and an overreliance on biomedical approaches.[15] There is also concern about a rebound surge in the epidemic in sub-Saharan Africa, particularly among adolescent girls and young women.[16] Nevertheless, in many ways, there is reason to hope that the global health community has reached a turning point in the history of the AIDS pandemic.[17]

The history of the global response to AIDS has given us valuable insights into how to forge a coordinated and effective response to future pandemics. When one reflects on the logarithmic magnitude by which the global response to AIDS has increased in recent years, it is startling to realize that some 20 years ago, before the existence of the Global Fund, PEPFAR, or the World Bank Multi-Country AIDS Programs, international AIDS assistance from donor governments to low- and middle-income countries hovered around $250 million annually. This is a minute

---

[15] A UNAIDS-Lancet Commission on Defeating AIDS-Advancing Global Health," *Lancet*, 11 July, 2015; 386(9989): 171–218.

[16] Leaders from around the world are ALL In to end the AIDS epidemic among adolescents. Unicef 2015. Accessed on May 5 at https://www.unicef.org/media/media_79820.html

[17] Richard. Horton, "Offline: Ending the AIDS epidemic," *The Lancet*, 384(9941):388, 2 August, 2014.

fraction of the $8.5 billion in assistance provided in 2013[18] and the $8.6 billion in 2014.[19] While donor funding declined to $7.5 billion in 2015 (a 13% decline), (Fig. 19.1), some of this decrease was due to currency fluctuations and a number of disbursement timing issues (making the actual decline 8%).[20] Fortunately, low- and middle-income countries are providng more domestic resources. Domestic funding reached an estimated $19.2 billion in 2015, accounting for 57% of total AIDS funding that year. This, as well as private sector funding, needs to continue to increase as donors (particularly in Europe) implement fiscal austerity measures and shift much of their development assistance to programs dealing with the influx of refugees to Europe from the Middle East. Unfortunately, these changing financial commitments are coming when there is an estimated $11 billion annual price tag for meeting the 90-90-90 targets[21] and still major gaps in funding for HIV prevention. At the time of this writing, for example, only 20% of global AIDS resources target prevention services.[22]

What lessons have we learned from the history of the global response to AIDS? We have identified at least seven, though we are confident that there are more.[23] The first lesson is that the world is capable of responding to new pandemics like AIDS. However, the history of GPA and of UNAIDS demonstrates that, when responding, donor countries can be impulsive (when launching and supporting new programs) and impatient (when demanding results), and tend to shift strategies to pursue short-term solutions for complex problems. As Jim Sherry has suggested, global governance around AIDS has often been reactive, rather than intentional and farsighted.[24] Donor nations in the fifth year of the pandemic established the WHO's

---

[18] Jennifer Kates, Adam Wexler, Eric Lief, Carlos Avila, and Benjamin Gobet, "Financing the Response to AIDS in Low- and Middle-Income Countries: International Assistance from Donor Governments in 2010," Menlo Park, CA and Geneva: Kaiser Family Foundation and UNAIDS, 2011, 7347-07; Jennifer Kates, Adam Wexler, Eric Lief, "Financing the Response to HIV in Low- and Middle-Income Countries: International Assistance from Donor Governments in 2013," Menlo Park, CA and Geneva: Kaiser Family Foundation and UNAIDS, 2014 https://kaiserfamilyfounda-tion.files.wordpress.com/2014/07/7347-10-financing-the-response-to-hiv-in-low-and-middle-income-countries.pdf.

[19] Kaiser Family Foundation and UNAIDS, Financing the Response to HIV in Low and Middle Income Countries, International Assistance from Donor Governments 2014, July 2015.

[20] Jennifer Kates, Adam Wexler, Eric Lief, "Financing the Response to HIV in Low- and Middle-Income Countries: International Assistance from Donor Governments in 2015," Kaiser Family Foundation and UNAIDS, 2016. http://files.kff.org/attachment/report-financing-the-response-to-aids-in-low-and-middle-income-countries-international-assistance-from-donor-gov-ernments-in-2014.

[21] Granich, Reuben, et al. "90-90-90 and ending AIDS: necessary and feasible," *The Lancet* 390.10092 (2017): 341–343.

[22] *Prevention GAP report.* Geneva: UNAIDS 2016 http://www.unaids.org/sites/default/files/media_asset/2016-prevention-gap-report_en.pdf.

[23] See, for example, Ronald O. Valdiserri, ed., *Dawning Answers: How the HIV/AIDS Epidemic Has Helped to Strengthen Public Health,* New York: Oxford University Press, 2003.

[24] Jim Sherry, Interview by Michael Merson, Geneva, October, 2001.

Special Programme on AIDS, which quickly evolved into GPA, and provided it with an unprecedented amount of financial support. At its pinnacle, GPA was the largest international health program in history. Yet, only 8 years later, the same donors reacted to the perceived failure of GPA by dissolving it to create a new, more complex, though highly innovative joint and cosponsored United Nations Program, UNAIDS. Seven years after the launch of UNAIDS, the same donors reacted once again in part to the perceived shortcomings of UNAIDS, by creating the Global Fund to Fight AIDS, Tuberculosis and Malaria, giving it a budget twenty times larger than UNAIDS (rather than creating, for example, an AIDS fund managed by UNAIDS). Shortly after that, the United States government launched PEPFAR, the largest single health program in its history of foreign assistance and one that is dedicated to AIDS prevention, treatment, and care, now funneling less than 1% of its budget to UNAIDS.[25] At the same time, donors encouraged WHO to reenter the AIDS field with the launch of a new "3 by 5" initiative, which, though unable to meet its goals in time, did return WHO as a major player in the global response.

An important question to ask is whether the dissolution of GPA was necessary to achieve a stronger coordinated response to the AIDS pandemic. How much was this decision a result of the donor community's dissatisfaction with the overall performance of Hiroshi Nakajima as WHO Director-General and his controversial reelection in 1992? How much of it was a consequence of the donor community's unrealistic expectations of what GPA could achieve in such a short period of time against such a complex disease? How much of it was a result of the donor community's realization of WHO's limitations as an agency, particularly at regional and country level, especially in Africa? Also, was it a poor decision to create UNAIDS without ensuring it had a strong link to WHO? These questions are important because UNAIDS has found it difficult to create the hoped-for unified and well-coordinated global response among UN agencies, much less among donors, civil society, foundations, and the private sector. Moreover, the transition that occurred between GPA and UNAIDS was far from smooth. Most importantly, it created a crisis in many heavily affected countries, particularly in Africa, where national programs were abruptly devoid of crucial GPA support.

There are no simple right or wrong answers to these questions, but they deserve serious consideration. Had HAART therapy been available 3 years earlier, it is tempting to speculate that the donor community might have wanted GPA to maintain its leadership in the global response, strongly encouraging it to strengthen its efforts in coordination among UN agencies. In any event, donor nations should not underestimate the significant consequences of abolishing a global program, abruptly

---

[25] Congressional Budget Justification Supplement. President's Emergency Plan for AIDS Relief (PEPFAR). Fiscal year 2017. http://www.pepfar.gov/documents/organization/259634.pdf; See also Jennifer Kates, Adam Wexler, and Eric Lief, *Financing the Response to HIV in Low- and Middle-Income Countries: International Assistance from Donor Governments in 2012*. Menlo Park, CA: The Henry J. Kaiser Family Foundation, September 2013, http://www.unaids.org/sites/default/files/en/media/unaids/contentassets/documents/document/2013/09/20130923_KFF_UNAIDS_Financing.pdf.

turning off the "response faucet," and transferring responsibilities to a new agency, particularly when confronting a quickly expanding global pandemic of a fatal disease. Before closing down an organization, one must be sure one can do better. If transitions like the one between GPA and UNAIDS occur again, they should be carried out carefully, responsibly, and with a clear understanding of the potential negative and unintended consequences such a decision may have, bearing in mind the challenges and resources required to mount a global response.[26]

Despite its well-known limitations, we expect the UN system will continue to be a key resource for governments. Consequently, and as we have seen in the history of UNAIDS, a second lesson learned (related to the first), is that donor nations need to more fully understand the realities and limitations of achieving a coordinated UN system. The experience of GPA and UNAIDS has shown us how the varying constituencies, mandates, histories, and governance structures of the UN agencies pose great challenges and obstacles for their successful collaboration. However, nations should encourage the UN system to operate more efficiently and effectively, which may on occasion require the establishment or dissolution of programs or agencies.

Our third lesson learned (also related to the first), concerns accountability. This book has provided a number of examples where the tail wagged the dog: that is, where personal animosities at the institutional level influenced or hindered the shape of the global response. As an example, UNAIDS understood that Nakajima and WHO had given their full cooperation and support to its establishment, and then within mere months, WHO sought to sabotage the new organization at global and regional levels. Another example was the ongoing effort by UNDP to maintain its own independent HIV program at all costs even after the creation of UNAIDS. These behaviors were enabled by the donors as they failed to provide the appropriate oversight that was required once they formed UNAIDS. Granted such supervision likely would have been diplomatically difficult and may not necessarily have been in their national interest. However, by not intervening, donors allowed these relationships to become poisonous and to negatively impact the global response. The lesson here is that international organizations and the donor community need to live up to their commitments, lest these institutional dysfunctions, as we have seen in the case of AIDS, wreak havoc on the lives of vulnerable people around the world.

There is consensus now that we cannot approach AIDS with an emergency response that only includes short-term "fixes."[27] Rather, we need to frame our global response as a struggle that will be with us for the foreseeable future. Mechanisms should exist which ensure organizations work closely together, synergistically rather than competitively or duplicatively. UNAIDS should resolve

---

[26] S. M. Bertozzi, T.E. Martz, P. Piot. "The evolving HIV/AIDS response and the urgent tasks ahead." *Health Affairs*. 2009 Nov–Dec;28(6):1578–90.

[27] Jennifer Kates, Adam Wexler, and Eric Lief, *Financing the Response to HIV in Low- and Middle-Income Countries: International Assistance from Donor Governments in 2012*. Menlo Park, CA: The Henry J. Kaiser Family Foundation, September 2013.

differences on strategic and technical issues, work within the UN architecture to continue to set targets for ending the AIDS pandemic by 2030, monitor progress in meeting the 90-90-90 targets, and assess the impact of the various components of the UN's response under its United Budget, Results, and Accountability Framework. PEPFAR should continue its efforts to help accelerate prevention and treatment efforts in countries, and the Global Fund should function primarily as a financing institution, maintaining the strong transparency and accountability mechanisms they both have in place. While these organizations have demonstrated greater collaboration recently, this would be the time for them to join together in a new and energized alliance of all the global actors to achieve the 2030 goal.[28]

The history of the global response to AIDS also demonstrates that the reaction to complex, global health crises like AIDS must be comprehensive, balanced, and evidence based. It is unlikely that we will have a magic bullet for AIDS or for many other future global health threats. Consequently, a fourth lesson is that programs which address these large-scale threats need to address the entire continuum, from prevention and control to therapy and care, with research conducted as needed along the way. Programs need to carefully plan each step in the continuum to ensure positive, long-term outcomes. In most contexts, prevention is a slow process, and it becomes even more difficult when providers lack an effective vaccine and the disease itself evokes panic and discrimination. In the case of AIDS, prevention efforts must receive the same level of program support as treatment, with the goal of reducing the number of new infections (rather than just measuring process outcomes such as the number of condoms distributed).[29] Combination prevention often offers the best hope for success.[30] Also, mechanisms must be in place to ensure that new prevention technologies and drugs are accessible and affordable to those in greatest need. Finally, throughout all these steps we must continue to create supportive environments to fight the discrimination that AIDS still engenders.[31] This will ensure that infected persons and those at risk for infection can safely and openly seek prevention and treatment services.

A poignant and fifth lesson is the value in seeking a polyphonic, multifaceted response. An old Chinese proverb says that "one who is good with a hammer thinks everything is a nail." No doubt, in the case of AIDS, the clashes between proponents of the "biomedical model," the "human rights" model, and the "development" model certainly hardened the intransigence of those in each camp to collaborate with those in the other. The history of the global AIDS response has demonstrated that interventions addressing the sociostructural determinants of disease risk take considerable time to show results. Rather than viewing this as a sign of ineffectiveness, policy-makers should exhibit patience in waiting for their desired effect. In conjunction with these more structural interventions, public health practitioners

---

[28] End AIDS Coalition Creates Unprecedented Collaboration at 'Tipping Point' in AIDS Epidemic," End AIDS Coalition, July 25, 2017.

[29] Ibid.

[30] Ibid.

[31] Charles E. Rosenberg, "What Is an Epidemic? AIDS in Historical Perspective," *Daedalus*, Living with AIDS (Spring, 1989), 118(2):1–17.

must employ shorter term, biomedical or technical responses as a means to slow down transmission. To advocate for one of these responses at the expense of the other is folly. The SDGs open up greater possibilities for bringing tougher action inside and outside the health sector in addressing the social and economic drivers of HIV infection, as well as many other health problems.

A sixth lesson is the indispensable need for contextualized programs within a global response. AIDS may be a global phenomenon, but all epidemics are local: "The so-called 'global AIDS epidemic' is, in reality, an amalgamation of multiple local epidemics that often differ markedly from one another," noted the aids2031 Consortium.[32] This means that while some principles and technologies apply to AIDS everywhere—whether they be "the value of a rights-based approach" or the use of ARVs—no "carbon copy" strategy will work in every location. "Generic responses to heterogeneous problems waste money," notes Bertozzi et al.[33] We would add that they also waste lives because they often miss the target they are hoping to achieve. The epidemiological footprint of HIV in South Africa was and is different than the one in Romania, and what works in urban San Francisco may not work in rural North Carolina, much less in the slums of Sao Paolo.[34] The history of the global response illustrates the need to tailor HIV prevention responses to those most at risk,[35] and that those populations will differ—demographically and culturally—in their various regions and countries.

A seventh and final lesson from the history of the global AIDS response is that the inclusion of civil society is often essential to the appropriate tailoring of effective actions in a given locale. This has certainly been the case with AIDS. While the appropriate participatory role of non-governmental groups and persons living with HIV has differed for each society, this principle has been essential to the success of any AIDS strategy, whether local, national, or global. However, we stress that this inclusion must be "balanced" because we have also learned that support to non-governmental organizations (NGOs) must compliment and not come at the expense of support to government health systems.[36] Moreover, activists and health professionals must strike the appropriate balance between advocacy and public health delivery. Finding that right balance requires tradeoffs depending on the context, and may change over time as local epidemics evolve.

All these lessons place considerable weight on public health practitioners and policy-makers to strengthen their health systems and place priority on strong program

---

[32] The aids2031 Consortium. *AIDS: Taking a Long-Term View*. Upper Saddle River, NJ: FT Press Science, 2011, 6.

[33] S. M. Bertozzi, T.E. Martz, P. Piot. "The evolving HIV/AIDS response and the urgent tasks ahead." *Health Affairs*. 2009 Nov–Dec;28(6):1578–90.

[34] Stephen Inrig. *North Carolina and the Problem of AIDS*. Chapel Hill, NC: University of North Carolina Press, 2011; S. M. Bertozzi, T.E. Martz, P. Piot. "The evolving HIV/AIDS response and the urgent tasks ahead." *Health Affairs*. 2009 Nov–Dec;28(6):1578–90; The aids2031 Consortium. *AIDS: Taking a Long-Term View*. Upper Saddle River, NJ: FT Press Science, 2011, 6.

[35] S. M. Bertozzi, T.E. Martz, P. Piot. "The evolving HIV/AIDS response and the urgent tasks ahead." *Health Affairs*. 2009 Nov–Dec;28(6):1578–90.

[36] J Pfeiffer et al., "The End of AIDS and the NGO Code of Conduct," *The Lancet*, 384(9944), 639–640.

management. Solid management decisions allow programs to operate efficiently, anticipate the spread of the disease, and appropriately allocate resources. Today, with treatment playing such a crucial role in care and prevention, national AIDS programs must train management and staff to address what is now a chronic disease and implement a "planning horizon" that is longer than 5 years and includes providers along the hierarchy of the health system. The needs of an increasingly complex pandemic require that managers ensure adequate linkages between individuals and their system of care.[37] Countries need to take ownership of the response to their epidemic if their effort is to be successful and sustainable.[38] Programs should also build evaluation into their structure on the front end, so they can generate evidence of their outcomes to justify their continued funding, ensure effectiveness, and enable future program implementers to learn from their successes and failures.

We cannot close without addressing the question as to the future of WHO. Until recently, most believed that it is the international agency which should lead the global response against infectious diseases that threaten global security, diseases like AIDS, SARS, avian influenza, and Ebola.[39] The failure of WHO to respond adequately to the 2014 Ebola outbreak in West Africa brought about numerous and profound criticisms of the agency that significantly damaged its reputation.[40] Its poor Ebola response severely dented the belief that WHO is competent to deliver results and lead a full emergency public health response.[41] The truth is that, faced with declining contributions to its budget, hampered by an archaic regional structure, and crowded by an ever growing field of global health actors, WHO has struggled greatly for the past two decades—since around the time of the dissolution of GPA—to locate its place in the field of global health governance. It has scrambled to reform itself into a more efficient and focused organization, but the effects of these changes have yet to materialize.[42] It is certainly not the organization with the reputation and prestige that it had when I first joined it in 1978.

---

[37] S. M. Bertozzi, T.E. Martz, P. Piot. "The evolving HIV/AIDS response and the urgent tasks ahead." *Health Affairs*. 2009 Nov–Dec;28(6):1578–90.

[38] Michele Sidibe et al., "AIDS governance; best practices for a post-2015 world," *The Lancet*, 2013 381, 2147–2149.

[39] Harvey V. Fineberg, "Pandemic Preparedness and Response—Lessons from the H1N1 Influenza of 2009," *New England Journal of Medicine* 2014; 370:1335–1342, April 3, 2014; Margaret Chan, "WHO Reform: Progress Report on Reform Implementation, Report by the Director-General, Sixty-Seventh World Health Assembly, Provisional Agenda Item 11.1," Geneva: World Health Organization, 8 May, 2014, A67/4 http://apps.who.int/gb/ebwha/pdf_files/WHA67/A67_4-en.pdf.

[40] "World Health Organization, Too bit to ail," *The Economist*, Dec 13, 2014; Somini Sengupta "Effort on Ebola Hurt WHO Chief," *the New York Times*, January 6, 2015.

[41] Report of the Ebola Assessment Panel, WHO, July 2015; "Our systems simply couldn't copy," *Lancet* 385: 2447, June 20, 2015; "Solving WHO's "persistent weakness" (part 1)," *Lancet*, 385:100, Jan 10, 2015.

[42] Mark. Dybul et al., Reshaping Global Health, Policy Review, 2012 No. 173, Hoover Institutions, Stanford University; "An irreversible change in global health governance." *Lancet* 385: 2536, May 30, 2015.

The unfortunate reality today is that WHO is not capable of providing the leadership required within the UN system to confront acute epidemic threats. However, as we saw during the Ebola outbreak, it is not evident from where this leadership should come. There have been a number of proposals. Some have called for strengthening WHO country and regional offices and establishing a new and dedicated WHO Center for Emergency Preparedness with an independent Board that publishes an annual report on global health security.[43] An independent panel convened by the Harvard School of Public Health and the London School of Hygiene and Tropical Medicine (LSHTM) recommended the formation of a WHO Standing Emergency Committee. A Commission on a Global Health Risk Framework for the Future convened by the United States National Academy of Medicine advocated for the creation of a WHO Center for Health Emergency Preparedness and Response. Still others have proposed that more leadership in this area be provided by the UN Secretary General's Office in UN headquarters in New York.[44]

Indeed, in May 2016, the World Health Assembly approved the establishment of a new WHO Health Emergencies Program to address a wide range of health emergencies—disease outbreaks, natural disasters, man-made disasters, and conflicts—with an agreed upon budget of $494 million, reflecting an increase of $160 million to WHO's current budget for emergency work. The Program would have a common results framework to standardize planning, budgeting, staffing, monitoring, and feedback across all levels of the organization.[45] An eight-member expert committee has been appointed to oversee and monitor the program. Time will tell whether WHO is able to raise the necessary funds for the program and, if it does, whether the program is sufficient to rectify the problems seen during the Ebola outbreak. To date, WHO's advice on and response to the expanding spread of the Zika virus, while not without controversy, has been viewed positively.

While improving its ability to respond to acute emergencies is no doubt essential, it is even more important to consider how to best restore WHO's overall credibility and address its more than 20-year decline as the world's leader in health.[46] It is because of this decline that WHO has a limited amount of flexible funding. By 2014, 80% of WHO's budget comprised of earmarked funds, which essentially

---

[43] Report of the Ebola Assessment Panel, WHO, July 2015; Suerie Moon, Devi Sridhar, Muhammad A Pate, Ashish K Jha, Chelsea Clinton, Sophie Delaunay, Valnora Edwin, Mosoka Fallah, David P Fidler, Laurie Garrett, Eric Goosby, Lawrence O Gostin, David L Heymann, Kelley Lee, Gabriel M Leung, J Stephen Morrison, Jorge Saavedra, Marcel Tanner, Jennifer A Leigh, Benjamin Hawkins, Liana R Woskie, Peter Piot, "Will Ebola change the game? Ten essential reforms before the next pandemic. The report of the Harvard-LSHTM Independent Panel on the Global Response to Ebola," *Lancet*, 386:2204–2221, 2015.

[44] Peter Sands, Carmen Mundaca-Shah, and Victor J. Dzau, "The Neglected Dimension of Global Security—A Framework for Countering Infectious-Disease Crises," *New England Journal of Medicine* 2016; 374:1281–1287 March 31, 2016 DOI: 10.1056/NEJMsr1600236.

[45] Reform of WHO's work in health emergency management, WHO Health Emergencies Program, Report by the Director-General, 69th World Health Assembly, Document 169/30, May 2016.

[46] Enhancing the Performance of International Health Institutions", Harvard Center for Population and Development Studies, February 1996.

makes it a donor driven organization, answering to donor agendas and priorities rather than the World Health Assembly[47]. Some have recommended a set of far more extensive reforms within WHO than it has proposed, reforms that would more radically change its governance structure (such as eliminating the regional offices and establishing more authority and budget control centrally), which is at the root of many of its operational problems.[48] Others have suggested the establishment of UN-HEALTH, a multi-stakeholder, governing body to provide global guidance in terms of norms, standards, and policies, and information on health trends and outcomes (similar but wider reaching than UNAIDS). Another proposed option is the formation of a UN Health Commission forum to enhance coordination between major global health agencies including the UN agencies, NGOs, and the private sector.[49] Some have even called for a Bretton Woods type conference to devise a new global health governance structure entirely.[50] Reaching a global consensus on the best way to organize and financially support a response to global threats could be included in any such deliberations.

Our own preference is the first of these options—for WHO to take the bold steps of genuinely reforming itself to be a true and trusted leader in global health and global health security, as agreed at the G7 Summit in Germany in June, 2015.[51] As proposed by the Harvard-LSHTM panel mentioned above, WHO should focus its future activities on its core functions as determined by a fundamental review of its constitution and mandate, develop a sustainable financial model that supports these core functions, and perhaps outsource some of its key activities to other global health organizations.[52] The newly elected Director-General, Tedros Ghebreyesus, will need to exhibit strong leadership, pay special attention to issues around WHO organizational structure, improve its transparency with regards to funding, and carry out the necessary reforms.[53] Our hope is that WHO and its Member States find the courage and political will to make the needed reforms and to do so very soon. If they

[47] Chelsea Clinton and Devi Sridhar. *Governing global health: who runs the world and why?* Oxford Univeristy Press, 2017, p. 185.

[48] "World Health Organization, Heal Thyself," *The Economist*, Dec. 13, 2014; Charles Clift "What's the World Health Organization For?" *Chatham House Report*, May 2014; Suerie Moon, Devi Sridhar, Muhammad A Pate, Ashish K Jha, Chelsea Clinton, Sophie Delaunay, Valnora Edwin, Mosoka Fallah, David P Fidler, Laurie Garrett, Eric Goosby, Lawrence O Gostin, David L Heymann, Kelley Lee, Gabriel M Leung, J Stephen Morrison, Jorge Saavedra, Marcel Tanner, Jennifer A Leigh, Benjamin Hawkins, Liana R Woskie, Peter Piot, "Will Ebola change the game? Ten essential reforms before the next pandemic. The report of the Harvard-LSHTM Independent Panel on the Global Response to Ebola," *Lancet*, 386:2204–2221, 2015.

[49] Marco Schaferhoff, Elina Suzuki, Philip Angelides, Steven Hoffman, "Rethinking the Global Health System, Chatam House," *Royal Institute of International Affairs*, September 2015.

[50] Richard Horton, "Offline: Global Health—an end of term report," *The Lancet* 2912, 379, 1934; K Abbasi, "The World Health Organization: no game of thrones," *BMJ* 2014; 348:g4265.

[51] Schloss Elmau, "Leaders' Declaration G-7 Summit, 7–8 June, 2015, G7 Germany 2015.

[52] J. Negin and R. Dhillon, "Outsourcing: how to reform WHO for the 21st Century." *BMJ Global Health* 2016;1:e000047. doi 10.1136/bmjgh-2016-000047.

[53] Elizabeth Fee. "Whither WHO? Our Global Health Leadership." *American Journal of Public Health*: November 2016, 106(11): 1903–1904. doi: 10.2105/AJPH.2016.303481.

do not, the global health community may require more radical actions, since the world cannot afford to wait any longer for WHO to lead effectively in addressing the many global health challenges before us now and in the future. As an example, the UN has launched an Interagency Coordination Group on Antimicrobial Resistance to coordinate the global response to antimicrobial resistance. While WHO co-chairs the group, it could become another example of WHO losing prime leadership in global health.[54]

Beyond WHO, we believe the history of AIDS and the manner in which the world responded has much to teach 21st century global health planners and policymakers about global health governance. Comprehensive and thoughtful planning can better prepare the global health community to respond to the short- and long-term needs created by such health crises. The risk in pandemics and other emergencies is that, it is only once the situation "is thoroughly out of hand", that we often belatedly respond with remedies, solutions, and interventions which have been garnered from other providers, during other emergencies, at other times. I had the privilege of working alongside many of those in the WHO Global Programme on AIDS—people who, returning to the words of former United States President Barack Obama, "are focused on how they can help people that they've never met; people who define themselves not by what makes them different from other people but by the humanity that we hold in common."[55] We have striven in this book to lift up and affirm the lives and efforts of many who have served during the AIDS pandemic, many whose work has until now not received the attention it deserves, and many more whose names could not be mentioned here because of page limitations. As we learn from their successes and their failures it is our hope that we can magnify their influence to, in some small way, reduce the cost, pain, and suffering that pandemics like AIDS inflict upon humankind.

---

[54] UN announces interagency group to coordinate global fight against antimicrobial resistance. UN News Centre. March 16, 2017. Available at http://www.un.org/apps/news/story.asp?NewsID=56365#.WPpKd_nyvcv

[55] Barack Obama, "The President Makes a Statement on Ukraine," Whitehouse.gov, July 18, 2014, https://www.whitehouse.gov/photos-and-video/video/2014/07/18/president-makes-statement-ukraine.

Appendix 1
Background on the Formation and Structure of the World Health Organization

Much of what is referred to as international or global health governance emerged in the twentieth century, beginning with the International Sanitary Office of the American Republics in 1902 (which addressed Western hemisphere nations); *l'Office Internationale d'Hygiene Public* in 1907 (which addressed "quarantinable" diseases); and the League of Nations Health Organization (LNHO) in 1920 (which advised League of Nations Member States on health matters).[1] This latter organization was particularly important for the publication, beginning in 1926, of its *Weekly Epidemiological Record* (WER), along with its scientific and technical reports, programs, and commissions. Schools of public health along with public health research institutes and foundation-supported public health programs began to emerge at this time (like Johns Hopkins School of Hygiene and Public Health, London School of Hygiene & Tropical Medicine, *l'Institut Pasteur*, and the Rockefeller Foundation's International Health Commission, respectively). Each of these efforts increased awareness about the complex interaction between poverty, poor nutrition, social deprivation, and negative health outcomes.

Global health became a much more organized and expansive field after World War II. The war caused substantial social, political, and economic destruction, both in the combatant nations and their colonial holdings. Various governments agreed, in the years after the war, to address reconstruction efforts and orchestrate development projects in Europe and strategic low- and middle-income countries by establishing or enlarging bilateral development agencies, and by creating or expanding existing inter-governmental organizations. At the national level, this meant that many high-income nations launched, strengthened, or overhauled their national disease control efforts, like the United States Centers for Disease Control and Prevention (CDC), and their development aid agencies such as the United States Agency for International

[1] Elizabeth Fee and Theodore M. Brown, "100 Years of the Pan American Health Organization," *Am J Public Health*. December 2002; 92(12): 1888–1889; Theodore M. Brown, Marcos Cueto, and Elizabeth Fee, "The World Health Organization and the Transition From "International" to "Global" Public Health," *Am J Public Health*. January 2006; 96(1): 62–72.

© Springer International Publishing AG 2018
M. Merson, S. Inrig, *The AIDS Pandemic*, DOI 10.1007/978-3-319-47133-4

Development (USAID), Norwegian Agency for Development Cooperation (NORAD), and the Japan International Cooperation Agency (JICA). At the international level, this meant many countries coming together to launch institutions like the World Bank (formally known as the International Bank for Reconstruction and Development), the International Monetary Fund, the United Nations Children's Fund (UNICEF), and the World Health Organization (WHO).

The United Nations (UN) system today is made up of the UN itself and many affiliated programs, funds, and specialized agencies, all with their own membership, leadership, and budget. The UN Specialized Agencies are autonomous organizations integrated into the UN system through negotiated agreements (see Appendix 2 for the UN structure). WHO is a specialized UN agency focused on global health. Member States held the first World Health Assembly (WHA) in Geneva in June 1948, whereby they formally merged three pre-existing entities—the *Office Internationale d'Hygiène Publique*, LNHO, and the United Nations Relief and Rehabilitation Administration (UNRRA)—into one new entity: WHO.

Based in Geneva, WHO has a multitiered structure (Fig. 1), with three governing entities: the WHA, an Executive Board, and six Regional Committees, and has its own membership and assessed budget. As a UN specialized agency, WHO ultimately reports to the UN's supreme governing body, the United Nations Economic and Social

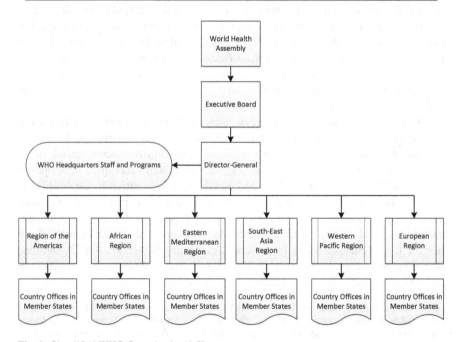

Structure and Operations of the World Health Organization

Fig. 1 Simplified WHO Organizational Chart

Council (ECOSOC), though ECOSOC has limited authority over WHO's governance, which primarily rests in the WHA. The WHA is made up of its Member States (currently 194), and it determines WHO's main organizational policies, approves its budget, and appoints its Director-General. Composed today of 34 members—each of whom is expected to be technically qualified in health—the Executive Board advises the WHA, gives effect to the WHA's decisions and policies, and generally facilitates its work. The Executive Board also nominates up to three candidates for the Director-General for consideration by the WHA, and a candidate requires a two-thirds majority to win the election. Up until 2017 the Executive Board selected a single candidate for Director-General, chosen through a secret ballot, whose name was passed to the World Health Assembly for confirmation.

The Director-General possesses a strong amount of autonomy and directs WHO operations from WHO's headquarters in Geneva. The Director-General is head of the Secretariat, is the chief technical and administrative officer of WHO, serves for a 5-year term, and—under today's governance rules—may stand once thereafter for reelection; several Directors-General have served for multiple terms during WHO's history.[2] Sitting under the Director-General are two more tiers in WHO's bureaucratic hierarchy: the WHO's regional offices and WHO's country offices. Each of the six regional offices—led by a Regional Director who is elected by the Member States in the region—coordinates, implements, and oversees WHO's regional programs. These Regional Directors hire all the regional office staff and have considerable influence over the shape of WHO activities at regional and national levels. The development of regional offices evolved in the late 1940s and the early 1950s. At first, Africa was not included in the regions; its office was only created after complex negotiations with colonial powers in Europe.

The WHO Country Representative directs the WHO country offices and advises each Member State's Ministry of Health on health policy, management, and technical issues. Country Representatives are usually professionals from countries in the region, most often physicians who previously served their government in some capacity. They give WHO direct access to a country's health ministry, while allowing the health ministry access to WHO's regional office and global programs.[3] Policy-making and implementation within WHO occur at all these levels in a variety of ways as discussed in greater detail throughout this book.

There is much to be commended about this decentralized structure, but many observers would agree that—as with many bureaucratic systems—it has several functional limitations. For example, the autonomy of the Regional Directors greatly restrains the authority of the Director-General. In addition, the politically influenced, recruitment process WHO has put in place has historically generated a cadre of staff in the regional and country offices with varied technical competence and uneven commitment to WHO's overall objectives. Also, WHO's limited country-level authority and resource allocation can constrain the ability of Country Representatives

---

[2] Dr. B. Chisholm served only one term, but Drs. M.G. Candau and H. Mahler served multiple terms.

[3] Fiona Godlee, "WHO at Country Level – A Little Impact, No Strategy." *BMJ* 1994, 309:1636-9.

to implement WHO goals. These and other factors have meant that WHO's promise of improving global health, while impressive in many respects, has not been fully realized and its influence and reputation over the past 20 years has gradually declined.[4]

Many of WHO's earliest global health efforts sidestepped these deficiencies by focusing on specific diseases (such as smallpox eradication) and by supporting programs that addressed these diseases through specialized extrabudgetary programs. By the late 1970s, however, the global health community recognized that many global health challenges required stronger health systems at the national level. Consequently, WHO began examining how it could help build up health systems in Member States. In 1978, a conference jointly sponsored by WHO and UNICEF in Alma Ata, USSR, called for "Health for All by the Year 2000" through the establishment and/or extension of primary health care capacity in low- and middle-income countries. By adapting this strategy, WHO transitioned from its focus primarily on specific diseases to one also concerned about health system structure and delivery.[5] Moreover, the Organization gradually and more substantially leveraged the perspective and experience of local and international non-governmental organizations in its health promotion and disease alleviation efforts. WHO also articulated an expanded concept of public health through its "Ottawa Charter for Health Promotion," a statement that emerged from WHO's International Conference on Health Promotion, held in Ottawa, Canada, in 1986.[6] The Ottawa Charter called for a more coordinated and expanded vision of global health and came just at the cusp of two important global transitions, the advent of the AIDS pandemic and the end of the Cold War. It is within this context that the events related in our story begin.

---

[4] Reference: Chatham House Report, Charles Clift, What's the World Health Organization for? May 2014, Chatham House, London.

[5] Kevin M. De Cock, S.B. Lucas, D. Mabey, E. Parry. "Tropical medicine for the 21st century." *BMJ*. 1995 Sep 30;311(7009):860-2.

[6] Ottawa Charter for Health Promotion, First International Conference on Health Promotion, Ottawa, 21 November 1986 - WHO/HPR/HEP/95.1 http://www.who.int/hpr/NPH/docs/ottawa_charter_hp.pdf.

Appendix 2
Structure of the United Nations

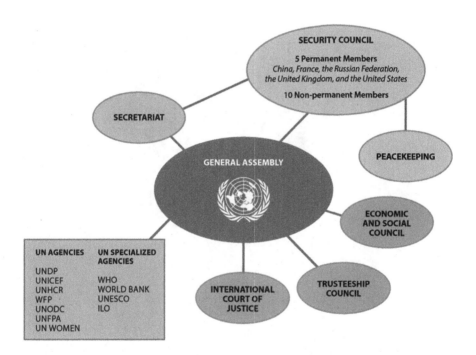

© Springer International Publishing AG 2018
M. Merson, S. Inrig, *The AIDS Pandemic*, DOI 10.1007/978-3-319-47133-4

Appendix 3
Interviews

Mohamed Abdelmoumene, Interview by Michael Merson, Geneva, October 28, 2014

Peter Aggleton, Interview by Michael Merson, October 23, 2001*

_____, Interview by Michael Merson, NH, September 21, 2001

Denis Altman, Interview by Michael Merson, November 2, 2001*

George Alleyne, Interview by Michael Merson, New Haven, CT, August, 2002

George Annas, Interview by Stephen Inrig, Dallas, TX, May 3, 2010

Fawsia Assaad, Interview by Michael Merson, New Haven, CT, July, 2002

_____, Interview by Stephen Inrig, Dallas, TX, December 23, 2010

_____, Interview by Stephen Inrig, Dallas, TX, October 5, 2010

Joe Asvall, Interview by Michael Merson, January, 2002

Seth Berkley, Interview by Michael Merson, New Haven, CT, August 21, 2002

Ken Bernard, Interview by Michael Merson, New Haven, CT, February, 2002

Stefano Bertozzi, Interview by Michael Merson, New Haven, NC, December, 2002

_____, Interview by Michael Merson, Cuernavaca, May 15, 2005

_____, Interview by Stephen Inrig, November 9, 2010

_____, Interview by Stephen Inrig, October 22, 2010

Christopher Beyrer, Interview by Stephen Inrig, Dallas, TX, October 18, 2010

Bob Black, Interview by Michael Merson, New Haven, CT, August, 2002

Ann Blackwood, Interview by Michael Merson, New Haven, CT, January, 2002

Neil Boyer, Interview by Michael Merson, New Haven, CT, January, 2002

Richard Butler, Interview by Michael Merson, New Haven, CT, February, 2002

Manuel Carballo, Interview by Michael Merson, New Haven, CT, November, 2002

Lisa Carty, Interview by Michael Merson, Durham, NC, October 8, 2012

V. Chanda-Mouli, Interview by Michael Merson, New Haven, CT, September, 2001

Suzanne Cherney, Interview by Michael Merson, August 13, 2013*

Hu Ching Li, Interview by Michael Merson, New Jersey, August, 2002

Claire Chollat-Troquet, Interview by Michael Merson, New Haven, CT, August 12, 2002

Thomas Coates, Interviewed by Michael Merson, New Haven, CT, February, 2002

© Springer International Publishing AG 2018

M. Merson, S. Inrig, *The AIDS Pandemic*, DOI 10.1007/978-3-319-47133-4

Joshua Cohen, Interviewed by Michael Merson, New Haven, CT, August, 2002
Sally Cowal, Interview by Michael Merson, New Haven, CT, February, 2002
Kathleen Cravero, Interview by Michael Merson, Geneva, October, 2001
James Curran, Interview by Michael Merson, New Haven, CT, March 9, 2002
_____, Interview by Michael Merson, New Haven, CT, September 3, 2002
Marjorie Dam, Interview by Michael Merson, New Haven, CT, September 29, 2001
Albina du Boisrouvray, Interview by Michael Merson, New Haven, CT, 2001
Kevin De Cock, Interview by Stephen Inrig, Dallas, TX, October 13, 2010
Joe Decosas, Interview by Michael Merson, New Haven, CT, October, 2001
Paul Delay, Interview by Michael Merson, New Haven, CT, December, 2002
Qhing Qhing Dhlamani, Interview by Michael Merson, New Haven, CT, August 14, 2002
Walt Dowdle, Interview by Michael Merson, New Haven, CT, August, 2002
_____, Interview by Stephen Inrig, August 10, 2010
Olavi Elo, Interview by Michael Merson, Geneva, September 21, 2001
Gunilla Ernberg, Interview by Michael Merson, New Haven, CT, August, 2002
Jose Esparza, Interview by Michael Merson, Seattle, WA, October, 2001
Harvey Fineberg, Interview by Stephen Inrig, Dallas, TX, October 8, 2010
Olivier Fontaine, Interview by Michael Merson, Geneva, October 29, 2014
Joseph Foumbi, Interview by Michael Merson, New Haven, CT, August, 2002
Helene Gayle, Interview by Michael Merson, New Haven, CT, February, 2002
_____, Interview by Michael Merson, August 10, 2014*
Duff Gillespie, Interview by Michael Merson, New Haven, CT, October, 2002
Tore Godal, Interview by Michael Merson, Geneva, October, 2001
Larry Gostin, Interview by Michael Merson, New Haven, CT, September, 2002
_____, Interview by Stephen Inrig, Dallas, TX, July 7, 2010
_____, Interview by Stephen Inrig, Dallas, TX, June, 2010
Michael Grodin, Interview by Stephen Inrig, Dallas, TX, 2010
Sophia Gruskin, Interview by Stephen Inrig, July 28, 2010
Aleya Hammad, Interview by Michael Merson, New Haven, CT, April, 2004
S.T. Han, Interview by Michael Merson, New Haven, CT, August 30, 2012
Catherine Hankins, Interview by Michael Merson, New Haven, CT, January 13, 2005
_____, Interview by Michael Merson, October 14, 2014*
Robert Hecht, Interview by Michael Merson, New Haven, CT, January, 2002
Ralph Henderson, Interview by Michael Merson, NH, February, 2003
_____, Interview by Stephen Inrig, Dallas, TX, November 8, 2010
David Heymann, Interview by Michael Merson, Geneva, October, 2001
Robert Hogan, Interview by Michael Merson, New Haven, CT, August, 2002
Gillian Holmes, Interview by Michael Merson, Geneva, October, 2001
King Holmes, Interview by Michael Merson, New Haven, CT, September, 2002
Vincent Iacopino, Interview by Stephen Inrig, Dallas, TX, October 4, 2010
Ralf Jurgens, Interview by Stephen Inrig, Dallas, TX, July 25, 2010
Noreen Kaleeba, Interview by Michael Merson, Geneva, October, 2001
Lars Kallings, Interview by Michael Merson, New Haven, CT, September, 2002

Nils Kastberg, Interview by Michael Merson, New York City, September, 2002
Kathleen Kay, Interview by Michael Merson, New Haven, CT, 2002
Ann Kern, Interview by Michael Merson, New Haven, CT, October, 2001
Ann Marie Kimball, Interview by Michael Merson, New Haven, CT, November, 2001
Melinda Kimble, Interview by Michael Merson, Washington, DC, February, 2002
Stuart Kingma, Interview by Michael Merson, Geneva, October, 2001
Jean Louis Lamboray, Interview by Michael Merson, Geneva, October, 2001
Peter Lamptey, Interview by Michael Merson, Washington, DC, December, 2002
Joep Lange, Interview by Michael Merson, New Haven, CT, September, 2002
Brad Langmaid, Interview by Michael Merson, New Haven, CT, September, 2002
Helge Larsen, Interview by Michael Merson, Geneva, October, 2001
J.W. Lee, Interview by Michael Merson, Geneva, October, 2001
Halfdan Mahler, Interview by Michael Merson, Geneva, October, 2001
Purnima Mane, Interview by Michael Merson, New Haven, CT, January, 2002
Mina Mauerstein-Bail, Interview by Michael Merson, New Haven, CT, September, 2002
_____, Interview by Michael Merson, New Haven, CT, October, 2001
Thierry Mertens, Interview by Michael Merson, Geneva, January 13, 2005
Hans Moerkerk, Interview by Michael Merson, New Haven, CT, August, 2002
Jane Moss, Interview by Michael Merson, Durham, NC, October 24, 2002
David Nabarro, Interview by Michael Merson, Geneva, October, 2001
Hiroshi Nakajima, Interview by Michael Merson, Poitiers, October 13, 2002
Ross Noble, Interview by Michael Merson, Geneva, October, 2001
Jeff O'Malley, Interview by Michael Merson, New Haven, CT, September, 2002
Kevin O'Reilly, Interview by Michael Merson, Geneva, January 13, 2005
June Osborne, Interview by Michael Merson, New Haven, CT, October 26, 2002
William Parra, Interview by Stephen Inrig, Dallas, TX, August 13, 2010
_____, Interview by Stephen Inrig, Dallas, TX, October 14, 2010
Joseph Perriens, Interview by Michael Merson, Geneva, September, 2001
_____, Interview by Michael Merson, Geneva, January, 2005
Anthony Piel, Interview by Michael Merson, Sharon, CT, December 22, 2001
Peter Piot, Interview by Stephen Inrig, Dallas, TX, February 2, 2011
_____, Interview by Michael Merson, New Haven, CT, October 26, 2002
Thomas Quinn, Interview by Stephen Inrig, Dallas, TX, December 9, 2011
_____, Interview by Stephen Inrig, Dallas, TX, February 3, 2011
_____, Interview by Michael Merson, New Haven, CT, August, 2002
Timothy Rothermel, Interview by Stephen Inrig, Dallas, TX, October 15, 2010
_____, Interview by Michael Merson, New York, August, 2002
Robin Ryder, Interview by Michael Merson, New Haven, CT, August, 2002
Geoffrey Schilds, Interview by Michael Merson, New Haven, CT, September, 2002
Doris Schopper, Interview by Michael Merson, Geneva, October, 2001
_____, Interview by Michael Merson Geneva, October 28, 2004
Bernhard Schwartlander, Interview by Michael Merson, January 3, 2015*
Jim Sherry, Interview by Michael Merson, Geneva, October, 2001

Gary Slutkin, Interview by Michael Merson, New Haven, CT, February 3, 2003
Gus Speth, Interview by Michael Merson, New Haven, CT, 1999
Todd Summers, Interview by Michael Merson, Washington, DC, July, 2012
Daniel Tarantola, Interview by Michael Merson, New Haven, CT, October, 2001
Susan Timberlake, Interview by Michael Merson, New Haven, CT, August, 2002
Tom Topping, Interview by Michael Merson, New Haven, CT, 2004
Eric Van Praag, Interview by Michael Merson, New Haven, CT, July, 2002
Mechai Viravaidya, Interview by Michael Merson, Barcelona, July, 2002
Gill Walt, Interview by Stephen Inrig, Dallas, TX, September 23, 2010
Roy Widdus, Interview by Michael Merson, New Haven, CT, October, 2001
Phil Wilson, Interview by Michael Merson, New Haven, CT, August, 2002
Fernando Zacarias, Interview by Michael Merson, New Haven, CT, January, 2002
Debrework Zewdie, Interview by Michael Merson, New Haven, CT, September, 2002

* Indicates email interview.

Appendix 4
Establishment of the Joint United Nations Programme on HIV/AIDS (UNAIDS) Timeline

November, 1989	GPA Management Committee (GMC) agrees to undertake external review of GPA
April, 1990	GMC sets up working group to prepare terms of reference and select committee for the external review
June, 1992	External review report submitted to GMC
November, 1992	GMC creates Task Force on HIV/AIDS Coordination
March, 1993	Meeting of GPA donors in London
May, 1993	WHA Resolution requesting WHO to study feasibility of establishing joint and cosponsored program on AIDS
May, 1993	First interagency meeting convened in New York with UN potential cosponsors
May and June 1993	Governing bodies of other cosponsors (except for the World Bank) pass resolutions to study the feasibility of establishing a joint and cosponsored program on AIDS
October, 1993	Cosponsors put forward three options for the structure of new program
November, 1993	Heads of all six cosponsors meet with Secretary General in New York and decide on Option A: The Strong Secretariat option
November, 1993	GMC's Task Force on HIV/AIDS Coordination also supports Option A
January, 1994	WHO Executive Board adopts Resolution recommending new program with Option A
July, 1994	ECOSOC approves Resolution calling for the establishment of new joint and cosponsored program (UNAIDS)
September, 1994	Committee of Cosponsoring Organizations (CCO) formed to oversee the implementation of new program and recruit new Executive Director
September, 1994	Search for UNAIDS Executive Director starts
December, 1994	Secretary General appoints Peter Piot as UNAIDS Executive Director
March, 1995	Michael Merson departs GPA and Stef Bertozzi appointed Interim GPA Director
July, 1995	UNAIDS Programme Coordinating Board holds first meeting
December, 1995	GPA closes
January, 1996	UNAIDS opens

© Springer International Publishing AG 2018
M. Merson, S. Inrig, *The AIDS Pandemic*, DOI 10.1007/978-3-319-47133-4

Appendix 5
World Health Organization 1993 Study of a Joint and co-sponsored United Nations Programme on HIV/AIDS: Synopsis of Options at Global Level

Annex 1

Joint and co-sponsored United Nations Programme on HIV/AIDS: synopsis of options at global level

	Option A	Option B	Option C
A. Program direction			
Level of program head	Program director	Program director	Program director
Selection process	Agreement of co-sponsors	Agreement of co-sponsors	Agreement of co-sponsors
Appointment process	Secretary-General upon recommendation of Director-General, WHO	Secretary-General	Secretary-General upon recommendation of Director-General, WHO

(continued)

© Springer International Publishing AG 2018

M. Merson, S. Inrig, *The AIDS Pandemic*, DOI 10.1007/978-3-319-47133-4

(continued)

	Option A	Option B	Option C
B. Secretariat			
1. Functions: Overall management and/or coordination *for:*	Information exchange	Information exchange	Information exchange
	Policy and strategic planning	Policy and strategic planning	Policy and strategic planning
	Monitoring all aspects of pandemic	Monitoring responses to and impact of the pandemic	Monitoring responses to and impact of the pandemic
	Advocacy	Advocacy	Advocacy
	Promotion of human rights	Promotion of human rights	Promotion of human rights
	Reporting key trends	Reporting key trends	Reporting key trends
	Fund-raising	Fund-raising	Fund-raising
	External relations	External relations	
	Public information	Public information	
	Evaluation approaches and frameworks	Evaluation approaches and frameworks	
	Research	Research (transsectoral)	
	Direct technical and financial support to countries through program staff	Support to countries through individual co-sponsors	
2. Staffing (all options assume total staff of 100 in secretariat of program and individual co-sponsors)	Approximately 90 (see paragraph 47)	Approximately 35 (see paragraph 76)	Approximately 10 (see paragraph 104)
3. Relationship to United Nations system	Administered by WHO/Geneva	To be determined (including possibility of administration by WHO)	Administered by WHO/Geneva
4. Authority	Establishes policy and technical guidelines, and provides policy and technical support to co-sponsors and other organizations of the United Nations system	Coordinating authority, provides policy and technical guidance, arbitrates areas of overlap within United Nations system	Coordinating authority, provides policy and technical guidance

(continued)

(continued)

	Option A	Option B	Option C
C. Activities of Co-sponsors			
	Individual co-sponsors continue to convey program guidance and advice to staff, and to ensure integration of HIV/AIDS issues into their broader health and socioeconomic activities	Development of institutional policies and programs that respond to their mandates, within a global policy and coordination framework	Development of institutional policies and programs that respond to their mandates, within a global policy and coordination framework
D. Achieving/Promoting Consensus			
1. Goal	Development of common policies, strategies, and approaches	Development of common policies, strategies, and approaches	Harmonization of policies and strategies
2. Method	Through program governance and management structure; continuing dialogue and exchange of information	Through governance and management structures of the co-sponsors; continuing dialogue and exchange of information	Through program governance structure; continuing dialogue and exchange of information
E. Governing/Advisory Bodies			
1. Principal governing body	Programme coordinating board	Joint coordinating board on AIDS	Joint coordinating board on AIDS
2. Terms of reference of principal governing body	Board approves budget and activities of program at global, regional, and country levels, reviews overall United Nations response at all levels, resolves programmatic issues affecting coordination	Board approves budget and activities of global secretariat, reviews overall United Nations response at all levels, resolves programmatic issues affecting coordination	Board approves budget and activities of global secretariat, reviews overall United Nations response at global level, resolves programmatic issues affecting coordination
3. Relationship to governing body of co-sponsors	Co-sponsors report to their respective governing bodies	Board representatives and co-sponsors report to their respective governing bodies	Board representatives and co-sponsors report to their respective governing bodies
4. Advisory Bodies	Inter-Agency Advisory Group on AIDS	Inter-Agency Advisory Group on AIDS	Inter-Agency Advisory Group on AIDS
	Committee of co-sponsoring organizations	Committee of co-sponsoring organizations	
	Technical advisory group		

(continued)

(continued)

	Option A	Option B	Option C
5. Reporting *vis-à-vis* other United Nations bodies	Report submitted to Economic and Social Council, on request	Report submitted to Economic and Social Council, on request	Report submitted to Economic and Social Council, on request
F. Funding			
	Organization of budget according to program areas, with activities of other bodies identified as appropriate; includes direct support to countries (e.g., ministries of health)	Consolidated annual appeal covering core functions of global secretariat and co-sponsors; coordination of individual fund-raising efforts of co-sponsors for special needs	Consolidated annual appeal covering core functions of global secretariat and co-sponsors; coordination of individual fund-raising efforts of co-sponsors for special needs
G. Relationship to country programming			
1. Relationship to national AIDS program	Operates under national guidelines and framework	Operates under national guidelines and framework	Operates under national guidelines and framework
	• Provides technical and financial support through program secretariat and individual co-sponsors	• Provides technical and financial support through individual co-sponsors	• Provides technical and financial support through individual co-sponsors
		• Operations decentralized to country level	
2. Relationship to interagency staff	Line manages program country staff member • Mutual exchange: policy and program guidance to and information and ideas from program country staff member	• Mutual exchange: policy and program guidance to and information and ideas from program country staff member	No program country staff

Reprinted from World Health Organization Executive Board 93rd Session, 21 December 1993 Study of a joint and co-sponsored United Nations Programme on HIV/AIDS.

Appendix 6
World Health Organization 1993 Study of a Joint and co-sponsored United Nations Programme on HIV/AIDS: Synopsis of Options at Country Level

Joint and co-sponsored United Nations[1] Programme on HIV/AIDS: synopsis of options at country level

	Option A	Option B	Option C
A. Role of Resident Coordinator	• Ensures coordination	• Ensures coordination	• Ensures coordination
	• Establishes committee or theme group on HIV/AIDS (and, if appropriate, task-oriented subgroups)	• Establishes committee or theme group on HIV/AIDS	• Establishes committee or theme group on HIV/AIDS
	• May designate organization to coordinate activities of United Nations system related to HIV/AIDS	• May designate organization to coordinate activities of United Nations system related to HIV/AIDS	• May designate organization to coordinate activities of United Nations system related to HIV/AIDS

(continued)

---

[1] This document was called ANNEX 2 in the Executive Board Ninety-third Session Provisional Agenda

© Springer International Publishing AG 2018
M. Merson, S. Inrig, *The AIDS Pandemic*, DOI 10.1007/978-3-319-47133-4

(continued)

	Option A	Option B	Option C
B. Stalling			
1. Category	• Program country staff member	• Program country staff member	• Technical staff recruited by individual organizations
	• Technical staff recruited by individual co-sponsors or, when requested by committee, by the program	• Technical staff recruited by individual co-sponsors	
2. Management	First-level supervision by Resident Coordinator or designated organization representative; second-level supervision by program director	Line managed by the Resident Coordinator or designated organization representative; reports to program director through standardized information/reporting mechanisms	No program country staff
C. Funding	• Support to medium-term plan	• Support to medium-term plan	• Support to medium-term plan
D. Interaction among co-sponsors	• Joint planning and consultation	• Joint planning and consultation	• Joint planning and consultation
	• Possibility of joint programs	• Possibility of joint programs	• Possibility of joint programs
	• Information exchange	• Information exchange	• Information exchange

Reprinted from World Health Organization Executive Board 93rd Session, 21 December, 1993 Study of a joint and co-sponsored United Nations Programme on HIV/AIDS.

Appendix 7

United Nations Economic and Social Council Resolution 1994/24 on Joint and co-sponsored Programme on Human Immunodeficiency Virus/Acquired Immunodeficiency Syndrome

"Resolution on Joint and Co-Sponsored Programme on Human Immunodeficiency Virus/Acquired Immunodeficiency Syndrome, HIV/AIDS"

United Nations ECOSOC resolution 1994/24, 29 July 1994 Economic and Social Council 44th plenary meeting, 26 July 1994 1994/24. Joint and co-sponsored United Nations programme on human immunodeficiency virus/acquired immunodeficiency syndrome (HIV/AIDS)

The Economic and Social Council,

Recalling its resolution 1993/51 on the coordination of United Nations activities related to HIV/AIDS,

Taking note of the decisions of the United Nations Development Programme, the United Nations Children's Fund, the United Nations Population Fund, the World Health Organization, the United Nations Educational, Scientific and Cultural Organization, and the World Bank to undertake a joint and -sponsored United Nations programme on HIV/AIDS, on the basis of co-ownership, collaborative planning and execution, and an equitable sharing of responsibility,

Noting that the World Health Organization is to be responsible for the administration in support of the program, including during the transition period,

Emphasizing that the global HIV/AIDS epidemic affects every country of the world and that its magnitude and impact are greatest in developing countries,

Emphasizing also the urgent need to mobilize fully all United Nations system organizations and other development partners in the global response to HIV/AIDS, in a coordinated manner and according to the comparative advantages of each organization,

1. Endorses the establishment of a joint and co-sponsored United Nations programme on HIV/AIDS, as outlined in the annex to the present resolution, subject to further review by April 1995 of progress made towards its implementation

2. Calls for the full implementation of the program by January 1996, and requests that a report confirming its implementation be submitted to the Economic and Social Council at its organizational session for 1996

© Springer International Publishing AG 2018
M. Merson, S. Inrig, *The AIDS Pandemic*, DOI 10.1007/978-3-319-47133-4

3. Notes that further details of the program are being developed by the Inter-Agency Working Group that has been established by the six co-sponsors

4. Invites the six co-sponsors to take immediate steps to transform the Inter-Agency Working Group into a formally constituted Committee of Co-sponsoring Organizations, comprising the heads of those organizations or their specifically designated representatives, which would function under a rotational chairmanship, establish a transition team, and assume interim responsibility, inter alia, for overseeing the transition process leading to the full implementation of the program

5. Also invites the six co-sponsors, through the Committee, to initiate action to fill the position of director of the joint and co-sponsored program as soon as possible, through an open, wide-ranging search process, including consultation with Governments and other concerned parties, and to submit their nominee to the Secretary-General, who will make the appointment

6. Urges the six co-sponsors, through the Committee, to initiate, as soon as possible, program activities at the country level, as well as any other program elements on which there is already full consensus

7. Stresses that priority should be given to the program's activities at the country level, where the response to the urgent needs and problems posed by HIV/AIDS should be focused, and underlines the importance of the program's country-level operations' functioning within the framework of national plans and priorities and a strengthened resident coordinator system, in accordance with General Assembly resolution 47/199

8. Also stresses that during the transition process, the ongoing HIV/AIDS activities of each of the six co-sponsors should be maintained and/or enhanced, bearing in mind the need for these activities to fit within national AIDS programs and the general framework of the joint and co-sponsored program

9. Requests the six co-sponsors, through the Committee, to produce the following by January 1995, for the consideration of the Economic and Social Council and other concerned parties: a comprehensive proposal specifying the program's mission statement and the terms and conditions of co-ownership, and detailing the program's organizational, programmatic, staffing, administrative, and financial elements, including proposed budgetary allocations, and to attach to this proposal an annex containing the proposed legal document that the six co-sponsors will sign to establish the program formally

10. Encourages the active involvement of the Task Force on HIV/AIDS Coordination during the program's detailed development phase, through the direct provision of assistance to the Committee, in accordance with the Committee's requirements

11. Requests the President of the Economic and Social Council to organize, in cooperation with the Committee of Co-sponsoring Organizations, informal open-ended consultations to be held as soon as possible for the purpose of deciding on the specific composition of the programme coordinating board that will govern the program, interacting periodically with the Committee during the transition period to facilitate progress towards program implementation,

and reviewing the detailed program proposal after it is received from the Committee, with a view to making appropriate recommendations on the proposal not later than April 1995

44th plenary meeting, 26 July 1994

Annex

I. Program Outline

1. The co-sponsored United Nations programme on HIV/AIDS represents an internationally coordinated response to the HIV/AIDS pandemic. The program comprises the following United Nations system organizations: the United Nations Development Programme, the United Nations Children's Fund, the United Nations Population Fund, the World Health Organization, the United Nations Educational, Scientific and Cultural Organization, and the World Bank. The program has been formally endorsed by the Executive Boards of the World Health Organization (resolution EB93.R5) and the United Nations Educational, Scientific and Cultural Organization (resolution 144EX-5.1.5); the other four co-sponsors have also committed themselves to full participation.
2. The fundamental characteristics that define the program are set out below.

II. Objectives

3. The objectives of the program are to:
   a. Provide global leadership in response to the epidemic
   b. Achieve and promote global consensus on policy and programmatic approaches
   c. Strengthen the capacity of the United Nations system to monitor trends and ensure that appropriate and effective policies and strategies are implemented at the country level
   d. Strengthen the capacity of national Governments to develop comprehensive national strategies and implement effective HIV/AIDS activities at the country level
   e. Promote broad-based political and social mobilization to prevent and respond to HIV/AIDS within countries, ensuring that national responses involve a wide range of sectors and institutions
   f. Advocate greater political commitment in responding to the epidemic at the global and country levels, including the mobilization and allocation of adequate resources for HIV/AIDS-related activities

4. In fulfilling these objectives, the program will collaborate with national Governments, intergovernmental organizations, non-governmental organizations, groups of people living with HIV/AIDS, and United Nations system organizations.

III. Co-sponsorship

5. The HIV/AIDS epidemic is a global concern. Interagency cooperation is vital for ensuring the mobilization of resources and the effective implementation of a coordinated program of activities throughout the United Nations system.
6. The program will draw upon the experience and strengths of the six co-sponsors to develop its strategies and policies, which will be incorporated in turn into their programs and activities. The co-sponsors will share responsibility for the development of the program, contribute equally to its strategic direction, and receive from it policy and technical guidance relating to the implementation of their HIV/AIDS activities. In this way, the program will also serve to harmonize the HIV/AIDS activities of the co-sponsors.
7. The program will be managed by a director, who will focus on the program's overall strategy, technical guidance, research and development, and the global budget. The co-sponsors will contribute to the resource needs of the program at levels to be determined. The World Health Organization will be responsible for the administration in support of the program.
8. Other United Nations system organizations concerned with the HIV/AIDS epidemic may be encouraged to join the program as co-sponsors in the future.

IV. Functional Responsibilities

9. The program will build on the capacities and comparative advantages of the co-sponsors. At the global level, the program will provide support in policy formulation, strategic planning, technical guidance, research and development, advocacy and external relations. This will include normative activities relating to HIV/AIDS in areas such as social and economic planning, population, culture, education, community development and social mobilization, sexual and reproductive health, and women and adolescents.
10. At the country level, the program will provide support to the resident coordinator system. Co-sponsors will incorporate the normative work undertaken at the global level on policy, strategy, and technical matters into their HIV/AIDS activities, consistent with national plans and priorities. An important function of the program will be to strengthen national capacities to plan, coordinate, implement, and monitor the overall response to HIV/AIDS. The participation in the program of six organizations of the United Nations system will ensure the provision of technical and financial assistance to national activities in a

coordinated multisectoral manner. This will strengthen intersectoral coordination of HIV/AIDS activities and will facilitate further incorporation of these activities in national program and planning processes.

11. While the program will not have a uniform regional structure, it will support intercountry or regional activities that may be required in response to the epidemic, utilizing regional mechanisms of the co-sponsors where appropriate.

V. Flow of Program Funds

12. Funds for program activities at the global level will be obtained through appropriate common global means. Contributions to the program will be channelled in accordance with the global budget and work plan.

13. Funding for country-level activities will be obtained primarily through the existing fund-raising mechanisms of the co-sponsors. These funds will be channelled through the disbursement mechanisms and procedures of each organization.

VI. Field-Level Coordination

14. It is recognized that national Governments have the ultimate responsibility for the coordination of HIV/AIDS issues at the country level. To this end, the arrangements of the program for coordinating HIV/AIDS activities will complement and support national development planning.

15. The coordination of field-level activities will be undertaken through the United Nations resident coordinator system within the framework of General Assembly resolutions 44/211 and 47/199. This will involve a theme group on HIV/AIDS established by the resident coordinator and comprising representatives of the six co-sponsors and other United Nations system organizations. The chairperson of the theme group will be selected by consensus from among the United Nations system representatives. It is intended that the theme group will help the United Nations system integrate more effectively its efforts with national coordination mechanisms. To support the coordination process, in a number of countries the program will recruit a country staff member, who will assist the chairperson of the theme group in carrying out his or her functions.

VII. Organizational Structure

16. A program director will be appointed by the Secretary-General upon the recommendation of the co-sponsors. This will follow a search process undertaken by the co-sponsors which will include consultation with Governments and other interested parties. The director will report directly to the programme coordinating board,

which will serve as the governance structure for the program. Annual reports prepared by the director will be submitted to the board and will also be made available to the governing body of each of the co-sponsors.

17. The composition of the programme coordinating board will be determined on the basis of open-ended consultations, as outlined in operative paragraph 11 of the present resolution. In exercising its governance role, the board will have ultimate responsibility for all policy and budgetary matters. It will also review and decide upon the planning and execution of the program. Its detailed responsibilities and meeting schedule will be specified in a document containing its terms of reference, which is currently being prepared.

18. The program will also have a committee of co-sponsoring organizations, which will serve as a standing committee of the board. It will comprise one representative from each of the co-sponsors. The committee will meet regularly and will facilitate the input of the co-sponsors into the strategy, policies, and operations of the program.

19. Through consultation with interested non-governmental organizations, a mechanism will be established to ensure their meaningful participation in the program, so that they can provide information, perspectives, and advice to the board, based on their experience and involvement with HIV/AIDS issues.

Appendix 8
UNAIDS Technical Support Division of Labor, Summary and Rationale 2005: Division of Responsibility Among UNAIDS co-sponsors

Division of Responsibility among UNAIDS Cosponsors		
Technical Support Areas	Lead Organization	Main Partners
1. STRATEGIC PLANNING, GOVERNANCE AND FINANCIAL MANAGEMENT		
HIV/AIDS, development, governance and mainstreaming, including instruments such as PRSPs, and enabling legislation, human rights and gender	UNDP	ILO, UNAIDS Secretariat, UNESCO, UNICEF, WHO, World Bank, UNFPA; UNHCR
Support to strategic, prioritized and costed national plans; financial management; human resources; capacity and infrastructure development; impact alleviation and sectoral work	World Bank	ILO, UNAIDS Secretariat, UNDP, UNESCO, UNICEF, WHO
Procurement and supply management, including training	UNICEF	UNDP, UNFPA, WHO, World Bank
HIV/AIDS workplace policy and programmes, private-sector mobilization	ILO	UNESCO, UNDP
2. SCALING UP INTERVENTIONS		
Prevention		
Prevention of HIV transmission in healthcare settings, blood safety, counselling and testing, sexuallytransmitted infection diagnosis and treatment, and linkage of HIV prevention with AIDS treatment services	WHO	UNICEF, UNFPA, ILO
Provision of information and education, condom programming, prevention for young people outside schools and prevention efforts targeting vulnerable groups (except injecting drug users, prisoners and refugee populations)	UNFPA	ILO, UNAIDS Secretariat, UNESCO, UNICEF, UNODC, WHO
Prevention of mother-to-child transmission (PMTCT)	UNICEF, WHO	UNFPA, WFP
Prevention for young people in education institutions	UNESCO	ILO, UNFPA, UNICEF, WHO, WFP
Prevention of transmission of HIV among injecting drug users and in prisons	UNODC	UNDP, UNICEF, WHO, ILO
Overall policy, monitoring and coordination on prevention	UNAIDS Secretariat	All Cospnsors
Treatment, care and support		
Antiretroviral treatment and monitoring, prophylaxis and treatment for opportunistic infections (adults and children)	WHO	UNICEF
Care and support for people living with HIV, orphans and vulnerable children, and affected households.	UNICEF	WFP, WHO, ILO
Dietary/nutrition support	WFP	UNESCO, UNICEF, WHO
Addressing HIV in emergency, reconstruction and security settings		
Strengthening HIV/AIDS response in context of security, uniformed services and humanitarian crises	UNAIDS Secretariat	UNHCR, UNICEF, WFP, WHO, UNFPA
Addressing HIV among displaced populations (refugees and IDPs)	UNHCR	UNESCO, UNFPA, UNICEF, WFP, WHO, UNDP
3. MONITORING AND EVALUATION, STRATEGIC INFORMATION, KNOWLEDGE SHARING AND ACCOUNTABILITY		
Strategic information, knowledge sharing and accountability, coordination of national efforts, partnership building, advocacy, and monitoring and evaluation, including estimation of national prevalence and projection of demographic impact	UNAIDS Secretariat	ILO, UNDP, UNESCO, UNFPA, UNHCR, UNICEF, UNODC, WFP, WHO, World Bank
Establishment and implementation of surveillance for HIV, through sentinel/population-based surveys	WHO	UNAIDS Secretariat

Reprinted from UNAIDS Technical Support Division of Labour. Summary and Rationale. UNAIDS 2005.

© Springer International Publishing AG 2018
M. Merson, S. Inrig, *The AIDS Pandemic*, DOI 10.1007/978-3-319-47133-4

Reference

1. Fee, E., Cueto, M., & Brown, T. M. (2016). At the roots of the World Health Organization's challenges: Politics and regionalization. *American Journal of Public Health, 106*(11), 1912–1917. doi:10.2105/AJPH.2016.303480.

Glossary of Terms

ACHAP	African Comprehensive HIV/AIDS Partnership
ACT UP	AIDS Coalition to Unleash Power
ADG	Assistant Director-General
AFRO	World Health Organizational Regional Office for Africa
AIDSCOM	The AIDS Public Health Communication Project
AIDSTECH	AIDS Technical Support
AMFAR	The American Foundation for AIDS Research
ARI	Acute Respiratory Infections Programme
ART	Antiretroviral therapy
ARV	Antiretroviral drugs
AZT	Azidothymidine
CCM	Country coordinating mechanisms
CCO	Committee of Cosponsoring Organizations
CDC	United States Centers for Disease Control and Prevention
CDD	Diarrheal Diseases Control Programme
CESCR	United Nations Committee on Economic Social and Cultural Rights
CIDA	Canadian International Development Agency
CPA	Control Programme on AIDS
CPP	Committee of Participating Parties
DGIP	Division of Global and Interregional Programs
DIESA	Department of International Economic and Social Affairs
EB	Epidemiological Bulletin
ECOSOC	United Nations Economic and Social Council
EPI	Expanded Programme on Immunization
ERC	External Review Committee
EURO	World Health Organization Regional Office for Europe
FAO	Food and Agriculture Organization
FDA	Food and Drug Administration

© Springer International Publishing AG 2018

M. Merson, S. Inrig, *The AIDS Pandemic*, DOI 10.1007/978-3-319-47133-4

G7	Group of Seven
G8	Group of Eight
GAO	United States Government Accountability Office
GAPC	Global AIDS Policy Coalition
GAVI	Global Alliance for Vaccines and Immunizations
GBSI	Global Blood Safety Initiative
GCA	Global Commission on AIDS
GCWA	Global Coalition on Women and AIDS
GHESKIO	Haitian Study Group on Kaposi's Sarcoma and Opportunistic Infections
GMC	Global Programme on AIDS Management Committee
GNP+	Global Network of People Living with HIV/AIDS
GOBI	Growth monitoring, oral rehydration therapy, breastfeeding, and immunization
GOBI FFF	Growth monitoring, oral rehydration therapy, breastfeeding, immunization food supplements, family spacing, and female education
GPA	Global Programme on AIDS
GTT	Global Task Team
HAART	Highly Active Antiretroviral Therapy
HRP	Special Programme of Research, Development and Research Training in Human Reproduction
IAAG	Interagency Advisory Group
IAS	International AIDS Society
IAVI	International AIDS Vaccine Initiative
ICASO	International Council of AIDS Service Organizations
IDU	Injection drug user
ILO	International Labour Organization
IMF	International Monetary Fund
IOM	Institute of Medicine
ITM	Institute of Tropical Medicine
JICA	Japan International Cooperation Agency
KABP/PR	Knowledge, attitude, belief and practice/partner surveys
KEMRI	Kenya Medical Research Institute
LFA	Local Fund Agents
LNHO	League of Nations Health Office
LSHTM	London School of Hygiene & Tropical Medicine
MAP	Multi-Country HIV/AIDS Program for Africa
MSM	Men who have sex with men
MTP	Medium term plan
NACO	National AIDS Control Organization
NACP	National AIDS Control Program
NBA	National Basketball Association
NGO	Non-governmental organization

NIAID	National Institutes of Allergy and Infectious Diseases
NIH	National Institutes for Health
NORAD	Norwegian Agency for Development Cooperation
OAU	Organization of African Unity
ODA	Overseas Development Administration
PAHO	Pan American Health Organization
PCB	Programme Coordinating Board
PEPFAR	President's Emergency Plan for AIDS Relief
PLWA	Person living with AIDS
PrEP	Pre-exposure prophylaxis
RCF	Red Cross Federation
SIDA	Swedish International Development Authority
SPA	Special Programme on AIDS
STD	Sexually transmitted disease
STP	Short term plan
TASO	The AIDS Support Organization
TDR	Special Programme for Research and Training in Tropical Diseases
The Global Fund	Global Fund to Fight AIDS, Tuberculosis, and Malaria
UBRAF	Unified Budget Results and Accountability Framework
UN	United Nations
UNAIDS	Joint United Nations Programme on HIV/AIDS
UNDP	United Nations Development Programme
UNESCO	United Nations Educational Scientific and Cultural Organization
UNFPA	United Nations Population Fund
UNGASS	United Nations General Assembly Special Session
UNHCR	United Nations High Commission for Refugees
UNICEF	United Nations Children's Emergency Fund
UNODC	United Nations Office on Drugs and Crime
UNRRA	United Nations Relief and Rehabilitation Administration
US	United States of America
USAID	United States Agency for International Development
USPHS	United States Public Health Service
USSR	Union of Soviet Socialist Republics
VDT	Venereal Transmitted Diseases
WER	Weekly Epidemiological Record
WFP	World Food Programme
WHA	World Health Assembly
WHO	World Health Organization
WPRO	World Health Organization Regional Office for the Western Pacific

Index

© Springer International Publishing AG 2018
M. Merson, S. Inrig, *The AIDS Pandemic*, DOI 10.1007/978-3-319-47133-4

Printed in the United States
By Bookmasters